Computational Drug Discovery and Design

Computational Drug Discovery and Design

Editor: Pamelia Clarkson

AMERICAN
MEDICAL PUBLISHERS
www.americanmedicalpublishers.com

AMERICAN
MEDICAL PUBLISHERS
www.americanmedicalpublishers.com

Cataloging-in-Publication Data

Computational drug discovery and design / edited by Pamelia Clarkson.
p. cm.
Includes bibliographical references and index.
ISBN 979-8-88740-016-7
1. Drug development--Data processing. 2. Drugs--Design--Data processing.
3. Drug development. 4. Drugs--Design. 5. Pharmacology--Data processing.
I. Clarkson, Pamelia.
RM301.25 .C66 2023
615.19--dc23

American Medical Publishers,
41 Flatbush Avenue,
1st Floor, New York,
NY 11217, USA

ISBN 979-8-88740-016-7 (Hardback)

Contents

Preface

It is often said that books are a boon to mankind. They document every progress and pass on the knowledge from one generation to the other. They play a crucial role in our lives. Thus I was both excited and nervous while editing this book. I was pleased by the thought of being able to make a mark but I was also nervous to do it right because the future of students depends upon it. Hence, I took a few months to research further into the discipline, revise my knowledge and also explore some more aspects. Post this process, I begun with the editing of this book.

Computer-aided drug discovery and design technologies have played a critical role in the development of therapeutically important small compounds. These technologies involve computational tools and sources which are used for storing, managing, analyzing and modeling compounds. These approaches can be divided into two categories: structure-based and ligand-based. Computer-aided drug design (CADD) is an important tool for speeding up and saving money in the expensive and time-consuming process of drug discovery and development. There has been a surge in protein and ligand structural data in recent years. As a result, the number of databases and bioinformatics tools available to handle and process the data has increased dramatically. For the discovery and development of new medications, the best use of the broad array of available computational techniques is critical. This book is a compilation of research works that discuss the emerging trends in computational drug discovery and design. It will help the readers in keeping pace with the rapid changes taking place in this field.

I thank my publisher with all my heart for considering me worthy of this unparalleled opportunity and for showing unwavering faith in my skills. I would also like to thank the editorial team who worked closely with me at every step and contributed immensely towards the successful completion of this book. Last but not the least, I wish to thank my friends and colleagues for their support.

Editor

1

Design, Synthesis and Evaluation of Dihydrobenzo[*cd*]indole-6-sulfonamide as TNF-α Inhibitors

Xiaobing Deng[1,2], *Xiaoling Zhang*[2], *Bo Tang*[3], *Hongbo Liu*[1], *Qi Shen*[2], *Ying Liu*[2,3]* and *Luhua Lai*[1,2,3]*

[1] *Peking–Tsinghua Center for Life Sciences, Peking University, Beijing, China,* [2] *Center for Quantitative Biology, Academy for Advanced Interdisciplinary Studies, Peking University, Beijing, China,* [3] *BNLMS, State Key Laboratory for Structural Chemistry of Unstable and Stable Species, College of Chemistry and Molecular Engineering, Peking University, Beijing, China*

Correspondence:
Ying Liu
liuying@pku.edu.cn
Luhua Lai
lhlai@pku.edu.cn

Tumor necrosis factor-α (TNF-α) plays a pivotal role in inflammatory response. Dysregulation of TNF can lead to a variety of disastrous pathological effects, including auto-inflammatory diseases. Antibodies that directly targeting TNF-α have been proven effective in suppressing symptoms of these disorders. Compared to protein drugs, small molecule drugs are normally orally available and less expensive. Till now, peptide and small molecule TNF-α inhibitors are still in the early stage of development, and much more efforts should be made. In a previously study, we reported a TNF-α inhibitor, **EJMC-1** with modest activity. Here, we optimized this compound by shape screen and rational design. In the first round, we screened commercial compound library for **EJMC-1** analogs based on shape similarity. Out of the 68 compounds tested, 20 compounds showed better binding affinity than **EJMC-1** in the SPR competitive binding assay. These 20 compounds were tested in cell assay and the most potent compound was 2-oxo-N-phenyl-1,2-dihydrobenzo[*cd*]indole-6-sulfonamide (**S10**) with an IC_{50} of 14 μM, which was 2.2-fold stronger than **EJMC-1**. Based on the docking analysis of **S10** and **EJMC-1** binding with TNF-α, in the second round, we designed **S10** analogs, purchased seven of them, and synthesized seven new compounds. The best compound, **4e** showed an IC_{50}-value of 3 μM in cell assay, which was 14-fold stronger than **EJMC-1**. **4e** was among the most potent TNF-α organic compound inhibitors reported so far. Our study demonstrated that 2-oxo-N-phenyl-1,2-dihydrobenzo[*cd*]indole-6-sulfonamide analogs could be developed as potent TNF-α inhibitors. **4e** can be further optimized for its activity and properties. Our study provides insights into designing small molecule inhibitors directly targeting TNF-α and for protein–protein interaction inhibitor design.

Keywords: TNF-α inhibitor, dihydrobenzo[*cd*]indole-6-sulfonamide, virtual screening, synthesis, structure activity analysis

INTRODUCTION

Tumor necrosis factor-α (TNF-α), an important cytokine mediator involved in inflammatory responses, is commonly used as a marker for many inflammatory disorders (Wajant et al., 2003). Antibodies that directly targeting TNF-α have achieved success in the treatment of inflammatory disorders such as rheumatoid arthritis, Crohn's disease, and ulcerative colitis (Bongartz et al., 2005; Jacobi et al., 2006). However, these biologics possess the possibility to cause anti-antibody immune responses and weaken the immune system to opportunistic infections (Scheinfeld, 2004; Ai et al., 2015).

Thus, developing inhibitors to block TNF-α is still of great importance. Zhu et al. have reported several rationally designed proteins that directly bound to TNF-α. They grafted three key residues from a virus viral 2L protein to a *de novo* designed small protein DS119, and then optimized their residues at the interface, which provided some small proteins that bind TNF-α with sub-micromolar affinities (Zhu et al., 2016). Other than small proteins, bicyclic peptides and helical peptides were also designed as peptidic antagonists of TNF-α (Lian et al., 2013; Zhang et al., 2013).

In addition to peptide inhibitors, small molecular inhibitors that directly targeting TNF-α have also been discovered (Leung et al., 2012; Davis and Colangelo, 2013; Shen et al., 2014). Suramin was thought to be the first small compound inhibitor that directly disrupts the interactions between TNF-α and its receptor (TNFR) (Grazioli et al., 1992). But its potency was too low to be used in clinic (Alzani et al., 1993). No breakthrough was made until 2005, when SPD304 was reported as the first potent small molecule inhibitor that directly targeting TNF-α, with an IC_{50} of 22 μM by ELISA. And the co-crystal structure of SPD304 in complex with TNF-α dimer was solved (He et al., 2005). However, as the 3-alkylindole moiety of SPD304 can be metabolized by cytochrome P450s to produce toxic electrophilic intermediates, its further applications *in vivo* is limited (Sun and Yost, 2008). After that, several novel TNF-α inhibitors were discovered using structure-based virtual screening (VS) of different chemical libraries. Chan et al. identified two compounds using high-throughput ligand-docking-based VS (**Figure 1**, **quinuclidine 1** and **indoloquinolizidine 2**), and their experimental tests showed that **quinuclidine 1** is more effective than **indoloquinolizidine 2** in inhibition of TNF-α induced NF-κB signaling in HepG2 cells, with IC_{50}-values of 5 and >30 μM, respectively (Chan et al., 2010). Choi and colleagues discovered a series of pyrimidine-2,4,6-trione derivatives from a 240,000-compound library. The best compound (**Figure 1**, **Oxole-1**) showed 64% inhibition at 10 μM (Choi et al., 2010). Leung et al. reported a novel iridium(III)-based direct inhibitor of TNF-α (**Figure 1**, **$[Ir(ppy)_2(biq)]PF_6$**; Leung et al., 2012). Mouhsine et al. used combined *in silico/in vitro/in vivo* screening approaches to identify orally available TNF-α inhibitors with IC_{50} of 10 μM (**Figure 1**, **Benzenesulfonamide-1**; Mouhsine et al., 2017). Other efforts to develop TNF-α inhibitors were also reported (Mancini et al., 1999; Buller et al., 2009; Leung et al., 2011; Hu et al., 2012; Alexiou et al., 2014; Ma et al., 2014; Kang et al., 2016). However, due to the low potency and high cytotoxicity, small molecule TNF-α inhibitors still have a long way to go for clinical applications (Davis and Colangelo, 2013). Highly active TNF-α inhibitors with novel chemical structures need to be developed. In a previous study, we have discovered a compound (**Figure 1**, **EJMC-1**) that directly bound TNF-α (Shen et al., 2014). The scaffold of the compound, 2-oxo-N-phenyl-1,2-dihydrobenzo[*cd*]indole-6-sulfonamide, has been reported as inhibitors of West Nile virus (Gu et al., 2006), RORγ inhibitors (Zhang et al., 2014), and BET bromodomain inhibitors (Xue et al., 2016; Mouhsine et al., 2017). Considering the good druggability of this scaffold, its analogs may be valuable for developing potent TNF-α inhibitors. In the present study, we used the scaffold of compound **EJMC-1** to perform similarity-based virtual screen and experimental testing. Top-ranking compounds were first tested for their abilities to reduce TNF-α binding with TNFR using surface plasmon resonance (SPR). Then the cell-based NF-κB reporter gene assay was used to test the activities of the compounds to reduce TNF-α induced signaling. New compounds were further designed, synthesized, and tested. The structure-activity relationship of these compounds was analyzed.

MATERIALS AND METHODS

General Information

HEK293T cells were received as a gift from Professor Jincai Luo (Peking University, China). The extracellular domain of the TNF receptor 1 (TNFR1-ECD) was purchased from R&D Systems. The selected compounds were purchased from the SPECS database with purity higher than 90% and for most compounds >95% (confirmed by the supplier, using NMR or LC-MS data available through the website). Other biochemistry reagents were from Sigma Aldrich unless indicated otherwise. The organic reagents and solvents were commercially available and purified according to conventional methods. All reactions were monitored by thin layer chromatography (TLC), using silica gel 60 F-254 aluminum sheets and UV light (254 and 366 nm) for detection. All title compounds gave satisfactory ^{1}H NMR, ^{13}C NMR, and mass spectrometry analyses. The ^{1}H NMR and ^{13}C NMR spectra were measured on a Bruker-400 M spectrometer using TMS as internal standard. High resolution mass spectra were recorded on a Bruker Apex IV FTMS mass spectrometer using ESI (electrospray ionization).

Synthesis

Benzo[*cd*]indol-2(*1H*)-one 2

2 was prepared based on the adoption of method by Kamal et al. (2012). Napthalic anhydride (1.98 g, 10 mmol), hydroxylamine hydrochloride (0.69 mg, 10 mmol), and dry pyridine (5 ml) were added to dried three-necked flask. Heating was discontinued after reflux for 1 h, than benzenesulfonyl chloride (5 g) was added portion wise to cause controlled boiling. Finally, heating was resumed for 1 h, and the hot mixture was poured into water (30 ml). The crystalline precipitate was collected, washed with 0.5 N NaOH and water. The crystals were boiled with water (15 ml) and ethanol (5 ml) containing sodium hydroxide (5 g) for 2 h, during the second of which, ethanol was allowed to distill

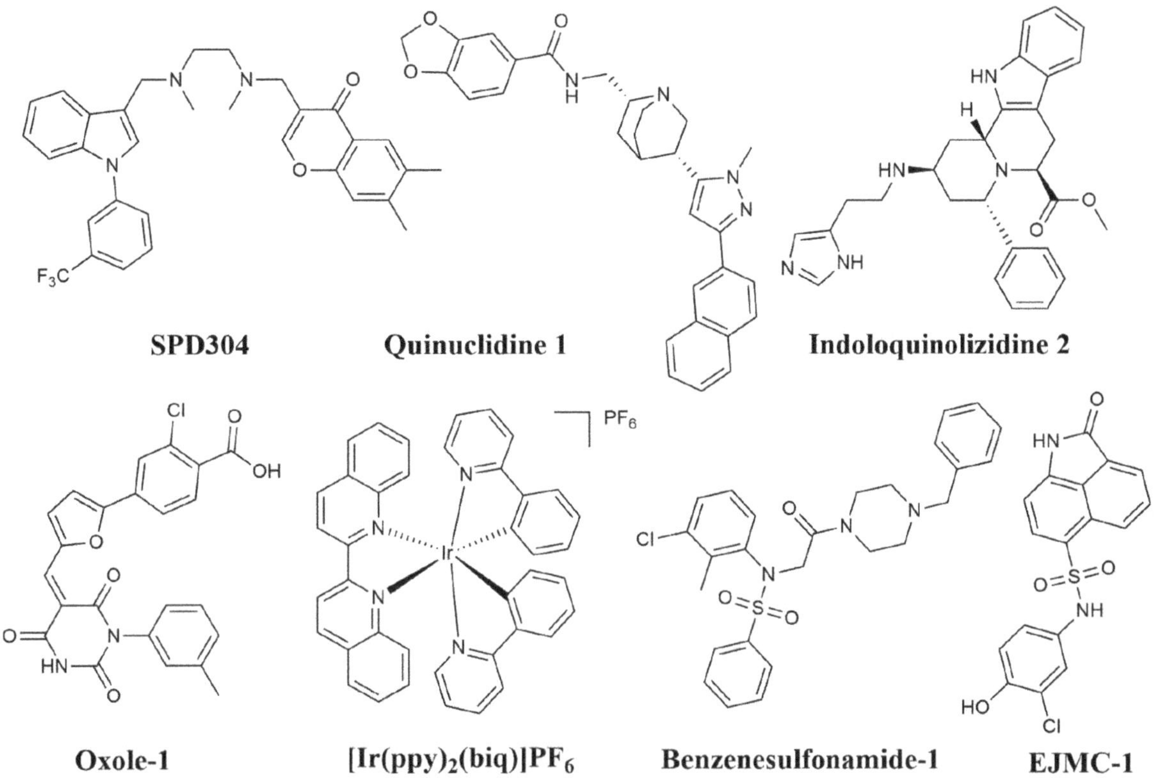

FIGURE 1 | Structures of small molecule inhibitors of TNF-α.

out. The solution was acidified with concentrated hydrochloric acid (3 ml), carbon dioxide being evolved and yellow crystals deposited. Next day, the crystals were washed, and dried to give light yellow needles (1.25 g, 74%). Mp175–179°C; ^{1}H NMR (DMSO, 300 MHz, DMSO-d_6) δ 8.05 (d, 1H, J = 6.7 Hz), 8.01 (d, 1H, J = 8.3 Hz), 7.75–7.70 (m, 1H), 7.53 (d, 1H, J = 8.3 Hz), 7.40 (dd, 1H, J = 7.5, 6.7 Hz), 6.94 (d, 1H, J = 6.7 Hz).

2-oxo-1,2-dihydrobenzo[*cd*]indole-6-sulfonyl Chloride 3

3 was prepared based on the adoption of method by Talukdar et al. (2010). Chlorosulfonic acid (3.2 ml) was added slowly to **2** (1.0 g, 5.9 mmol). The reaction mixture was stirred at 0°C for 1 h and at room temperature for 2 h. The mixture was then poured into ice water (20 ml). The precipitate was washed with water (2 × 10 ml) and dried to give product as yellow solid (0.66 g, 38%). Used without further purification.

General Procedure for N-Substituted 2-oxo-N-phenyl-1,2-dihydrobenzo[*cd*]indole-6-sulfonamides 4

A mixture of 2-oxo-1,2-dihydrobenzo[*cd*]indole-6-sulfonyl chloride (100 mg, 0.37 mmol), 0.37 mmol aniline, 0.4 ml Et_3N, 20 mg DMAP was dissolved in 5 ml DMF, the reaction mixture was stirred at room temperature, the reaction was detected by TLC, after the reaction was finished, extracted with 50 ml ethyl acetate and 20 ml water, washed with water 20 ml three times, then 20 ml saturated NH_4Cl aqueous, 20 ml brine. The organic layer was dried by Na_2SO_4, and the solvent was removed *in vacuo*. The residue was purified by Column chromatography.

N-(5-aminonaphthalen-1-yl)-2-oxo-1,2-dihydrobenzo[*cd*]indole-6-sulfonamide 4a

Seventy-six milligrams, yield 54%. ^{1}H NMR (400 MHz, DMSO-d_6) δ 5.66 (s, 2H), 6.52 (d, J = 7.5 Hz, 1H), 6.88 (t, J = 8.1 Hz, 1H), 6.92 (d, J = 7.6 Hz, 1H), 7.04 (d, J = 8.4 Hz, 1H), 7.11 (d, J = 7.3 Hz, 1H), 7.18 (t, J = 7.9 Hz, 1H), 7.87 (dd, J = 7.9, 4.0 Hz, 3H), 8.07 (d, J = 7.0 Hz, 1H), 8.65 (d, J = 8.4 Hz, 1H), 10.18 (s, 1H), 11.07 (s, 1H). ^{13}C NMR (101 MHz, DMSO-d_6) δ 168.70, 144.73, 142.65, 132.68, 132.01, 130.51, 130.23, 129.48, 128.50, 126.64, 126.46, 125.92, 124.71, 124.56, 123.29, 122.84, 122.76, 121.03, 110.30, 107.63, 104.54. HRMS (ESI): calcd for $C_{21}H_{16}N_3O_3S$, [(M+H)$^+$], 391.0912, found 390.0896.

N-(3-aminonaphthalen-2-yl)-2-oxo-1,2-dihydrobenzo[*cd*]indole-6-sulfonamide 4b

Thirty-four milligrams, yield 26%. ^{1}H NMR (400 MHz, DMSO-d_6) δ 1.20–1.29 (m, 2H), 4.67–5.36 (m, 2H), 6.79 (s, 1H), 6.95 (d, J = 7.6 Hz, 1H), 7.05 (ddd, J = 8.1, 6.7, 1.2 Hz, 1H), 7.22 (ddd, J = 8.2, 6.8, 1.3 Hz, 1H), 7.35 (s, 1H), 7.41 (d, J = 8.2 Hz, 1H), 7.46 (d, J = 8.2 Hz, 1H), 7.85 (dd, J = 8.4, 7.0 Hz, 1H), 7.95 (d, J = 7.6 Hz, 1H), 8.08 (d, J = 7.0 Hz, 1H), 8.65 (d, J = 8.4 Hz, 1H), 11.12 (s, 1H). ^{13}C NMR (101 MHz, DMSO-d_6)

δ 169.10, 143.82, 142.21, 132.68, 132.21, 130.81, 130.01, 129.31, 128.65, 126.66, 126.45, 125.87, 124.63, 124.53, 123.39, 122.81, 122.77, 121.03, 110.60, 106.63, 103.59. HRMS (ESI): calcd for $C_{21}H_{16}N_3O_3S$, $[(M+H)^+]$, 390.0912, found 390.0896.

2-oxo-N-(1,2,3,4-tetrahydronaphthalen-1-yl)-1,2-dihydrobenzo[*cd*]indole-6-sulfonamide 4c

Sixty-eight milligrams, yield 48%. ^{1}H NMR (400 MHz, DMSO-d_6) δ 1.31–1.42 (m, 2H), 1.55–1.74 (m, 2H), 2.55–2.70 (m, 2H), 4.33 (dd, J = 9.7, 5.3 Hz, 1H), 6.93–6.97 (m, 2H), 7.02 (s, 1H), 7.08 (d, J = 7.4 Hz, 2H), 7.90–7.95 (m, 1H), 8.14 (t, J = 6.9 Hz, 2H), 8.35 (d, J = 8.4 Hz, 1H), 8.72 (d, J = 8.4 Hz, 1H), 11.16 (s, 1H). ^{13}C NMR (101 MHz, DMSO-d_6) δ 169.31, 142.98, 137.57, 136.86, 132.65, 130.89, 130.37, 130.12, 129.17, 128.95, 127.41, 127.35, 126.67, 126.10, 125.31, 124.82, 105.17, 51.51, 30.68, 28.87, 19.68. HRMS (ESI): calcd for $C_{42}H_{36}N_4NaO_6S_2$, $[(2M+Na)^+]$, 779.1974, found 799.1939.

N-(naphthalen-1-ylmethyl)-2-oxo-1,2-dihydrobenzo[*cd*]indole-6-sulfonamide 4d

Fifteen milligrams, yield 10%. ^{1}H NMR (400 MHz, DMSO-d_6) δ 4.43 (d, J = 5.7 Hz, 2H), 6.94 (d, J = 7.5 Hz, 1H), 7.25–7.36 (m, 3H), 7.41 (ddd, J = 8.1, 6.8, 1.2 Hz, 1H), 7.72–7.76 (m, 1H), 7.82 (d, J = 8.1 Hz, 1H), 7.85–7.90 (m, 2H), 7.98 (d, J = 7.5 Hz, 1H), 8.08 (d, J = 7.0 Hz, 1H), 8.40 (t, J = 5.9 Hz, 1H), 8.65 (d, J = 8.3 Hz, 1H), 11.10 (s, 1H). ^{13}C NMR (101 MHz, DMSO-d_6) δ 169.29, 133.54, 132.94, 132.84, 131.08, 130.74, 130.04, 128.93, 128.69, 128.47, 127.29, 126.52, 126.33, 126.07, 125.47, 125.13, 124.74, 123.89, 104.98, 44.73. HRMS (ESI): calcd for $C_{44}H_{33}N_4O_6S_2$, $[(2M+H)^+]$, 777.1842, found 777.1804.

N-(1H-indol-6-yl)-2-oxo-1,2-dihydrobenzo[*cd*]indole-6-sulfonamide 4e

Ninety-one milligrams, yield 68%. ^{1}H NMR (300 MHz, DMSO-d_6) δ 6.21–6.27 (m, 1H), 6.67 (dd, J = 8.4, 2.0 Hz, 1H), 6.95 (d, J = 7.7 Hz, 1H), 7.05 (d, J = 1.7 Hz, 1H), 7.17–7.22 (m, 1H), 7.27 (d, J = 8.5 Hz, 1H), 7.91 (dd, J = 8.4, 7.0 Hz, 1H), 7.97 (d, J = 7.6 Hz, 1H), 8.08 (d, J = 6.9 Hz, 1H), 8.74 (d, J = 8.3 Hz, 1H), 10.20 (s, 1H), 10.91 (s, 1H), 11.11 (s, 1H). ^{13}C NMR (101 MHz, DMSO-d_6) δ 169.15, 143.24, 136.18, 133.83, 131.41, 130.96, 129.77, 128.07, 127.28, 126.38, 125.87, 125.29, 124.90, 120.64, 114.44, 105.02, 104.61, 101.32. HRMS (ESI): calcd for $C_{38}H_{27}N_6O_6S_2$, $[(2M+H)^+]$, 727.1433, found 727.1428.

N-(3-(1-methyl-1H-pyrazol-4-yl)phenyl)-2-oxo-1,2-dihydrobenzo[*cd*]indole-6-sulfonamide 4f

Seventy-six milligrams, yield 51%. ^{1}H NMR (300 MHz, DMSO-d_6) δ 3.84 (s, 3H), 6.80 (dt, J = 5.4, 2.8 Hz, 1H), 7.04 (d, J = 7.6 Hz, 1H), 7.09 - 7.13 (m, 2H), 7.19 (s, 1H), 7.64 (s, 1H), 7.90 - 7.95 (m, 1H), 7.98 (s, 1H), 8.09 (d, J = 7.0 Hz, 1H), 8.19 (d, J = 7.7 Hz, 1H), 8.72 (d, J = 8.3 Hz, 1H), 10.59 (s, 1H), 11.16 (s, 1H). ^{13}C NMR (101 MHz, DMSO-d_6) δ 169.25, 143.33, 136.18, 133.83, 133.56, 131.41, 130.96, 130.51, 129.77, 128.07, 127.28, 126.38, 125.87, 125.29, 124.90, 124.64, 119.44, 117.82, 117.61, 114.32, 40.51. HRMS (ESI): calcd for $C_{21}H_{17}N_4O_3S$, $[(M+H)^+]$, 405.1021, found 405.1086.

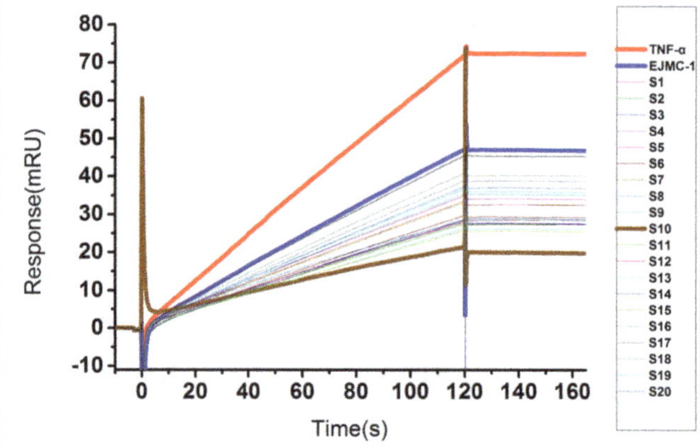

FIGURE 2 | SPR competitive binding curves of compounds from shape screening of **EJMC-1**. Compounds showed competitive binding to TNF-α. The Red curve was TNF-α binding with TNFR1-ECD alone, and the other curves were TNF-α TNFR1-ECD in the presence of compounds at 100 μM. The reference compound **EJMC-1** was colored blue and the best compound in SPR assay **S10** was colored brown.

6-((1H-benzo[d]imidazol-1-yl)sulfonyl)benzo[*cd*]indol-2(1H)-one 4g

Eighty milligrams, yield 62%. ^{1}H NMR (400 MHz, DMSO-d_6) δ 7.16 (d, J = 7.8 Hz, 1H), 7.37-7.31 (m, 2H), 7.69–7.75 (m, 1H), 7.82 (dt, J = 8.3, 0.9 Hz, 1H), 7.93–8.03 (m, 1H), 8.12 (d, J = 7.0 Hz, 1H), 8.71 (d, J = 7.8 Hz, 1H), 8.76 (d, J = 8.4 Hz, 1H), 9.19 (s, 1H), 11.35 (s, 1H). ^{13}C NMR (101 MHz, DMSO-d_6) δ 168.46, 145.77, 143.47, 142.38, 136.22, 132.11, 129.83, 127.72, 127.05, 126.04, 125.57, 125.46, 124.71, 123.50, 122.77, 120.65, 112.18, 104.85. HRMS (ESI): calcd for $C_{36}H_{23}N_6O_6S_2$, $[(2M+H)^+]$, 699.1120, found 699.1135.

Competitive Binding Assay Using SPR

Binding interactions between TNF-α and TNFR1-ECD in the presence/absence of small molecule inhibitors were examined on the SPR-based Biacore T200 instrument (GE Healthcare). TNFR1-ECD was immobilized on a CM5 sensor chip using standard amine-coupling at 25°C with 1X running buffer PBS-P (GE Healthcare). A reference flow cell was activated and blocked in the absence of TNFR1-ECD. All experiments were performed in phosphate-buffered saline (PBS)-EP buffer (10 mM NaH_2PO_4/Na_2HPO_4, 150 mM NaCl, 3.7 mM EDTA, 0.05% surfactant P20, pH 7.4) at 25°C with a flow rate of 50 μl/min. A final concentration of 20 nM TNF-α was mixed with each compound at various concentrations (as indicated in section Results) in PBS-EP and the mixture was injected. Equal amounts of TNF-α mixed with PBS-EP were used as a control. Regeneration was achieved by extended washing with glycine hydrochloride buffer (10 mM Glycine-HCl, pH 2.1) after each sample injection.

Cell Based NF-κB Reporter Assay

The cellular assay were carried out as described previously (Zhang et al., 2013). HEK293T cells were grown to

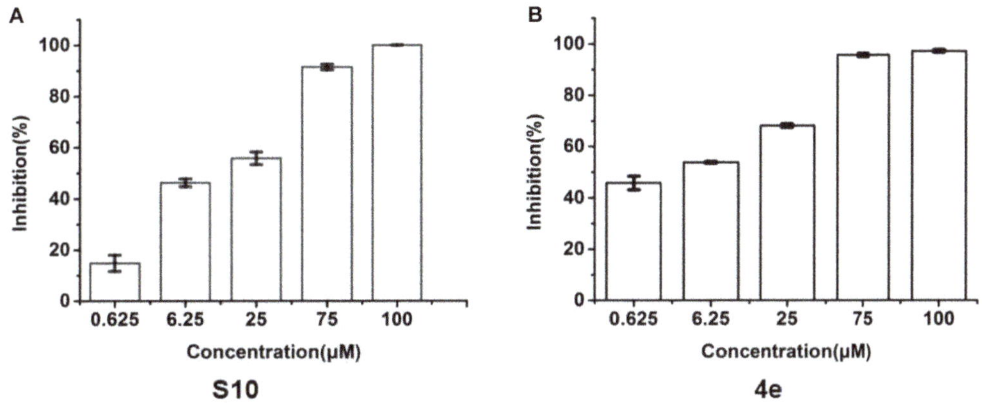

FIGURE 3 | Inhibition of TNF-α induced NF-κB transcription activity. **(A)** Dose-response of compounds S10 in the cell based assay in 293T cell line. **(B)** Dose-response of compounds **4e** in the cell based assay in 293T cell line. The data was reported as means ± errors from three independent experiments.

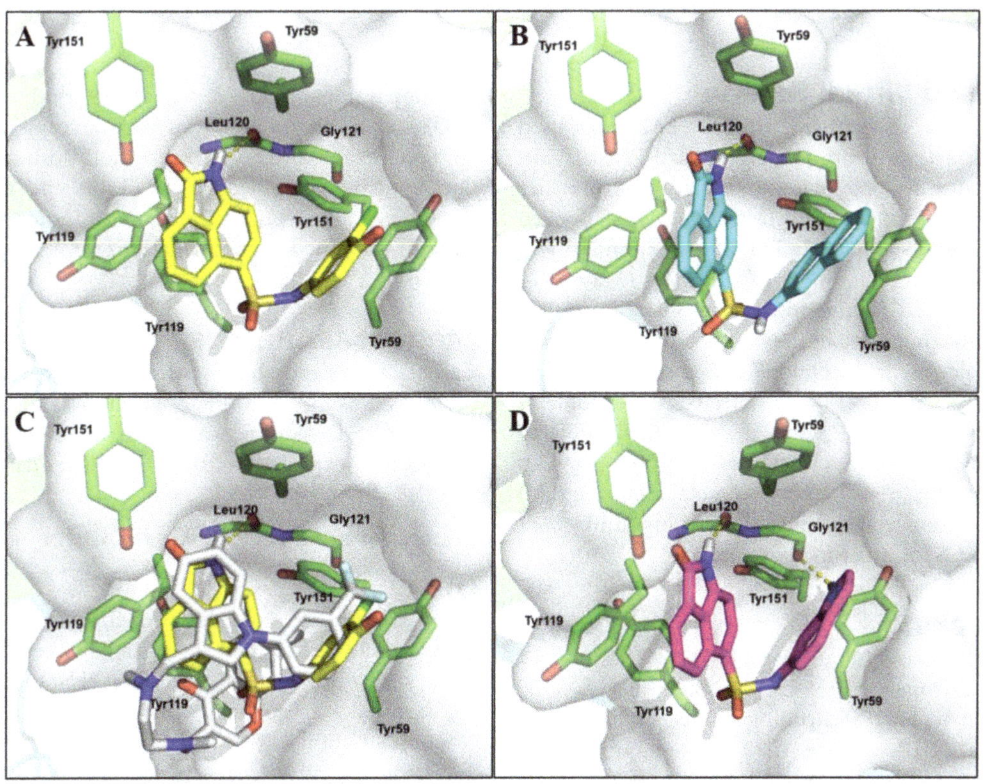

FIGURE 4 | The predicted binding modes of TNF-α inhibitors. Predicted binding mode of compounds **EJMC-1** and **4e** to TNF-α. The binding site was shown as surface, the key residues were shown as sticks (green). **(A)** compound **EJMC-1** (yellow). **(B)** Compound **S10** (cyan). **(C) EJMC-1** compare to **SPD304** (gray). **(D)** compound **4e** (magenta).

70% confluence in 6 cm dish at 37°C in Dulbecco's modified Eagle's medium supplemented with 10% fetal bovine serum (FBS; Gibco), then transfected with purified plasmids 0.6 μg pGL4.32 (luc2P/NF-κB-RE/Hygro plasmid) and 0.4 μg pGL4.74 (hRluc/TK) with ViaFect transfection reagent (Promega). After 24 h, the transfected cells were seeded in 96-wells plate, 40,000 cells per well. Twelve hours later, 100 μL pre-incubated mixture of TNF-α and small molecules was added to stimulate the cells for 6 h and the luciferase assays were carried out using the Dual-Glo Luciferase Assay System (Promega) with a BioTek synergy 4 Multi-Mode Microplate Reader. The final concentration of TNF-α in each well was 10 ng/ml. Equal amounts of TNF-α without small molecular were added to the cells as a negative control to calculate the percentage of activity inhibition.

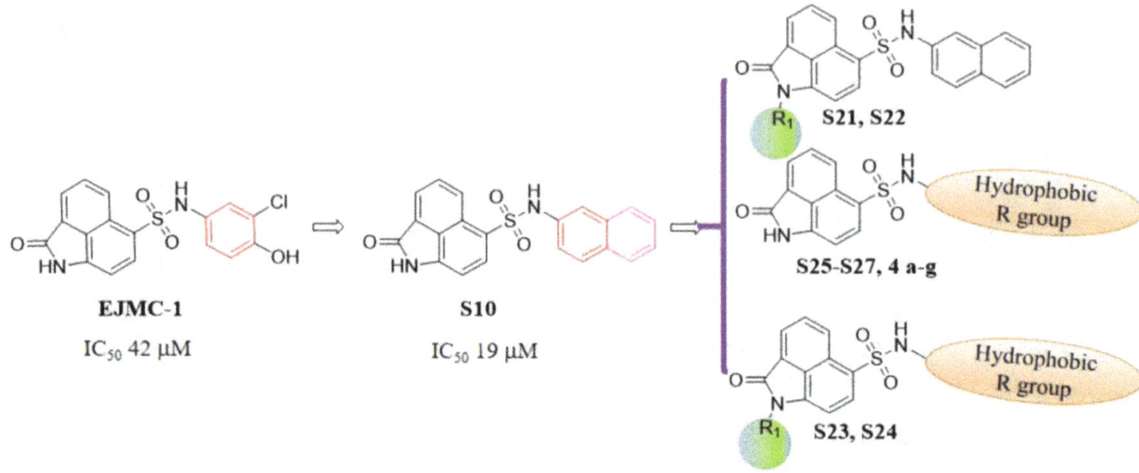

FIGURE 5 | Designed TNF-α inhibitors.

Similarity-Based Virtual Screen

The crystal structure of TNF-α dimer (PDB code: 2AZ5) was used for grid generation. The program Glide Standard Precise (SP) mode was used to do the molecular docking studies (Friesner et al., 2004; Halgren et al., 2004). **EJMC-1** was first docked to TNF-α dimer, and its conformation in the complex was used for Shape Screening of the SPECS library (May 2013 version for 10 mg; 197,276 compounds). The Shape Similarity indexes between each compound in the library and the reference compound were calculated. A total of 587 compounds with indexes between 0.8 and 0.99 were selected as candidates for the second round manual selection with the following selection criteria: (a) containing at least one ring which provides hydrophobic interaction; (b) containing no metal atoms; and (c) shared in multiple structures. A total of 68 compounds were purchased from SPECS for experimental testing.

Molecular Docking

The complex structure of TNF-α with SPD304 (PDB code: 2AZ5) was retrieved from the Protein Data Bank and docking was performed with maestro (Schrödinger, Inc., version 10.2). Compound **EJMC-1, S10,** and **4e** were docked into TNF-α dimer protein using Glide Docking module (Friesner et al., 2004; Halgren et al., 2004). The details of the docking workflow are listed below: (1) Protein was prepared using the "Protein Preparation Wizard" workflow. All water molecules were removed from the structure of the complex. Hydrogen atoms and charges were added during a brief relaxation. After optimizing the hydrogen bond network, the crystal structure was minimized using the OPLS_2005 force field with the maximum root mean square deviation (RMSD) value of 0.3 Å. (2) The ligand was prepared with LigPrep module in Maestro, including adding hydrogen atoms, ionizing at a pH range from 7.2 to 7.4, and producing the corresponding low-energy 3D structure. (3) Pose prediction mode of Glide Docking modules were adopted to dock the molecules into the SPD304-binding site with the default parameters. The center of the grid box was defined with SPD304. The top-ranking poses of molecule **EJMC-1, S10,** and **4e** were retained. The LigPrep mol2 format output was also docked using AutoDock Vina (Trott and Olson, 2010) with standard protocols. The computed binding free energies and structures for the top conformations were saved for post-docking analysis.

Statistical Analysis

Cell assay was repeated for three times. Statistical analysis was performed using OriginPro 9.1, data was fit by DoseResp using Origin 9.1. DoseResp was a three-parameter Hill equation. Results were expressed as mean ± *SD* (standard deviation value).

RESULTS AND DISCUSSION

Chemistry

Seven derivatives of dihydrobenzo[*cd*]indole-6-sulfonamide were synthesized using a three-step synthetic route (**Scheme 1**) with yields between 10 and 68%. Napthalic anhydride was transformed to benzo[*cd*]indol-2(*1H*)-one by aminolysis reaction smoothly, with a yield of 74%. Then, benzo[*cd*]indol-2(*1H*)-one underwent nucleophile substitution reaction with chlorosulfonic acid to get key intermediate 2-oxo-1,2-dihydrobenzo[*cd*]indole-6-sulfonyl chloride (**3**), with a yield of 38%. Reactions of compound **3** with various amines in the presence of a catalyst system consisting of DMAP, Et_3N, afforded **4** and derivatives in good yields. The original spectra of featured compounds shown in Supplementary Image 1.

Compounds From Similarity Search of EJMC-1 Block TNF-α Binding to TNFR

We used compound **EJMC-1** as the reference compound for similarity search (**Figure 1**). The binding conformation of **EJMC-1** with TNF-α was generated using molecular docking and used in pharmacophore based shape screening over the SPECS library.

TABLE 1 | The structure and activities of **S10** analogs.

Compound	Structure	IC_{50} in cell assay (μM)[a]	Source
EJMC-1	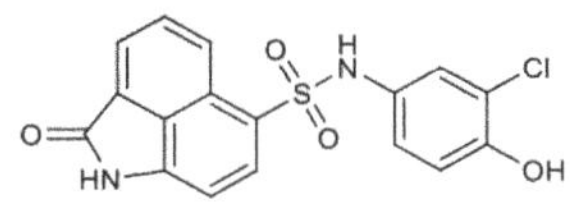	43.2 ± 2.6	SPECS
S10	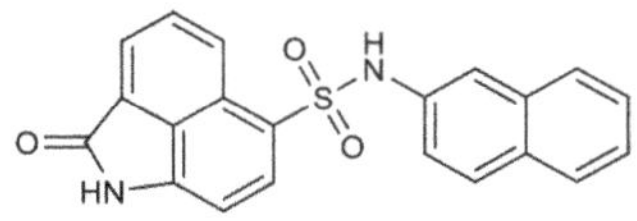	19.1 ± 2.2	SPECS
S21	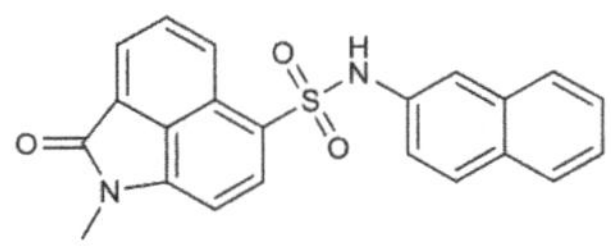	28.8 ± 3.1	SPECS
S22	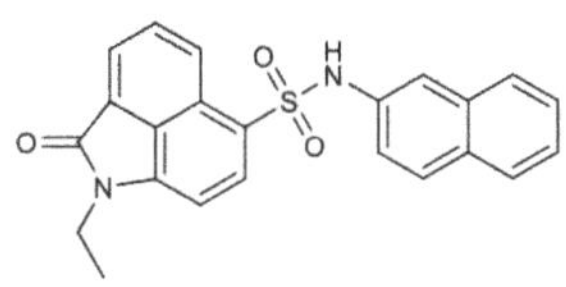	16.0 ± 1.8	SPECS
S23	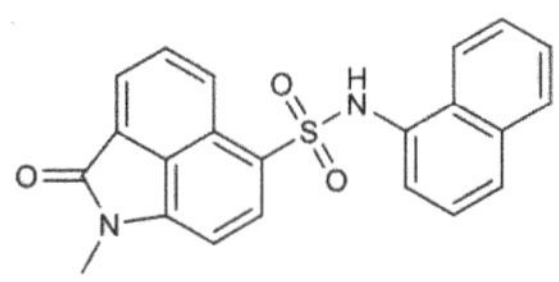	24.6 ± 2.1	SPECS
S24	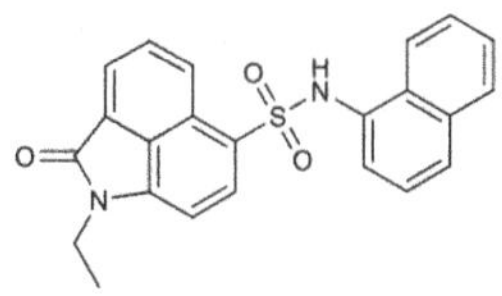	19.8 ± 1.5	SPECS
S25	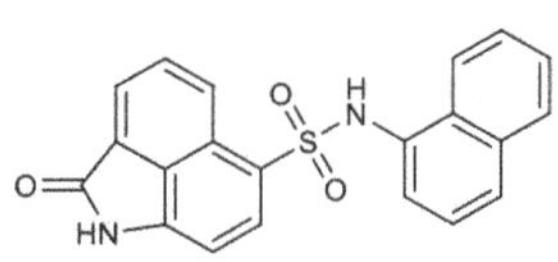	14.0 ± 2.3	SPECS
S26	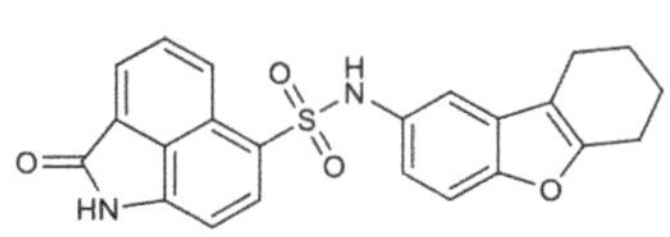	16.0 ± 2.3	SPECS
S27	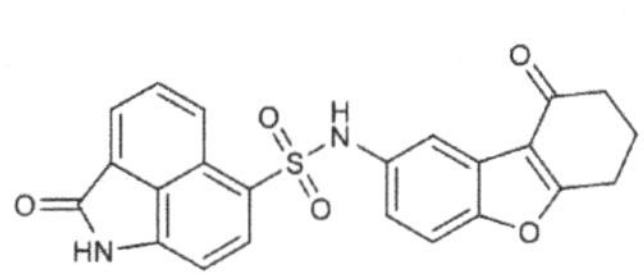	28.5 ± 3.8	SPECS
4a	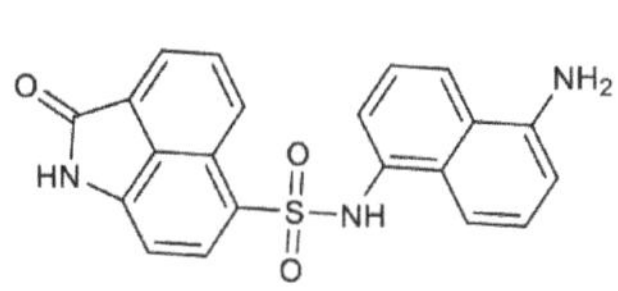	>100	Synthesis
4b	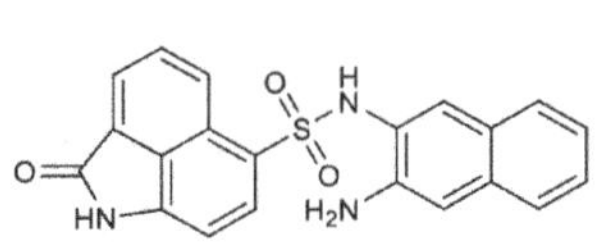	>100	Synthesis
4c	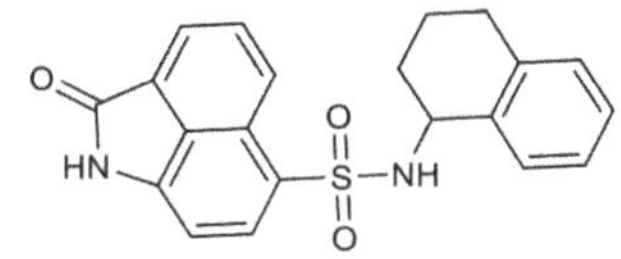	12.5 ± 1.6	Synthesis
4d	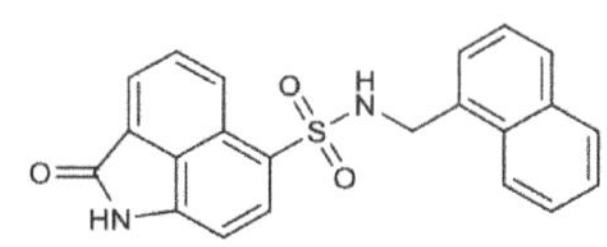	>100	Synthesis
4e	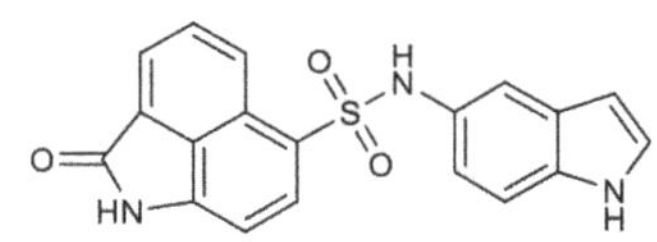	3.0 ± 0.8	Synthesis
4f	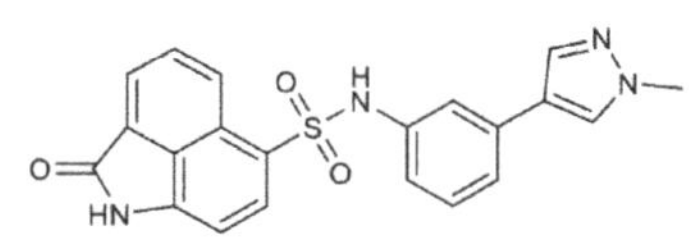	6.2 ± 1.3	Synthesis
4g	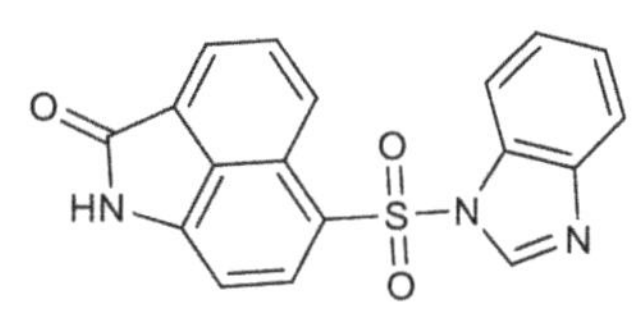	>100	Synthesis
SPD304	6.4 ± 0.6		

[a]*Data shown represent the mean (n = 3).*

Compounds with similarity index between 0.80 and 0.99 with **EJMC-1** were subjected to further manual selection. A total of 68 compounds were selected for experimental testing (Table S1). The chemical structures of these compounds fall into two classes, sulfonates and sulfonamides. The sulfonamides contain both N-aryl sulfonamides and N-alkylsulfonamides, with or without substituted aminocarbonyl group (Table S1).

We used a SPR competitive assay to test whether these compounds can more efficiently block TNF-α and TNFR binding than **EJMC-1**. TNF-α with or without compounds flowed over the chip surface where the extracellular domain of TNFR was immobilized. At the concentration of 100 μM, 20 of the 68 compounds reduced the TNF-α binding signal compared to **EJMC-1** (**Figure 2**). These 20 candidates were selected for further cell-based inhibition studies. The specs ID of these 20 compounds were listed in Table S2, and the corresponding chemical structures were in supporting information. All the sulfonamide derivatives of **EJMC-1** showed competitive binding with TNF-α against TNFR1, while sulfonates could not.

EJMC-1 Analogs Inhibit TNF-α Induced NF-κB Gene Expression

To explore whether these compounds with enhanced abilities to reduce TNF-α binding with receptor were active under cellular environment, we used a luciferase assay to monitor

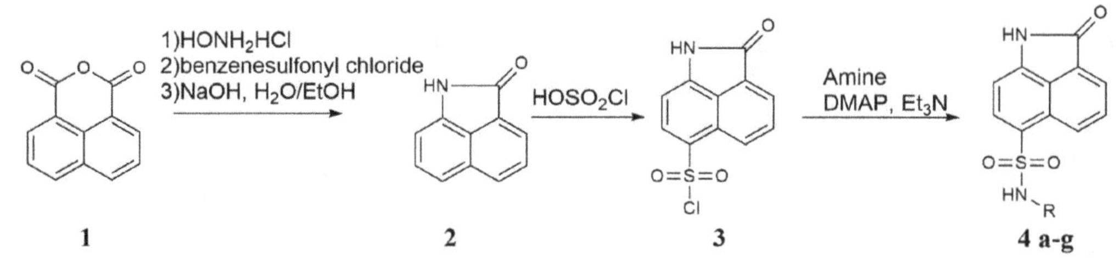

SCHEME 1 | Synthesis of 2-oxo-1,2-dihydrobenzo[*cd*]indole-6-sulfonamide derivatives.

their influences on NF-κB transcriptional activity. In this assay, in transfected cells, TNF-α induces NF-κB activation through TNFR1, which then drives the expression of the luciferase. The cell-level inhibitory effects of these 20 compounds were measured using the Dual-Glo Luciferase Assay System. With two dose screen, two compounds, **S3 and S10** showed better activity than **EJMC-1** (Table S2). The best compound, **S10**, suppressed NF-κB transcriptional activity dose-dependently (**Figure 3A**) with an IC_{50} of 19.1 ± 2.2 μM. The positive control, SPD304, displayed an IC_{50} of 6.4 ± 0.6 μM in the side-by-side experiment.

Docking Analysis and Compound Design

Molecular docking gave clues on rational designing compounds with potential enhanced activities and understanding SAR. In the complex structure of TNF-α with SPD304, SPD304 bound to a pocket in the TNF-α dimer (He et al., 2005; Shen et al., 2014). **EJMC-1** was shown to bind with the same site (He et al., 2005; Shen et al., 2014). Both Glide and AutoDock Vina were used in the docking study. We first tested whether the binding pose of SPD304 can be reproduced. We have tried many times with different parameters, but was unable to get a binding pose that is close to that in the crystal structure (with the minimum RMSD up to 4 Å). We then used AutoDock Vina to dock SPD 304 to the TNF-α dimer and the lowest binding free energy conformation obtained was closed to its crystal conformation with a RMSD of 0.70 Å. Despite of the different binding conformations obtained for SPD304 by using two docking software, the top ranking conformations of **EJMC-1** were almost the same from the docking runs using both Glide and AutoDock Vina. These differences might due to the flexibility of SPD304, which adopted a U shape conformation, and the conformational sampling preference of the docking software. As there are no essential differences in the docking poses of the compounds other than SPD304, we used the Glide docking poses of these compounds to compare to SPD304 in the crystal structure. Compared to **EJMC-1**, **S10** had increased hydrophobic interaction with the Tyr59 residue (**Figures 4A,B**). In addition to the nonpolar interactions with TNF-α as in the case of SPD304, the scaffold of **EJMC-1** and **S10** provide further polar interactions, strengthening the specificity and activity (**Figure 4C**). As **EJMC-1** is smaller than that of SPD304 with unoccupied hydrophobic space in the pocket (**Figure 4C**), several analogs with larger substituted group of sulfonamide of 2-oxo-1,2-dihydrobenzo[*cd*]indole-6-sulfonamide were designed and docked to this site. Compound **4e,** with larger hydrophobic group size and additional H-bond donor, interacts favorably with TNF-α and might be more potent (**Figure 4D**). Based on the docking analysis, the designed analogs were purchased or synthesized for cell assay.

Optimization of Compound S10 and Structure-Activity Analysis

As shown in the cell assay, the inhibition activity of **S10** increased about 2-fold than that of **EJMC-1.** The introduction of the naphthalene ring provides stronger hydrophobic interactions. Based on the docking analysis and increased activity of **S10**, we try to: (1) Keep naphthalene ring, changed N-substituted groups of dihydrobenzo[*cd*]indole, (2) Keep N-H of dihydrobenzo[*cd*]indole, optimize the hydrophobic R group, (3) optimize both N-substituted groups of dihydrobenzo[*cd*]indole and the hydrophobic R group (**Figure 5**). Seven commercially available analogs of **S10** were purchased for testing (**Table 1**). The SPECS ID of these seven **S10** analogues were listed in Table S3. We further synthesized seven new compounds in three steps from 1,8-Naphthalic anhydride through conventional reactions (**Scheme 1** and **Figure 5**). All compounds passed the PAINS (pan assay interference compounds) remover, which filters out compounds that appear as frequent hitters (promiscuous compounds) in many biochemical high throughput screens (Baell and Holloway, 2010).

All the compounds were tested using the TNF-α induced NF-κB reporter assay. The structures and activities were listed in **Table 1**. For **S10**, methyl or ethyl group substitution on the amide of 2-oxo-1,2-dihydrobenzo[*cd*]indole-6-sulfonamide had no obviously enhanced inhibition (**S21** and **S22**), and the α or β substitution of the naphthyl group did not affect the inhibition (**S23, S24,** and **S25**). The size of the N-substituted groups of sulfonamide was important for inhibition activity (**EJMC-1, S10,** and **S27**). The flexibility and aromaticity of the N-substituted two-ring group of sulfonamide played dominant role, too rigid or too flexible dramatically reduced the activity (**4g, 4d**). The fact that N-(5-aminonaphthalen-1-yl) and N-(3-aminonaphthalen-1-yl) group substituted compounds lost functions might be caused by the conformation change due to additional amino group on the naphthalene ring. Introducing heterocycle significantly increases the inhibition activity (**4e and 4f**). The N-(*1H*-indol-6-yl) substituted sulfonamides (**4e**) were 6-fold more potent than

S10, even better than SPD304 (**Table 1**, **Figure 3B**). Though **S10** and **4e** had similar size of substitution group on sulfonamide, **4e** shown better inhibition activity than **S10** might due to the additional H-bond that **4e** forms with the backbone carbonyl of Gly121 (**Figure 4C**). Meanwhile, the indolyl group of **4e** was also deeper in the binding pocket than that of naphthyl group on **S10** (**Figure 4D**).

CONCLUSION

We have optimized a previously reported TNF-α inhibitor **EJMC-1** using similarity-based VS and rational design. An analog of **EJMC-1**, **S10** was found with 2-fold TNF-α increased inhibition activity. Based on the structures of **EJMC-1**, **S10**, and their interactions with TNF-α, we designed derivatives of 2-oxo-1,2-dihydrobenzo[*cd*]indole-6-sulfonamide. Several commercially available ones were purchased and seven new compounds were synthesized for SAR study. After two rounds of design, we obtained **4e** with an IC_{50} of $3.0 \pm 0.8\,\mu M$, which is one of the most potent TNF-α small molecule inhibitors reported so far. Compound **4e** provides a good starting point for developing more potent TNF-α small molecule inhibitors.

AUTHOR CONTRIBUTIONS

LL and YL designed and guided this study; XD designed the research, performed molecular docking and similarity search, and conducted the chemical synthesis; XZ performed the cell assay; HL and QS participated in the cell assay; BT performed the SPR binding assay; XD, LL, and YL analyzed the data and wrote the manuscript with input from all authors; XD and XZ have equal contribution of this work.

ACKNOWLEDGMENTS

This work was supported in part by the Ministry of Science and Technology of China (2016YFA0502303, 2015CB910300) and the National Natural Science Foundation of China (21633001, 21573012).

REFERENCES

Ai, J. W., Zhang, S., Ruan, Q. L., Yu, Y. Q., Zhang, B. Y., Liu, Q. H., et al. (2015). The risk of tuberculosis in patients with rheumatoid arthritis treated with tumor necrosis factor-alpha antagonist: a metaanalysis of both randomized controlled trials and registry/cohort studies. *J. Rheumatol.* 42, 2229–2237. doi: 10.3899/jrheum.150057

Alexiou, P., Papakyriakou, A., Ntougkos, E., Papaneophytou, C. P., Liepouri, F., Mettou, A., et al. (2014). Rationally designed less toxic SPD-304 analogs and preliminary evaluation of their TNF inhibitory effects. *Arch. Pharm.* 347, 798–805. doi: 10.1002/ardp.201400198

Alzani, R., Corti, A., Grazioli, L., Cozzi, E., Ghezzi, P., and Marcucci, F. (1993). Suramin induces deoligomerization of human tumor necrosis factor alpha. *J. Biol. Chem.* 268, 12526–12529.

Baell, J. B., and Holloway, G. A. (2010). New substructure filters for removal of Pan Assay Interference Compounds (PAINS) from screening libraries and for their exclusion in bioassays. *J. Med. Chem.* 53, 2719–2740. doi: 10.1021/jm901137j

Bongartz, T., Matteson, E. L., and Orenstein, R. (2005). Tumor necrosis factor antagonists and infections: the small print on the price tag. *Arth. Rheum.* 53, 631–635. doi: 10.1002/art.21471

Buller, F., Zhang, Y. X., Scheuermann, J., Schäfer, J., Bühlmann, P., and Neri, D. (2009). Discovery of TNF inhibitors from a DNA-encoded chemical library based on diels-alder cycloaddition. *Chem. Biol.* 16, 1075–1086. doi: 10.1016/j.chembiol.2009.09.011

Chan, D. S., Lee, H. M., Yang, F., Che, C. M., Wong, C. C., Abagyan, R., et al. (2010). Structure-based discovery of natural-product-like TNF-α inhibitors. *Angew Chem. Int. Ed. Engl.* 49, 2860–2864. doi: 10.1002/anie.2009 07360

Choi, H., Lee, Y., Park, H., and Oh, D. S. (2010). Discovery of the inhibitors of tumor necrosis factor alpha with structure-based virtual screening. *Bioorg. Med. Chem. Lett.* 20, 6195–6198. doi: 10.1016/j.bmcl.2010.08.116

Davis, J. M., and Colangelo, J. (2013). Small-molecule inhibitors of the interaction between TNF and TNFR. *Future Med. Chem.* 5, 69–79. doi: 10.4155/fmc.12.192

Friesner, R. A., Banks, J. L., Murphy, R. B., Halgren, T. A., Klicic, J. J., Mainz, D. T., et al. (2004). Glide: a new approach for rapid, accurate docking and scoring. 1. Method and assessment of docking accuracy. *J. Med. Chem.* 47, 1739–1749. doi: 10.1021/jm0306430

Grazioli, L., Alzani, R., Ciomei, M., Mariani, M., Restivo, A., Cozzi, E., et al. (1992). Inhibitory effect of suramin on receptor binding and cytotoxic activity of tumor necrosis factor alpha. *Int. J. Immunopharmacol.* 14, 637–642. doi: 10.1016/0192-0561(92)90125-5

Gu, B. H., Ouzunov, S., Wang, L. G., Mason, P., Bourne, N., Cuconati, A., et al. (2006). Discovery of small molecule inhibitors of West Nile virus using a high-throughput sub-genomic replicon screen. *Antiviral Res.* 70, 39–50. doi: 10.1016/j.antiviral.2006.01.005

Halgren, T. A., Murphy, R. B., Friesner, R. A., Beard, H. S., Frye, L. L., Pollard, W. T., et al. (2004). Glide: a new approach for rapid, accurate docking and scoring. 2. Enrichment factors in database screening. *J. Med. Chem.* 47, 1750–1759. doi: 10.1021/jm030644s

He, M. M., Smith, A. S., Oslob, J. D., Flanagan, W. M., Braisted, A. C., Whitty, A., et al. (2005). Small-molecule inhibition of TNF-α. *Science* 310, 1022–1025. doi: 10.1126/science.1116304

Hu, Z., Qin, J., Zhang, H., Wang, D., Hua, Y., Ding, J., et al. (2012). Japonicone A antagonizes the activity of TNF-α by directly targeting this cytokine and selectively disrupting its interaction with TNF receptor-1. *Biochem. Pharmacol.* 84, 1482–1491. doi: 10.1016/j.bcp.2012.08.025

Jacobi, A., Mahler, V., Schuler, G., and Hertl, M. (2006). Treatment of inflammatory dermatoses by tumour necrosis factor antagonists. *J. Eur. Acad. Dermatol. Venereol.* 20, 1171–1187. doi: 10.1111/j.1468-3083.2006.01733.x

Kamal, A., Ramakrishna, G., Lakshma Nayak, V., Raju, P., Subba Rao, A. V., Viswanath, A., et al. (2012). Design and synthesis of benzo[c,d]indolone-pyrrolobenzodiazepine conjugates as potential anticancer agents. *Bioorg. Med. Chem.* 20, 789–800. doi: 10.1016/j.bmc.2011.12.003

Kang, T. S., Mao, Z., Ng, C. T., Wang, M., Wang, W., Wang, C., et al. (2016). Identification of an iridium(III)-based inhibitor of tumor necrosis factor-α. *J. Med. Chem.* 59, 4026–4031. doi: 10.1021/acs.jmedchem.6b00112

Leung, C. H., Chan, D. S. H., Kwan, M. H. T., Cheng, Z., Wong, C. Y., Zhu, G. Y., et al. (2011). Structure-based repurposing of FDA-approved drugs as TNF-α inhibitors. *ChemMedChem* 6, 765–768. doi: 10.1002/cmdc.201100016

Leung, C. H., Zhong, H. J., Yang, H., Cheng, Z., Chan, D. S., Ma, V. P., et al. (2012). A metal-based inhibitor of tumor necrosis factor-α. *Angew. Chem. Int. Ed. Engl.* 51, 9010–9014. doi: 10.1002/anie.201202937

Lian, W. L., Upadhyaya, P., Rhodes, C. A., Liu, Y. S., and Pei, D. H. (2013). Screening bicyclic peptide libraries for protein-protein interaction inhibitors:

discovery of a tumor necrosis factor-α antagonist. *J. Am. Chem. Soc.* 135, 11990–11995. doi: 10.1021/ja405106u

Ma, L., Gong, H., Zhu, H., Ji, Q., Su, P., Liu, P., et al. (2014). A novel small-molecule tumor necrosis factor alpha inhibitor attenuates inflammation in a hepatitis mouse model. *J. Biol. Chem.* 289, 12457–12466. doi: 10.1074/jbc.M113.521708

Mancini, F., Toro, C. M., Mabilia, M., Giannangeli, M., Pinza, M., and Milanese, C. (1999). Inhibition of tumor necrosis factor-alpha (TNF-alpha)/TNF-alpha receptor binding by structural analogues of suramin. *Biochem. Pharmacol.* 58, 851–859. doi: 10.1016/S0006-2952(99)00150-1

Mouhsine, H., Guillemain, H., Moreau, G., Fourati, N., Zerrouki, C., Baron, B., et al. (2017). Identification of an *in vivo* orally active dual-binding protein-protein interaction inhibitor targeting TNFα through combined *in silico/in vitro/in vivo* screening. *Sci. Rep.* 7:3424. doi: 10.1038/s41598-017-03427-z

Scheinfeld, N. (2004). A comprehensive review and evaluation of the side effects of the tumor necrosis factor alpha blockers etanercept, infliximab and adalimumab. *J. Dermatolog. Treat.* 15, 280–294. doi: 10.1080/09546630410017275

Shen, Q., Chen, J., Wang, Q., Deng, X., Liu, Y., and Lai, L. (2014). Discovery of highly potent TNFalpha inhibitors using virtual screen. *Eur. J. Med. Chem.* 85, 119–126. doi: 10.1016/j.ejmech.2014.07.091

Sun, H., and Yost, G. S. (2008). Metabolic activation of a novel 3-substituted indole-containing TNF-alpha inhibitor: dehydrogenation and inactivation of CYP3A4. *Chem. Res. Toxicol.* 21, 374–385. doi: 10.1021/tx700294g

Talukdar, A., Morgunova, E., Duan, J., Meining, W., Foloppe, N., Nilsson, L., et al. (2010). Virtual screening, selection and development of a benzindolone structural scaffold for inhibition of lumazine synthase. *Bioorg. Med. Chem.* 18, 3518–3534. doi: 10.1016/j.bmc.2010.03.072

Trott, O., and Olson, A. J. (2010). AutoDock Vina: improving the speed and accuracy of docking with a new scoring function, efficient optimization and multithreading. *J. Comput. Chem.* 31, 455–461. doi: 10.1002/jcc.21334

Wajant, H., Pfizenmaier, K., and Scheurich, P. (2003). Tumor necrosis factor signaling. *Cell Death Differ.* 10, 45–65. doi: 10.1038/sj.cdd.4401189

Xue, X. Q., Zhang, Y., Liu, Z. X., Song, M., Xing, Y. L., Xiang, Q. P., et al. (2016). Discovery of benzo[*cd*]indol-2(*1H*)-ones as potent and specific BET bromodomain inhibitors: structure-based virtual screening, optimization, and biological evaluation. *J. Med. Chem.* 59, 1565–1579. doi: 10.1021/acs.jmedchem.5b01511

Zhang, C. S., Shen, Q., Tang, B., and Lai, L. H. (2013). Computational design of helical peptides targeting TNFα. *Angew. Chem. Int. Ed. Engl.* 52, 11059–11062. doi: 10.1002/anie.201305963

Zhang, Y., Xue, X., Jin, X., Song, Y., Li, J., Luo, X., et al. (2014). Discovery of 2-oxo-1,2-dihydrobenzo[*cd*]indole-6-sulfonamide derivatives as new RORγ inhibitors using virtual screening, synthesis and biological evaluation. *Eur. J. Med. Chem.* 78, 431–441. doi: 10.1016/j.ejmech.2014.03.065

Zhu, C., Zhang, C., Zhang, T., Zhang, X., Shen, Q., Tang, B., et al. (2016). Rational design of TNFα binding proteins based on the *de novo* designed protein DS119. *Protein Sci.* 25, 2066–2075. doi: 10.1002/pro.3029

2

Discovery of Natural Products as Novel and Potent FXR Antagonists by Virtual Screening

Yanyan Diao[1]*, Jing Jiang*[1]*, Shoude Zhang*[1]*, Shiliang Li*[1]*, Lei Shan*[2]*, Jin Huang*[1]*, Weidong Zhang*[2] *and Honglin Li*[1]*

[1] *Shanghai Key Laboratory of New Drug Design, State Key Laboratory of Bioreactor Engineering, School of Pharmacy, East China University of Science and Technology, Shanghai, China,* [2] *Department of Phytochemistry, School of Pharmacy, Second Military Medical University, Shanghai, China*

Correspondence:
Honglin Li
hlli@ecust.edu.cn

Farnesoid X receptor (FXR) is a member of nuclear receptor family involved in multiple physiological processes through regulating specific target genes. The critical role of FXR as a transcriptional regulator makes it a promising target for diverse diseases, especially those related to metabolic disorders such as diabetes and cholestasis. However, the underlying activation mechanism of FXR is still a blur owing to the absence of proper FXR modulators. To identify potential FXR modulators, an in-house natural product database (NPD) containing over 4,000 compounds was screened by structure-based virtual screening strategy and subsequent hit-based similarity searching method. After the yeast two-hybrid (Y2H) assay, six natural products were identified as FXR antagonists which blocked the CDCA-induced SRC-1 association. The IC_{50} values of compounds **2a**, a diterpene bearing polycyclic skeleton, and **3a**, named daphneone with chain scaffold, are as low as 1.29 and 1.79 μM, respectively. Compared to the control compound guggulsterone ($IC_{50} = 6.47\ \mu$M), compounds **2a** and **3a** displayed 5- and 3-fold higher antagonistic activities against FXR, respectively. Remarkably, the two representative compounds shared low topological similarities with other reported FXR antagonists. According to the putative binding poses, the molecular basis of these antagonists against FXR was also elucidated in this report.

Keywords: FXR, antagonist, virtual screening, molecular docking, similarity searching, natural product

INTRODUCTION

The farnesoid X receptor (FXR, NR1H4), a member of the metabolic nuclear receptor superfamily, regulates the expressions and activities of a broad spectrum of genes. Since 1995 when FXR was isolated from a rat cDNA library for the first time (Forman et al., 1995), the studies on the physiological functions of FXR have been appealing and challenging. FXR is conserved from teleost fish to human beings (Maglich et al., 2003) and is abundantly expressed in liver, intestine, and kidney. As the endogenous receptor of bile acids, FXR can be activated by chenodeoxycholic acid (CDCA), lithocholic acid (LCA), deoxycholic acid (DCA), and many other bile acids (Makishima et al., 1999). In addition, FXR is also reported to exert regulatory roles in lipoprotein and glucose homeostasis, fatty acid and triglyceride synthesis, liver regeneration, and bacterial growth in the intestine (Lee et al., 2006; Wang et al., 2008). All these accumulating data make FXR a promising pharmaceutical target for multiple diseases, especially those related to metabolic disorders such as diabetes and cholestasis (Schaap et al., 2014; Gonzalez et al., 2016; Yuan and Li, 2016; Filho et al., 2017).

As a typical nuclear receptor, FXR shares common structural characteristics with other members of this superfamily, which comprises a highly conserved DNA-binding domain (DBD), a moderately conserved ligand-binding domain (LBD), and a ligand-dependent transcriptional activation domain (AF-2) (Pellicciari et al., 2005).Upon the binding of proper ligand to the LBD, FXR will undergo a conformational change, which is critical to determine whether a coactivator or a corepressor binds efficiently to the AF-2 motif. If activated by appropriate agonists, the recruitment of coactivators (such as SRC-1, DRIP, and PRMT) to FXR occurs, which further up- or down-regulates the expressions of certain target genes. While for antagonists, the association of FXR with activators will be hindered (Lew et al., 2004). Although it is widely accepted that FXR participates in many biological processes, owing to the diversity and complexity of target genes involved in the FXR signaling pathways (Zhang and Edwards, 2008), the physiological functions of FXR haven't been clearly defined. Therefore, it is still an essential step to identify potential FXR modulators, which may contribute to the elucidation of physiological effects of FXR and provide novel opportunities for the treatment of metabolic diseases by targeting FXR.

Apart from the natural bile acid ligands with steroidal skeleton, over 700 structurally diverse FXR modulators have also been identified (Gaulton et al., 2017), most of which function as agonists (Carotti et al., 2014). Obeticholic acid (6α-ethyl-chenodeoxycholic acid, 6-ECDCA), a semi-synthetic bile acid analog with highly potent FXR agonistic activity (EC_{50} = 0.099 μM) (Pellicciari et al., 2002), is the first FDA-approved drug that is used for treating primary biliary cholangitis (PBC) (Nevens et al., 2016). In contrast, the development of FXR antagonists, which are also useful chemical tools to unravel the physiological roles and relative clinical significance of FXR (Li et al., 2013), does not seem to be satisfactory due to the scanty number of potent FXR antagonists that have been reported so far. Guggulsterone, a natural product extracted from the resin of the guggul tree, is the most described FXR antagonist, with the ability of blocking the agonist-induced coactivator recruitment and decreasing the hepatic cholesterol in wild-type mice (Urizar et al., 2002). However, the researches on guggulsterone are still confined to preclinical and academic studies because of the complexity of its mechanism of action (Fiorucci et al., 2010; Yamada and Sugimoto, 2016). Although other natural or synthetic FXR antagonists have also been developed (**Figure 1**; Wu et al., 2002; Dussault et al., 2003; Nam et al., 2007; Choi et al., 2011; Huang et al., 2012; Xu et al., 2015), further pharmaceutically relevant activities were rarely reported. Herein, six natural products were identified as antagonists from an in-house natural product database (NPD) through virtual screening strategy and subsequent biological experiment validation. In the yeast two-hybrid (Y2H) assay (Fields and Sternglanz, 1994; Lin and Lai, 2017), these compounds could abolish CDCA-induced FXR activation at micromolar level. We hope the natural products revealed in this study will offer novel scaffolds for uncovering new FXR regulatory mechanism and provide insights into potential development for further discovery of FXR modulators.

MATERIALS AND METHODS

Structure-Based Virtual Screening

Protein Preparation

The crystal structures of FXR-LBD in complex with 6-ECDCA (Mi et al., 2003) (PDB code 1OSV, a dimer and chain B was used) and fexaramine (Downes et al., 2003) (PDB code 1OSH, monomer) were obtained from the Protein Data Bank. The synthetically modified bile acid ligand 6-ECDCA was derived from the structure of CDCA, but showed almost 100-fold more potent FXR agonistic activity than CDCA and did not activate other nuclear receptors. Fexaramine is a synthetic non-steroidal FXR agonist, which was identified by optimization of a benzopyrane-based combinatorial derived library. The coactivators and all the water molecules were removed. Hydrogen atoms and charges were added during a brief relaxation performed using the "Protein Preparation Wizard" workflow in Maestro 10.1. After the hydrogen bond network was optimized, the crystal structure was minimized until the root-mean-square deviation (RMSD) between the minimized structure and the starting structure reached 0.3 Å with OPLS_2005 force field.

Glide Docking

The grid-enclosing box was placed on the centroid of the crystallographic ligand in the optimized protein structure and defined to enclose residues located within 15.0 Å of the binding pocket. A scaling factor of 0.8 was set to van der Waals (VDW) radii of those receptor atoms with partial atomic charges of less than 0.15 to soften the nonpolar parts of the receptor. After addition of hydrogen atoms and ionization at a pH range of 5.0-9.0, the three-dimensional structures of compounds in the NPD were generated with Ligprep v3.3 module. Standard precision (SP) and extra precision (XP) approaches of Glide (Friesner et al., 2004; Halgren et al., 2004) were respectively adopted to dock the molecules into the binding site with the default parameters, and only the top one pose for each molecule were retained. After parallel Glide SP scorings using two different protein structures (PDB codes 1OSV and 1OSH), the top 500 docking poses were reserved for each docking calculation and subjected to XP calculation with a more precise scoring function, and the top 200 docking poses were retained, respectively, for further visual observation.

Hit-Based Similarity Searching

The similarity searching process was accomplished in Pipeline Pilot v7.5, and two of the most potent FXR antagonists **2a** and **3a** were used as query molecules, respectively. The Tanimoto coefficient (Tc) of similarity between the query molecule and the target molecule was calculated using SciTegic functional connectivity fingerprints of radius 4 (FCFP_4) (Bender et al., 2009). The minimum Tc was set to a low value of 0.3, to maximize the number of obtained analogs.

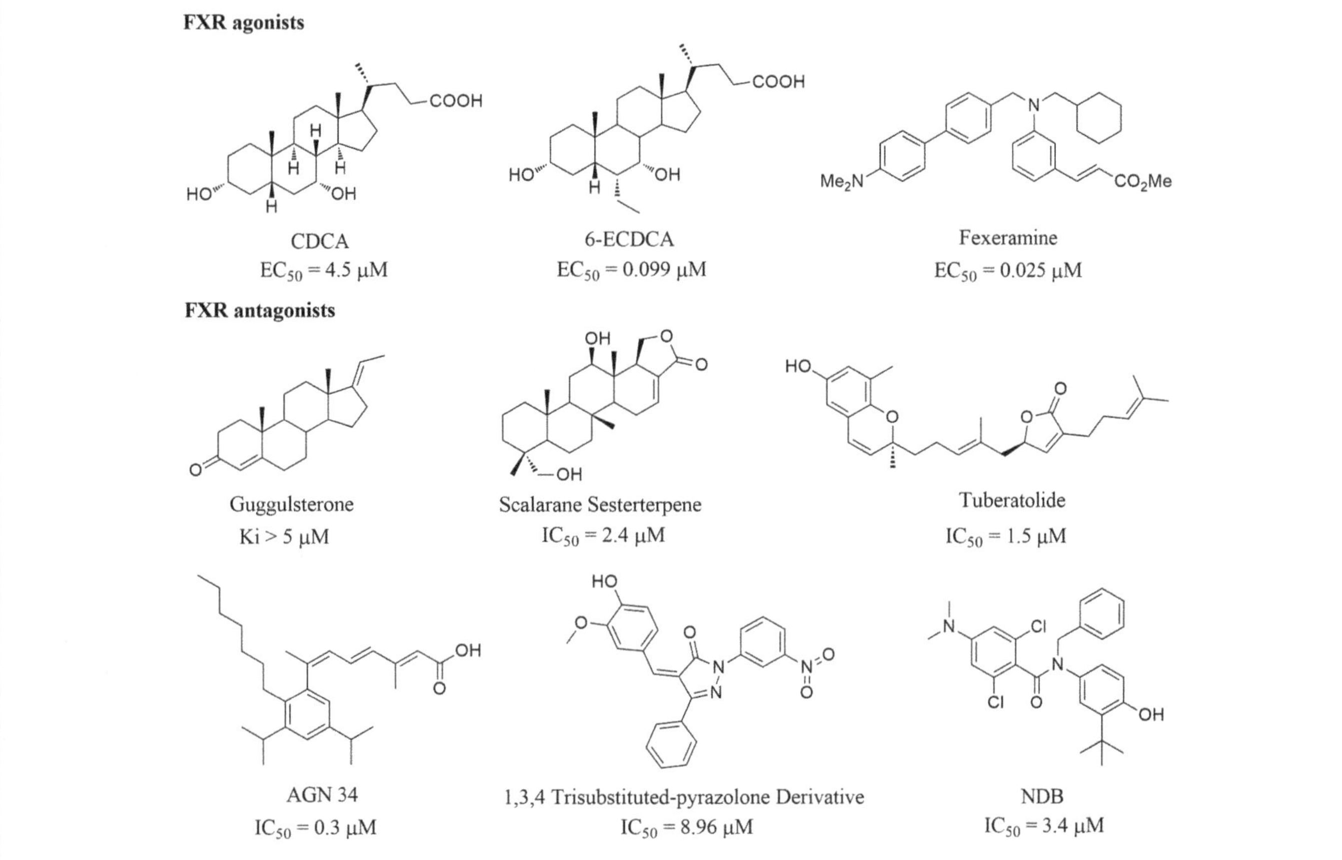

FIGURE 1 | Selected structures of the reported FXR modulators.

SRC-1 Recruitment Assay

Materials

The restriction and modification enzymes in this work were obtained from New England Biolabs (Beijing, China). *P*-nitrophenyl α-D-galactopyranoside (PNP-α-Gal), yeast nitrogen base without amino acids, agar, PEG3350, dimethyl sulfoxide (DMSO), lithium acetate, and glucose were all purchased from Sigma (Shanghai, China). The yeast expression plasmids pGADT7 and pGBKT7 were from Clontech (Palo Alto, CA), and CDCA was from Merck. The dropout supplement free from leucine and tryptophan (-Leu/-Trp DO supplement) was bought from Takara, and Salmon Sperm DNA was obtained from invitrogen. The yeast strain AH109 was purchased from Clontech (Palo Alto, CA).

Plasmid Construction

Based on the genome sequences of FXRα (GenBank accession no. NC 000012.10), human FXRα-LBD (200-473 AA) was sub-cloned into vector pGBKT-7 using NdeI and BamHI restrict enzyme sites. The primers used for PCR amplification were listed as follows: FXRα-LBD (sense) 5′-ATCATATG-GAAATTCAGTGTAAATCTAAGCG-3′, (anti-sense) 5′-ATGGATCCTCACTGCA-CGTCCCA-3′. The combination plasmid pGADT7-SRC-1 was prepared as described previously (Lin et al., 2008), by amplifying with the following primers: (sense) 5′-CAGAATTC-CATAACAATGACAGACTTTCA-3′ and (anti-sense) 5′-AAGGATCCCACCTTTA- CATCATCCAGGCT-3′.

Y2H System Construction

We constructed the Y2H for FXR by yeast co-transformation with pGBKT7-FXR LBD (BD) and pGADT7-SRC-1 (AD) according to the lithium acetate method. Briefly, 500 ng of BD and AD were added to 50 μL of the yeast competent cells and mixed with 36 μL of lithium acetate, 240 μL of 50% PEG3350, and 50 ng single-strain DNA at 30°C for 30 min, followed by heat-shock (250 rpm) at 42°C for 30 min. The mixture was subsequently spread on a drop-out-agar plate without leucine and tryptophan (6.7 g/L yeast nitrogen base without amino acids, 1.54 g/L -Leu/-Trp DO supplement, 20 g/L glucose, 20 g/L agar). The plates were incubated at 30°C for 48 h for yeast growth and the PCR method was used to confirm the successful transformation.

Y2H Assay

We performed Y2H assay to determine the agonistic or antagonistic activities of the compounds. Yeast transformations were incubated with either a control vehicle (DMSO) or the indicated compounds for 24 h in an hFXR agonist testing, and in antagonist assays treated with tested compounds plus 10 μM

CDCA. The quantitative α-galactosidase activity assays were carried out by using PNP-α-Gal as the substrate according to the Clontech manual. Each experiment was repeated three times independently.

1. Vortex the overnight culture tube for 0.5–1 min to disperse cell clumps and then each sample needs 200 μL to record the exact OD_{600}.
2. Centrifuge the tube at 14,000 rpm (10,000 × g) for 30 s. Incubate 16 μL cell culture medium supernatant with 48 μL PNP-α-Gal at 30°C for 60 min. Be sure to cover microtiter plates with a lid or parafilm to prevent evaporation.
3. Terminate the reaction by adding 136 μL of 1 μM sodium carbonate. Record the optical density of each sample at 410 nm.

The α-galactosidase activity was calculated according to the following formula:

$$\alpha - \text{galactosidase activity}[\text{milliunits}/(\text{mL} \times \text{cell})] = \frac{OD_{410} \times V_f \times 1000}{(\varepsilon \times b) \times t \times V_i \times OD_{600}}$$

where t is the elapsed time of incubation (min), V_f is the final volume of assay (200 μL), V_i is the volume of culture medium supernatant added (16 μL), OD_{600} is the optical density of overnight culture, and $\varepsilon \times b$ is the *p*-nitrophenol molar absorptivity at 410 nm×the light path (cm) = 10.5 mL/μmol (Yeast Protocols Handbook PT3024-1, Clontech).

The agonistic activation and inhibition rates (%) were calculated as follows:

$$\text{agonistic activation} = \frac{GA_{treated}}{GA_{DMSO}}$$

$$\text{inhibition rate}(\%) = \frac{GA_{CDCA} - GA_{treated}}{GA_{CDCA} - GA_{DMSO}}$$

where *GA* indicates α-galactosidase activity.

Chemistry

The NPD is our in-house collection of over 4,000 natural products isolated from about 100 plants and their structures were established by extensive spectroscopic. The purities of all compounds were checked by using NMR and HPLC (purities ≥ 95%). The detailed data of the natural products mentioned in the report are listed as follows.

1a: Abiesatrine B, isolated from *Abies georgei*; amorphous powder; ESI-MS: *m/z* 491 [M + Na]$^+$; ^{1}H-NMR (600 MHz, CD_3OD, δ): 2.28 (m), 1.83 (m), 1.95 (m), 1.58 (m), 3.39 (m), 1.45 (m), 1.92 (m), 5.66 (m), 1.42 (m), 2.25 (m), 1.81 (dd, *J* =14.7, 2.4 Hz), 5.56 (dd, *J* = 8.4, 2.4 Hz), 1.45 (m), 1.92 (m), 0.96 (s), 0.95 (s), 2.21 (m), 0.88 (d, *J* = 6.3 Hz), 2.92 (dd, *J* =14.1, 1.8 Hz), 2.23 (m), 6.86 (d, *J* = 1.5 Hz), 2.16 (d, *J* = 1.5 Hz), 0.94 (s), 0.92 (s), 1.20 (s). ^{13}C-NMR (150 MHz, CD_3OD, δ): 30.7, 26.5, 77.2, 38.0, 39.4, 24.3, 120.1, 147.5, 52.6, 36.0, 29.1, 123.8, 157.4, 51.2, 37.9, 39.2, 47.6, 25.4, 22.8, 40.2, 16.2, 49.4, 205.5, 129.7, 149.1, 15.9, 174.6, 28.9, 23.6, 26.6.

1b: (24Z)-3,23-Dioxo-9βH-lanosta-7,24-dien-27-oic acid, isolated from *Abies georgei*; amorphous powder; ESI-MS: *m/z* 467 [M - H]$^-$; ^{1}H-NMR (300 MHz, CD_3OD, δ): 5.67 (1H, dt, *J* = 7.5, 2.7 Hz), 1.94 (3H, d, *J* = 1.2 Hz), 1.08 (3H, s), 1.07 (3H, s), 1.05(3H, s), 0.99 (3H, s), 0.95 (3H, d, *J* = 6.0 Hz), 0.82 (3H, s); ^{13}C-NMR (75 MHz, CD_3OD, δ): 35.2, 35.3, 221.7, 48.1, 53.7, 24.0, 122.8, 149.9, 46.8, 37.0, 21.9, 35.6, 45.2, 53.2, 34.2, 29.5, 54.7, 22.9, 23.5, 34.2, 20.8, 50.1, 200.0, 128.1, 150.2, 173.6, 28.4, 21.7, 27.9.

1c: Abiesatrine D, isolated from *Abies georgei*; amorphous powder; ESI-MS: *m/z* 477 [M + H]$^+$; ^{1}H-NMR (600 MHz, CD_3OD, δ): 1.73 (m), 1.61(m), 2.50 (dt, *J* = 7.5, 1.8 Hz), 1.42 (dt, *J* = 12.0, 1.2 Hz), 1.94 (m), 1.89 (m), 5.65 (dt, *J* = 7.8, 2.7 Hz), 2.21 (m), 1.64 (m), 1.85 (m), 1.72 (m), 1.60 (m), 1.43 (m), 1.96 (m), 1.29 (m), 1.54 (m), 0.79 (m), 1.00 (s), 1.42 (m), 0.92 (d, *J* = 6.6 Hz), 1.63 (m), 1.58 (m), 2.24 (m), 2.15 (m), 6.19 (dt, *J* = 7.5, 1.2 Hz), 1.85 (brs), 1.10 (s), 1.11 (s), 1.03 (s). ^{13}C-NMR (150 MHz, CD_3OD, δ): 34.2, 34.3, 219.1, 47.0, 52.4, 23.0, 121.5, 148.7, 45.5, 35.8, 20.9, 34.4, 44.0, 51.9, 33.1, 29.7, 53.0, 22.4, 23.1, 36.1, 18.2, 34.6, 26.0, 145.7, 126.6, 172.6, 12.0, 28.0, 21.3, 27.4.

2a: 15-Hydroxy-7-oxo-8,11,13-abietatrien-18-oic acid, isolated from *Abies georgei*; amorphous powder; ESI-MS: *m/z* 329 [M - H]$^-$; ^{1}H-NMR (300 MHz, CD_3OD, δ): 8.06 (1H, d, *J* = 2.1 Hz), 7.72 (1H, d, *J* =8.4, 2.1 Hz), 7.43 (1H, d, *J* = 8.4 Hz), 1.51 (6H, s), 1.31 (3H, s), 1.27 (3H, s); ^{13}C-NMR (75 MHz, CD_3OD, δ): 39.1, 19.5, 38.2, 48.2, 45.7, 38.6, 201.5, 131.4, 155.9, 38.6, 124.9, 132.2, 149.1, 124.0, 72.6, 31.7, 31.7, 183.4, 17.4, 23.8.

2b: 17-Nor-7,15-dion-8,11,13-abietatrien-18-oic acid, isolated from *Abies georgei*; amorphous powder; ESI-MS: *m/z* 313 [M - H]$^-$; ^{1}H-NMR (600 MHz, CD_3OD, δ): 2.48 (m), 1.61 (dt, *J* = 6.9, 3.0 Hz), 1.81 (m), 1.80 (m), 2.68 (dd, *J* = 14.2, 3.0 Hz), 2.86 (dd, *J* = 17.6, 14.2 Hz), 7.63 (d, *J* = 8.4 Hz), 8.18 (dd, *J* = 8.4, 2.1 Hz), 8.52 (d, *J* = 2.1 Hz), 2.61 (s), 1.35 (s), 1.32 (s). ^{13}C-NMR (150 MHz, CD_3OD, δ): 38.2, 19.1, 37.8, 47.5, 45.0, 38.8, 199.5, 132.0, 161.8, 39.5, 125.9, 134.5, 136.6, 128.5, 199.3, 26.7, 181.0, 16.9, 23.5.

3a: Daphneone, isolated from *Daphne odora* Thunb. var. *marginata*; white powder; ESI-MS: *m/z* 255 [M + H]$^+$; ^{1}H-NMR (500 MHz, DMSO-d6, δ): 2.92 (2H, t, *J* = 6.0Hz), 1.61 (2H, t, *J* = 3.0 Hz), 1.61 (2H, t, *J* = 3.0 Hz), 2.60 (2H, t, *J* = 6.0 Hz), 7.84 (2H, d, *J* = 9.0 Hz), 6.85 (2H, d, *J* = 9.0 Hz), 6.85 (2H, d, *J* = 9.0 Hz), 7.84 (2H, d, *J* = 9.0 Hz), 7.18 (m), 7.27 (m), 7.18 (m), 7.27 (m), 7.18 (m), 10.28 (s); ^{13}C-NMR (125 MHz, DMSO-d6, δ): 23.7, 30.5, 34.9, 37.1, 115.1, 115.1, 128.3, 128.2, 128.1, 125.5, 128.1, 128.2, 130.3, 130.3, 142.0, 161.8, 198.1.

3b: Daphneolon, isolated from *Daphne odora* Thunb. var. *marginata*; white powder; EI-MS: *m/z* 270 [M]; ^{1}H-NMR (500 MHz, CD_3OD, δ): 1.80 (2H, m); 2.72 (1H, m); 3.00 (1H, m); 3.08 (1H, m), 3.09 (1H, m), 4.14 (1H, m), 6.80 (2H, d, *J* = 7.0 Hz), 7.11 (1H, m), 7.15 (4H, m), 7.84 (2H, d, *J* = 7.0 Hz); ^{13}C-NMR (125 MHz , CD_3OD, δ): 31.0, 38.3, 44.6, 66.9, 114.3, 124.8, 127.4, 127.5, 128.5, 130.1, 141.5, 161.9, 198.1.

3c: Daphnenone, isolated from *Daphne tangutica* Maxim; white powder; EI-MS: m/z 252 [M]$^+$; ^{13}C-NMR (125MHz, DMSO-d6, δ): 187.3, 125.9, 146.7, 33.5, 33.7, 128.7, 130.9, 115.3, 162.0, 115.3, 130.9, 141.0, 128.3, 128.3, 125.8, 128.3, 128.3.

3d: P-coumaric acid, isolated from *Incarvillea mairei* var. *grandiflora* (Wehrhahn) Grierson; white amorpuous powder; ESI-MS: *m/z* 164 [M]$^+$; ^{1}H NMR (600 MHz ,CD_3OD, δ): 6.32

(1H, d, J = 16.0 Hz), 7.37 (1H, d, J = 16.0 Hz), 7.35 (2H, d, J = 8.5 Hz), 6.77 (2H, d, J = 8.5 Hz), 5.0 (4-OH), 6.41 (-H), 6.77 (3-H,5-H), 7.35 (2-H,6-H), 7.37 (7-H), 11.0 (-H); ^{13}C-NMR (150 MHz ,CD_3OD, δ): 128.7 (s), 130.1 (d), 116.6 (d), 159.8 (s), 116.6 (d), 130.1 (d), 141.5 (d), 122.6 (d), 171.5 (s).

3e: Ethylparaben, isolated from *Aeschynanthus bracteatus*; Colloidal; ESI-MS: m/z 175 $[M + Na]^+$; ^{1}H-NMR (300 MHz, CD_3OD, δ): 7.97 (1H, d, J = 9.0 Hz), 6.87 (1H, d, J = 9.0 Hz), 6.87 (1H, d, J = 9.0 Hz), 7.97 (1H, d, J = 9.0 Hz), 4.35 (2H, d, J = 7.2 Hz), 1.26 (3H, s); ^{13}C-NMR (75 MHz ,CD_3OD, δ): 123.1, 131.9, 115.1, 159.7, 115.1, 131.9, 162.9, 60.7, 14.4.

RESULTS AND DISCUSSIONS

Protein Structure Selection and Redocking Validation

The binding of proper modulators to LBD is the molecular basis for FXR activation that triggers the conformational change of FXR, the subsequent coactivators association, and the final target genes regulation. Previous studies have shown that FXR can be activated by structurally diverse agonists, and an array of crystal structures of FXR-LBD complexed with agonists have been solved. The agonist-binding pocket is positioned in the interior of the LBD, and agonists with different skeletons display enormously distinct binding features (Maloney et al., 2000; Soisson et al., 2008; Flatt et al., 2009; Jin et al., 2013). Computational studies, along with crystallographic experiments (Xu et al., 2015), support the notion that the agonist-binding pocket can also be occupied by antagonists (Meyer et al., 2005). Given the variability of the binding pockets occupied by distinct modulators, it is necessary to use different FXR crystallographic models in the virtual screening process, in order to maximize the diversity of hit compounds. At the time when we initiated this study, there were in total 27 crystal structures of FXR in complex with different modulators in the Protein Data Bank. After deleting the structures bound with structurally analogous ligands and those without published biological data, 10 unique protein structures were reserved for further analysis.

Protein flexibility has vital influence on ligand recognition, and even subtle protein conformational changes can significantly affect the results of docking simulations (Kitchen et al., 2004). Nevertheless, the receptor is usually held rigid for most docking procedures, including Glide used in this study, to speed up virtual screening of large databases. To compensate for the limitations of rigid protein conformation, as well as to simply the computational simulations, we decided to select two receptors representing dramatically dissimilar conformations to the other reported crystal structures to perform two independent docking calculations. Both the binding site similarity and ligand similarity profiles were taken into consideration for docking model selection. On the one hand, pairwise binding pocket similarities among the 10 structures were calculated using our in-house program PocketShape, which is designed for computational evaluation of the binding site similarity based on pocket shape and property and could be accessed through the webserver SiteMapper (http://lilab.ecust.edu.cn/). Residues within 5Å distance around the ligand were extracted as the binding site for each structure. Typically, two binding sites with a score value over than 0.8 are considered similar. On the other hand, pairwise molecular similarities among the 10 crystallographic ligands were calculated with SciTegic FCFP_4 fingerprints in Pipeline Pilot v7.5, and a Tc cutoff value of 0.6 was set to define similarity.

The binding pocket and ligand similarity values of the 10 unique crystal structures were plotted in Figure S1. Meanwhile, for each model, the average pocket and ligand similarity values were calculated, respectively, to evaluate its uniqueness. Four crystal structures 1OSH, 1OSV, 3OLF, and 4WVD were considered, as all of them have top five minimum average values ranked by either pocket or ligand similarity calculations. Although both the pocket and ligand similarity values of 4WVD scatter in a low range, its ligand ivermectin is a large macrocyclic lactone (Jin et al., 2013), making the ligand binding pocket expand to a volume of 1081 Å^3 (Dundas et al., 2006), which is likely to cause artificial enrichment of molecules with large sizes and high molecular weights in docking procedure (Verdonk et al., 2004). Therefore, we did not choose 4WVD. The Tc values of the FXR agonist 6-ECDCA in 1OSV to other ligands are relatively low with predominant scattering below 0.2, and its binding pocket also reveals uniqueness with the average similarity value of 0.62. Moreover, 6-ECDCA is the only FDA-approved FXR modulator so far. Therefore, the 1OSV model was first selected for docking simulation (Mi et al., 2003). After thoroughly analyzing the binding interactions, the biological activities against FXR, as well as the X-ray crystal parameters, the second model of 1OSH was preferentially reserved, the ligand of which has a lower Tc value to 6-ECDCA than that of 3OLF (0.13 vs. 0.15).

Alignment of the 6-ECDCA and fexaramine binding sites exhibited substantial differences in both shape and surrounded residues (Figure S2A). And the tremendous dissimilarities of the two ligands in terms of topological structures and induced binding conformations render them extend to non-overlapping space. To evaluate the docking accuracy of Glide, the two cocrystallized ligands were redocked into the active pocket using Glide XP scoring for each structure. Superimposition of the best redocked poses and the experimental structures (Figures S2B,C) gave the RMSD values of 0.53 Å for 6-ECDCA and 0.65 Å for fexaramine, indicating the robustness of Glide in accurately reproducing the bioactive conformations of the ligands for our two docking models. Cross-docking calculations were also carried out where each crystal structure ligand was docked into the binding pocket of the other. The ligand 6-ECDCA could be docked into 1OSH by Glide XP mode, but the predicted binding pose deviated greatly from the crystallized bioactive conformation (Figure S2D). In agreement with the enormous differences of the two binding sites, fexaramine could not be accommodated by the smaller 6-ECDCA-binding site of 1OSV, hence no proposed docking pose was obtained.

Virtual Screening

To search for potent FXR modulators, structure-based virtual screening strategy, an effective method to identify novel ligands

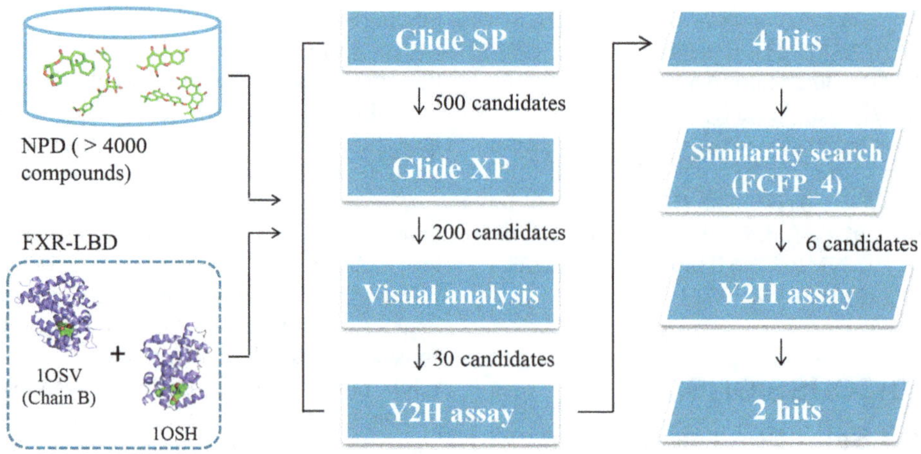

FIGURE 2 | Schematic representation of the whole strategy adopted in this study to identify potential FXR modulators.

based on predicted binding poses and docking scores, was executed using Glide v6.6 (Maestro v10.1, Schrödinger Inc.). And we speculated that if the docking pose of a certain compound to the agonist-binding pocket was computationally favorable, it could be an effective FXR modulator, either an agonist or an antagonist. The screened natural products database is a collection of over 4000 natural products isolated from about 100 plants, the structures of which have been validated by our researchers. After hierarchical virtual screenings independently implemented with Glide (**Figure 2**) by using two crystal structures of the receptor, a total of 400 top-ranking compounds were retrieved as candidates from the NPD. These candidates were then subjected to visual inspection to remove those that are likely to be nonbinders. With consideration of key interactions observed from the crystal structures, such as predominant VDW complementarity and some critical hydrogen bonds with polar residues, each docked pose of these candidates was carefully checked to delete the inappropriate compounds. Meanwhile, a specific focus was put on the sizes of the candidates, and those compounds with relatively large groups protruding out of the binding pocket were not considered. Additionally, the compounds with the same scaffold were reserved with a maximum of three to maximize the structural diversity. A total of 30 candidates were finally selected for further bioactivity assay. In the coactivator-recruitment assay based on the Y2H system, none of the 30 compounds could enhance the association of SRC-1 to FXR-LBD, thus no agonist was found. Intriguingly, four compounds (**1a, 2a, 3a, 3c**) strongly inhibited the CDCA-induced SRC-1 recruitment with the inhibition rate higher than 50% in the concentration of 25 μM, displaying apparent FXR antagonistic profiles. The IC_{50} values of the four compounds were determined (**Table 1,** Figure S4), and guggulsterone was used as the reference compound.

Starting from the potent FXR antagonists **2a** and **3a** as hit compounds, the in-house NPD was re-screened using similarity searching method, to obtain more potent derivatives as well as to establish underlying structure-activity relationships (SAR). A prior minimum Tc value of 0.6 was first set to retrieve analogous compounds. Unfortunately, only several derivatives were obtained for each hit compound, probably owing to the heterogeneity of the in-house NPD. We, thus, chose a relatively low threshold of 0.3 to maximize the number of obtained analogs. Subsequently, the analogs were also manually checked, and only compounds possessing the same skeleton to the hit compound and with proper sizes were selected. After further *in vitro* Y2H assay, two compounds **3d** and **3e** with the Tc values of 0.4 and 0.41, respectively, to compound **3a**, were found to display moderate antagonistic activities against FXR. As illustrated in **Table 1**, compounds **3d** and **3e** share the phenol moiety with compound **3a**, and their IC_{50} values were 14.1 and 19.3 μM, respectively.

To evaluate the performance of the virtual screening strategy adopted in this study, the rankings and docking scores of the newly identified natural products were retrospectively examined. The distribution of docking scores of the top ranking candidates reserved from Glide calculations were presented in Figure S3. The natural compounds bearing different scaffolds, including **1c, 2a, 2b, 3b,** and **3c,** could be ranked in the top 500 candidates during the Glide SP docking process using both crystal structures 1OSV and 1OSH, whereas the Glide XP results are totally different. As shown in **Table 2,** compounds containing similar chemical skeleton to the crystallographic ligand tend to score higher. Moreover, none of the identified FXR antagonists could be simultaneously ranked in the top 200 candidates by the two Glide XP calculations, confirming the rationality of using two distinct crystal structures for structure-based virtual screening. Despite of the confirmed moderate antagonistic effects against FXR, compounds **3d** and **3e** with smaller sizes were excluded after the initial Glide SP screening, which may be ascribed to the recognized bias of structure-based virtual screening method toward high molecular weight compounds (Pan et al., 2003). The results also demonstrate that 2D molecular similarity search method is a powerful and complementary approach to structure-based virtual screening, which could retrieve biologically active compounds that are regarded as false-negatives by docking simulations.

TABLE 1 | Chemical structures and activities of FXR antagonists and their analogs reported in this study[a].

Compd.	Structure	Inhibition rate % (25 μM)	IC_{50} (μM)[b]	Agonistic activation (25 μM)
1a	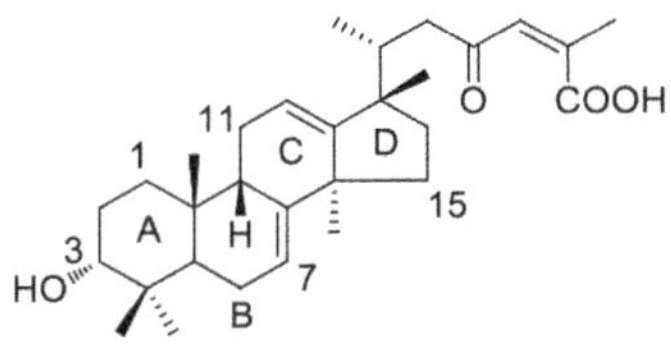	67.35	13.5	1.09
1b	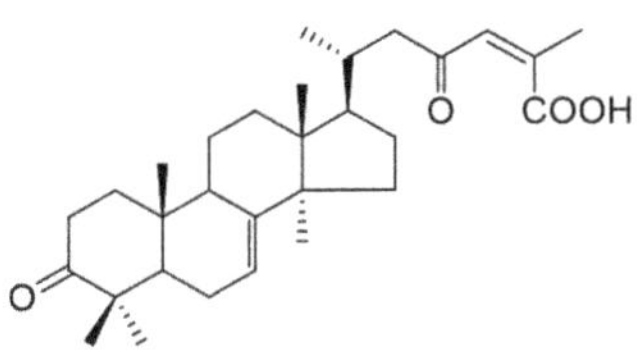	22.66	>25	1.12
1c	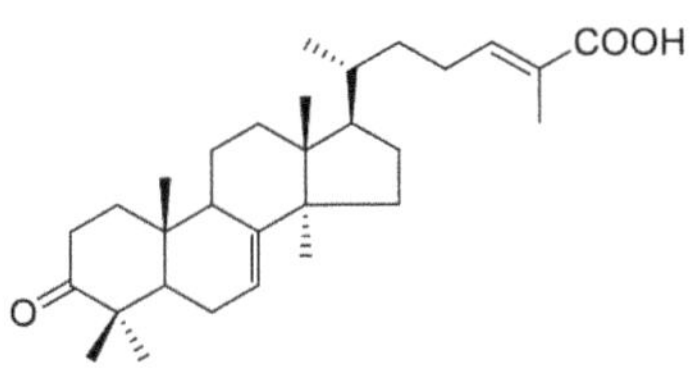	12.84	>25	0.93
2a	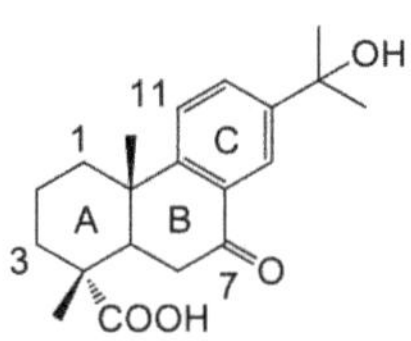	82.16	1.29	1.05
2b	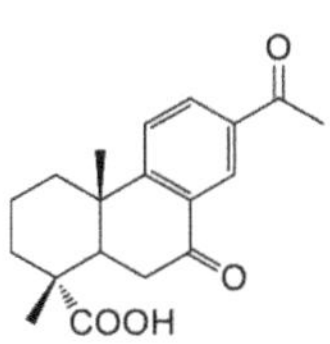	10.05	>25	0.90
3a	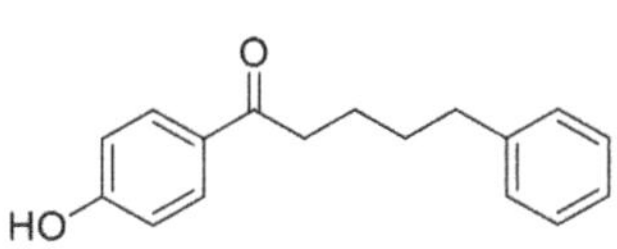	84.45	1.79	1.03
3b	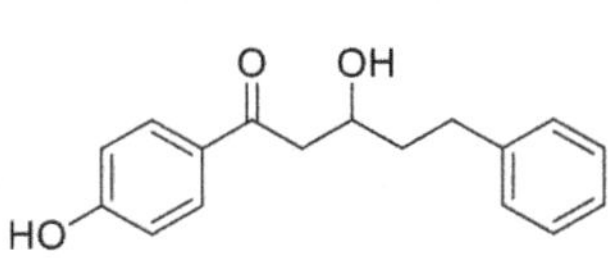	41.4	>25	0.76

(Continued)

TABLE 1 | Continued

Compd.	Structure	Inhibition rate % (25 μM)	IC_{50} (μM)[b]	Agonistic activation (25 μM)
3c	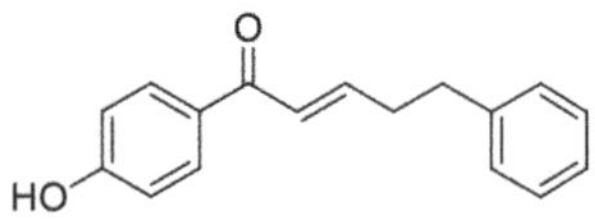	54.9	5.46	1.29
3d	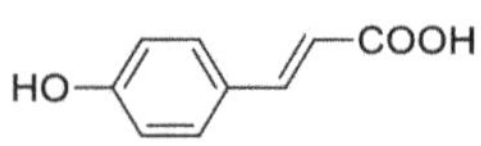	52.8	14.1	1.08
3e	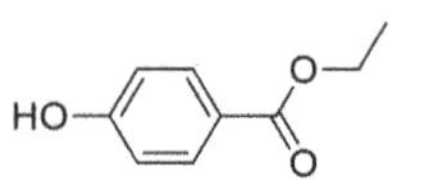	60.1	19.3	0.93
DMSO		0	–	1.00
CDCA		–	–	2.70
Guggulsterone		60.72	6.47	–

[a] *Data shown are the average values of triplicate measurements determined by Y2H assays. This system employs the interaction between hFXR-LBD and the coactivator SRC-1.*
[b] *Attempts to determine IC_{50} values were made if the inhibition rate at 25 μM was larger than 50%.*

TABLE 2 | The rankings and docking scores of the natural products.

Compd.[a]	Glide SP (kcal/mol)				Glide XP (kcal/mol)			
	1OSV		1OSH		1OSV		1OSH	
	Rank	Score	Rank	Score	Rank	Score	Rank	Score
1a	20	−10.02	–	–	2	−15.1	–	–
1b	37	−9.52	–	–	13	−13.2	–	–
1c	395	−7.99	309	−8.16	42	−12.01	–	–
2a	59	−9.16	292	−8.23	70	−11.41	–	–
2b	93	−8.91	381	−7.87	171	−10.34	–	–
3a	–	–	177	−8.61	–	–	142	−10.55
3b	488	−7.83	120	−8.85	–	–	139	−10.57
3c	390	−8.00	133	−8.80	–	–	195	−10.05
3d*	–	–	–	–	–	–	–	–
3e*	–	–	–	–	–	–	–	–

[a] *Compounds that were ruled out by structure-based virtual screening process but recovered using similarity searching method are labeled with *.*

Structural Novelty Assessment

The six natural products were first reported to show FXR antagonistic activity. To evaluate their structural novelty with respect to known FXR antagonists, the pairwise Tc values of chemical similarity were calculated based on the FCFP_4 fingerprints. The Tc value between the similar compounds **3a** and **3c** is 0.67, a Tc cutoff value of 0.6 was therefore set to define similarity. 15 structurally diverse FXR antagonists including seven natural products (compounds **4–21**, Table S1) were collected from literatures, among which the maximum Tc value is 0.46. As shown in **Figure 3**, all the Tc values of the six newly identified hits to the known 15 FXR antagonists were below 0.4, and the maximum Tc values of compounds **1a**, **2a**, and **3a** were 0.38, 0.25, and 0.31 (Table S2), respectively. Accordingly, the six natural products could be considered to be structurally novel as FXR antagonists.

Analysis of Predicted Binding Poses

From the structural point of view, the six antagonists can be simply categorized into two classes: terpenes possessing polycyclic skeletons and phenols with chain scaffolds. In order to better delineate SAR, their inactive analogs were also displayed and analyzed in this study.

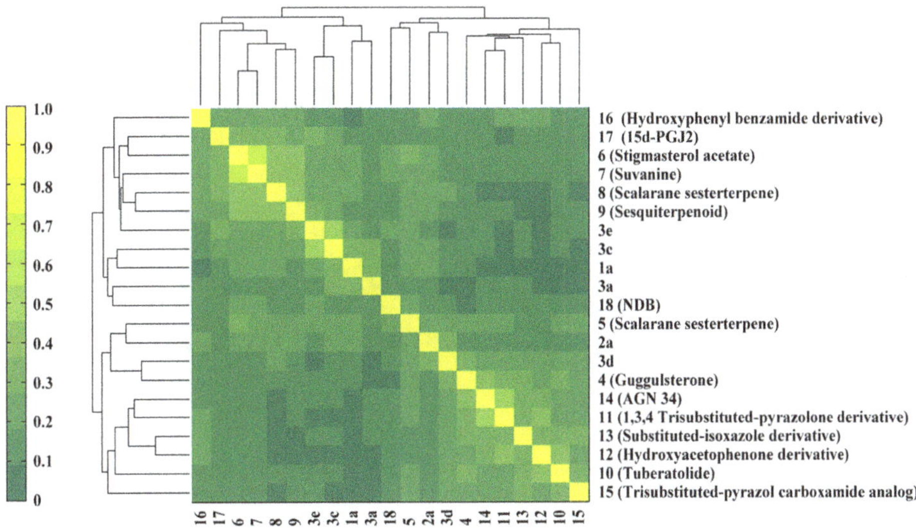

FIGURE 3 | Heatmap presentation of topological similarities of the six natural products to the 15 reported FXR antagonists.

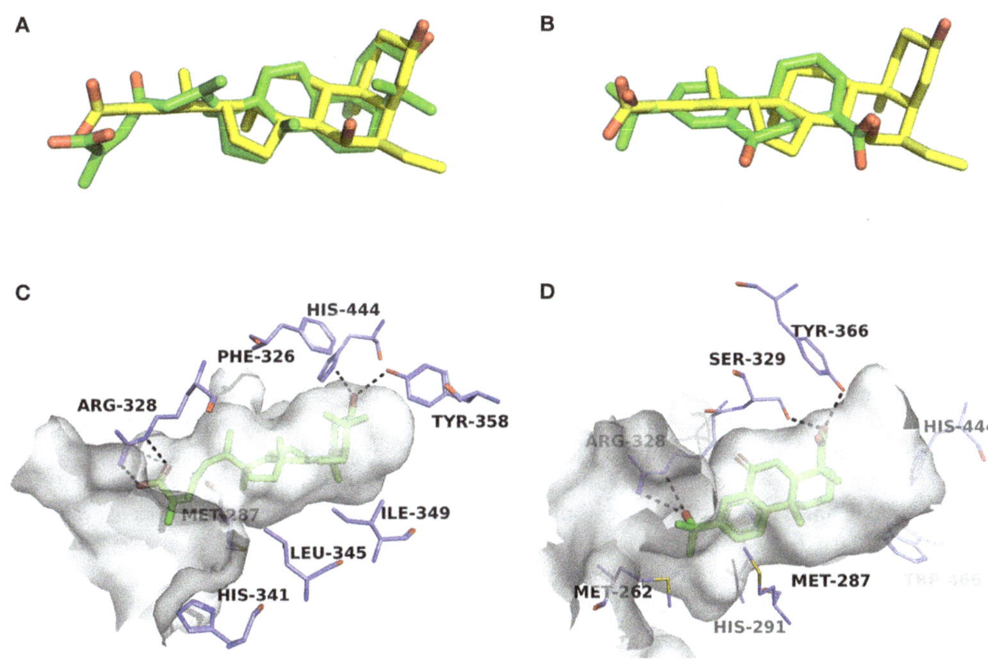

FIGURE 4 | Superposition of docking poses of compounds **1a** and **2a** onto 6-ECDCA **(A,B)** and their proposed interactions with FXR **(C,D)**. The conformation of 6-ECDCA (yellow sticks) was extracted from the crystal structure 1OSV. Compounds **1a** and **2a** are shown as green sticks and hydrogen bonds are highlighted as black dashes. Key residues around the binding pocket are shown as blue lines.

Terpenes

Compounds **1a** and **2a** belong to triterpenes and diterpenes, respectively (Yang et al., 2010), and both of them are isolated from *Abies georgei* which grows exclusively in China. In a previous study, compound **1a** was reported to have moderate agonistic effect against estrogen receptor (ER). The polycyclic ring skeletons of the two compounds are much similar to that of the bile acids, especially for the tetracyclic triterpene compound **1a**. However, the Tc values between compounds **1a** and **2a** and 6-ECDCA are as low as 0.36 and 0.28, respectively. Intriguingly, despite the opposite activities against FXR, the proposed binding poses of the two compounds closely resemble that of 6-ECDCA when interacting with FXR (**Figure 4**). Similar to 6-ECDCA, compound **1a** adopts *cis*-orientation in the A/B rings linkage, which is considered to be a unique feature for bile acids. The ring skeleton fits the binding pocket well through favorable VDW

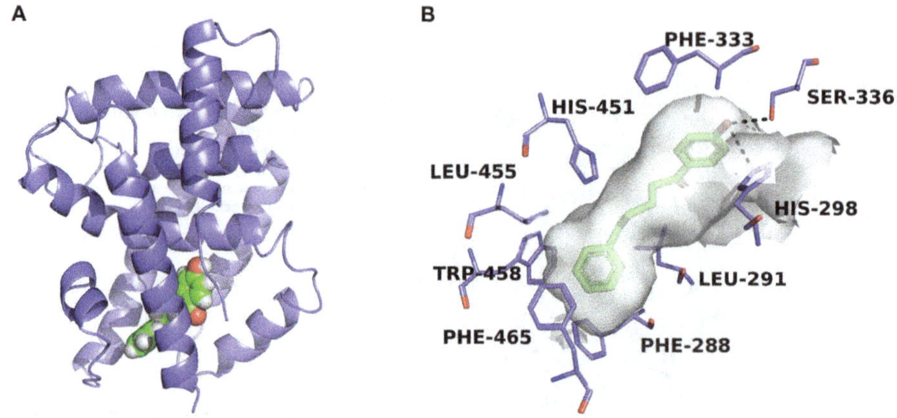

FIGURE 5 | Predicted binding pose of compound **3a** against FXR. **(A)** Overall view. The X-ray crystal structure of the FXR-LBD (PDB ID: 1OSH) is shown in cartoon, and the docked inhibitor is represented by spheres. **(B)** Detailed binding interactions of compound **3a** with FXR. Key residues around the binding pocket are displayed as green lines, and the hydrogen bonds are presented as black dashed lines.

contacts and hydrophobic effects with adjacent residues. The 3α-OH group extends to the space between helix 7 and helix 10/11 and putatively participates in hydrogen bond interactions with residues Tyr358 and His444. Additionally, the terminal carboxyl group could interact with residue Arg328, located at the entrance of the binding pocket, through salt bridge or hydrogen bond interactions. All the interactions described above are beneficial to the binding of compound **1a** to FXR. However, the hydrogen bond formed between the 7α-OH of 6-ECDCA and Tyr366 is absent for compound **1a** due to its structural variation on ring B. Under the physical-shape discrimination mechanism employed by FXR (Mi et al., 2003), bile acids without a 7α-OH group, such as LCA and DCA, showed extremely weak affinity with FXR, which may also cause the moderate antagonistic activity of compound **1a** against FXR.

For the analogs where the 3α-OH groups are replaced by carbonyl groups (compounds **1b** and **1c**), no detectable antagonistic activity was found in the coactivator recruitment assay. The planarity of the double bond may restrict the carbonyl oxygen atom to a position distant from residues Tyr358 and His444, and the absence of corresponding hydrogen bond interactions presumably results in the loss of agonistic effects against FXR.

Compared with compound **1a**, compound **2a** has a relatively smaller volume, but displayed 10-fold stronger antagonistic activity. Apparently, compound **2a** doesn't fit the canonical mechanism that nuclear receptors' antagonists are usually voluminous than agonists (Meyer et al., 2005). In the proposed binding pose with FXR, compound **2a** reveals the same amphipathic properties as the bile acid ligands. The oxygen atom of the carboxyl group putatively forms hydrogen bond interactions with residues Ser329 and Tyr366. At the other end of compound **2a**, hydrogen bond interactions could also form between the hydroxyl group and Arg328. The hydroxyl group seems to be essential for the antagonistic activity of compound **2a**, as its analog with an acetyl group (compound **2b**) exhibited no observed activity against FXR. Owing to the methyl group located at the10α-position, the carboxyl-substituted hydrocarbon ring A protrudes from the benzene ring panel, making VDW contacts and hydrophobic effects with Met325 on helix 5. Besides, the sequential ring structure could interact with loop H1-H2 (Met262), helix 3 (His291 and Met287), and helix 6 (Leu345) by favorable hydrophobic and VDW interactions.

Because of the relatively smaller volume, compound **2a** is not able to extend to the pocket that is occupied by rings A and B of 6-ECDCA, hence no direct interactions with helix 10/11 and helix 12 were observed. Previous studies have suggested that the π-cation interaction between His444 on helix 10/11 and Trp466 on helix 12 plays a critical role for the active conformation of helix 12 induced by endogenous bile acids (Mi et al., 2003; Pellicciari et al., 2005). Steroid agonists with 3α-OH group could facilitate the π-cation interaction by providing appropriate disposition of His444 through the steric restriction of hydrogen bonds formed between 3α-OH and residues His444 and Tyr358. Consequently, without the ability of establishing the triad of Tyr358, His444, and Trp466, compound **2a** couldn't secure helix 12 in the active conformation, thus preventing the recruitment of coactivators.

Phenols

Compounds **3a** and **3c**, named daphneone and daphnenone respectively (Zhang et al., 2006), are constituents of *Daphne odora* Thunb. var. *marginata*, an ornamental plant whose growth is restricted to the south of China. The two compounds, together with their simple structures and small volume, are extraordinarily peculiar to present antagonistic effects against the CDCA-induced SRC-1 association with FXR. Moreover, it is difficult to find common structural features between the two compounds and known agonists or antagonists. Accordingly, we turned to the initial docking poses to probe the structural basis of the FXR antagonistic profiles of this chemical series (**Figure 5**).

The two compounds were selected from the virtual screening process using the crystal structure of FXR-fexaramine complex. Compound **3a** is sandwiched in the cleft enclosed by helices 5, 7, and 10/11, partially overlapping with the fexaramine-binding pocket. The hydroxyl group points toward helix 5 and

TABLE 3 | *In silico* predicted properties of the six FXR antagonists.

Compd.	MW[a]	donorHB[b]	accptHB[c]	#rotor[d]	QPlogS[e]	QPlogPo/w[f]	QPPCaco[g]	Rule of five[h]	Rule of three[i]
1a	468.67	2.0	5.7	7	−6.60	5.52	142.21	1	1
2a	330.42	2.0	4.75	3	−4.23	3.03	82.62	0	0
3a	254.32	1.0	2.75	7	−4.27	3.92	1315.91	0	0
3c	252.31	1.0	2.75	6	−4.33	3.59	1160.27	0	0
3d	164.16	2.0	2.75	4	−1.55	1.38	68.09	0	0
3e	166.17	1.0	2.75	3	−2.27	2.46	1083.37	0	0
6-ECDCA	420.63	3.0	5.40	7	−5.36	4.28	48.73	0	0

The recommended ranges by QikProp are as follows:
[a]Molecular weight, 130.0–725.0.
[b]Number of hydrogen bond donors, 0.0–6.0.
[c]Number of hydrogen bond acceptors, 2.0–20.0.
[d]Number of non-trivial rotatable bonds, 0–15.
[e]Predicted aqueous solubility, −6.5–0.5.
[f]Predicted octanol/water partition coefficient, −2.0–6.5.
[g]Predicted apparent Caco-2 cell permeability in nm/sec, <25 poor, >500 great.
[h]Number of violations of Lipinski's rule of five, maximum is 4.
[i]Number of violations of Jorgensen's rule of three, maximum is 3.

may form hydrogen bonds with residues Ser336 and His298. On the other terminal, the benzene ring moiety extends to the aromatic residues-rich groove formed by Phe288 (helix 7), Trp458 (helix 10/11), and Phe465 (loop H10/11-H12), and probably contacts with these residues by advantageous π-stacking interactions. The linker between the two benzene rings fits the pocket by hydrophobic interactions and VDW contacts with surrounding residues such as Leu291, Met294, Ile356, and Ile361.

Previous molecular dynamics simulation studies assumed that the intrinsically unstable loop H10/11-12 controlled the flexibility of helix 12 (Costantino et al., 2005). Through offset face-to-face π-stacking interaction between the benzene ring and Phe465, both compounds **3a** and **3c** could contact with the loop directly, which may interfere with the conformation of the loop and push helix 12 away from its active conformation. For compound **3c** which has a double bond in the linker region, the antagonistic effect in the SRC-1-recruinment assay is slightly weaker. Presumably, the relatively flexible hydrocarbon linker is more suitable for the binding process with FXR-LBD, hence compound **3a** displayed stronger antagonistic activity. When a hydroxyl group was introduced into the hydrocarbon linker, the antagonistic activity of compound **3b** markedly decreased, displaying an IC_{50} value higher than 25 μM. Whereas the much smaller compounds **3d** and **3e**, which share the phenolic moiety with **3a**, exhibited moderate antagonistic effects against FXR. Compounds **3d** and **3e** were docked to FXR by Glide XP mode using the crystal structure 1OSH. As illustrated in Figure S5, the two small molecules occupy merely a fraction of the fexeramine-binding pocket. Hydrophobic effects and shape complementarities presumably dominate the interactions with FXR, as no hydrogen bond was detected in their proposed binding poses.

Notably, compounds **3a** and **3c** have been previously reported to show cytotoxic activities against a variety of human tumor cell lines, including K562, A549, MCF-7, LOVO, HepG2, and A375-S2, with the IC_{50} values ranging from 3.12 to 51.0 μM (Zhang et al., 2006; Wang et al., 2012). Besides, the agonistic profiles of compounds **3d** and **3e** against ER have also been described in a previous study (Cao et al., 2013). The phenol FXR antagonists identified in this study are relatively small, especially for compounds **3d** and **3e**, which probably have effects on other targets in living cells. Further thorough investigations are ongoing to better elucidate the exact mechanisms of action of the newly identified natural FXR antagonists and their implications regarding *in vivo* pharmacological effects.

Druglikeness Evaluation

To assess the drug-like profiles of the six natural products, an *in silico* prediction of ADME properties was performed using QikProp v4.3 module integrated into Maestro 10.1, and 6-ECDCA was used as the reference compound (**Table 3**). All physically significant descriptors and pharmaceutically relevant properties of the natural FXR antagonists, except for compound **1a**, fall into the recommended ranges of 95% of known drugs, suggesting remarkable potential of druglikeness. The QPlogPo/w and QPlogS values of compound **1a** exceed the limits of either Lipinski's rule of five or Jorgensen's rule of three, therefore the aqueous/lipid solubility should be taken into consideration if further structural optimization was carried out based on the tetracyclic triterpene compound **1a**.

CONCLUSION

In summary, we have established a small NPD containing over 4,000 compounds that were previously isolated from about 100 medicinal plants. From the database, six FXR antagonists were identified by strategic virtual screening method, which validated the feasibility of virtual screening to explore the potential targets of natural products. Although procured on the basis of known agonist-binding pocket, two of the most potent compounds **2a** and **3a** could antagonize the CDCA-induced SRC-1 recruitment to FXR-LBD with the IC_{50} values of 1.29 μM and 1.79 μM, respectively. The predicted docking mode of the diterpene **2a** against FXR exhibited partially similar binding interactions to those of the crystallographic ligand 6-ECDCA bound to FXR, whereas the daphneone **3a** showed noncanonical proposed binding mode, which may directly contact with the intrinsically unstable loop H10/11-12 by π-stacking interactions with the aromatic residue Phe465. Moreover, as assessed by QikProp, most of the natural FXR antagonists displayed comparable drug-like properties to that of 95% of known drugs. We hope our discovery will provide promising chemical scaffolds for further hit-to-lead optimization and for the study of FXR-related biological mechanisms.

AUTHOR CONTRIBUTIONS

HL, WZ, and LS conceived the study. YD and SL performed molecular simulations. YD analysed the data and drafted the manuscript. JJ, SZ, and JH carried out experimental studies. HL reviewed and revised the manuscript. All authors have read and approved the final manuscript.

FUNDING

The research is supported in part by the National Key Research and Development Program (Grant 2016YFA0502304), Special Program for Applied Research on Super Computation of the NSFC-Guangdong Joint Fund (the second phase) under Grant No. U1501501 and the Fundamental Research Funds for the Central Universities. SL is also sponsored by Shanghai Sailing Program (No. 18YF1405100).

REFERENCES

Bender, A., Jenkins, J. L., Scheiber, J., Sukuru, S. C., Glick, M., and Davies, J. W. (2009). How similar are similarity searching methods? A principal component analysis of molecular descriptor space. *J. Chem. Inf. Model.* 49, 108–119. doi: 10.1021/ci800249s

Cao, X., Jiang, J., Zhang, S., Zhu, L., Zou, J., Diao, Y., et al. (2013). Discovery of natural estrogen receptor modulators with structure-based virtual screening. *Bioorg. Med. Chem. Lett.* 23, 3329–3333. doi: 10.1016/j.bmcl.2013.03.105

Carotti, A., Marinozzi, M., Custodi, C., Cerra, B., Pellicciari, R., Gioiello, A., et al. (2014). Beyond bile acids: targeting Farnesoid X Receptor (FXR) with natural and synthetic ligands. *Curr. Top. Med. Chem.* 14, 2129–2142. doi: 10.2174/1568026614666141112094058

Choi, H., Hwang, H., Chin, J., Kim, E., Lee, J., Nam, S. J., et al. (2011). Tuberatolides, potent FXR antagonists from the Korean marine tunicate botryllus tuberatus. *J. Nat. Prod.* 74, 90–94. doi: 10.1021/np100489u

Costantino, G., Entrena-Guadix, A., Macchiarulo, A., Gioiello, A., and Pellicciari, R. (2005). Molecular dynamics simulation of the ligand binding domain of farnesoid X receptor. Insights into helix-12 stability and coactivator peptide stabilization in response to agonist binding. *J. Med. Chem.* 48, 3251–3259. doi: 10.1021/jm049182o

Downes, M., Verdecia, M. A., Roecker, A. J., Hughes, R., Hogenesch, J. B., Kast-Woelbern, H. R., et al. (2003). A chemical, genetic, and structural analysis of the nuclear bile acid receptor FXR. *Mol. Cell* 11, 1079–1092. doi: 10.1016/S1097-2765(03)00104-7

Dundas, J., Ouyang, Z., Tseng, J., Binkowski, A., Turpaz, Y., and Liang, J. (2006). CASTp: computed atlas of surface topography of proteins with structural and topographical mapping of functionally annotated residues. *Nucleic Acids Res.* 34, W116–W118. doi: 10.1093/nar/gkl282

Dussault, I., Beard, R., Lin, M., Hollister, K., Chen, J., Xiao, J., et al. (2003). Identification of gene-selective modulators of the bile acid receptor FXR. *J. Biol. Chem.* 278, 7027–7033. doi: 10.1074/jbc.M209863200

Fields, S., and Sternglanz, R. (1994). The two-hybrid system: an assay for protein-protein interactions. *Trends Genet.* 10, 286–292. doi: 10.1016/0168-9525(90)90012-U

Filho, C. D. D., Downes, M., and Evans, R. M. (2017). Farnesoid X receptor an emerging target to combat obesity. *Digest. Dis.* 35, 185–190. doi: 10.1159/000450909

Fiorucci, S., Mencarelli, A., Distrutti, E., Palladino, G., and Cipriani, S. (2010). Targeting farnesoid-X-receptor: from medicinal chemistry to disease treatment. *Curr. Med. Chem.* 17, 139–159. doi: 10.2174/092986710790112666

Flatt, B., Martin, R., Wang, T. L., Mahaney, P., Murphy, B., Gu, X. H., et al. (2009). Discovery of XL335 (WAY-362450), a highly potent, selective, and orally active agonist of the farnesoid X receptor (FXR). *J. Med. Chem.* 52, 904–907. doi: 10.1021/jm8014124

Forman, B. M., Goode, E., Chen, J., Oro, A. E., Bradley, D. J., Perlmann, T., et al. (1995). Identification of a nuclear receptor that is activated by farnesol metabolites. *Cell* 81, 687–693. doi: 10.1016/0092-8674(95)90530-8

Friesner, R. A., Banks, J. L., Murphy, R. B., Halgren, T. A., Klicic, J. J., Mainz, D. T., et al. (2004). Glide: a new approach for rapid, accurate docking and scoring. 1. Method and assessment of docking accuracy. *J. Med. Chem.* 47, 1739–1749. doi: 10.1021/jm0306430

Gaulton, A., Hersey, A., Nowotka, M., Bento, A. P., Chambers, J., Mendez, D., et al. (2017). The ChEMBL database in 2017. *Nucleic Acids Res.* 45, D945–D954. doi: 10.1093/nar/gkw1074

Gonzalez, F. J., Jiang, C. T., and Patterson, A. D. (2016). An intestinal microbiota-farnesoid X receptor axis modulates metabolic disease. *Gastroenterology* 151, 845–859. doi: 10.1053/j.gastro.2016.08.057

Halgren, T. A., Murphy, R. B., Friesner, R. A., Beard, H. S., Frye, L. L., Pollard, W. T., et al. (2004). Glide: a new approach for rapid, accurate docking and scoring. 2. Enrichment factors in database screening. *J. Med. Chem.* 47, 1750–1759. doi: 10.1021/jm030644s

Huang, H., Yu, Y., Gao, Z., Zhang, Y., Li, C., Xu, X., et al. (2012). Discovery and optimization of 1,3,4-trisubstituted-pyrazolone derivatives as novel, potent, and nonsteroidal farnesoid Xreceptor (FXR) selective antagonists. *J. Med. Chem.* 55, 7037–7053. doi: 10.1021/jm3002718

Jin, L., Feng, X., Rong, H., Pan, Z., Inaba, Y., Qiu, L., et al. (2013). The antiparasitic drug ivermectin is a novel FXR ligand that regulates metabolism. *Nat. Commun.* 4:1937. doi: 10.1038/ncomms2924

Kitchen, D. B., Decornez, H., Furr, J. R., and Bajorath, J. (2004). Docking and scoring in virtual screening for drug discovery: methods and applications. *Nat. Rev. Drug Discov.* 3, 935–949. doi: 10.1038/nrd1549

Lee, F. Y., Lee, H., Hubbert, M. L., Edwards, P. A., and Zhang, Y. (2006). FXR, a multipurpose nuclear receptor. *Trends Biochem. Sci.* 31, 572–580. doi: 10.1016/j.tibs.2006.08.002

Lew, J. L., Zhao, A., Yu, J., Huang, L., de Pedro, N., Pelaez, F., et al. (2004). The farnesoid X receptor controls gene expression in a ligand-and promoter-selective fashion. *J. Biol. Chem.* 279, 8856–8861. doi: 10.1074/jbc.M306422200

Li, F., Jiang, C. T., Krausz, K. W., Li, Y., Albert, I., Hao, H., et al. (2013). Microbiome remodelling leads to inhibition of intestinal farnesoid X receptor signalling and decreased obesity. *Nat. Commun.* 4:2384. doi: 10.1038/ncomms3384

Lin, J. S., and Lai, E. M. (2017). Protein-protein interactions: yeast two-hybrid system. *Methods Mol. Biol.*. 1615, 177–187. doi: 10.1007/978-1-4939-7033-9_14

Lin, Z., Shen, H., Huang, J., Chen, S., Chen, L., Chen, J., et al. (2008). Butyl 4-(butyryloxy) benzoate functions as a new selective estrogen receptor [beta]

agonist and induces GLUT4 expression in CHO-K1 cells. *J. Steroid Biochem.* 110, 150–156. doi: 10.1016/j.jsbmb.2008.03.028

Maglich, J. M., Caravella, J. A., Lambert, M. H., Willson, T. M., Moore, J. T., and Ramamurthy, L. (2003). The first completed genome sequence from a teleost fish (Fugu rubripes) adds significant diversity to the nuclear receptor superfamily. *Nucleic Acids Res.* 31, 4051–4058. doi: 10.1093/nar/gkg444

Makishima, M., Okamoto, A. Y., Repa, J. J., Tu, H., Learned, R. M., Luk, A., et al. (1999). Identification of a nuclear receptor for bile acids. *Science* 284, 1362–1365.

Maloney, P. R., Parks, D. J., Haffner, C. D., Fivush, A. M., Chandra, G., Plunket, K. D., et al. (2000). Identification of a chemical tool for the orphan nuclear receptor FXR. *J. Med. Chem.* 43, 2971–2974. doi: 10.1021/jm0002127

Meyer, U., Costantino, G., Macchiarulo, A., and Pellicciari, R. (2005). Is antagonism of E/Z-guggulsterone at the farnesoid X receptor mediated by a noncanonical binding site? A molecular modeling study. *J. Med. Chem.* 48, 6948–6955. doi: 10.1021/jm0505056

Mi, L. Z., Devarakonda, S., Harp, J. M., Han, Q., Pellicciari, R., Willson, T. M., et al. (2003). Structural basis for bile acid binding and activation of the nuclear receptor FXR. *Mol. Cell* 11, 1093–1100. doi: 10.1016/S1097-2765(03)00112-6

Nam, S. J., Ko, H., Ju, M. K., Hwang, H., Chin, J. W., Ham, J., et al. (2007). Scalarane sesterterpenes from a marine sponge of the genus spongia and their FXR antagonistic activity. *J. Nat. Prod.* 70, 1691–1695. doi: 10.1021/np070024k

Nevens, F., Andreone, P., Mazzella, G., Strasser, S. I., Bowlus, C., Invernizzi, P., et al. (2016). A placebo-controlled trial of obeticholic acid in primary biliary cholangitis. *N. Engl. J. Med.* 375, 631–643. doi: 10.1056/NEJMoa1509840

Pan, Y., Huang, N., Cho, S., and MacKerell, A. D. Jr. (2003). Consideration of molecular weight during compound selection in virtual target-based database screening. *J. Chem. Inf. Comput. Sci.* 43, 267–272. doi: 10.1021/ci020055f

Pellicciari, R., Costantino, G., and Fiorucci, S. (2005). Farnesoid X receptor: from structure to potential clinical applications. *J. Med. Chem.* 48, 5383–5403. doi: 10.1021/jm0582221

Pellicciari, R., Fiorucci, S., Camaioni, E., Clerici, C., Costantino, G., Maloney, P. R., et al. (2002). 6 alpha-ethyl-chenodeoxycholic acid (6-ECDCA), a potent and selective FXR agonist endowed with anticholestatic activity. *J. Med. Chem.* 45, 3569–3572. doi: 10.1021/jm025529g

Schaap, F. G., Trauner, M., and Jansen, P. L. (2014). Bile acid receptors as targets for drug development. *Nat. Rev. Gastro. Hepat.* 11, 55–67. doi: 10.1038/nrgastro.2013.151

Soisson, S. M., Parthasarathy, G., Adams, A. D., Sahoo, S., Sitlani, A., Sparrow, C., et al. (2008). Identification of a potent synthetic FXR agonist with an unexpected mode of binding and activation. *Proc. Natl. Acad. Sci. U.S.A.* 105, 5337–5342. doi: 10.1073/pnas.0710981105

Urizar, N. L., Liverman, A. B., Dodds, D. T., Silva, F., Ordentlich, P., Yan, Y., et al. (2002). A natural product that lowers cholesterol as an antagonist ligand for FXR. *Science* 296, 1703–1706. doi: 10.1126/science.1072891

Verdonk, M. L., Berdini, V., Hartshorn, M. J., Mooij, W. T., Murray, C. W., Taylor, R. D., et al. (2004). Virtual screening using protein-ligand docking: avoiding artificial enrichment. *J. Chem. Inf. Comp. Sci.* 44, 793–806. doi: 10.1021/ci034289q

Wang, L. B., Dong, N. W., Wu, Z. H., and Wu, L. J. (2012). Two new compounds with cytotoxic activity on the human melanoma A375-S2 cells from Daphne giraldii callus cells. *J. Asian Nat. Prod. Res.* 14, 1020–1026. doi: 10.1080/10286020.2012.701206

Wang, Y. D., Chen, W. D., Moore, D. D., and Huang, W. (2008). FXR: a metabolic regulator and cell protector. *Cell Res.* 18, 1087–1095. doi: 10.1038/cr.2008.289

Wu, J., Xia, C. S., Meier, J., Li, S. Z., Hu, X., and Lala, D. S. (2002). The hypolipidemic natural product guggulsterone acts as an antagonist of the bile acid receptor. *Mol. Endocrinol.* 16, 1590–1597. doi: 10.1210/mend.16.7.0894

Xu, X., Xu, X., Liu, P., Zhu, Z. Y., Chen, J., Fu, H. A., et al. (2015). Structural basis for small molecule NDB (N-benzyl-N-(3-(tert-butyl)-4-hydroxyphenyl)-2,6-dichloro-4-(dimethylamino) benzamide) as a selective antagonist of farnesoid X receptor alpha (FXR alpha) in stabilizing the homodimerization of the receptor. *J. Biol. Chem.* 290, 19888–19899. doi: 10.1074/jbc.M114.630475

Yamada, T., and Sugimoto, K. (2016). Guggulsterone and its role in chronic diseases. *Adv. Exp. Med. Biol.* 929, 329–361. doi: 10.1007/978-3-319-41342-6_15

Yang, X. W., Feng, L., Li, S. M., Liu, X. H., Li, Y. L., Wu, L., et al. (2010). Isolation, structure, and bioactivities of abiesadines AY, 25 new diterpenes from Abies georgei Orr. *Bioorg. Med. Chem.* 18, 744–754. doi: 10.1016/j.bmc.2009.11.055

Yuan, Z. Q., and Li, K. W. (2016). Role of farnesoid X receptor in cholestasis. *J. Digest. Dis.* 17, 501–509. doi: 10.1111/1751-2980.12378

Zhang, W., Zhang, W. D., Liu, R. H., Shen, Y., Zhang, C., Cheng, H., et al. (2006). Two new chemical constituents from Daphne odora Thunb. *var. marginata. Nat. Prod. Res.* 20, 1290–1294. doi: 10.1080/14786410601101860

Zhang, Y., and Edwards, P. (2008). FXR signaling in metabolic disease. *FEBS Lett.* 582, 10–18. doi: 10.1016/j.febslet.2007.11.015

3

Supramolecular Organization of Nonstoichiometric Drug Hydrates: Dapsone

Doris E. Braun and Ulrich J. Griesser*

Institute of Pharmacy, University of Innsbruck, Innsbruck, Austria

***Correspondence:**
Doris E. Braun
doris.braun@uibk.ac.at

The observed moisture- and temperature dependent transformations of the dapsone (4,4′-diaminodiphenyl sulfone, DDS) 0. 33-hydrate were correlated to its structure and the number and strength of the water-DDS intermolecular interactions. A combination of characterization techniques was used, including thermal analysis (hot-stage microscopy, differential scanning calorimetry and thermogravimetric analysis), gravimetric moisture sorption/desorption studies and variable humidity powder X-ray diffraction, along with computational modeling (crystal structure prediction and pair-wise intermolecular energy calculations). Depending on the relative humidity the hydrate contains between 0 and 0.33 molecules of water per molecule DDS. The crystal structure is retained upon dehydration indicating that DDS hydrate shows a non-stoichiometric (de)hydration behavior. Unexpectedly, the water molecules are not located in structural channels but at isolated-sites of the host framework, which is counterintuitively for a hydrate with non-stoichiometric behavior. The water-DDS interactions were estimated to be weaker than water-host interactions that are commonly observed in stoichiometric hydrates and the lattice energies of the isomorphic dehydration product (hydrate structure without water molecules) and (form **III**) differ only by $\sim$1 kJ mol^{-1}. The computational generation of hypothetical monohydrates confirms that the hydrate with the unusual DDS:water ratio of 3:1 is more stable than a feasible monohydrate structure. Overall, this study highlights that a deeper understanding of the formation of hydrates with non-stoichiometric behavior requires a multidisciplinary approach including suitable experimental and computational methods providing a firm basis for the development and manufacturing of high quality drug products.

Keywords: dapsone, hydrate, crystal structure prediction, temperature and moisture dependent stability, intermolecular energy

INTRODUCTION

The vast majority of drugs is formulated and administered in a solid (mostly crystalline) form, since this aggregation state assures the highest chemical and storage stability of the drug compound. However, a drug compound may occur in a variety of different solid state forms, which is subsumed under the general term "polymorphism" comprising one component forms (polymorphs, amorphous form) and multicomponent phases (hydrates, solvates, co-crystals). The statement "*Many people think that polymorphism and solid state chemistry is the hardest thing to get right in drug development*" (Byrn, 2004) clearly reflects on the challenges encountered and efforts to be undertaken in pre-formulation to guarantee that the best solid form is used in a drug formulation. The molecular structure of a drug compound determines its biological/pharmacological properties and is thus an invariant, i.e., cannot be changed in order to optimize the physicochemical and biopharmaceutical properties of a drug. The only strategy to improve such properties at the molecular level is the formation of bioreversible derivatives of the drug compound (prodrugs), which are transformed to the active molecules by metabolic principles in the organism (Rautio et al., 2008, 2017). The molecular features of a drug (molecular size, shape, flexibility, hydrogen bond donors/acceptors, etc.,) determine the potential of a drug to occur in different "supramolecular" states (solid state forms) which may exhibit significantly different physicochemical properties that are critical for the adjustment of an optimal performance of a pharmaceutical product. The most critical parameters are equilibrium solubility and dissolution rate but also differences in density, hardness, melting point, mechanical strength, chemical stability etc. may affect manufacturing processes and are relevant for shelf-life stability and finally the bioavailability of a final dosage form. Thus, identifying solid state forms of a drug and understanding their phase relationships, interconversion pathways and properties is a key concern in modern drug development (Byrn et al., 1999; Bernstein, 2002; Hilfiker, 2006; Brittain, 2009). Multiple solid forms, including salts, co-crystals and solvates, have been found for 90% of molecules (Stahly, 2007) and therefore, considerably extend the range of solid form options available for delivering drugs.

The past experience of late-appearing, more stable forms, as in the case of ritonavir (Chemburkar et al., 2000) or rotigotine (Perez-Lloret et al., 2013), has not only triggered the awareness of the issue of solid forms but also led to the implementation of polymorphism screenings, a survey of crystallization conditions designed to find and identify solid forms of a drug substance, as a routine in the pre-formulation phase. Experimental solid form screens may encompass up to thousands of crystallization experiments and need to be tailored to the properties of the investigated molecule (Newman, 2013; Cruz-Cabeza Aurora et al., 2015). The wide range of methods that have led to the discovery of novel forms (Llinàs and Goodman, 2008) highlight, however, that there is no standard recipe for comprehensive experimental solid form screening. Furthermore, the problem that there is no endpoint in experimental solid form screening, a computational method ensuring that all relevant forms have been found is in high demand. To this end, crystal structure prediction (CSP) on smaller pharmaceuticals has shown high promise in complementing experimental solid form screening, helping to rationalize and unify experimental observations on polymorphs, hydrates and solvates (Cruz-Cabeza et al., 2008; Campeta et al., 2010; Braun et al., 2011a, 2014a,b, 2016; Baias et al., 2013; Bhardwaj et al., 2013; Ismail et al., 2013; Kendrick et al., 2013; Price et al., 2014, 2016; Singh and Thakur, 2014; Braun and Griesser, 2016b; Price and Reutzel-Edens, 2016). The aim of an experimental polymorph screen is the identification of those solid state forms which are relevant for a product development, and the main expectation of a CSP study is the confirmation that those forms are among the lowest energy structures. Yet, computing the crystal energy landscapes of larger drug molecules including its hydrates and solvates is still too complex and computationally very (time) demanding. For multi-component systems host (drug molecule) and different guest molecules in different stoichiometric ratios would have to be considered separately.

Generating knowledge of how water (vapor) is associated with a specific material and how it affects the stability of a product is a crucial task in pre-formulation studies, because water inevitably appears in the manufacturing and storage process of pharmaceutical products. Knowledge about hydrate formation (water adducts) is of importance, as hydrates can be the most stable solid form at relevant production and storage conditions and it is well-known that at least one-third of organic (drug) molecules (Stahly, 2007; Braun, 2008; Cruz-Cabeza Aurora et al., 2015) form hydrates. A transformation to a hydrate may be unavoidable. In a hydrate the water molecules occupy regular positions in the crystal lattice of the parent substance. The water can either fill structural voids or be an integral part of the structure. Based on the moisture sorption/desorption behavior hydrates can be subdivided into two main classes (Gal, 1968; Griesser, 2006). "Stoichiometric" hydrates are regarded as molecular compounds. Dehydration always leads to a different structure or the amorphous state. "Non-stoichiometric" hydrates incorporate a range of water levels as a function of temperature and water vapor pressure. The latter often host water molecules in open structural voids that allow for reversible water uptake/release without significant changes in the crystal structure. The water in non-stoichiometric hydrates is often rather weakly bound and may interact with other components compromising the stability and performance of formulated products. Thus, knowledge of hydrate formation, moisture and temperature dependent stability is crucial for the development of a high quality fine chemical product.

Dapsone (4,4′-diaminodiphenyl sulfone; DDS, **Figure 1**) has been chosen in this study as a model compound for evaluating the value of computational chemistry in solid form screening and characterization of a pharmaceutical hydrate. The compound itself has been synthesized for the first time over 100 years ago (Fromm and Wittmann, 1908) and its microbial activity and therapeutic use for leprosy has already been studied in the 1940s. DDS has reinvented itself as a drug many times and has been in use for numerous indications, treatment of leprosy, dermatitis herpetiformis, malaria, prophylaxis of pneumocytosis etc. (Wolf and Orni-Wasserlauf, 2000; Wozel and Blasum, 2014).

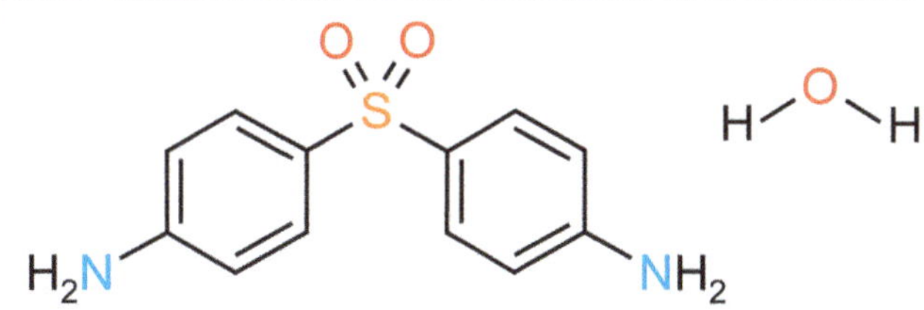

FIGURE 1 | Molecular diagram of 4,4′-diaminodiphenyl sulfone (DDS, dapsone) hydrate.

Today, it is mainly used as first-line drug in the treatment of leprosy in combination with rifampicin and clofazimine. As such, it is listed in the WHO's List of Essential Medicines (medications satisfying the priority health care needs in humans) (World Health Organization, 2017). The compound is known to be polymorphic (anhydrate forms **I–IV**), with form **III** being reported to be the most stable form (Brandstaetter-Kuhnert et al., 1963; Kuhnert-Brandstatter and Moser, 1979). Single crystal structures are known for anhydrate forms **III** (Dickinson et al., 1970; Deo et al., 1980; Bocelli and Cantoni, 1990; Su et al., 1992; Bertolasi et al., 1993) and **II** (Braun et al., 2017). It is also known that DDS forms solvates with dichloromethane, 1,4-dioxane and tetrahydrofuran (Babashkina et al., 2012; Lemmer et al., 2012). Furthermore, several crystal structure determinations of a hydrate with the unusual DDS:water stoichiometry of 3:1 (0.33-hydrate) have been reported (Kuz'mina et al., 1981; Bel'skii et al., 1983; Yathirajan et al., 2014). Apart from these structure reports no other information about the hydrate can be found in the literature.

The aim of this study was to unravel the molecular/structural reasons for hydrate formation in DDS, the structural and thermodynamic relationship between the **0.33-Hy** and water-free DDS forms and their interconversion pathways as a function of temperature and humidity/water activity through a combination of computational and experimental methods. A range of experimental techniques (crystallization, slurry experiments, thermal analysis and X-ray diffraction), along with CSP and pair-wise intermolecular energy calculations were applied to explore the solid forms at an atomistic level. The applied method for estimating the intermolecular interaction energies (CE-B3LYP), best described as a hybrid method, did perform surprisingly well compared to B3LYP-D2/6-31G(d,p) counterpoise-corrected energies, but in considerable less computation time (Turner et al., 2014). However, calculating water interactions in organic (drug) hydrates represents a big challenge as the balance of host (organic molecule)-host, host-water, and water-water intermolecular interactions has to be modeled accurately. Most simple water potentials have been parametrized against a wide range of liquid properties (Guillot, 2002). A potential for studying ices and amorphous water, which reparametrized the TIP4P potential to reproduce the density of several forms of ice, has been developed by Abascal et al. (2005). Very recently it has been demonstrated (in lead optimization), that accurately modeling intermolecular interactions involving water requires the incorporation of three-body terms and nanoscale treatment of the dielectric response of confined frustrated water molecules (Fernández, 2016, 2017; Fernandez and Scott, 2017). Nevertheless, in our study we decided to test the applicability of the readily available and transferable CE-B3LYP method, which was not explicitly developed for hydrate structures. We address the role of CSP in hydrate screening and modeling and investigate whether it is possible to derive information about hydrate stability and dehydration mechanism based on structural classifications and simple intermolecular interaction energy estimations (i.e., estimating the strengths of host-host, water-host and water-water interactions).

MATERIALS AND METHODS

Computational Generation of the Monohydrate Crystal Energy Landscape

The global energy minimum of DDS, obtained using Gaussian09 (Frisch et al., 2009), was used in the CSP searches. 350,000 $Z' = 1$ monohydrate structures were generated using CrystalPredictor2.0 (Karamertzanis and Pantelides, 2005, 2007; Habgood et al., 2015) in 48 common space groups for organic molecules (Supplementary Material). The molecules were held rigid and the lattice energy was evaluated by an exp-6 potential with atomic charges derived using the CHELPG scheme (Breneman and Wiberg, 1990) and minimized. The 10,000 lowest energy crystal structures were used as starting points for optimizing the intermolecular lattice energy (U_{inter}), with an improved model for the intermolecular forces. This was calculated using the FIT exp-6 potential parameters (Coombes et al., 1996), the sulfur potential derived by Scheraga (Day et al., 2009) and the distributed multipoles (Stone, 2005) derived from the PBE0/6-31G(d,p) charge density using GDMA2 (Stone, 2010).

The optimal proton positions of the amino group and orientation of the phenyl groups, in all crystal structures within 15 kJ mol^{-1} of the global minimum (116 structures), were determined using the CrystalOptimizer database method (Kazantsev et al., 2011). This was done by minimizing the lattice energy (E_{latt}), calculated as the sum of the intermolecular contributions (U_{inter}) and the conformational energy penalty paid for distortion of the molecular geometry to improve the hydrogen bonding geometries. Conformational energy penalties (ΔE_{intra}, with respect to the pyramidal global conformational energy minimum) and isolated molecule charge densities were computed at the PBE0/6-31G(d,p) level, for each conformation considered in the minimization of E_{latt}. All isolated-molecule wave function calculations were performed using Gaussian09 (Frisch et al., 2009) and intermolecular lattice energies using DMACRYS (Price et al., 2010).

The 100 most stable structures (within 30 kJ mol^{-1} of the global minimum) were used as starting points for periodic electronic structure calculations. The DFT-D calculations were carried out with the CASTEP plane wave code (Clark et al., 2005) using the Perdew-Burke-Ernzerhof (PBE) generalized gradient approximation (GGA) exchange-correlation density functional (Perdew et al., 1996) and ultrasoft pseudopotentials (Vanderbilt, 1990), with the addition of a semi-empirical dispersion correction developed by Tkatchenko and Scheffler (TS) (Tkatchenko Scheffler and Scheffler, 2009). Brillouin zone integrations were performed on a symmetrized Monkhorst–Pack k-point grid with the number of k-points chosen to provide a maximum spacing of 0.07 Å^{-1} and a basis set cut-off of 780 eV. The self-consistent field convergence on total energy was set to $1\text{x}10^{-5}$ eV. Energy minimizations were performed using the Broyden–Fletcher–Goldfarb–Shanno optimization scheme within the space group constraints. The optimizations were considered complete when energies were converged to better than 2×10^{-5} eV per atom, atomic displacements converged to 1×10^{-3} Å, maximum forces to 5×10^{-2} eV Å^{-1}, and maximum stresses were converged to 1×10^{-1} GPa. Isolated molecule minimizations to compute the isolated DDS and water energy (U_{gas}) were performed by placing a single molecule in a fixed cubic $35 \times 35 \times 35$ Å^3 unit cell and optimized with the same settings as used for the crystal calculations.

The experimental hydrate, lower hydrates and forms **II** and **III** of DDS, as well as other selected hydrates (Supplementary Material), were minimized with CASTEP and the same settings were used as described for generating the monohydrate crystal energy landscape.

Crystal Explorer Calculations

The pair-wise energy contributions to **0.33-Hy** and other well-characterized hydrate structures, have been calculated using CrystalExplorer V17 (Turner et al., 2014, 2015; Mackenzie et al., 2017). The optimized atomic positions (PBE-TS) have been used in all subsequent intermolecular interaction energy calculations. The model energies have been calculated between all unique nearest neighbor molecular pairs. The used model (termed CE-B3LYP) uses B3LYP/6-31G(d,p) molecular wave functions calculated by applying the molecular geometries extracted from the crystal structures. This approach uses electron densities of unperturbed monomers to obtain four separate energy components: electrostatic (E_E), polarization (E_P), dispersion (E_D), and exchange-repulsion (E_R). Each energy term was scaled independently to fit a large training set of B3LYP-D2/6-31G(d,p) counterpoise-corrected energies from both organic and inorganic crystals. The CE-B3LYP energies reproduced the training set energies with a mean absolute deviation of ~1 kJ mol^{-1} (Turner et al., 2014).

Conformational Analysis

Conformational energy scans were performed at the B3LYP/6-31G(d,p) level of theory using Gaussian09 (Frisch et al., 2009), allowing the two torsion angles defining the position of the phenyl rings, C–C–S–C, to rotate by 360° in 20° steps.

Materials and Preparation of DDS Hydrate

Dapsone form **III** (purity 97%) was purchased from Aldrich. The obtained sample was recrystallized from a hot-saturated methanol solution. The solid product was isolated by filtration and consisted of form **III**. The organic solvents used were all of analytical grade and purchased from Aldrich or Fluka.

DDS **0.33-Hy** was prepared as follows: (i) a slurry of DDS form **III** in water was stirred in the temperature range from 10 to 30°C for 1 week. The suspension was filtered and the solid was stored at ambient conditions. (ii) A hot saturated solution of form **III** in water (close to the boiling point) was cooled to room temperature (RT). Within 2 days large elongated **0.33-Hy** crystals were obtained.

Thermal Analysis

For hot-stage thermomicroscopic (HSM) investigations a Reichert Thermovar polarization microscope, equipped with a Kofler hot-stage (Reichert, A), was used. Photographs were taken with an Olympus DP71 digital camera (Olympus, A).

Differential Scanning Calorimetry (DSC) thermograms were recorded on a Diamond DSC (Perkin-Elmer Norwalk, Ct., USA) controlled by the Pyris 7.0 software. Using a UM3 ultramicrobalance (Mettler, Greifensee, CH), samples of ~5–7 mg were weighed into perforated or sealed aluminum pans. The samples were heated using rates in between 1 and 20°C min^{-1} and cooled using a rate of 5 or 10°C min^{-1} with dry nitrogen as the purge gas (purge: 20 mL min^{-1}). The instrument was calibrated for temperature with pure benzophenone (mp 48.0°C) and caffeine (236.2°C), and the energy calibration was performed with indium (mp 156.6°C, heat of fusion 28.45 J g^{-1}). The errors on the stated temperatures (extrapolated onset temperatures) and enthalpy values were calculated at the 95% confidence interval (CI) and are based on at least five measurements.

Thermogravimetric Analysis (TGA) was carried out with a TGA7 system (Perkin-Elmer, Norwalk, CT, USA) using the Pyris 2.0 Software. Approximately 7–10 mg of sample was weighed into a platinum pan. Two-point calibration of the temperature was performed with ferromagnetic materials (Alumel and Ni, Curie-point standards, Perkin-Elmer). Heating rates of 5 and 10°C min^{-1} were applied and dry nitrogen was used as a purge gas (sample purge: 20 mL min^{-1}, balance purge: 40 mL min^{-1}).

Powder X-Ray Diffraction (PXRD)

PXRD patterns were obtained using an X'Pert PRO diffractometer (PANalytical, Almelo, NL) equipped with a θ/θ coupled goniometer in transmission geometry, programmable XYZ stage with well plate holder, Cu-K$\alpha_{1,2}$ radiation source with a focusing mirror, a 0.5° divergence slit, a 0.02° Soller slit collimator on the incident beam side, a 2 mm antiscattering slit, a 0.02° Soller slit collimator on the diffracted beam side and a solid state PIXcel detector. The patterns were recorded at a tube voltage of 40 kV and tube current of 40 mA, applying a step size of $2\theta = 0.013°$ with 200 s per step in the 2θ range between 2° and 40°. For non-ambient RH measurements, a VGI stage (VGI 2000M, Middlesex, UK) was used.

The diffraction patterns were indexed using the first 20 peaks with DICVOL04 and the space group was determined based on a statistical assessment of systematic absences (Markvardsen et al., 2001) as implemented in the DASH structure solution package (David et al., 2006). Pawley fits (Pawley, 1981) and Rietveld refinements (Rietveld, 1969) were performed with Topas Academic V5 (Coelho, 2012). The background was modeled with Chebyshev polynomials and the modified Thompson-Cox-Hastings pseudo-Voigt function was used for peak shape fitting. For the Rietveld refinements the DDS and water molecules were treated as rigid body molecules using the PBE-TS optimized conformations of the **0.33-Hy** structure.

Gravimetric Moisture Sorption/Desorption Experiments

Moisture sorption and desorption studies were performed with the automatic multisample gravimetric moisture sorption analyser SPS23-10μ (ProUmid, Ulm, D). Approximately 500–750 mg of sample was used for each analysis. The measurement cycles were started at 60% with an initial stepwise desorption (decreasing humidity) to 0%, followed by a sorption cycle (increasing humidity) up to 90% relative humidity (RH), a desorption cycle to 0% RH and a final sorption cycle to 90% RH. The RH changes were set to 2% and the equilibrium condition for each step was set to a mass constancy of ± 0.001% over 60 min and a maximum time limit of 48 h per step.

Water Activity Measurements (Slurry Method)

DDS form **III** was stirred (500 r.p.m.) in 1.5–2.5 mL of each methanol and water mixture [each containing a different mole fraction of water corresponding to a defined water activity Zhu et al., 1996, Supplementary Material] at 25.0 ± 0.1°C for 21 days. Samples were withdrawn, filtered and the resulting phase was determined using PXRD.

RESULTS AND DISCUSSION

Computational Screening for DDS Monohydrates

The fact that the asymmetric unit of **0.33-Hy** (Kuz'mina et al., 1981; Bel'skii et al., 1983; Yathirajan et al., 2014) consists of four crystallographically distinct molecules (three DDS and one water) makes CSP studies for the experimental stoichiometry too time-consuming. Therefore, we decided to generate the monohydrate crystal energy landscape (one DDS and one water molecule) with the aim to estimate whether water molecules can compete against the DDS-DDS intermolecular interactions and form strong DDS-water contacts. In **Figure 2** the computed monohydrate structures are plotted according to lattice energy, which equals the energy that would be required to separate the molecules to infinity, against packing index.

To estimate whether any of the hypothetical monohydrate structure is competitive in energy with form **III**, we compared the lattice energy of the hydrate (E_{latt}-Hy) to the lattice energies of the anhydrate (E_{latt}-III) and ice (E_{latt}-ICE). If E_{latt}-Hy < E_{latt}-III + E_{latt}-ICE (we assume that hydrate formation is thermodynamically driven), then the hydrate is more stable than the anhydrate. Using the lattice energies of **0.33-Hy**, form **III** (**Table 1**) and a value of −59 kJ mol^{-1} (Whalley, 1957, 1976) for ice, as the used functional is known to overbind the ice crystal structures (Thierfelder et al., 2006; Beran and Nanda, 2010), then only one structure, 01_1963, was calculated to be more stable than **III**. The most stable hypothetical monohydrate was estimated to be 12.38 kJ mol^{-1} more stable than form **III**, which is a respectable potential energy differences ($\Delta_{trs}U$) for a monohydrate with respect to an anhydrate. Thus, the CSP study clearly indicates hydrate formation.

Furthermore, $\Delta_{trs}U$ for the **0.33-Hy** to form **III** was calculated to be 15.37 kJ mol^{-1}, indicating that the experimental hydrate is 3 kJ mol^{-1} more stable than the computed lowest energy monohydrate structure and rationalizing why the stable 0.33-hydrate and not a monohydrate is formed experimentally.

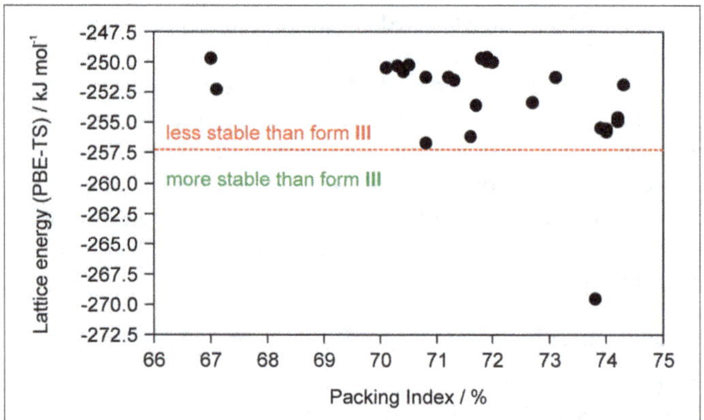

FIGURE 2 | Summary of crystal structure prediction for DDS monohydrate ($Z' = 1$), with each symbol denoting a crystal structure by its lattice energy and packing index. The vertical red dotted line separates the monohydrate structure that was calculated to be more stable than form III and ice from other computed hydrate structures that are less stable.

Experimental Screening for DDS Hydrate(s)

To confirm that **0.33-Hy** is indeed the stable DDS hydrate form and that 01_1963 is not a yet undiscovered monohydrate we subjected DDS to an experimental hydrate screening program. Evaporative crystallization experiments of DDS from a saturated (20°C) aqueous solution, as well as cooling crystallization experiments from hot (boiling) saturated solutions in water at 5°, 25°, 50°, and 75°C resulted in **0.33-Hy** crystals in the form of elongated plates. In contrast, evaporation experiments of a hot-saturated solution of DDS in water resulted in a mixture of **0.33-Hy** and form **III**. Slurry experiments in water, isothermal or cycling between 5° and 50°C, always yielded the **0.33-Hy**.

Another successful way to produce hydrates are moisture sorption experiments. Therefore, form **III** and **V** (see section Moisture Dependent Stability of the Hydrate) were subjected to automated and manual water vapor sorption experiments. Neither form **III**, nor form **V** showed a transformation in the RH range up to 90%. Furthermore, no transformation was observed in long-time storage experiments of the two anhydrous DDS forms over saturated KOAc (24% RH), K_2CO_3 (43% RH), NaCl (75% RH), KNO_3 solutions (92% RH) or water (100% RH) within 3 months (end of experiments) at RT and 8°C. Similarly, also **0.33-Hy** did not dehydrate or transform to another hydrate if stored under the same conditions over the same time period.

TABLE 1 | Lattice energy calculations (E_{latt}) of **0.33-Hy**, 01_1963, forms **II** and **III** and the isomorphic dehydrate structure (**0.33-Hy** without water molecules, **Hy**$_{dehy}$) and potential energy differences ($\Delta_{trs}U$) with respect to form **III**.

Form	E_{latt}/kJ mol^{-1}	$\Delta_{trs}U_{x-III}$/kJ mol^{-1}
0.33-Hy	−222.95	15.37[a]
Hy$_{dehy}$	−197.26	−0.90[b]
01_1963	−269.54	12.38[a]
Form **II**	−194.92	−3.25[b]
Form **III**	−198.16	0[b]

[a]Calculated according to: $-\Delta_{trs}U_{x-III} = E_{latt}\text{-}x - (E_{latt}\text{-}\mathbf{III} + E_{latt}\text{-}ICE)$. [b] $-\Delta_{trs}U_{x-III} = E_{latt}\text{-}x - E_{latt}\text{-}\mathbf{III}$.

Characterization of the DDS Hydrate

DDS Hydrate Structure and Intermolecular Interaction Energies

To identify the key interactions in the DDS hydrate the pair-wise CE-B3LYP intermolecular energies were estimated starting from the PBE-TS optimized hydrate with the CSD Refcode ANSFON02 (Yathirajan et al., 2014). The intermolecular energies are subdivided into classical electrostatic (E_E), polarization (E_P), dispersion (E_D) and exchange-repulsion energies (E_R) and can be graphically represented by their "energy frameworks" (Turner et al., 2014, 2015; Mackenzie et al., 2017).

The hydrate crystallizes in the monoclinic space group $C2/c$ with three DDS and one water molecule in the asymmetric unit, rationalizing the 3:1 stoichiometry (Kuz'mina et al., 1981; Bel'skii et al., 1983; Yathirajan et al., 2014). The three crystallographically independent DDS molecules (color coded in the packing diagram shown in **Figure 3A**) exhibit very similar conformations. The first DDS molecule (mol A, shown in red in **Figure 3A**) does not show any interaction with the hydrate water (**Table 1**), but forms two strong intermolecular interactions with itself, denoted with 2 and 4, mediated by inversion and 2-fold symmetry, respectively (**Figure 3B**). Furthermore, mol A forms classical hydrogen bonded interactions with neighboring DDS molecules

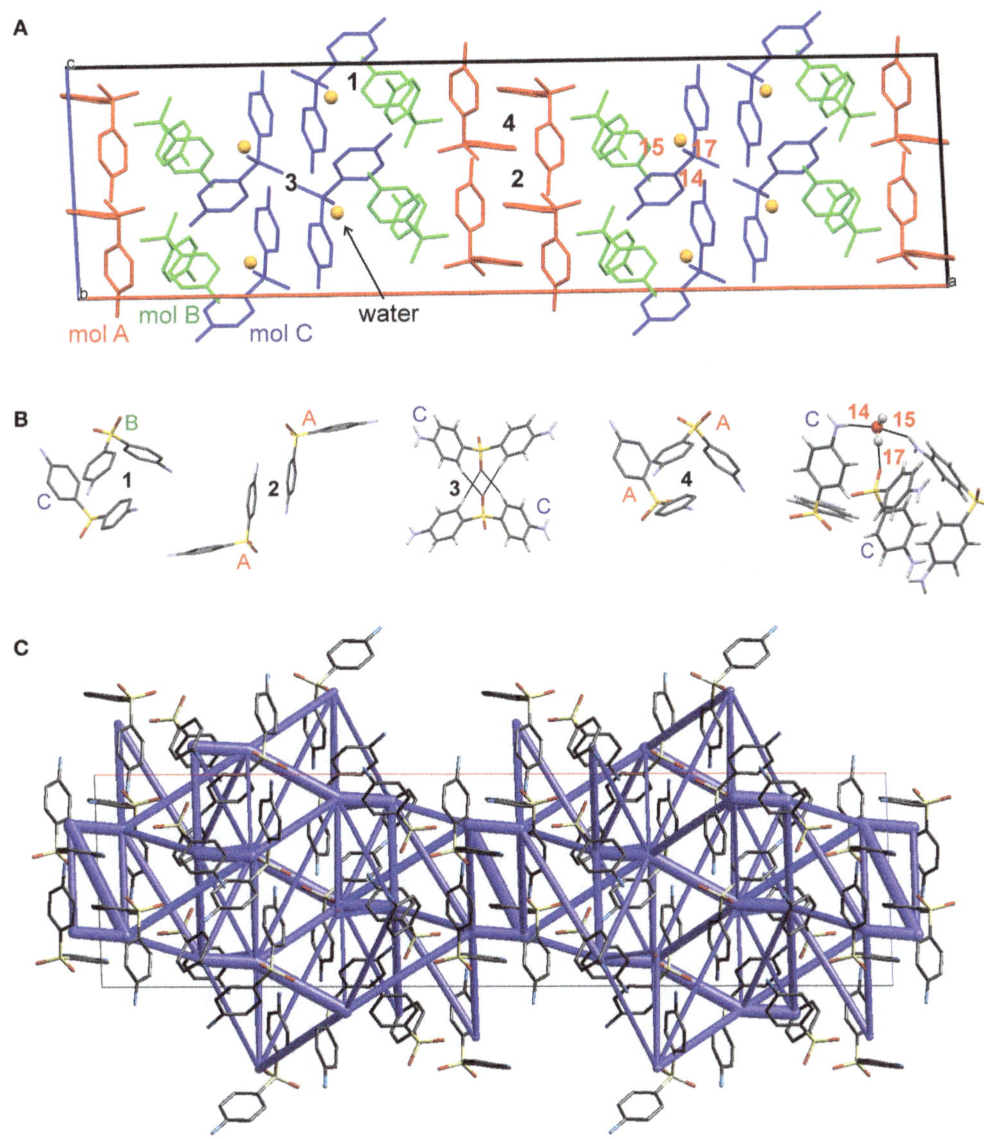

FIGURE 3 | (A) Packing diagram of DDS **0.33-Hy** (ANSFON02, Yathirajan et al., 2014) viewed along the crystallographic *b* axis. The symmetry independent molecules are color coded and hydrogen atoms have been omitted for clarity. Numbers denote key pair-wise intermolecular interactions, which are enlarged in **(B)** and listed in **Table 2**. Hydrogen bonding is indicated with black lines. **(C)** Energy frameworks (total energy) for **0.33-Hy**, viewed along the crystallographic *b* axis. The energy scale factor is 80, and interaction energies with magnitudes smaller than 15 kJ mol^{-1} have been omitted. For additional views see Supplementary Material.

(interactions 5, 7, and 11; **Table 2**). In contrast to interactions 2 and 4, which have dispersion as the strongest contributor to the energy (π···π stacks), Coulomb interactions are the reason for the stability of the latter three (also true for 3, 6, 8, 9, 14, 15, 16, and 21). Molecule B (green) and C (blue) form the strongest pair-wise interaction (1, **Figure 3B**), which can be related to interaction 4. The third most stable interaction (3) involves mol C and is formed of four C–H···O close contacts. The strongest classical hydrogen bonded interaction (5, **Table 2**), N–H···O, is significantly less stable than interactions 1–4.

The water molecule, interacting only with mol B and mol C, forms three hydrogen bonds, two N–H···O_{water} and one O_{water} – H···O. Thus, the water molecule shows the water environment type DAA (Infantes et al., 2007), with A corresponding to hydrogen bonding acceptor and D to hydrogen bonding donor. According to Morris and Rodriguez-Hornedo (Morris and Rodriguez-Hornedo, 1993; Brittain et al., 2009) the DDS hydrate can be classified as an isolated-site hydrate, which retains water in segregated pockets in the crystal structure. The strongest pair-wise water-DDS interaction was calculated to be −22.5 kJ mol^{-1}, which is distinctly weaker than the strongest pair-wise DDS-DDS interaction (−53.9 kJ mol^{-1}).

The presence of an isolated-site hydrate could be confirmed by calculating the total energy of the hydrate and lower hydrate structures thereof, i.e., structures which were generated by systematically removing water molecules from the packing presented in **Figure 3** (using the P1 cell). **Figure 4** shows that a plot of the energy contributions from the water molecules to the hydrate structure vs. the water content gives a linear relationship. This clearly indicates that the water molecule interacts solely with DDS molecules in the **0.33-Hy**, which is a characteristic feature of an isolated-site hydrate.

Temperature Dependent Stability of the Hydrate

Key information for handling and storing hydrates is knowledge about temperature- and moisture-dependent stability. The dehydration process of **0.33-Hy** was monitored with HSM (**Figure 5**), DSC and TGA (**Figure 6**). To investigate the impact of the atmospheric conditions on the dehydration behavior and associated processes, different experimental conditions were applied: dry and silicon oil preparations (HSM), heating of the sample in perforated or sealed DSC crucibles and using different heating rates. The obtained thermodynamic data are summarized in **Table 3**.

The dehydration of **0.33-Hy** occurs in the temperature range from 40 to 90°C. With HSM (dry preparation, **Figure 5**) hardly any change is observed during the dehydration process of the **0.33-Hy** to the isostructural dehydrate (**Hy**$_{dehy}$). However, with TGA and DSC the dehydration is well observable. Under N_2 purge (TGA) the dehydration process starts immediately and a mass loss of ~0.3 mol of water per mol DDS was determined. In DSC investigations (1a, 2a), the dehydration appears as a broad endothermic event which partly overlaps with a second endothermic process at a heating rate of 10°C min^{-1}. Using lower heating rates (not shown) the two thermal events can be separated and the heat of dehydration, $\Delta_{dehy}H_{Hy-dehy}$ of 10.60 kJ mol^{-1}(sample contained 0.18 mol water per mol DDS)

TABLE 2 | Pair-wise intermolecular interaction energies[a] (**Figure 3C**) of DDS **0.33-Hy**.

ID[b]	Mol[c]	Mol[c]	N[d]	Symmetry operation	d[e]	E_E	E_P	E_D	E_R	E_{tot}	Interaction
					Å	kJ mol^{-1}					
1	mol B	mol B	1	–	3.84	−16.0	−5.2	−76.1	53.7	−53.9	π···π
2	mol A	mol A	1	−x, −y, −z	8.37	−35.4	−6.6	−39.7	38.0	−53.3	
3	mol C	mol C	1	−x+1/2, −y+1/2, −z	5.72	−47.1	−15.7	−29.0	54.0	−53.3	4xC–H···O
4	mol A	mol A	1	−x, y, −z+1/2	3.58	−11.5	−5.4	−89.5	75.9	−47.2	π···π
5	mol A	mol C	1	–	8.83	−33.6	−9.6	−12.7	32.4	−33.7	N–H···O
6	mol C	mol C	2	−x+1/2, y+1/2, −z+1/2	8.31	−28.1	−7.9	−13.6	22.4	−33.5	N–H···O
7	mol A	mol A	1	–	9.03	−29.5	−8.4	−10.1	23.5	−31.7	N–H···O
8	mol B	mol B	2	x, −y, z+1/2	8.46	−28.7	−7.2	−10.4	21.5	−31.5	N–H···O
9	mol B	mol B	2	x, −y, z+1/2	8.84	−27.1	−10.1	−13.7	29.1	−30.1	N–H···O
10	mol B	mol A	1	–	6.58	−16.6	−6.4	−32.0	32.9	−29.9	
11	mol A	mol A	2	x, −y, z+1/2	9.53	−33.1	−10.8	−14.9	42.9	−29.6	N–H···O
12	mol A	mol A	2	x, −y, z+1/2	7.86	−15.4	−4.7	−19.4	20.6	−23.9	N–H···N
13	mol B	mol C	1	–	9.2	−12.2	−4.5	−16.3	10.7	−23.8	
14	mol C	water	1	–	7.08	−25.9	−6.2	−6.1	23.7	−22.5	N–H···O_W
15	mol B	water	1	–	6.62	−16.7	−2.9	−5.7	8.6	−19.5	N–H···O_W
16	mol C	mol C	1	−x+1/2, −y+1/2, −z	11.23	−9.4	−2.2	−11.0	2.8	−19.4	
17	mol C	water	1	–	5.25	−33.8	−7.2	−4.4	41.4	−19.2	O_W-H···O
18	mol B	mol C	1	–	10.37	−20.0	−5.1	−12.6	27.5	−18.9	N–H···N
19	mol C	mol C	2	x, −y, z+1/2	8.13	−6.5	−3.8	−9.3	3.9	−15.4	

[a]*Electrostatic (E_E), polarization (E_P), dispersion (E_D) and exchange-repulsion energy (E_R) contributions. $E_{tot} = k_E E_E + k_P E_P + k_D E_D + k_R E_R$, with k being scale factors (Mackenzie et al., 2017)* [b]*Interaction ID;* [c]*molecule according to* ***Figure 3A;*** [d]*N – number of times interaction is present.* [e]*Centroid distances.*

was determined. The known enthalpy value for the vaporization of water at the dehydration temperature ($T_{dehy} \approx 60°C$, $\Delta_{vap}H$ H_2O = 42.482 kJ mol^{-1} (Riddick and Bunger, 1986) can be subtracted from the measured heat of dehydration ($\Delta_{dehy}H$), according to Equation (1), resulting in an estimation of the heat change ($\Delta_{trs}H$) upon hydrate to anhydrate transformation. The enthalpy of this reaction was calculated to be 2.95 ± 0.09 kJ mol^{-1} (**Table 3**).

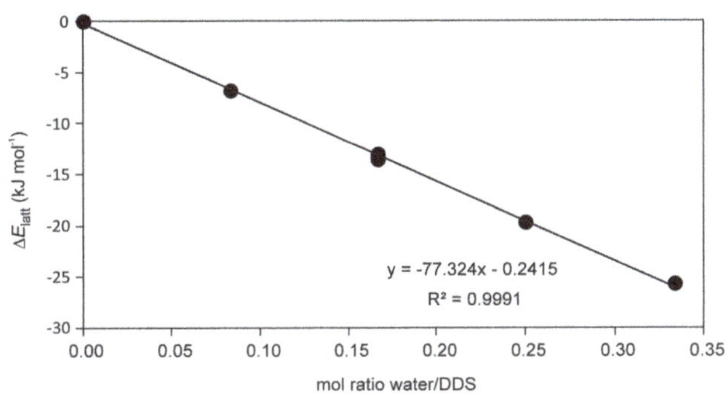

FIGURE 4 | Energetic contribution (ΔE_{latt}, see Supplementary Table 5) of the water to the DDS hydrate structure in dependency of water occupancy (mol ratio water/DDS) in **0.33-Hy**.

$$\Delta_{trs}H_{Hy-dehy} = \Delta_{dehy}H_{Hy-dehy} - 0.18 \cdot \Delta_{vap}H_{H2O} \quad (1)$$

The second endotherm of the DSC traces (perforated crucibles) with an onset temperature of 103.6°C corresponds to the solid-solid phase transformation of **Hy**$_{dehy}$ to form **II** (1.08 kJ mol^{-1}). In HSM investigations an increase in birefringence is observable during the transformation process. Upon further heating, form **II** melts at 177.2°C (1a) and concomitantly form **I** crystalizes, which then melts at 179°C. Upon cooling the melt of DDS (1b) spontaneous crystallization of form **II** occurs around 110°C. The presence of form **II** is confirmed by the occurrence of the exothermic event at 75°C (cooling curve), indicating the transformation of form **II** to form **III**. The measured enthalpy value of −2.02 kJ mol^{-1} agrees with the enthalpy value of the transformation **III** → **II** (2.06 kJ mol^{-1}), which can be determined on reheating. A more detailed study of this transformation has been reported just recently by us (Braun et al., 2017). In a separate experiment, the DSC heating run of **0.33-Hy** was stopped above the **Hy**$_{dehy}$ → **II** transition peak (2a) and the subsequent cooling curve shows the exothermic **II** → **III** transition (2b). The temperature range and enthalpy of this spontaneous transition confirm unambiguously that mainly form **II** is present after the hydrate is heated to about 150°C. Form **III** transforms back to form **II** at 81°C (1c and 2c) just about 6°C

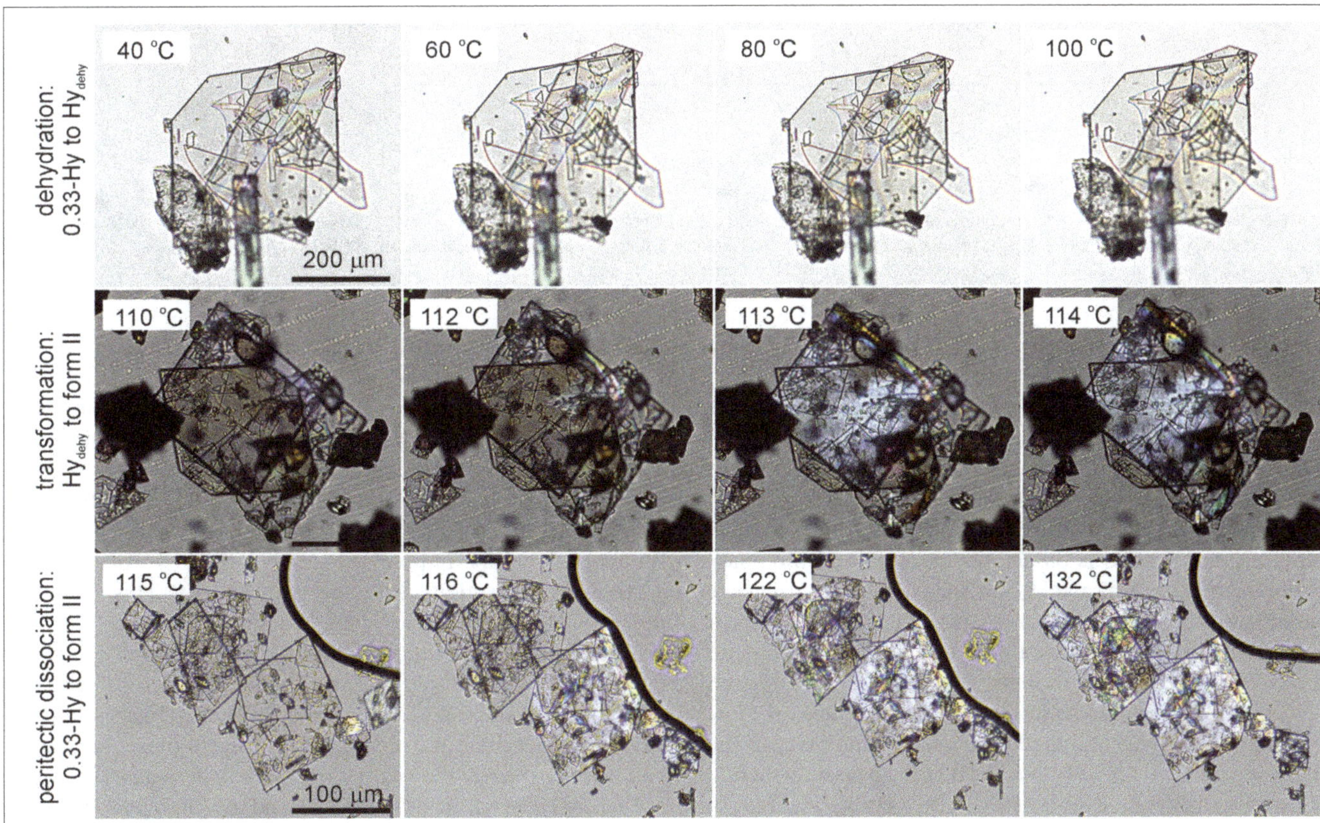

FIGURE 5 | Photomicrographs of DDS **0.33-Hy**. Dehydration in the temperature range 40°-100°C, **Hy**$_{dehy}$ to form **II** transformation in the temperature range 110°-114°C, and peritectic dissociation (crystals embedded in high-viscosity silicon oil) of **0.33-Hy** to form **II** in the temperature range 115°−132°C.

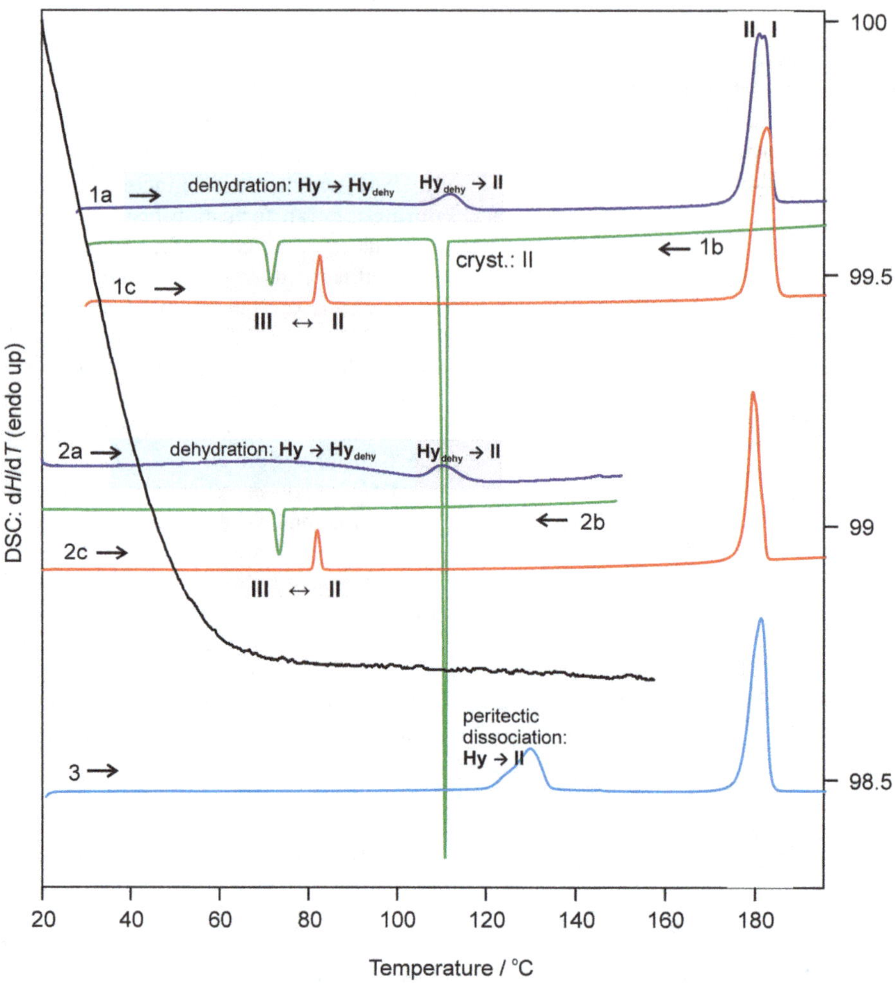

FIGURE 6 | Selected DSC and TGA thermograms of DDS **0.33-Hy**, recorded using a heating/cooling rate of 10°C min^{-1}. DSC curves 1 and 2 were measured using perforated DSC crucibles and curve 3 using a hermetically sealed 3bar DSC crucible. I, II, III-anhydrous forms **I**, **II**, and **III**; Hy, **0.33-Hy**; dehy, $\mathbf{Hy}_{dehy}$.

above the **II** → **III** transition peak highlighting the weak kinetic control of this reversible solid-solid transformation.

By embedding the hydrate crystals into high viscosity silicon oil (HSM, **Figure 5**) or using hermetically sealed DSC crucibles (3, **Figure 6**) the peritectic dissociation process of **0.33-Hy** to form **II** can be observed or recorded around 125°C, respectively. A fast nucleation and growth process of form **II** occurs, thus no clear melting process is observable by HSM and the phase transition is mainly indicated by an increase in birefringence (**Figure 5**). The measured heat of ~5 kJ mol^{-1} can be related to the **0.33-Hy** to form **II** transformation, but also includes an unknown contribution from the enthalpy of solution of a fraction of the dehydration product in the liberated water. Due to the low water solubility of DDS and the low water stoichiometry of the hydrate the measured **0.33-Hy** to form **II** enthalpy is only slightly higher than the sum of the heats of **0.33-Hy** to $\mathbf{Hy}_{dehy}$ and $\mathbf{Hy}_{dehy}$ to form **II** transformations of ~4 kJ mol^{-1}. Thus for DDS, it is possible to estimate the **0.33-Hy** to form **II** transition enthalpy directly in a hermetically sealed DSC crucible.

Moisture Dependent Stability of the Hydrate

The moisture sorption/desorption experiments of **0.33-Hy** (**Figure 7**) clearly indicate a non-stoichiometric hydration/dehydration behavior. The isotherm shows a continuous course and the water content of the hydrate adjusts quickly to a specific value if the RH is altered. It is particularly striking that the sorption and desorption isotherms are superimposable, i.e., that there is no hysteresis between the sorption and desorption curve. This fact and the short time to reach the equilibrium water content on changing RH suggests that the diffusion of water molecules into or out of the structure occurs without special constraints and without significant changes of the DDS framework. This observation is even more surprising because the water molecules are located at isolated-sites in the **0.33-Hy** structure (**Figure 3A**) and not in open structure voids (channels, layers), which is the commonly expected feature for hydrates with a non-stoichiometric dehydration behavior.

TABLE 3 | Thermochemical data of DDS solid forms (T, temperature; ΔH, enthalpy) obtained starting from the hydrate (**Hy: 0.33** mol water/mol DDS) compared with the CE-B3LYP energy estimation.

Process	DSC		CE-B3LYP
	T/°C	ΔH/kJ mol^{-1}	kJ mol^{-1}
DEHYDRATION			
Hy[a] → Hy_{dehy}	40–90	10.60 ± 0.10	
Hy → Hy_{dehy}		16.95 ± 0.13[b]	
Contribution of water to Hy structure			13.85
TRANSFORMATION			
Hy → Hy_{dehy}	40–90	2.95 ± 0.09	2.98[c]
Hy_{dehy} → II	103.6 ± 2.8	1.08 ± 0.05	
II → III	75.2 ± <0.1	−2.02 ± 0.08	
III → II	81.5 ± 0.2	2.06 ± 0.07	
PERITECTIC DISSOCIATION			
Hy → II	126.5 ± 0.5	4.98 ± 0.53	

[a] *Referred to a hydrate with 0.18 mol water/mol DDS.*
[b] *Estimated form 0.18-Hy.*
[c] *13.85 kJ mol^{-1}–10.87 kJ mol^{-1}.*

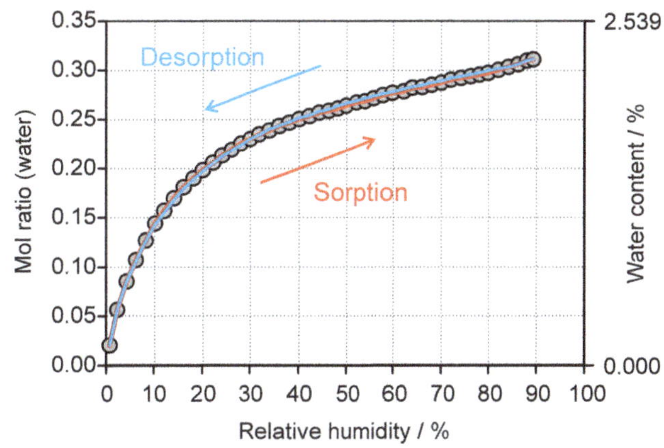

FIGURE 7 | Gravimetric moisture sorption/desorption isotherms of DDS **0.33-Hy** at 25°C. Circles represent data points recorded at equilibrium conditions (see experimental section).

The automated gravimetric moisture sorption/desorption analysis of **0.33-Hy** was complemented with longer-term drying experiments at 0% RH (storage over P_2O_5) at 25°, 50°, and 75°C to investigate whether $\mathbf{Hy_{dehy}}$ transforms to another DDS anhydrate polymorph. $\mathbf{Hy_{dehy}}$ is stable for at least 3 weeks at 25°C and for at least 10 days at 50°C. At 75°C the transformation to form **III** starts within 1 week at 0%. No new polymorph emerged in the drying studies.

The changes seen in the gravimetric moisture sorption/desorption studies (**Figure 7**) were correlated with structural changes to **0.33-Hy** using variable-humidity PXRD at 25°C (**Figure 8**, Supplementary Material for the PXRD patterns). In the case of the DDS hydrate only slight changes in peak positions and peak intensities can be observed with varying RH. Changes in lattice parameters were quantified by indexation and Rietveld refinement of the **0.33-Hy** PXRD patterns recorded at different RH values. The lattice parameters changed by max. 0.2% in the range 90% to 1%, and the cell volume by only 0.66%. Such small changes are in the range one would expect from a non-stoichiometric hydrate and they are for example of similar magnitude as measured for the non-stoichiometric hydrate HyA of brucine (Braun and Griesser, 2016a). Plotting the **0.33-Hy** cell volume in dependence of the RH (**Figure 8A**) perfectly reproduces the course of the sorption/desorption isotherms in **Figure 7**.

Using the optimized (PBE-TS) experimental structure as starting model, Rietveld refinements were performed with PXRD patterns of samples recorded in 10% RH steps during a desorption and sorption cycle. The aim of this study was to unravel whether the water position in the **0.33-Hy** varies depending on the RH conditions. **Figure 8C** exemplarily shows an overlay of the hydrate structures at 90 and 1% RH. The DDS molecules are superimposable and also the water shows hardly any positional variation with RH. The structures solved at different RH values differ solely in the fractional occupancy factor to which the water molecule refined to (**Figure 8B**). It is surprising that this method works so well even though the water is only a very minor contributor to the overall electron density of the hydrate structure. The lowest water content observed for **0.33-Hy** in the RH dependent PXRD experiments was 0.005(12) mol of water per three moles of DDS, which is in reasonable agreement with the value determined in the automatic gravimetric sorption/desorption measurements (0.02 mol water per mol DDS) determined at the same RH. No phase change was observed in the moisture dependent PXRD experiments.

The question remains why the water egress/ingress in the **0.33-Hy** is fast, which is not expected from a hydrate where the water molecules are located at isolated-sites. **Figure 9A** illustrates a possible escape route of water molecules parallel to [011]. However, this route requires cooperative movement of the diaminophenyl moieties of the DDS molecules to temporarily open up diffusion pathways, similar to that seen in hydrates of β-cyclodextrin (β-CD) (Steiner and Koellner, 1994), ciprofloxacin (Mafra et al., 2012) or DB7 (Braun et al., 2015). The potential energy surface scans of DDS reveal (**Figure 9B**) that considerable movement of the diaminophenyl moieties is possible with low energy cost (ΔE_{intra}), which we assume enables the local formation of the required diffusion pathways.

Sorption/desorption studies based on exposure of the solid material to various moisture conditions are controlled by kinetic parameters, which must be minimized in order to assess the thermodynamic equilibrium between the hydrate and a dehydrated state. This can be achieved for example by slurring the substance in solvents with different water activities, as has been demonstrated in previous studies (Ahlqvist and Taylor, 2002a,b; Braun et al., 2013; Braun and Griesser, 2016a). The most obvious indicator for the kinetic barrier is the hysteresis between the sorption and desorption curve observed in moisture sorption/desorption isotherms. The hysteresis can be extreme in stoichiometric hydrates and is usually small in hydrates with non-stoichiometric behavior. The isotherm of DDS **0.33-Hy** shows no hysteresis indicating that there is practically no kinetic barrier

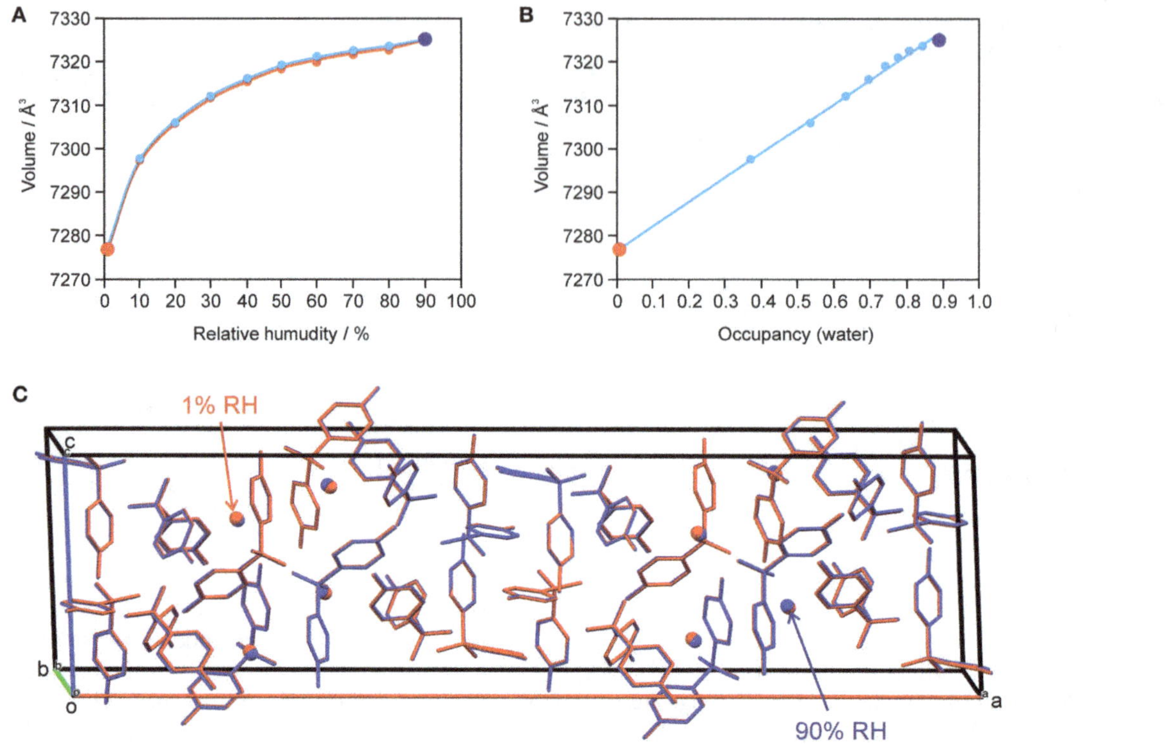

FIGURE 8 | Data derived from moisture-dependent PXRD measurements and Rietveld refinement showing **(A)** the change in cell volume with RH und **(B)** factional occupancy factor of the water molecule vs. cell volume in **0.33-Hy**. In **(C)** an overlay of the hydrate at 90% (in blue) and 1% RH (red) is shown. H-atoms are omitted for clarity.

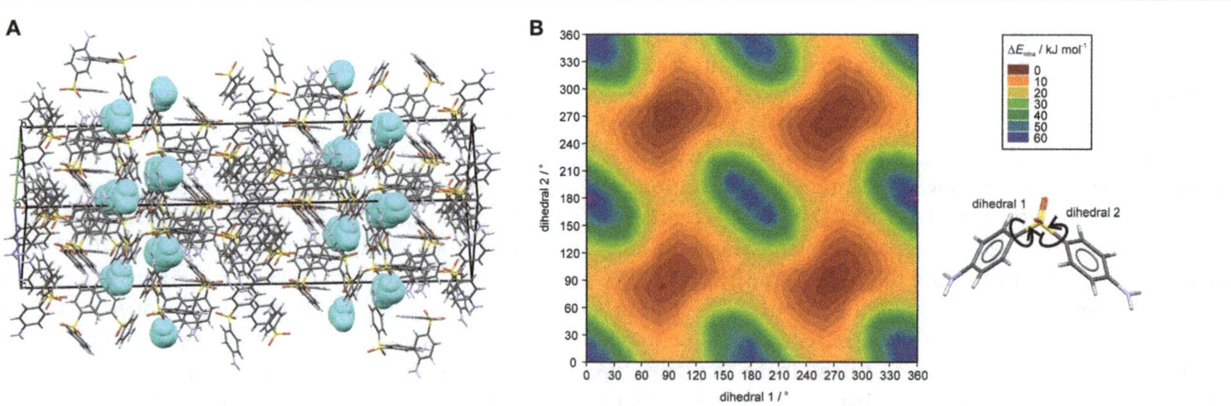

FIGURE 9 | (A) DDS **0.33-Hy** structure (ANSFON02, Yathirajan et al., 2014), with water molecules depicted as space-fill in turquois, showing a possible water egress/ingress route parallel to [011]. **(B)** Two dimensional potential energy surface scan for DDS with respect to dihedrals 1 and 2 at the B3LYP level of theory with the 6-31G(d,p) basis set using the optimized DDS conformation.

between the ingress or release processes of the water molecules to/from the crystal structure but also that the phase is maintained and no transformation to another form with different structural features occurs. To test the phase behavior under different "moisture conditions" (water activities) in solvent systems, we subjected DDS to a slurry study in methanol/water mixtures of various compositions, covering the water activity (a_W) range from 0 to 1.0 (corresponding to 0 to 100% RH) in 0.01 steps and the range 0.6 to 0.7 in 0.001 steps using form **III** as the starting form (**Figure 10**). Surprisingly, we obtained a new anhydrous form, named form **V** hereafter, which emerged as the only stable solid phase below a water activity of 0.64. At an $a_W > 0.66$, **0.33-Hy** was obtained, suggesting that this hydrate is the stable form at high water activities and that the equilibrium between the DDS form **V** and the **0.33-Hy**, lies at an a_W value of ~0.655 at 25°C.

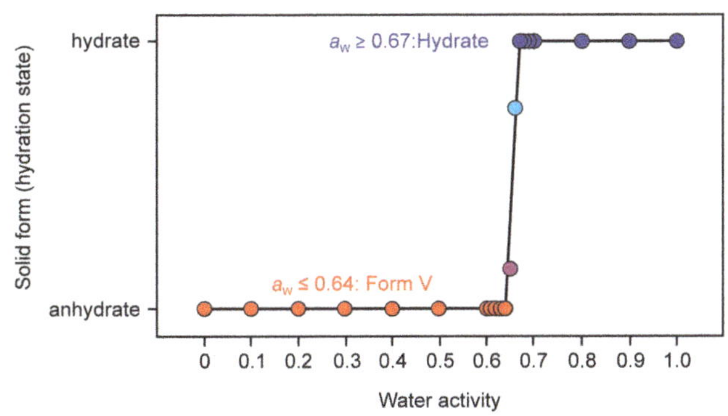

FIGURE 10 | Phase diagram after equilibration for 21 days showing the stability ranges of solid phases of DDS (**form V** and the **0.33-Hy**) as a function of water activity in methanol/water mixtures at 25°C. Anhydrous form **III** was used as a starting phase; the phase identity and composition was determined with PXRD.

Thermal analysis and PXRD characterization confirmed that the new form **V** does not correspond to any of the four known polymorphs (Brandstaetter-Kuhnert et al., 1963; Kuhnert-Brandstatter and Moser, 1979). A thorough characterization of the new form, which is obviously the thermodynamically most stable anhydrate form at RT, and phase interrelations to the known polymorphs will be addressed elsewhere.

Estimation of Host-Host, Host-Water, and Water-Water Interaction Energies in Organic Hydrates

To understand the nature and stability of a hydrate it is important to consider the location and interaction energies of the water molecules in the framework of the host structure. If water molecules are located in open structural voids (tunnels or connected pockets) the term channel hydrate (Brittain et al., 2009) is commonly used. In such hydrates the water molecules may be mobile and may readily escape through these tunnels on modest increase in temperature or decrease in relative humidity (RH). In contrast, if the water molecules are located at isolated-sites (Brittain et al., 2009), it is assumed that water egress is not as facile and requires a considerable rearrangement of the hydrate packing to allow the release of water molecules. This rearrangement results mostly in the formation of a different packing arrangement or in a partial or total collapse of the structure yielding a disordered or amorphous state upon dehydration. The non-stoichiometric behavior of hydrates, where the water content in the structure depends on the water vapor pressure of the surrounding medium (atmosphere), is normally observed in channel hydrates and not in isolated-site hydrates. However, as demonstrated above, DDS **0.33-Hy** shows clearly the typical features of an isolated-site hydrate (**Figure 3A**) but on the other hand shows a non-stoichiometric (de)hydration behavior (see **Figure 7**) which is a contradiction and questions the common relation between structural features and the stability of hydrates.

To further clarify why the hydrate water can escape easily from the "isolated sites" in the **0.33-Hy**, without disrupting the structure, we estimated the pair-wise interaction energies for DDS and water molecules in the **0.33-Hy** structure (**Table 2**). The use of the CE-B3LYP energies and not a specific water potential, not considering specific effects (nanoscale dielectric responses of water) and three-body energy terms were justified by the fact that the contribution of the water to **0.33-Hy** was found to be in reasonable agreement with the experiment (**Table 3**). The water interactions contribute -13.85 kJ mol^{-1} to the **0.33-Hy** lattice. The CE-B3LYP energies of **0.33-Hy** (-142.87 kJ mol^{-1}) and **Hy**$_{dehy}$ (-132.00 kJ mol^{-1}, optimized RT structures) differ by 10.87 kJ mol^{-1}, ignoring the conformational changes which are expected to account for $<$ 0.2 kJ mol^{-1} in the case of DDS. Thus, the sum of the interaction energies ($E_{cluster}$) roughly corresponds to the lattice energy. Furthermore, we calculated the intermolecular energies for water-host, water-water and host-host molecules for a series of well characterized organic hydrate systems (pharmaceuticals and model compounds) and contrasted the values to the DDS **0.33-Hy** (**Figure 11**, Supplementary Material). The chosen test set consists of stoichiometric and non-stoichiometric hydrates, as well as of channel and isolated-site hydrates. This analysis should indicate, whether it is possible to assess hydrate stability and/or the dehydration mechanism from general features of the hydrate structure and not the location of the water molecules in the structure alone.

In **Figure 11** the calculated interaction energies are grouped into contributions arising from host-host interactions and the incteractions including water molecules (host-water and water-water). Furthermore, the ratio between the host-host and water interactions has been calculated. The hydrates are ranked according to the compound:water ratio. For three of the chosen hydrates (dapsone, indinavir, and brucine) it is possible to remove the water molecules under maintaining the crystal structure, which is characteristic for a non-stoichiometric dehydration behavior. A grouping into channel and isolated-site hydrates is not always straight forward, in particular if more than one water molecule is present (di-, tri-hydrate, etc.,). However, based on the energetic contributions, host-water vs. water-water, such a classification is facilitated as it can be expected that in isolated-site hydrates the host-water and in channel hydrates the water-water interactions predominate, respectively. Furthermore, the sum of host-host interactions are stronger in isolated-site hydrates than in channel hydrates.

A requirement for maintaining the crystal lattice upon dehydration is that the hydrate structure exhibits strong and/or a predominance of host-host interactions. Indeed, the three non-stoichiometric hydrates of the test set show the highest percentage of host-host interactions, i.e., ~90% of the interaction energies for the DDS and indinavir hydrates. This value is lower for brucine (61.5%) but compared to dihydrates showing a stoichiometric behavior, brucine exhibits the most/strongest host-host interactions. The fact that the DDS and indinavir hydrates are isolated-site hydrates and brucine is a channel hydrate highlights that it is not possible to deduce whether a stoichiometic or non-stoichiometric dehydration mechanism

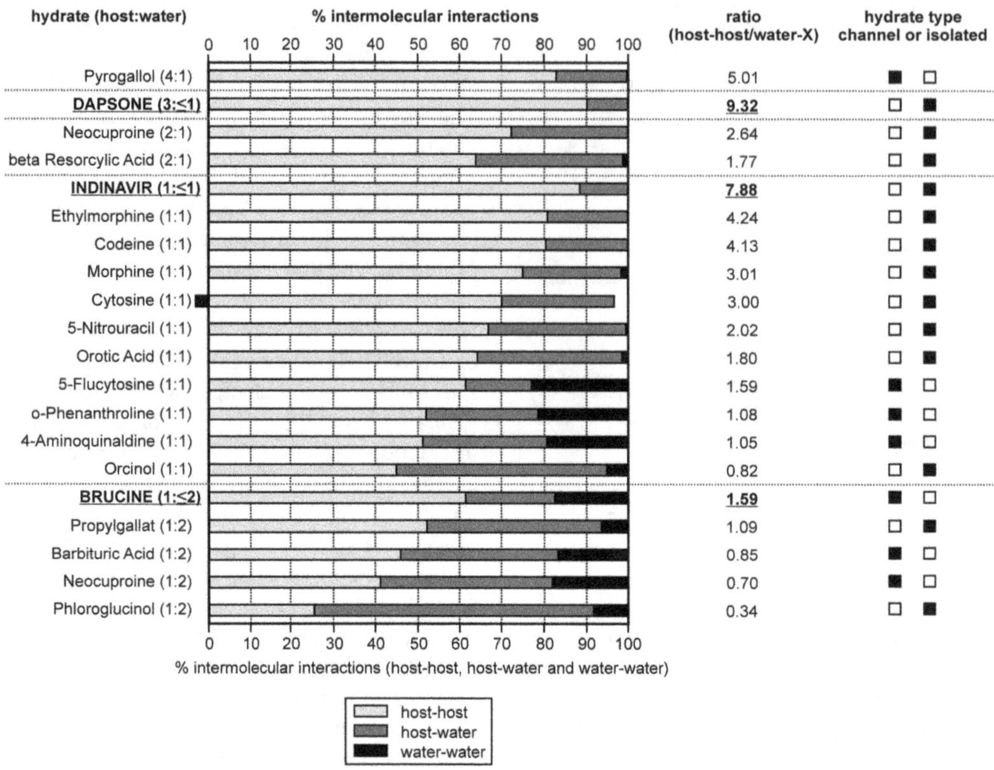

FIGURE 11 | Overall contribution of intermolecular interactions in hydrate structures grouped into host-host, host-water and water-water interactions. The hydrates are ranked according to their compound:water ratio and non-stoichiometric hydrates are indicated in bold and are underlined. The ratio given was calculated as: [(host-host interactions)/(host-water and water-water interactions)].

occurs from the location of the water molecules in the hydrate structure alone. Though, it is possible to rationalize a non-stoichiometric dehydration behavior from the energy contributions of the intermolecular interactions considering the compound:water ratios. On the other hand, the analysis shows that the moisture- or temperature dependent stability of hydrates cannot be derived from the interaction energy calculations. For example, the 5-flucytosine monohydrate (I) already dehydrates at RH values < 40%, whereas 4-aminoquinaldine monohydrate (Hy1A) dehydrates only at RH values below 10% (RT), but exhibits less energetic contributions from the host-host interactions than the 5-flucytosine monohydrate (I).

In the case of **0.33-Hy** the latter analysis (**Figure 10**) strongly indicates that water is only weakly bound and rationalizes the facile moisture- and temperature dependent dehydration behavior.

DISCUSSION

Molecular Level Understanding of the Dehydration Mechanism Derived from the Hydrate Structure

Knowledge of how water vapor is sorbed by a hygroscopic material and how moisture affects the physical and chemical stability of a (pharmaceutical) product is a crucial question in developing drug products or preparations produced from other fine chemicals. Failures and time delays in product developments can be minimized or avoided with knowledge compiled in thorough solid state investigations. Hydrates require a thorough evaluation of their composition and stability under production relevant conditions and additionally the transformation pathways between different solid state forms of a compound, as well as their stability ranges, should be elucidated. This is mandatory to select the ideal solid state form that guarantees an optimal product performance and stability. In general, non-stoichiometric hydrates are undesired solid forms because any change in water vapor pressure of the surrounding medium causes a change in the water content of the substance, which can be critical for weighing and dosing operations and may thus lead to errors in any analyses, which require exact sample amounts. Such variations in the water content are often difficult to avoid as it requires special efforts to precisely control temperature and humidity conditions during processing and storage. Furthermore, the water molecules which have been released from such a hydrate may interact with other excipients in a drug formulation. Gravimetric moisture sorption/desorption studies (**Figure 7**), combined with environmental PXRD experiments (Supplementary Material) are the preferred analytical techniques for unraveling this non-stoichiometric behavior of a hydrate.

DDS **0.33-Hy** is a prime example for an isolated site hydrate with non-stoichiometric dehydration behavior. The latter behavior may be expected for hydrates where the water is located in open voids such as channels or layers. Thus, this study highlights that the popular structural classification of hydrates into isolated-site hydrates (water molecules are isolated from direct contact), channel hydrates (chains of water molecules) and ion-associated hydrates (metal ions are coordinated with water) cannot be directly related to the dehydration behavior or dehydration mechanism of a hydrate. However, by complementing the structural features with intermolecular energy calculations the observed dehydration behavior can be rationalized. As shown for DDS **0.33-Hy** the water molecules are only weakly bound (**Figure 11**), allowing a facile water egress/ingress with changing environmental conditions. Furthermore, the energy difference between the isomorphic dehydrate structure and anhydrate polymorphs is small. The lattice energy difference between $\mathbf{Hy}_{dehy}$ and form **II** was calculated as 1.6 kJ mol^{-1} (PBE-TS, at −273°C) and the transition enthalpy between $\mathbf{Hy}_{dehy}$ and form **II** determined to be 1.08 ± 0.05 kJ mol^{-1} (experimentally measured at ~100°C). Thus, the calculations rationalize and indicate the non-stoichiometric dehydration mechanism.

Computational Modeling of Pharmaceutical Hydrates

Modeling and predicting hydrate structures of pharmaceuticals still represent a big challenge in computational chemistry. Numerous potentials have been developed for modeling water (Guillot, 2002), however, there exists no method that can sufficiently model all its abnormalities. In organic hydrates the water molecules may be described as confined at nanoscales, implying frustration in their hydrogen-bonding coordination. Consequently, accurately modeling the water molecules in a hydrate lattice requires modeling efforts which go well beyond the methods applied for modeling the organic solid state (Reilly et al., 2016). In lead optimization is has been demonstrated that incorporating the three-body energy terms, and modeling frustration and frustration-related dielectric responses, significantly improves the results (Fernández, 2016, 2017; Fernandez and Scott, 2017). Considering and modeling the latter can be expected to significantly increase the accuracy of lattice and intermolecular energy calculations of water containing species, albeit at the expense of computational cost.

A major difficulty with using CSP in hydrate solid form screening is the computational expense in time and resources to generate the crystal energy landscape for all possible hydrate stoichiometries (mono-, di-, etc.,). However, solid form modeling at the electronic and atomistic level can provide vital support for unraveling the solid state for a compound which may not be achieved with experiments alone. A CSP study answers the question what types of crystal packings are favorable for a specific molecule, unraveling the compromises between close packing efficiency, conformational preferences and the different types of intermolecular interactions that can lead to feasible structures for a molecule (polymorph) or multi-component system (salt, solvate, hydrate, co-crystal). It should be stressed that CSP aids the interpretation of the experimental data (Price et al., 2014) and can guide experimentalists to find new solid forms (Arlin et al., 2011; Braun et al., 2014b, 2016; Neumann et al., 2015; Srirambhatla et al., 2016).

To significantly reduce the computational cost, and to make the calculations feasible, we did not attempt to computationally screen for different hydrate stoichiometries (Braun et al., 2011b) for the chosen model compound DDS, but used the crystal energy landscape of the 1:1 stoichiometry (monohydrate) as a guidance for hydrate formation. The monohydrate crystal energy landscape (**Figure 2**) shows only one hydrate structure that is more stable than the non-solvated form **III** and thus indicates hydrate formation.

CONCLUSIONS

4,4′-Diaminodiphenyl sulfone (DDS) forms a non-stoichiometric hydrate, with a water content of 0–0.33 mol of water per mol of DDS. The upper limit of this ratio is obvious from the features of the crystal structure, but it is surprising that the structurally isolated and hydrogen bonded water molecules can easily leave and enter the structure, which is indicated by the continuous change in water content when the hydrate is exposed to different RH values. This observation highlights that it is not advisable to make assumptions about the dehydration behavior based on the location of the water molecules in the structure alone. However, supported by intermolecular energy interaction calculations (host-host, water-host and water-water) and by comparing the lattice energies of the isomorphic dehydrate (hydrate without water) and anhydrate polymorph(s) of the same compound it is possible to rationalize and to potentially predict a non-stoichiometric dehydration behavior. Furthermore, this study shows that even though CSP has been performed with only one hydrate stoichiometry (here monohydrate) the outcome may be sufficient to get insight into the hydrate formation potential of a compound. However, such a limited approach requires a thorough analysis of the computed structures.

In our opinion, a sound understanding of hydrates and their often complex behavior can only be achieved by a full multidisciplinary investigation, including structural, moisture- and temperature dependent studies combined with modeling. Such an understanding may be mandatory to avoid complications during processing, storing and handling of a hydrate.

AUTHOR CONTRIBUTIONS

DB conceived and designed the research and headed, wrote and revised the manuscript, while UG contributed to the writing and the revision of the article.

FUNDING

DB gratefully acknowledges funding by the Elise Richter program of the Austrian Science Fund (FWF, project V436-N34). The computational results presented have been achieved using the HPC infrastructure LEO of the University of Innsbruck.

ACKNOWLEDGMENTS

The authors are grateful to Profs. C. C. Pantelides and C. S. Adjiman (Imperial College London) for the use of the CrystalPredictor and CrystalOptimizer programs, Prof. S. L. Price (University College London) for the use of the DMACRYS program and Elisabeth Achammer for support in few of the calculations.

REFERENCES

Abascal, J. L. F., Sanz, E., Fernandez, R. G., and Vega, C. (2005). A potential for the study of ices and amorphous water: TIP4P/ice. *J. Chem. Phys.* 122:234511. doi: 10.1063/1.1931662

Ahlqvist, M. U. A., and Taylor, L. S. (2002a). Water diffusion in hydrated crystalline and amorphous sugars monitored using H/D exchange. *J. Pharm. Sci.* 91, 690–698. doi: 10.1002/jps.10068

Ahlqvist, M. U. A., and Taylor, L. S. (2002b). Water dynamics in channel hydrates investigated using H/D exchange. *Int. J. Pharm.* 241, 253–261. doi: 10.1016/S0378-5173(02)00242-9

Arlin, J. B., Price, L. S., Price, S. L., and Florence, A. J. (2011). A strategy for producing predicted polymorphs: catemeric carbamazepine form V. *Chem. Commun.* 47, 7074–7076. doi: 10.1039/c1cc11634g

Babashkina, M. G., Safin, D. A., Robeyns, K., Brzuszkiewicz, A., Kozlowski, H., and Garcia, Y. (2012). Thiophosphorylated bis-thioureas for competitive bulk liquid membrane transport of some metal ions. *CrystEngComm* 14, 1324–1329. doi: 10.1039/C1CE06244A

Baias, M., Dumez, J. N., Svensson, P. H., Schantz, S., Day, G. M., and Emsley, L. (2013). *De novo* determination of the crystal structure of a large drug molecule by crystal structure prediction-based powder NMR crystallography. *J. Am. Chem. Soc.* 135, 17501–17507. doi: 10.1021/ja4088874

Bel'skii, V. K., Chernikova, N. Y., Rotaru, V. K., and Kruchinin, M. M. (1983). Crystal and molecular structure of components of epoxy resins. II. 4,4′-diaminodiphenyl sulfone hydrate. *Kristallografiya* 28, 690–694.

Beran, G. J. O., and Nanda, K. (2010). Predicting organic crystal lattice energies with chemical accuracy. *J. Phys. Chem. Lett.* 1, 3480–3487. doi: 10.1021/jz101383z

Bernstein, J. (2002). *Polymorphism in Molecular Crystals*. Oxford: Clarendon Press.

Bertolasi, V., Ferretti, V., Gilli, P., and De Benedetti, P. G. (1993). Molecular structure and crystal packing of five 4-aminophenyl (4-substituted phenyl) sulfones. Correlations between structural distortions, spectroscopic parameters and electronic substituent effects. *J. Chem. Soc. Perkin Trans.* 2, 213–219. doi: 10.1039/p29930000213

Bhardwaj, R. M., Price, L. S., Price, S. L., Reutzel-Edens, S. M., Miller, G. J., Oswald, I. D. H., et al. (2013). Exploring the experimental and computed crystal energy landscape of olanzapine. *Cryst. Growth Des.* 13, 1602–1617. doi: 10.1021/cg301826s

Bocelli, G., and Cantoni, A. (1990). Stereochemical studies of oligomers. XXVII. reinvestigation of the structure of 4,4'-diaminodiphenyl sulfone. *Acta Crystallogr. Sect. C Cryst. Struct. Commun.* C46, 2257–2259. doi: 10.1107/S0108270190004991

Brandstaetter-Kuhnert, M., Kofler, A., and Hoffmann, R. (1963). Microscopic characterization and identification of pharmaceuticals. IV. *Sci. Pharm.* 31, 140–148.

Braun, D. E. (2008). *Crystal Polymorphism of Drug Compounds: Statistical Aspects, Analytical Strategies and Case Studies*. Ph.D. Thesis, University of Innsbruck.

Braun, D. E., Ardid-Candel, M., D'oria, E., Karamertzanis, P. G., Arlin, J. B., Florence, A. J., et al. (2011a). Racemic naproxen: a multidisciplinary structural and thermodynamic comparison with the enantiopure form. *Cryst. Growth Des.* 11, 5659–5669. doi: 10.1021/cg201203u

Braun, D. E., Bhardwaj, R. M., Arlin, J. B., Florence, A. J., Kahlenberg, V., Griesser, U. J., et al. (2013). Absorbing a little water: the structural, thermodynamic, and kinetic relationship between pyrogallol and its tetarto-hydrate. *Cryst. Growth Des.* 13, 4071–4083. doi: 10.1021/cg4009015

Braun, D. E., and Griesser, U. J. (2016a). Stoichiometric and non-stoichiometric hydration of brucine. *Cryst. Growth Des.* 16, 6111–6121. doi: 10.1021/acs.cgd.6b01231

Braun, D. E., and Griesser, U. J. (2016b). Why do hydrates (solvates) form in small neutral organic molecules? Exploring the crystal form landscapes of the alkaloids brucine and strychnine. *Cryst. Growth Des.* 16, 6405–6418. doi: 10.1021/acs.cgd.6b01078

Braun, D. E., Karamertzanis, P. G., and Price, S. L. (2011b). Which, if any, hydrates will crystallise? Predicting hydrate formation of two dihydroxybenzoic acids. *Chem. Commun.* 47, 5443–5445. doi: 10.1039/c1cc10762c

Braun, D. E., Koztecki, L. H., McMahon, J. A., Price, S. L., and Reutzel-Edens, S. M. (2015). Navigating the waters of unconventional crystalline hydrates. *Mol. Pharm.* 12, 3069–3088. doi: 10.1021/acs.molpharmaceut.5b00357

Braun, D. E., Krueger, H., Kahlenberg, V., and Griesser, U. J. (2017). Molecular level understanding of the reversible phase transformation between forms, III. and II of dapsone. *Cryst. Growth Des.* 17, 5054–5060. doi: 10.1021/acs.cgd.7b01089

Braun, D. E., McMahon, J. A., Koztecki, L. H., Price, S. L., and Reutzel-Edens, S. M. (2014a). Contrasting polymorphism of related small molecule drugs correlated and guided by the computed crystal energy landscape. *Cryst. Growth Des.* 14, 2056–2072. doi: 10.1021/cg500185h

Braun, D. E., Oberacher, H., Arnhard, K., Orlova, M., and Griesser, U. J. (2016). 4-Aminoquinaldine monohydrate polymorphism: prediction and impurity aided discovery of a difficult to access stable form. *CrystEngComm* 18, 4053–4067. doi: 10.1039/C5CE01758K

Braun, D. E., Orlova, M., and Griesser, U. J. (2014b). Creatine: polymorphs predicted and found. *Cryst. Growth Des.* 14, 4895–4900. doi: 10.1021/cg501159c

Breneman, C. M., and Wiberg, K. B. (1990). Determining atom-centered monopoles from molecular electrostatic potentials - the need for high sampling density in formamide conformational-analysis. *J. Comput. Chem.* 11, 361–373. doi: 10.1002/jcc.540110311

Brittain, H. G. (2009). *Polymorphism in Pharmaceutical Solids*. New York, NY; London: Informa Healthcare.

Brittain, H. G., Morris, K. R., and Boerrigter, S. X. M. (2009). "Structural aspects of solvatomorphic systems," in *Polymorphism in Pharmaceutical Solids, 2nd Edn.*, ed H. G. Brittain (New York, NY; London: Informa Healthcare), 233–281.

Byrn, S. R. (2004). *Presented at the International School of Crystallography*. Erice: Presented at the International School of Crystallography.

Byrn, S. R., Pfeiffer, R. R., and Stowell, J. G. (1999). *Solid-State Chemistry of Drugs*. West Lafayette, IN: SSCI, Inc.

Campeta, A. M., Chekal, B. P., Abramov, Y. A., Meenan, P. A., Henson, M. J., Shi, B., et al. (2010). Development of a targeted polymorph screening approach for a complex polymorphic and highly solvating API. *J. Pharm. Sci.* 99, 3874–3886. doi: 10.1002/jps.22230

Chemburkar, S. R., Bauer, J., Deming, K., Spiwek, H., Patel, K., Morris, J., et al. (2000). Dealing with the impact of ritonavir polymorphs on the late stages of bulk drug process development. *Org. Process Res. Dev.* 4, 413–417. doi: 10.1021/op000023y

Clark, S. J., Segall, M. D., Pickard, C. J., Hasnip, P. J., Probert, M. J., Refson, K., et al. (2005). First principles methods using CASTEP. *Zeitschrift fur Kristallographie* 220, 567–570. doi: 10.1524/zkri.220.5.567.65075

Coelho, A. A. (2012). *Topas Academic V5*. Brisbane, QLD: Coelho Software.

Coombes, D. S., Price, S. L., Willock, D. J., and Leslie, M. (1996). Role of electrostatic interactions in determining the crystal structures of polar organic molecules. A distributed multipole study. *J. Phys. Chem.* 100, 7352–7360. doi: 10.1021/jp960333b

Cruz-Cabeza, A. J., Day, G. M., and Jones, W. (2008). Towards prediction of stoichiometry in crystalline multicomponent complexes. *Chem. Eur. J.* 14, 8830–8836. doi: 10.1002/chem.200800668

Cruz-Cabeza Aurora, J., Reutzel-Edens Susan, M., and Bernstein, J. (2015). Facts and fictions about polymorphism. *Chem. Soc. Rev.* 44, 8619–8635. doi: 10.1039/C5CS00227C

David, W. I. F., Shankland, K., Van De Streek, J., Pidcock, E., Motherwell, W. D. S., and Cole, J. C. (2006). DASH: a program for crystal structure determination from powder diffraction data. *J. Appl. Crystallogr.* 39, 910–915. doi: 10.1107/S0021889806042117

Day, G. M., Cooper, T. G., Cruz-Cabeza, A. J., Hejczyk, K. E., Ammon, H. L., Boerrigter, S. X. M., et al. (2009). Significant progress in predicting the crystal structures of small organic molecules - a report on the fourth blind test. *Acta Crystallogr. B Struct. Sci.* 65, 107–125. doi: 10.1107/S0108768109004066

Deo, N., Tiwari, R. K., and Singh, T. P. (1980). Crystallization and x-ray crystal data of sulfonamides. *J. Sci. Res.* 2, 137–139.

Dickinson, C., Stewart, J. M., and Ammon, H. L. (1970). X-ray crystal structure of the antimalarial and antileprotic drug, 4,4′-diaminodiphenyl sulfone. *J. Chem. Soc. D* 920–921. doi: 10.1039/C29700000920

Fernándezz, A. (2016). Non-Debye frustrated hydration steers biomolecular association: interfacial tension for the drug designer. *FEBS Lett.* 590, 3481–3491. doi: 10.1002/1873-3468.12418

Fernández, A. (2017). Dielectric response of frustrated water down to a single-molecule contribution. *Ann. Phys.* 529:1600373. doi: 10.1002/andp.201600373

Fernandez, A., and Scott, L. R. (2017). Advanced modeling reconciles counterintuitive decisions in lead optimization. *Trends Biotechnol.* 35, 490–497. doi: 10.1016/j.tibtech.2016.12.003

Frisch, M. J., Trucks, G. W., Schlegel, H. B., Scuseria, G. E., Robb, J. M. A., Cheeseman, R., et al. (2009). *Gaussian 09.* Wallingford, CT: Gaussian Inc.

Fromm, E., and Wittmann, J. (1908). Derivatives of p-nitrothiophenol. *Ber. Dtsch. Chem. Ges.* 41, 2264–2273. doi: 10.1002/cber.190804102131

Gal, S. (1968). Phenomenological study of water vapor sorption isotherms of solid sorbents. *Chimia* 22, 409–425.

Griesser, U. J. (2006). "The importance of solvates," in *Polymorphism: In the Pharmaceutical Industry*, ed R. Hilfiker (Weinheim: Wiley-VCH), 211–233.

Guillot, B. (2002). A reappraisal of what we have learnt during three decades of computer simulations on water. *J. Mol. Liq.* 101, 219–260. doi: 10.1016/S0167-7322(02)00094-6

Habgood, M., Sugden, I. J., Kazantsev, A. V., Adjiman, C. S., and Pantelides, C. C. (2015). Efficient handling of molecular flexibility in Ab initio generation of crystal structures. *J. Chem. Theory Comput.* 11, 1957–1969. doi: 10.1021/ct500621v

Hilfiker, R. (2006). *Polymorphism in the Pharmaceutical Industry.* Weinheim: Wiley-VCH.

Infantes, L., Fabian, L., and Motherwell, W. D. S. (2007). Organic crystal hydrates: what are the important factors for formation. *CrystEngComm* 9, 65–71. doi: 10.1039/B612529H

Ismail, S. Z., Anderton, C. L., Copley, R. C. B., Price, L. S., and Price, S. L. (2013). Evaluating a crystal energy landscape in the context of industrial polymorph screening. *Cryst. Growth Des.* 13, 2396–2406. doi: 10.1021/cg400090r

Karamertzanis, P. G., and Pantelides, C. C. (2005). Ab initio crystal structure prediction-I. Rigid molecules. *J. Comput. Chem.* 26, 304–324. doi: 10.1002/jcc.20165

Karamertzanis, P. G., and Pantelides, C. C. (2007). Ab initio crystal structure prediction. II. Flexible molecules. *Mol. Phys.* 105, 273–291. doi: 10.1080/00268970601143317

Kazantsev, A. V., Karamertzanis, P. G., Adjiman, C. S., and Pantelides, C. C. (2011). Efficient handling of molecular flexibility in lattice energy minimization of organic crystals. *J. Chem. Theory Comput.* 7, 1998–2016. doi: 10.1021/ct100597e

Kendrick, J., Stephenson, G. A., Neumann, M. A., and Leusen, F. J. (2013). Crystal structure prediction of a flexible molecule of pharmaceutical interest with unusual polymorphic behavior. *Cryst. Growth Des.* 13, 581–589. doi: 10.1021/cg301222m

Kuhnert-Brandstatter, M., and Moser, I. (1979). Polymorphism of Dapson and ethambutoldihydrochloride. *Mikrochim. Acta* 1, 125–136. doi: 10.1007/BF01197529

Kuz'mina, L. G., Struchkov, Y. T., Novozhilova, N. V., and Tudorovskaya, G. L. (1981). Crystal structure of an aqueous solvate of p-diaminodiphenylsulfone. *Kristallografiya* 26, 695–701.

Lemmer, H., Stieger, N., Liebenberg, W., and Caira, M. R. (2012). Solvatomorphism of the antibacterial dapsone: X-ray structures and thermal desolvation kinetics. *Cryst. Growth Des.* 12, 1683–1692. doi: 10.1021/cg300019f

Llinàs, A., and Goodman, J. M. (2008). Polymorph control: past, present and future. *Drug Discov. Today* 13, 198–210. doi: 10.1016/j.drudis.2007.11.006

Mackenzie, C. F., Spackman, P. R., Jayatilaka, D., and Spackman, M. A. (2017). CrystalExplorer model energies and energy frameworks: extension to metal coordination compounds, organic salts, solvates and open-shell systems. *IUCrJ* 4, 575–587. doi: 10.1107/S205225251700848X

Mafra, L., Santos, S. M., Siegel, R., Alves, I., Almeida Paz, F. A., Dudenko, D., et al. (2012). Packing interactions in hydrated and anhydrous forms of the antibiotic ciprofloxacin: a solid-state, NMR. X-ray diffraction, and computer simulation study. *J. Am. Chem. Soc.* 134, 71–74. doi: 10.1021/ja208647n

Markvardsen, A. J., David, W. I. F., Johnson, J. C., and Shankland, K. (2001). A probabilistic approach to space-group determination from powder diffraction data. *Acta Crystallogr. Sect. A* 57, 47–54. doi: 10.1107/S0108767300012174

Morris, K. R., and Rodriguez-Hornedo, N. (1993). "Hydrates," in *Encyclopedia of Pharmaceutical Technology*, eds J. Swarbrick and J. Boylan (New York, NY: Marcel Dekker), 393–440.

Neumann, M. A., Van De Streek, J., Fabbiani, F. P. A., Hidber, P., and Grassmann, O. (2015). Combined crystal structure prediction and high-pressure crystallization in rational pharmaceutical polymorph screening. *Nat. Commun.* 6:7793. doi: 10.1038/ncomms8793

Newman, A. (2013). Specialized solid form screening techniques. *Org. Process Res. Dev.* 17, 457–471. doi: 10.1021/op300241f

Pawley, G. S. (1981). Unit-cell refinement from powder diffraction scans. *J. Appl. Crystallogr.* 14, 357–361. doi: 10.1107/S0021889881009618

Perdew, J. P., Burke, K., and Ernzerhof, M. (1996). Generalized gradient approximation made simple. *Phys. Rev. Lett.* 77, 3865–3868. doi: 10.1103/PhysRevLett.77.3865

Perez-Lloret, S., Rey, M. V., Ratti, P. L., and Rascol, O. (2013). Rotigotine transdermal patch for the treatment of Parkinson's Disease. *Fundam. Clin. Pharmacol.* 27, 81–95. doi: 10.1111/j.1472-8206.2012.01028.x

Price, L. S., McMahon, J. A., Lingireddy, S. R., Lau, S. F., Diseroad, B. A., Price, S. L., et al. (2014). A molecular picture of the problems in ensuring structural purity of tazofelone. *J. Mol. Struct.* 1078, 26–42. doi: 10.1016/j.molstruc.2014.01.014

Price, S. L., Braun, D. E., and Reutzel-Edens, S. M. (2016). Can computed crystal energy landscapes help understand pharmaceutical solids? *Chem. Commun* 52, 7065–7077. doi: 10.1039/C6CC00721J

Price, S. L., Leslie, M., Welch, G. W. A., Habgood, M., Price, L. S., Karamertzanis, P. G., et al. (2010). Modelling organic crystal structures using distributed multipole and polarizability-based model intermolecular potentials. *Phys. Chem. Chem. Phys.* 12, 8478–8490. doi: 10.1039/c004164e

Price, S. L., and Reutzel-Edens, S. M. (2016). The potential of computed crystal energy landscapes to aid solid-form development. *Drug Discov. Today* 21, 912–923. doi: 10.1016/j.drudis.2016.01.014

Rautio, J., Kärkkäinen, J., and Sloan, K. B. (2017). Prodrugs - Recent approvals and a glimpse of the pipeline. *Eur. J. Pharm. Sci.* 109, 146–161. doi: 10.1016/j.ejps.2017.08.002

Rautio, J., Kumpulainen, H., Heimbach, T., Oliyai, R., Oh, D., Jaervinen, T., et al. (2008). Prodrugs: design and clinical applications. *Nat. Rev. Drug Discovery* 7, 255–270. doi: 10.1038/nrd2468

Reilly, A. M., Cooper, R. I., Adjiman, C. S., Bhattacharya, S., Boese, A. D., Brandenburg, J. G., et al. (2016). Report on the sixth blind test of organic crystal structure prediction methods. *Acta Crystallogr. Sect. B* 72, 439–459. doi: 10.1107/S2052520616007447

Riddick, J. A., and Bunger, W. B. (1986). *Techniques of Chemistry, Vol. 2: Organic Solvents: Physical Properties and Methods of Purification. 4th Edn.* New York, NY: Wiley-Interscience.

Rietveld, H. M. (1969). A profile refinement method for nuclear and magnetic structures. *J. Appl. Crystallogr.* 2, 65–71. doi: 10.1107/S0021889869006558

Singh, S. S., and Thakur, T. S. (2014). New crystalline salt forms of levofloxacin: conformational analysis and attempts towards the crystal structure prediction of the anhydrous form. *CrystEngComm* 16, 4215–4230. doi: 10.1039/c4ce00263f

Srirambhatla, V. K., Guo, R., Price, S. L., and Florence, A. J. (2016). Isomorphous template induced crystallisation: a robust method for the targeted crystallisation of computationally predicted metastable polymorphs. *Chem. Commun.* 52, 7384–7386. doi: 10.1039/C6CC01710J

Stahly, G. P. (2007). Diversity in single- and multiple-component crystals. The search for and prevalence of polymorphs and cocrystals. *Cryst. Growth Des* 7, 1007–1026. doi: 10.1021/cg060838j

Steiner, T., and Koellner, G. (1994). Crystalline Î²-cyclodextrin hydrate at various humidities: fast, continuous, and reversible dehydration studied by X-ray diffraction. *J. Am. Chem. Soc.* 116, 5122–5128. doi: 10.1021/ja00091a014

Stone, A. J. (2005). Distributed multipole analysis: stability for large basis sets. *J. Chem. Theory Comput.* 1, 1128–1132. doi: 10.1021/ct050190

Stone, A. J. (2010). *GDMA: A Program for Performing Distributed Multipole Analysis of Wave Functions Calculated Using the Gaussian Program System. 2.2 Edn.* Cambridge: University of Cambridge.

Su, G., Pan, F., He, Y., and Guo, S. (1992). Crystal structure and NLO properties of 4,4′-diaminodiphenylsulfone (DAPS). *Jiegou Huaxue* 11, 293–296.

Thierfelder, C., Hermann, A., Schwerdtfeger, P., and Schmidt, W. G. (2006). Strongly bonded water monomers on the ice Ih basal plane: density-functional calculations. *Phys. Rev. B* 74. doi: 10.1103/PhysRevB.74.045422

Tkatchenko, A., and Scheffler, M. (2009). Accurate molecular van der waals interactions from ground-state electron density and free-atom reference data. *Phys. Rev. Lett.* 102:073005. doi: 10.1103/PhysRevLett.102.073005

Turner, M. J., Grabowsky, S., Jayatilaka, D., and Spackman, M. A. (2014). Accurate and efficient model energies for exploring intermolecular interactions in molecular crystals. *J. Phys. Chem. Lett.* 5, 4249–4255. doi: 10.1021/jz502271c

Turner, M. J., Thomas, S. P., Shi, M. W., Jayatilaka, D., and Spackman, M. A. (2015). Energy frameworks: insights into interaction anisotropy and the mechanical properties of molecular crystals. *Chem. Commun.* 51, 3735–3738. doi: 10.1039/C4CC09074H

Vanderbilt, D. (1990). Soft self-consistent pseudopotentials in a generalized eigenvalue formalism. *Phys. Rev. B* 41, 7892–7895. doi: 10.1103/PhysRevB.41.7892

Whalley, E. (1957). The difference in the intermolecular forces on H2O and D2O. *Trans. Faraday Soc.* 53, 1578–1585. doi: 10.1039/tf9575301578

Whalley, E. (1976). The hydrogen bond in ice. *Hydrogen Bond* 3, 1425–1470.

Wolf, R., and Orni-Wasserlauf, R. (2000). A century of the synthesis of dapsone: its anti-infective capacity now and then. *Int. J. Dermatol.* 39, 779–783. doi: 10.1046/j.1365-4362.2000.00739.x

World Health Organization (2017). *20th WHO Model List of Essential Medicines* [Online]. 847. Available online at: http://www.who.int/medicines/publications/essentialmedicines/en/ (Accessed September 18, 2017).

Wozel, G., and Blasum, C. (2014). Dapsone in dermatology and beyond. *Arch. Dermatol. Res.* 306, 103–124. doi: 10.1007/s00403-013-1409-7

Yathirajan, H. S., Nagaraja, P., Nagaraj, B., Bhaskar, B. L., and Lynch, D. E. (2014). *CCDC 255853: Experimental Crystal Structure Determination [Data set]*. Cambridge Crystallographic Data Centre. Available online at: https://doi.org/10.5517/cc8l7bd

Zhu, H., Yuen, C., and Grant, D. J. W. (1996). Influence of water activity in organic solvent + water mixtures on the nature of the crystallizing drug phase. 1. Theophylline. *Int. J. Pharm.* 135, 151–160. doi: 10.1016/0378-5173(95)04466-3

4

Pharmacophore Modeling and *In Silico/In Vitro* Screening for Human Cytochrome P450 11B1 and Cytochrome P450 11B2 Inhibitors

Muhammad Akram[1], *Watcharee Waratchareeyakul*[2], *Joerg Haupenthal*[3], *Rolf W. Hartmann*[3, 4] *and Daniela Schuster*[1*]

[1] *Institute of Pharmacy - Pharmaceutical Chemistry and Center for Molecular Biosciences Innsbruck (CMBI), University of Innsbruck, Innsbruck, Austria,* [2] *Department of Chemistry, Faculty of Science and Technology, Rambhai Barni Rajabhat University, Chanthaburi, Thailand,* [3] *Department of Drug Design and Optimization, Helmholtz Institute for Pharmaceutical Research Saarland, Saarbrücken, Germany,* [4] *Department of Pharmacy, Pharmaceutical and Medicinal Chemistry, Saarland University, Saarbrücken, Germany*

Correspondence:
Daniela Schuster
daniela.schuster@uibk.ac.at

Cortisol synthase (CYP11B1) is the main enzyme for the endogenous synthesis of cortisol and its inhibition is a potential way for the treatment of diseases associated with increased cortisol levels, such as Cushing's syndrome, metabolic diseases, and delayed wound healing. Aldosterone synthase (CYP11B2) is the key enzyme for aldosterone biosynthesis and its inhibition is a promising approach for the treatment of congestive heart failure, cardiac fibrosis, and certain forms of hypertension. Both CYP11B1 and CYP11B2 are structurally very similar and expressed in the adrenal cortex. To facilitate the identification of novel inhibitors of these enzymes, ligand-based pharmacophore models of CYP11B1 and CYP11B2 inhibition were developed. A virtual screening of the SPECS database was performed with our pharmacophore queries. Biological evaluation of the selected hits lead to the discovery of three potent novel inhibitors of both CYP11B1 and CYP11B2 in the submicromolar range (compounds **8–10**), one selective CYP11B1 inhibitor (Compound **11**, $IC_{50} = 2.5\ \mu M$), and one selective CYP11B2 inhibitor (compound **12**, $IC_{50} = 1.1\ \mu M$), respectively. The overall success rate of this prospective virtual screening experiment is 20.8% indicating good predictive power of the pharmacophore models.

Keywords: cushing's syndrome, wound healing, hypertension, congestive heart failure, myocardial fibrosis, pharmacophore modeling, model validation, virtual screening

INTRODUCTION

Cortisol is a glucocorticoid hormone that modulates many processes in the body such as blood sugar levels, immune system activity, metabolism of proteins, carbohydrates and fats, and bone formation (Cain and Cidlowski, 2017). Hypercortisolism in an unwanted increase in the secretion of cortisol and is the cause of many diseases such as Cushing's syndrome, metabolic disorders, and suppression of the immune system leading to delayed wound healing (Zhu et al., 2016). Cushing's syndrome is a condition that has symptoms like obesity, facial plethora, round face, decreased libido, thin skin, and easy bruising, impaired growth in children, menstrual irregularities, hypertension, hirsutism, depression, glucose intolerance, weakness, osteopenia, and nephrolithiasis

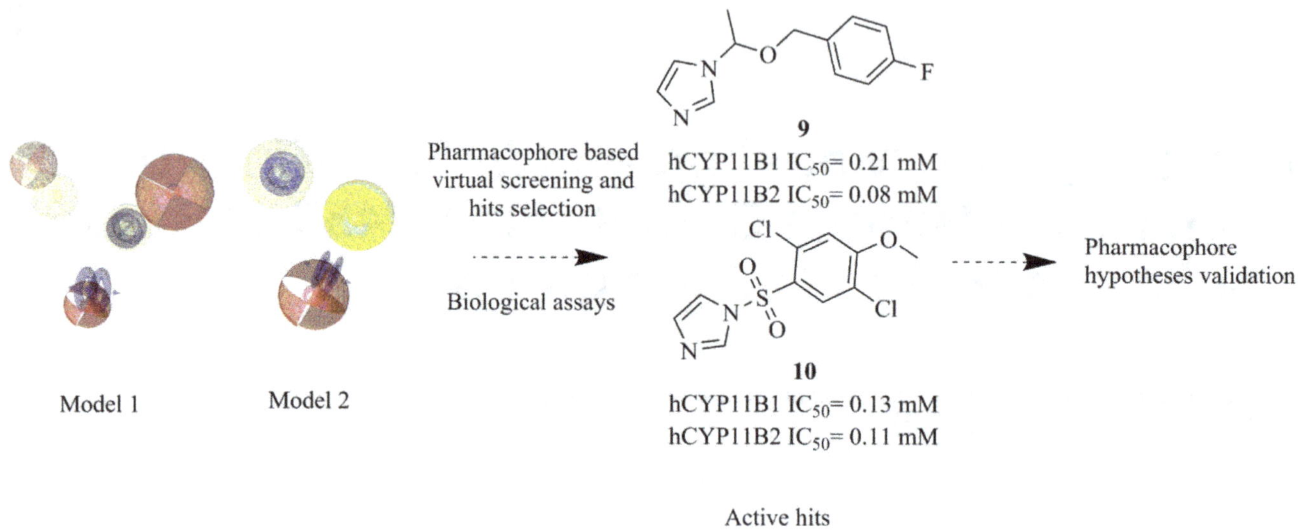

GRAPHICAL ABSTRACT| Novel CYP11B1 and 2 inhibitors identified by virtual screening.

in more than 50% of clinically observed patients (Newell-Price et al., 1998; Savage et al., 2001; Faggiano et al., 2003; Pecori Giraldi et al., 2003). A tumor of the pituitary or adrenal gland is the main reason for the over-secretion of cortisol. In most cases, a surgical removal or radiation therapy of the tumor is not applied, and instead the patients are treated with drugs (Tritos et al., 2011). The use of glucocorticoid receptor antagonists for treating this situation often comes with an increased secretion of cortisol, potentially due to the pituitary feedback mechanism (Orth, 1978). An alternative treatment could be the reduction of cortisol formation by inhibiting cytochrome P450 11B1. It catalyzes the final step in the formation of cortisol by hydroxylating 11-deoxycortisol in the zona fasciculate of adrenal cortex (**Figure 1**) (Sayers, 1950). This mechanism of action is expected not to cause the adverse effects observed for glucocorticoid receptor antagonists (Nieman, 2002).

Aldosterone is a potent mineralocorticoid hormone, which regulates blood pressure by increasing the reabsorption of sodium at the distal convoluted tubule in the kidney. Under normal conditions, aldosterone secretion is controlled by the renin-angiotensin-aldosterone-system (RAAS). In case of insufficient renal flow, excessive aldosterone is released by the activation of the RAAS pathway (Young and Funder, 2000). The increase in aldosterone levels causes an increase in blood volume that elevates blood pressure. An unwanted increase in plasma aldosterone levels results in various pathological conditions like hyperaldosteronism, congestive heart failure, myocardial fibrosis, cardiac hypertrophy, ventricular arrhythmia, and other adverse effects through triggering cardiac fibroblasts (Ramires et al., 1998; Brilla, 2000; Lijnen and Petrov, 2000; Briet and Schiffrin, 2010). CYP11B2 catalyzes the rate-limiting step in the formation of aldosterone from corticosterone in the zona glomerulosa of the adrenal cortex (Sayers, 1950; Lifton et al., 2001). The anti-mineralocorticoid spironolactone is used to treat hypertension and heart failure (Pitt et al., 1999). However, this therapy is accompanied by severe antiandrogenic adverse effects (Soberman and Weber, 2000). An alternative approach for the management of congestive heart failure and hypertension would be the inhibition of CYP11B2, probably leading to fewer adverse effects (Azizi et al., 2013).

Both CYP11B1 and CYP11B2 are mitochondrial enzymes and belong to the cytochrome P450 family. They use NADPH as a cofactor (Guengerich, 2007). After moving to the mitochondrial matrix, the enzymes length is reduced to 479 amino acids, of which 450 (93%) amino acids are identical in both of them (Belkina et al., 2001). The molecular mass of CYP11B1 is 50 kDa and for CYP11B2 is 48.5 kDa (Ogishima et al., 1991). Although their primary sequence is highly similar, they have different functionalities (Belkina et al., 2001).

Several potent inhibitors of CYP11B1 and CYP11B2 have been reported (**Figure 2**). Some of these compounds were discovered using rational SAR studies and molecular modeling approaches. In 2006, Ulmschneider et al. developed a ligand-based pharmacophore model for CYP11B2 inhibitors by superimposing previously synthesized active and inactive ligands for CYP11B2 from their research group (Ulmschneider et al., 2006). Their pharmacophore consisted of four points: three ring centroids and an aromatic nitrogen. The model had a steric inclusion area that mapped the active compounds and a

Abbreviations: kDa, kilodalton; CYP11B1, cytochrome p450 11B1; CYP11B2, cytochrome p450 11B2; ACTH, adrenocorticotrophic hormone; RAAS, renin-angiotensin-aldosterone-system; XVOL, exclusion volume; PAINS, pan-assay interference compounds; PDB, protein data bank, RMSD, root mean square deviation; Å, angstrom; Thr, threonine; Phe, phenylalanine; Ile, isoleucine; Trp, tryptophan; Met, methionine; Ala, alanine; Arg, arginine; IC_{50}, half maximal inhibitory concentration; 2D, two dimensional; CAS, chemical abstract service; VS, virtual screening; EtOH, ethyl alcohol; DMSO, dimethyl sulfoxide; min, minutes; rpm, revolutions per minute; HPLC, high performance liquid chromatography; HCl, hydrochloric acid; *E.coli*, Escherichia coli; NADPH, nicotinamide adenine dinucleotide phosphate.

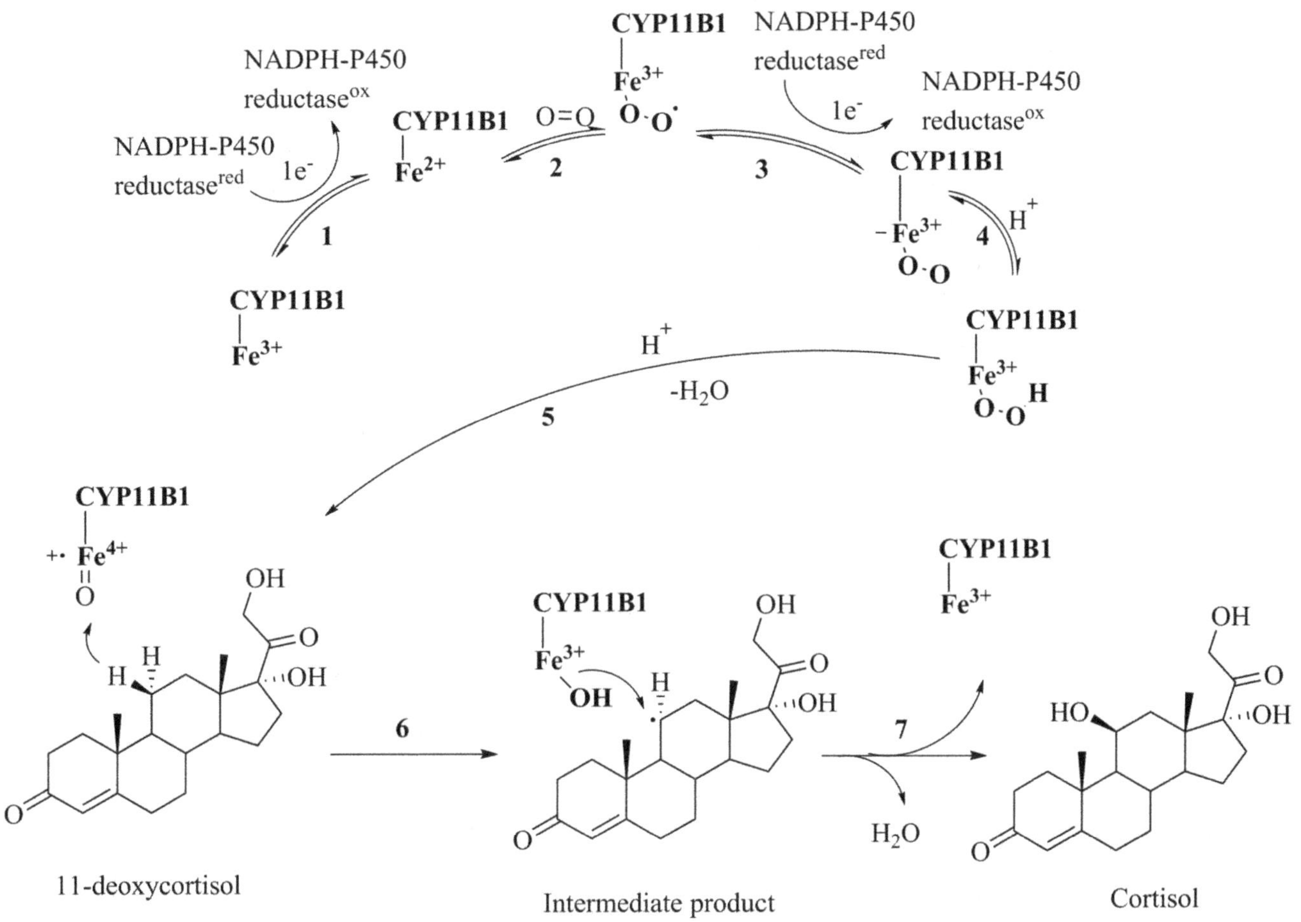

FIGURE 1 | Catalytic cycle of the conversion of 11-deoxycortisol to cortisol by CYP11B1(Guengerich, 2007). **(1)** Transfer of an electron from NADPH reductase to the heme iron resulting in the transformation of the ferric-form to the ferrous-form; **(2)** oxygen attachment to the ferrous-form producing an intermediate; **(3)** transfer of a second electron from NADPH reductase to the heme iron resulting in a peroxo-iron intermediate; **(4)** transfer of a proton producing its protonated form; **(5)** attachment of another proton to the intermediate and release of a water molecule producing a perferryl oxygen complex that immediately forms a free radical; **(6)** and **(7)** oxidation of 11-deoxycortisol to cortisol.

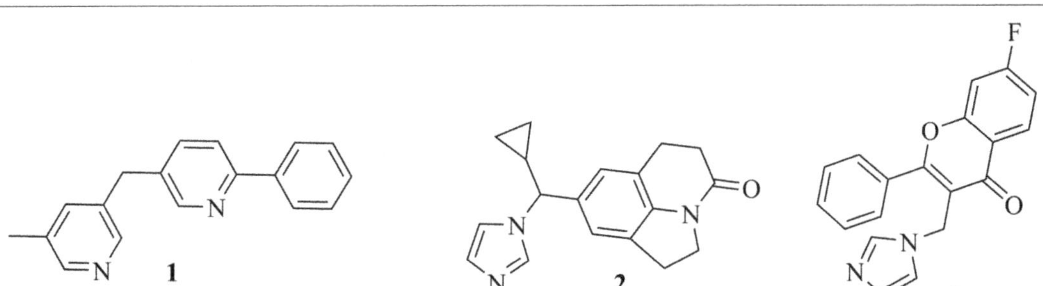

1

hCYP11B1 IC_{50} = 2 nM
hCYP11B2 IC_{50} = 33 nM

2

hCYP11B1 IC_{50} = 2.2 nM
hCYP11B2 IC_{50} = 24 nM

3

hCYP11B1 IC_{50} = 9.7 nM
hCYP11B2 IC_{50} = 94.9 nM

FIGURE 2 | Structures of previously published CYP11B1 and CYP11B2 inhibitors (Yin et al., 2012; Emmerich et al., 2013; Gobbi et al., 2016).

steric exclusion area that was derived from inactive compounds. They validated their pharmacophore model by designing and synthesizing acenaphthalene-based inhibitors of CYP11B2, followed by *in vitro* testing. In another study performed by

Lucas et al. (2008a), the authors designed and synthesized potential lead compounds for CYP11B2 inhibition with the help of a ligand-based pharmacophore model containing hydrophobic and hydrogen bond acceptor features. After the biological testing, the compounds were docked into a homology model of CYP11B2 (Lucas et al., 2008a). In 2011, the same group refined their previous ligand-based pharmacophore hypothesis based on diverse inhibitors. They added two hydrophobic features to their previous pharmacophore. Their final pharmacophore had four essential features, seven optional features, and five exclusion spheres. The refined pharmacophore of this study was validated by synthesizing and testing predicted inhibitors for CYP11B2 from the tetrahydropyrroloquinolinone scaffold, which led to potent compounds (Lucas et al., 2011). In addition to this, Gobbi et al. designed and synthesized several xanthone-based inhibitors of CYP11B1 and CYP11B2 based on the pharmacophore models by Lucas et al. (Lucas et al., 2011; Gobbi et al., 2013). The rationally designed inhibitors of CYP11B1 and CYP11B2 had a hydrophobic part in addition to the imidazolylmethyl ring, which was assumed to form a complex with the heme iron of CYP11B1 and CYP11B2 enzymes. This complexation is believed to play an important role for the inhibition of CYP11B1 and CYP11B2 enzymes (Gobbi et al., 2013).

All the above mentioned pharmacophore models have been successfully used to optimize already known active compound classes. However, none of them has been used to prospectively screen large, chemically diverse 3D molecular databases and identify novel active scaffolds. Our goal was therefore to create and validate an *in silico* model for future virtual screening (VS) experiments to find diverse inhibitors of either CYP11B1 or CYP11B2 or both, which could be used as pharmacological tool compounds. For this purpose, ligand-based pharmacophore queries of CYP11B1 and CYP11B2 inhibitors were generated. This method was chosen because of its frequently higher retrieval of active hits compared to docking (Chen et al., 2009) and because ligand-based models can often be better trained to recognize structurally diverse compounds binding to the same target compared to structure-based models (Schuster et al., 2010).

WORKFLOW

Datasets

Modeling Dataset

Data sets for model development were collected from the scientific literature (Table S1) (Dorr et al., 1984; Ulmschneider et al., 2005a,b, 2006; Voets et al., 2005, 2006; Heim et al., 2008; Lucas et al., 2008a,b, 2011; Adams et al., 2010; Roumen et al., 2010; Hille et al., 2011a,b; Stefanachi et al., 2011; Zimmer et al., 2011; Hu et al., 2012; Yin et al., 2012, 2013; Blass, 2013a,b; Emmerich et al., 2013; Ferlin et al., 2013; Gobbi et al., 2013; Meredith et al., 2013; Pinto-Bazurco Mendieta et al., 2013). As training-set compounds it is very important to select those compounds that are highly active, because VS commonly renders hits that are less active than the training compounds (Scior et al., 2012). For inactive compounds of the test set, a very high activity cut-off value must be chosen so that it is justified to refine the model according to the inactives. Therefore, the activity cut-off for active compounds of the test set was an IC_{50} of less than 2 μM and for inactive compounds, it was more than 100 μM, respectively. Finally, a test set of 386 active compounds (Dorr et al., 1984; Ulmschneider et al., 2005a,b, 2006; Voets et al., 2005, 2006; Heim et al., 2008; Lucas et al., 2008a,b, 2011; Adams et al., 2010; Roumen et al., 2010; Hille et al., 2011a,b; Stefanachi et al., 2011; Zimmer et al., 2011; Hu et al., 2012; Yin et al., 2012, 2013; Blass, 2013a,b; Emmerich et al., 2013; Ferlin et al., 2013; Gobbi et al., 2013; Meredith et al., 2013; Pinto-Bazurco Mendieta et al., 2013) was collected for the theoretical validation of the models. This data set contained compounds with IC_{50}s from 0.1 nM to 2 μM. Since no compound with an $IC_{50} > 100\,\mu$M was found in the literature, a decoy database representing the test set of putatively inactive compounds was assembled for theoretical validation purposes. Using the platform DecoyFinder (Cereto-Massagué et al., 2012), which extracts decoys from the ZINC (Irwin and Shoichet, 2005) database, 36 decoys per compound were generated based on the active compounds in the dataset. After removing duplicates, 15948 decoys remained in the database. The 2D structures of all active compounds were constructed in ChemBioDraw Ultra 14.0 (Cambridgesoft, 1986–2015). For conformational analysis, LigandScout 3.12 (Wolber and Langer, 2005) generated up to 500 conformers for each compound in the dataset with OMEGA-BEST (Hawkins et al., 2010; Hawkins and Nicholls, 2012) settings.

Pharmacophore Modeling

The espresso function of LigandScout was used to create ligand-based pharmacophores (Krautscheid et al., 2014). This workflow first assigns pharmacophore features to all of the conformations of the training compounds. Then, the features of the two most rigid training compounds are aligned to create intermediate common feature pharmacophore models. These intermediate models are ranked according to a selected scoring function. In this study, the default scoring function *pharmacophore fit and atom overlap* was used. The generated pharmacophore models usually profit from manual refinement to optimize their sensitivity (Equation 1) and specificity (Equation 2) (Vuorinen et al., 2014). The sensitivity of models can be improved by removing spatial restrictions, deleting features or marking them as optional, and adjusting the size of the features depending on the geometrical mapping of active compounds (Vuorinen et al., 2014).

$$Sensitivity = \frac{\text{actives found by model}}{\text{all actives in dataset}} \quad (1)$$

$$Specificity = \frac{\text{inactives not found by model}}{\text{all inactives in dataset}} \quad (2)$$

Prospective Virtual Screening

For prospective model validation, the commercial SPECS compound database was searched. The sd file containing 207976 compounds was downloaded from the SPECS webpage (www.specs.net, April_2015). The conformational analysis was performed with the same program and settings as the modeling databases. VS of the SPECS database was performed using the default settings of LigandScout 3.12.

PAINS Filtering

Pan-assay interfering substances (PAINS) appear as frequent hitters in many biological screening assays and are discussed as possible false positive hits in VS experiments for various reasons (Baell and Holloway, 2010). Therefore, PAINS filters were applied to the virtual hits obtained by the pharmacophore models. For this purpose, the sd files were submitted to the online server FAF-Drugs3 (Lagorce et al., 2015).

Hit Selection

In order to select diverse virtual hits for biological evaluation, a total number of 50 chemical clusters were generated from the hits obtained by model 1 using the *cluster ligands* protocol implemented in Discovery Studio 4.0 (Accelrys, 2015). For this purpose, we used the default predefined set known as Feature-Connectivity Fingerprint *FCFP_6*. FCFP generates clusters on the basis of pharmacophoric features instead of functional groups and six indicates the effective diameter of the largest feature and is equal to the double of iterations performed (Rogers and Hahn, 2010). For further processing, the top two hits from each cluster were selected based on their pharmacophore fit value.

Biological Testing

Preparation of Inhibitor Solution

The selected potential inhibitors were dissolved in DMSO at a concentration of 10 mM to generate stock solutions. Various aliquots were then made from fresh stock solutions and each aliquot was tested only once. All the selected inhibitors were diluted with 100% ethanol (negative control) to the desired concentration to observe their inhibition of CYP11B1 and CYP11B2.

CYP11B1 and CYP11B2 Inhibition Assays

The selected hits were evaluated for their inhibition of human CYP11B1 and CYP11B2 enzymes expressed in hamster V79MZh cells. Approximately 8000000 V79MZh cells were cultured in 24-well cell culture plates for 24 h. The area of each well was 1.9 cm^2. The cells were exposed to various concentrations of inhibitor solutions. The reactions were started by incubating the cells with $[^3H]$11-deoxycorticosterone. The incubation time for CYP11B1 cells was 15–60 and 50–120 min for CYP11B2 cells. The reactions were stopped by extracting the supernatant with cold ethyl acetate at 4°C. Samples were mixed (10 min), and centrifuged (12,500 rpm). The organic (upper) layer was separated into fresh Eppendorf tubes and dried. The steroids were re-dissolved in methanol-water (65–35%) and were analyzed by radio-HPLC (Denner et al., 1995a; Ehmer et al., 2002). Ketoconazole (Hille et al., 2011b) (CYP11B1 IC_{50} = 120 nM, CYP11B2 IC_{50} = 60 nM,) was used as positive control and ethanol was used as negative control.

CYP17 Inhibition Assay

The inhibition of CYP17 was investigated using the 5,000 g sediment of homogenized *Escherichia coli* (Ehmer et al., 2000). Human CYP17 along with NADPH-P450 reductase was used to perform the assay as described previously. The incubation time for the reaction was 30 min at 37°C. The reaction was started by adding $[^3H]$-progesterone, and was quenched with 1 M HCl. The reaction mixture was extracted twice with ethyl acetate at 4°C in order to avoid impurities. The samples were dried, prepared with methanol, and analyzed with radio-HPLC. DSMO was used as negative control. Abiraterone (IC_{50} = 100 nM) and ketoconazole (IC_{50} = 4 μM) were used as reference inhibitors (Sergejew and Hartmann, 1994).

Docking

The 2D structures were prepared for docking in ChemBioDraw Ultra 14.0 (Cambridgesoft, 1986–2015). The ChemBioDraw files were converted to structure data (sd) format using a protocol designed in Pipeline Pilot Client 2016 (Accelrys, 2011). The 3D starting conformation of each chemical structure was generated using OMEGA 2.3.2 from OpenEye (Hawkins et al., 2010; Hawkins and Nicholls, 2012). The X-ray crystal structure of CYP11B2 in complex with fadrozole (PDB entry 4FDH) (Strushkevich et al., 2013) was used for docking employing a genetic algorithm implemented in GOLD 5.2 (Jones et al., 1995, 1997). The binding site was defined by selecting the 6 Å space around the co-crystallized ligand. In order to obtain the best docking poses, the default docking template for CYP450 *Goldscore P450* was used. Gold's *Goldscore* was used as a scoring function to rank the docked poses of inhibitor compounds. For validating the docking experiment, the co-crystallized ligand was re-docked into the binding site, which resulted in an RMSD of 0.223 Å.

RESULTS

CYP11B1 and CYP11B2 Inhibitor Pharmacophore Models

Pharmacophore models for CYP11B1 and CYP11B2 inhibitors were derived from highly potent training compounds. These compounds are expected to form a complex of an aromatic nitrogen with the heme iron in the active site of the enzyme. This sort of complex inhibits the catalytic process of the enzyme by preventing oxygen binding to heme iron.

The ligand-based, common feature pharmacophore model 1 was generated from compounds **4** and **5** (**Figure 3A**) (Meredith et al., 2013). From the 10 reported pharmacophore queries, the model with the highest *pharmacophore-fit and atom overlap* score (0.9084) and highest *pharmacophore-fit* score of training compounds was selected for further refinement. This pharmacophore model was composed of two aromatic ring features (AR-1 and AR-2), three hydrophobic features (H-1, H-2, and H-3), three hydrogen bond acceptors (HBA-1, HBA-2, and HBA-3), and 47 XVOLs (**Figures 3B,C**). HBA-1 represents the heterocyclic nitrogen of the training compounds, which is hypothesized to form a complex with the heme of the CYP enzymes. The remaining pharmacophore features represent various common features of the training compounds. Pharmacophore model 1 was made more sensitive by; (1) increasing the feature tolerance of AR-1, AR-2, and HBA-3 from default 1–1.6, 1.3, and 1.75 Å, respectively, (2) and marking the H-1, H-2, H-3, and HBA-2 features as optional. The theoretically validated model 1 found 76 out of 384 active hits excluding the two training compounds and 77 out of 15946 decoys. The training compounds **4** and **5** mapped all the features of refined pharmacophore model 1 with *pharmacophore-fit* scores of 87.50 and 87.59, respectively.

Ligand-based pharmacophore model 2 was generated from training compounds **6** and **7** (Ulmschneider et al., 2005b; Hille et al., 2011b) (**Figure 4A**) using the same settings as for model 1. The model which achieved the highest *pharmacophore fit and atom overlap* score (0.9174) and highest *pharmacophore-fit* score for the training compounds was selected for further

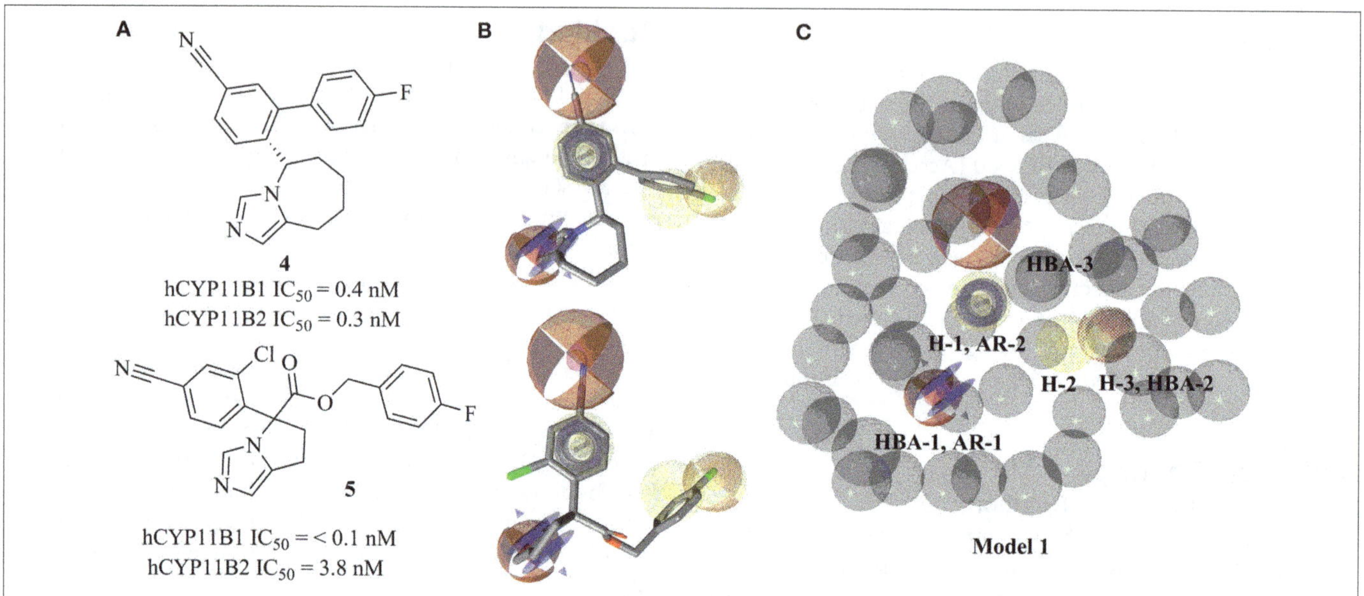

FIGURE 3 | Pharmacophore model 1 with training compounds **4** and **5**. **(A)** 2D training compounds with their IC_{50} values are drawn. **(B)** Training compounds mapped into the model. **(C)** Final pharmacophore model 1 with color-coded features (yellow—hydrophobic, blue rings—AR, red—HBA, dotted style—optional features). The model consisted of 3 hydrophobic features, 3 HBAs, 2 AR features, and 47 XVOLs.

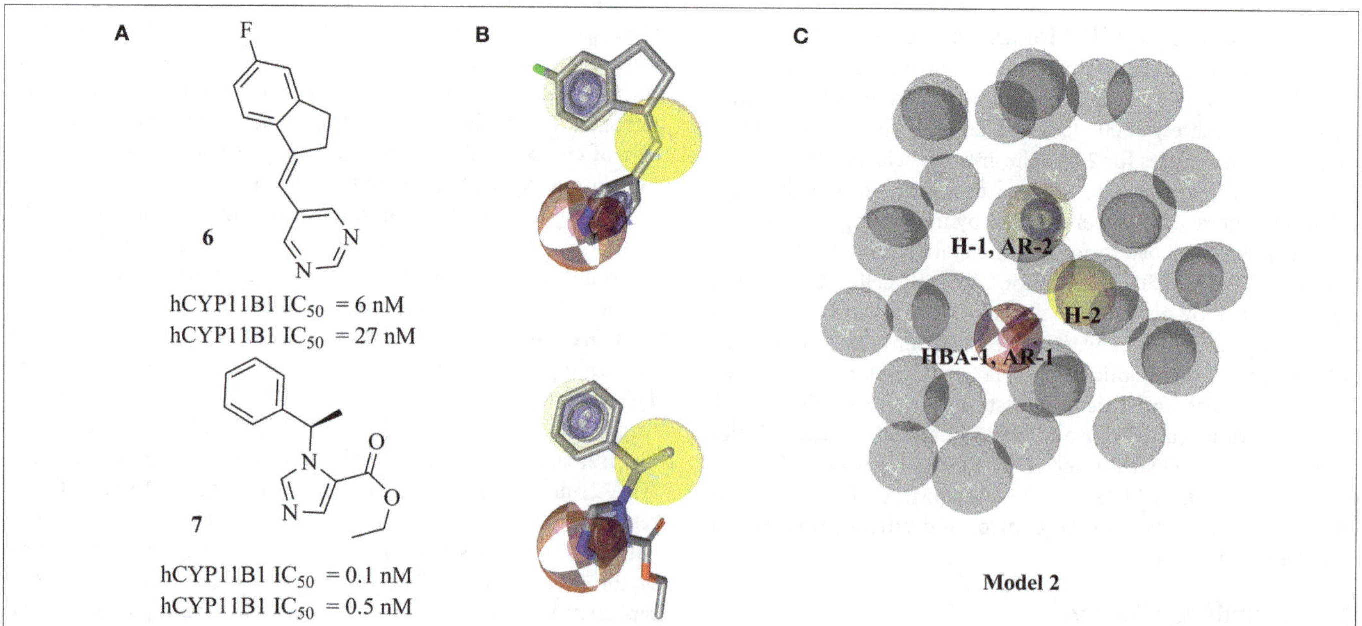

FIGURE 4 | Pharmacophore model 2 with its training compounds **6** and **7**. **(A)** Training compounds with their IC_{50} values are drawn. **(B)** Mapping of training compounds with the model are shown. **(C)** The pharmacophore model is shown. Pharmacophore features are marked by colors. Model 2 comprised of 2 hydrophobic features, 2 AR features, 1 HBA feature, and 33 XVOLs.

optimization. It consisted of two AR features (AR-1, AR-2), two hydrophobic (H-1 and H-2) features, one HBA (HBA-1), and 33 XVOLs (**Figures 4B,C**). The shared HBA feature of both of the training compounds was derived from the nitrogen of pyrimidine and imidazole rings. This model was made more sensitive by marking the hydrophobic feature H-1 as optional. In the validation screening, the final model found 36 active hits among 384 active compounds excluding the two training compounds and 10 out of 15946 decoys. The training compounds **6** and **7** mapped all the features of the refined model 2 and both got *pharmacophore-fit* score of 58.66, respectively.

The sensitivity values for both models 1 and 2 were calculated, which were 0.20 for model 1 and for model 2, respectively.

TABLE 1 | Inhibition of CYP11B1, CYP11B2, and CYP17 enzyme activity by the virtual hits.

Cpd.	CAS number	CYP11B1[a] IC_{50} (μM)[b]	CYP11B2[a] IC_{50} (μM)[b]	CYP17[c,d]	Fit value
8	839687-79-5	3.04 ± 0.72	2.77 ± 0.48	n.i.[e]	58.07 model 1
9	445402-94-8	0.21 ± 0.04	0.08 ± 0.005	n.i.	57.27 model 2
10	898644-65-0	0.13 ± 0.02	0.11 ± 0.02	n.i.	47.25 model 1, 46.42 model 2
11	489434-32-4	2.52 ± 0.28	15.58 ± 8.45	n.d.[f]	58.19 model 2
12	895332-29-3	33 ± 6%[d]	1.12 ± 0.22	n.i.	57.24 model 2

[a]*Human CYP11B1 and CYP11B2 enzymes expressed in hamster v79MZh cells.*
[b]*Mean value of at least three experiments.*
[c]*Human CYP17 enzyme isolated from Escherichia coli.*
[d]*Inhibition was measured at 10 μM concentration.*
[e]*n.i., not inhibited.*
[f]*n.d., not determined.*

Virtual Screening and Removal of False Positive Hits

Both pharmacophore models were employed for the VS of the drug discovery database SPECS (207,976 compounds) to find novel CYP11B1 and CYP11B2 inhibitors. The VS campaign resulted in 1,120 hits in total, including 1,023 hits found by model 1 and 97 hits found by model 2, respectively. A PAINS filter removed 65 compounds from the hit list obtained by model 1 and 4 from the hit list retrieved by model 2, respectively. First of all, we focused on consensus hits. Just one compound (**10**) was fitting to both pharmacophore models. Second, we aimed to validate each pharmacophore with a similar number of virtual hits in the biological testing. Because many of the hits that remained after virtual screening and PAINS filtering were derivatives of the same or similar scaffolds, we additionally performed a structural clustering to group the hits according to their chemical structure. The final selection was based on high fit values, chemical diversity, and the presence of an aromatic nitrogen in a ring system. Finally, 24 hits were submitted to *in vitro* evaluation including 11 hits found by model 1, 12 hits found by model 2, and 1 consensus hit (**Table 1**).

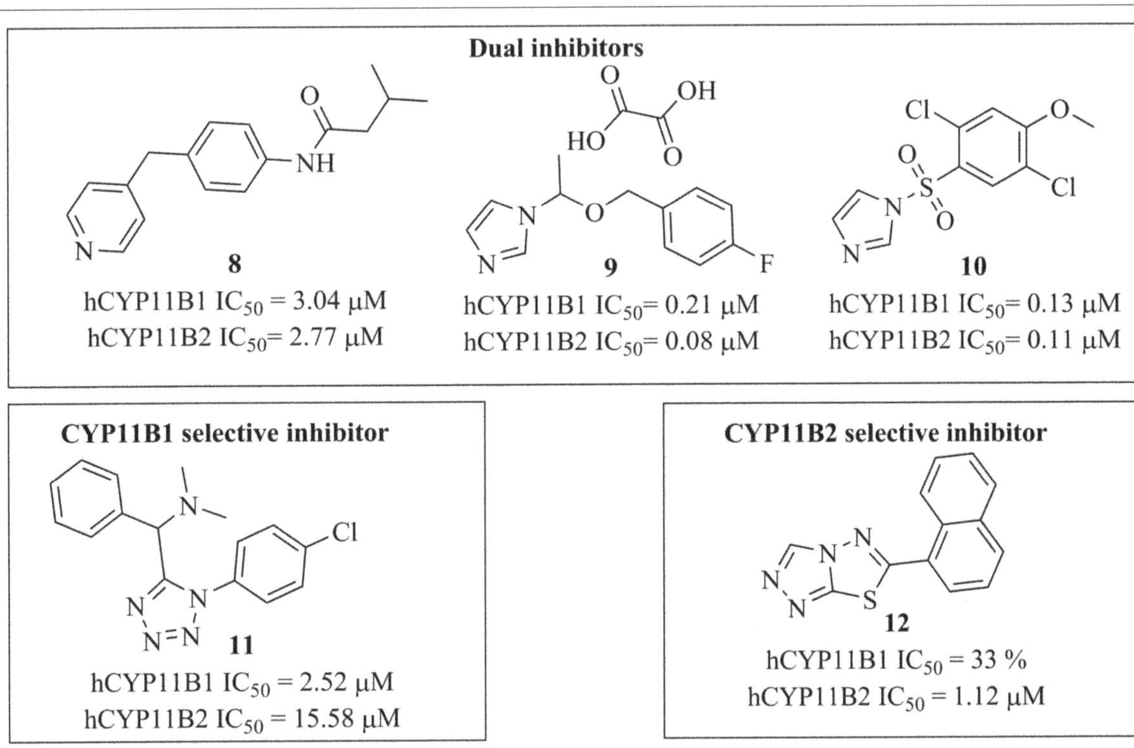

FIGURE 5 | Structures of the compounds **8–12** along with their IC_{50} values determined in cell-based assays.

Inhibition of Human CYP11B1 and CYP11B2 Enzymes

The selected 24 hits were analyzed for CYP11B1 and CYP11B2 inhibitory activities in a cell-based assay. In a first step, all hits were tested against both CYP11B1 and CYP11B2 at a concentration of 10 μM. Three compounds (**8**, **9**, and **10**) amongst the 24 tested hits showed more than 50% inhibition on both CYP11B1 and CYP11B2 at a concentration of 10 μM (**Table 1**) and were therefore dual inhibitors. Compound **11** inhibited CYP11B1 more potently than CYP11B2. Compound **12** selectively inhibited CYP11B2 (**Figure 5**). These five compounds were further evaluated for their IC_{50} values (**Table 1**). All of the newly discovered compounds that inhibited human CYP11B1 and CYP11B2 had a pyridine or pyrazole ring in their structures. The tested inactive compounds are showed in **Figure 6**.

Selectivity over Human CYP17 Enzyme

The four most active compounds **8–10** and **12** were analyzed for the inhibition of the steroidogenic enzyme CYP17. The inhibition values were measured at a concentration of 10 μM of inhibitor. None of the tested compounds inhibited CYP17 (**Table 1**).

Docking of Active Hits into CYP11B2 Binding Sites

Because a ligand-based virtual screening workflow was used for selecting the test compounds, a docking study was performed to propose binding modes for the inhibitors. Previous studies have suggested that binding affinity of the enzyme was highly dependent on the coordination geometry between the heme iron and the heterocyclic nitrogen of the inhibitor. Accordingly, an angle of 90° of the aromatic nitrogen-iron vector projected on the heme-porphyrin plane would lead to potent inhibition (Yin et al., 2014).

The docked pose of compound **9** showed the binding interaction of an imidazole-nitrogen with the heme iron at the binding site in a perpendicular way with an angle of 92°. The linker formed hydrophobic contacts with Thr318, Phe130, Ile488, Phe487, Phe231, and Trp116. The phenyl ring

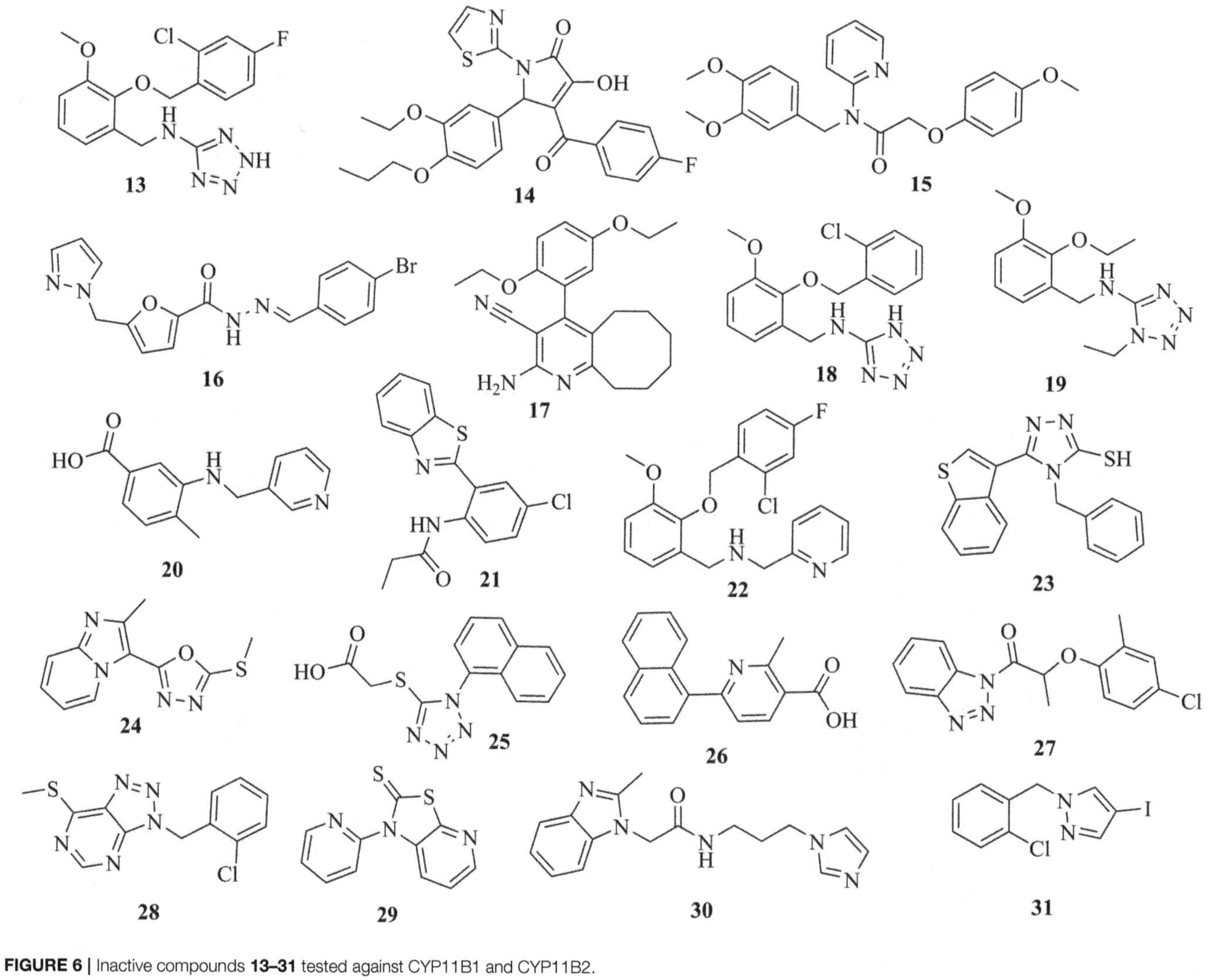

FIGURE 6 | Inactive compounds **13–31** tested against CYP11B1 and CYP11B2.

contacted Trp116, Met230, Trp260, and Ala313. Finally, the fluorine formed a bifurcated hydrogen bond with Arg120 and hydrophobic interactions with Trp260, Met309, and Ala313 (**Figure 7A**).

The imidazole nitrogen of compound **10** interacted with the heme iron in a perpendicular manner with an angle of 87°. The oxygen atoms of the sulfate formed a hydrogen bond with Thr318. The other marked interactions included hydrophobic interactions of halogens with Ile488, Phe130, Trp116, Phe130, and the heme porphyrin (**Figure 7B**).

Compound **12** inhibited CYP11B2 more selectively than CYP11B1. Two of the triazole nitrogen atoms were complexed

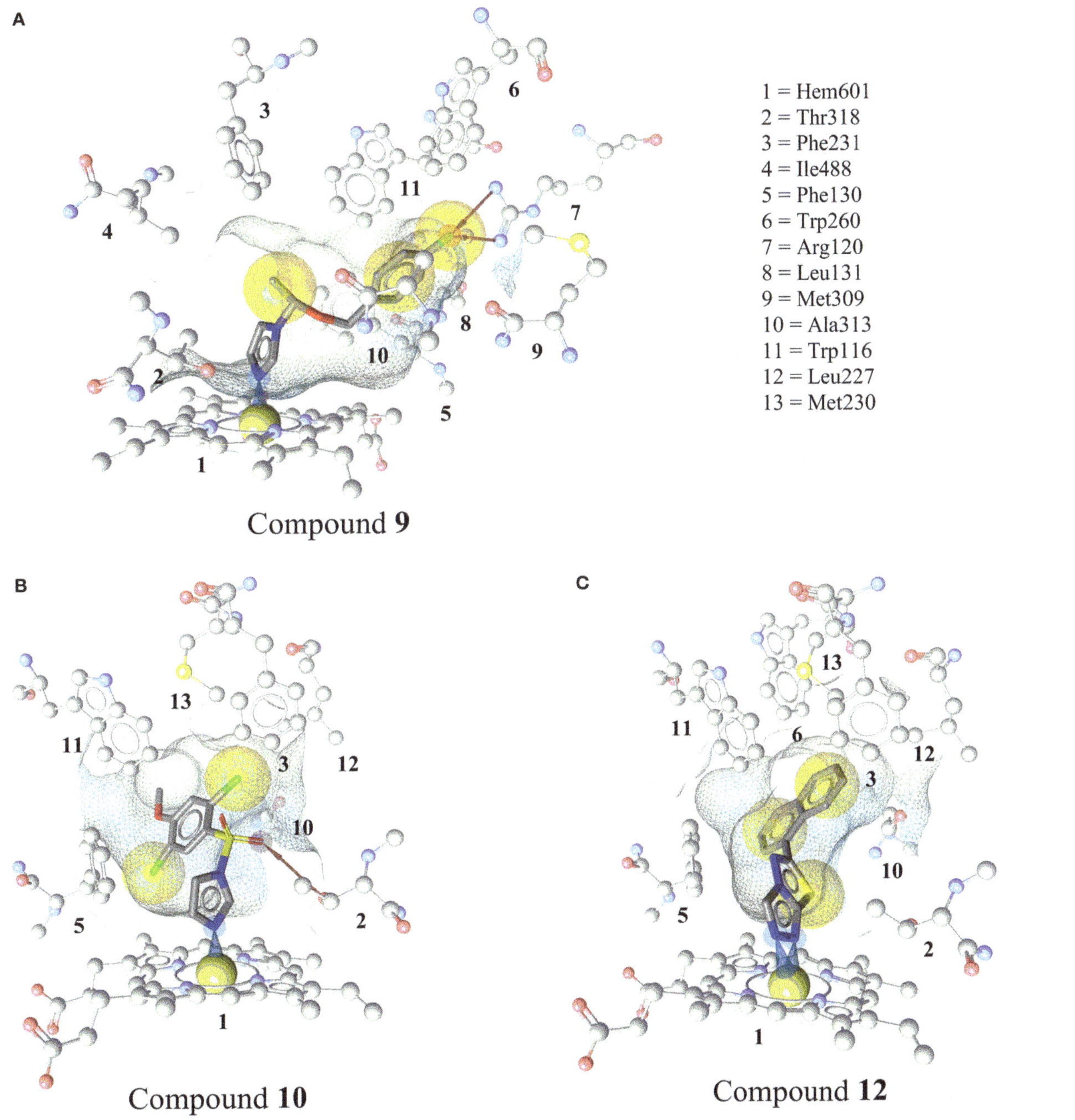

FIGURE 7 | Predicted binding modes of the newly discovered inhibitors **9, 10**, and **12** in CYP11B2 (PDB code = 4FDH). **(A)** Docking pose of compound **9** showing an iron complex of the imidazole-N with the heme iron and HBA interaction of the fluorine with Arg120. **(B)** The docking pose of compound **10** showing an iron binding interaction of the imidazole-N with the heme iron, a hydrogen bond between the sulfonamide and Thr318, and hydrophobic interactions of the halogens. **(C)** Docking pose of compound **12**, a selective CYP11B2 inhibitor. Two N atoms of the triazole ring formed iron-binding interactions with the heme iron. The wire frame network represented the binding pocket, and its surface is colored by aggregated lipophilicity (gray)/hydrophilicity (blue).

with the heme iron at angles of 84 and 77°, respectively. The biphenyl part interacted via hydrophobic interactions with Phe130, Ala313, Trp116, Trp260, Met230, Leu227, Phe231, and Thr318 (**Figure 7C**).

DISCUSSION

This study was performed to generate and validate novel pharmacophore models for CYP11B1 and CYP11B2 inhibitors (**Figures 3, 4**). The developed pharmacophore queries were experimentally validated by screening the SPECS database. After removing the 69 PAINS (Baell and Holloway, 2010) compounds from a total of 1,120 virtual hits, 24 were selected for *in vitro* testing. These hits were biologically evaluated on hamster V79MZh cells expressing human CYP11B1 or CYP11B2 (Denner et al., 1995a; Ehmer et al., 2002). Five out of 24 selected hits inhibited CYP11B1 and/or CYP11B2 (**Table 1**). The predictive power of both pharmacophore models was analyzed. Eleven out of 24 compounds were selected by model 1, of them compounds **8** and **10** inhibited both CYP11B1 and CYP11B2 *in vitro* (**Table 1**). This implies a success rate of 18%. Among the 13 compounds selected by model 2, compounds **9–11** inhibited both CYP11B1 and CYP11B2, and compound **12** showed selective inhibition of CYP11B2. This results in a success rate of 31%. Compound **10** was a consensus hit and inhibited both CYP11B1 and CYP11B2. Thus, an overall success rate of both pharmacophore models was 21%. These findings showed that both models 1 and 2 had adequate prospective, predictive power with success rates quite typical for this virtual screening method. According to a search of the SciFinder database, none of the compounds discovered in this study were reported as CYP11B1 and CYP11B2 inhibitors in literature before. Due to the 93.9% identical amino acid residues in CYP11B1 and CYP11B2 (Kawamoto et al., 1992; Taymans et al., 1998) it is challenging to generate selective pharmacophore models for CYP11B1 and CYP11B2 inhibition. Model 1 found compounds **8** and **10**, both are novel dual inhibitors of CYP11B1 and CYP11B2. The IC_{50} values for compounds **8** and **10** for CYP11B1 inhibition were 3.04 and 0.13 μM, respectively, and for CYP11B2 inhibition were 2.77 and 0.11 μM, respectively (**Table 1**). Model 2 found compounds **9–12**, of them **9** and **10** were dual inhibitors of CYP11B1 and CYP11B2. The IC_{50} value for compound **9** for CYP11B1 inhibition was 0.21 μM and for CYP11B2 inhibition was 0.08 μM, respectively The IC_{50} values of compound **11** (CYP11B1 = 2.52 μM, CYP11B2 = 15.58 μM) showed that it had a selectivity factor of 6 for CYP11B1 inhibition over CYP11B2. Compound **12** was a selective inhibitor of CYP11B2 with an IC_{50} = 1.12 μM, while it was a very weak inhibitor of CYP11B1 with an inhibition of 33% at a concentration of 10 μM.

An X-ray crystal structure of CYP11B1 has not been published yet; however the crystal structure of CYP11B2 was available from the PDB (Berman et al., 2000) (PDB ID = 4FDH) (Strushkevich et al., 2013). The positioning of the novel inhibitors into the binding pocket of CYP11B2, which is similar to the well-known inhibitor fadrozole, rationalizes their biological activities (**Figure 7**).

A close analysis of the mapping of the active hits and fadrozole into the pharmacophore models was performed. Combined aromatic ring-HBA features (AR-1 and HBA-1) of the respective pharmacophore models (**Figure 9**) mapped an aromatic nitrogen of all the novel inhibitors **8–12**. The angle and position of the aromatic nitrogen toward the heme iron is important for making an inhibition complex at the binding site. In the docking analysis, all active hits formed this interaction in an angle of around 90° (**Figure 7**).

According to the results obtained in this study, we compared our pharmacophore queries with previously reported pharmacophore models (Ulmschneider et al., 2006; Lucas et al., 2008a, 2011; Gobbi et al., 2013), Previously published studies used molecular modeling as a tool for designing optimized CYP11B1 and CYP11B2 inhibitors (Ulmschneider et al., 2006; Lucas et al., 2008a, 2011; Gobbi et al., 2013). Our pharmacophore queries were based on diverse training compounds (Ulmschneider et al., 2005a; Hille et al., 2011b; Meredith et al., 2013), and had different numbers and locations of pharmacophore features in space. In comparison to the previous models, our pharmacophores additionally include aromatic

TABLE 2 | Detailed analysis of pharmacophore features mapped by all novel inhibitors 8-12 of CYP11B1 and CYP11B2.

Model 1	Cpd.[a] 8	Cpd. 9	Cpd. 10	Cpd. 11	Cpd. 12	Model 2
HBA-1	Yes	Yes	Yes	Yes	Yes	HBA-1
HBA-2[b]	–	–	–	–	–	–
HBA-3	Yes	–	Yes	–	–	–
H-1[a]	Yes	Yes	–	Yes	Yes	H-1[a]
H-2[a]	–	–	–	–	–	–
H-3[a]	–	–	–	–	–	–
AR-1	Yes	Yes	Yes	Yes	Yes	AR-1
AR-2	Yes	Yes	Yes	Yes	Yes	AR-2
–	–	Yes	Yes	Yes	Yes	H-2

[a]*Compound.*
[b]*Optional feature.*

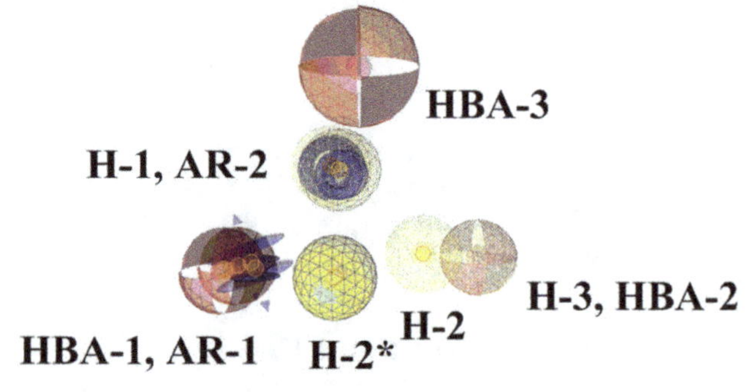

FIGURE 8 | Comparison of pharmacophore models 1 and 2. The highlighted features (wireframe) are from pharmacophore model 2. The pharmacophore features are color-coded. Yellow represents hydrophobic, blue denotes AR, and red shows the HBAs. Four pharmacophore features of both pharmacophores are common. H-2* is hydrophobic feature from model 2.

features (AR-1 and AR-2) (**Figure 9**, **Table 2**). The alignment of our pharmacophore models reveals that they have four features in common, including HBA-1, AR-1, AR-2, and H-1 (**Figure 8**). All the novel inhibitors found in this study were mapped to analyze the importance of different pharmacophore features. The alignment showed that HBA-1, HBA-3 AR-1, AR-2, H-1, H-2 were essential features in mapping the active compounds during virtual screening run (**Figure 9**, **Table 2**). All of the newly discovered inhibitors in this study have aromatic nitrogen-containing heterocycles and hydrophobic parts (**Figure 9**). The heterocyclic nitrogen part has a crucial role in forming an iron-binding interaction with heme of these CYP enzymes and was mapped by the HBA-1 and AR-1 features of the pharmacophores. This type of interaction inhibited the catalytic process of the target enzymes and has been reported earlier (Denner et al., 1995a,b; Hartmann et al., 2003; Bureik et al., 2004; Ulmschneider et al., 2005b; Hoyt et al., 2015).

Both active hits from model 1 did not map the two optional features of the model. This suggests that these features may be deleted from the model without losing active hits. A model with fewer and no optional features is much faster in screening virtual compound libraries. In future studies, a refined model 1 without those optional features can be applied for screening millions of compounds in a still reasonable time.

To compare the ligand-based features of the models to the protein-ligand interactions observed in the available X-ray structures of CYP11B2, the co-crystallized inhibitor fadrozole (4FDH) was aligned to pharmacophore model 1. Fadrozole mapped five features of the model (Figure S1), but also didn't map the two optional features supporting the hypothesis that those are not advantageous. A comparison of structure-based pharmacophore models derived from 4FDH (Strushkevich et al., 2013) and 4ZGX (Martin et al., 2015) co-crystallized structures is given in the supporting information (Figure S2). The general description about the generation of pharmacophore models has been previously outlined (Vuorinen et al., 2014; Akram et al., 2015; Kaserer et al., 2015).

During the validation of our pharmacophore models, three novel dual CYP11B1 and CYP11B2 inhibitors, one novel selective CYP11B1 inhibitor, and one novel selective CYP11B2 inhibitor were discovered. Compound **11** was a selective inhibitor of CYP11B1 that is the principal enzyme for the production of cortisol, which inhibition may be a strategy for the treatment of Cushing's syndrome and delayed wound healing (Nieman, 2002). Compound **12** was a selective CYP11B2 inhibitor, which is the key enzyme for the production of aldosterone, which inhibition is a potential target for the treatment of congestive heart failure, myocardial fibrosis, and hypertension. Compounds **8–10** are potent dual inhibitors of CYP11B1 and CYP11B2, which makes them interesting lead compounds for the development of drugs that could achieve a complete blockade of adrenal corticoid formation. Compounds **8–12** could be further chemically optimized to enhance their biological efficacies and selectivities by bioisosteric replacements or substitution of rings.

Compounds **8–10** and **12** were also tested for inhibition of human steroidogenic enzyme CYP17 (**Table 1**), because it belongs to the same class and has same inhibition mechanism

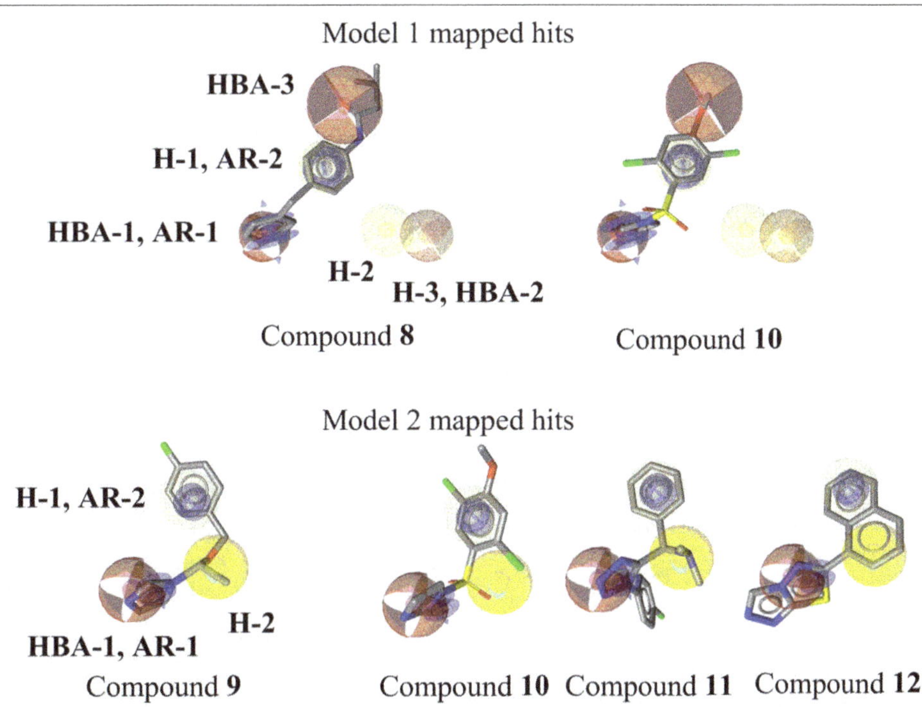

FIGURE 9 | Mapping of novel CYP11B1 and CYP11B2 inhibitors to pharmacophore models. Pharmacophore features are color-coded. Yellow represents hydrophobic, blue denotes AR, and red shows the HBAs. Optional features (dotted style) are not mapped by the virtual hits **8** and **10**.

as other CYP enzymes (Devore and Scott, 2012). None of the novel inhibitors showed inhibition of human CYP17 of more 3% at a concentration of 10 μM. This showed the selectivity of these novel inhibitors over CYP17.

The virtually selected hits **13–31** that showed no or only very weak inhibition during *in vitro* testing on human CYP11B1 and CYP11B2 might not be able to bind to the target, may have suffered from degradation or did not reach the binding site of the enzyme, and/or could have been pumped out of the cells via cellular efflux pumps (Johnstone et al., 2000). A precise conclusion for their inactivity is difficult to draw (**Figure 6**).

CONCLUSION

In the course of this study, ligand-based pharmacophore models for CYP11B1 and CYP11B2 inhibition were developed. For experimental validation of pharmacophore queries, the virtually selected hits were tested *in vitro*. This process resulted in the identification of new structural features advantageous for CYP11B inhibition (AR-1, AR-2, H-1, H-2, and HBA-3) and five novel CYP11B1 and/or CYP11B2 inhibitors. All of the novel inhibitors contained a heterocyclic nitrogen that is frequently present in CYP inhibitors. This project validated our pharmacophore model for future virtual screening campaigns. Regarding the quality of the pharmacophore models, model 2 gave more active hits than model 1. Both models will be refined further based on the biological testing to enhance their sensitivity and specificity.

AUTHOR CONTRIBUTIONS

DS planned and supervised the study. WW and MA created the pharmacophore models. MA performed the virtual screening and hits selection along with DS. MA conducted biological experiments under supervision of JH and RH. MA, JH, DS, and RH analyzed the data. All authors were involved in the preparation of the manuscript and approved the final version.

ACKNOWLEDGMENTS

This study was funded by the Austrian Science Fund FWF (P26782) and a Young Talents Grants from the University of Innsbruck. DS is an Ingeborg Hochmair Professor at the University of Innsbruck. MA is also grateful to Standortagentur Tirol for facilitating the ERASMUS+ program for performing *in vitro* assays at the Helmholtz Institute for Pharmaceutical Research Saarland (HIPS), Germany. We are thankful to InteLigand and OpenEye Inc. for providing LigandScout and OMEGA academic licenses. We acknowledge the help of Philipp Schuster and Grant Alexander Begg for proofreading the manuscript.

REFERENCES

Accelrys, I. (2011). *Pipeline Pilot*. San Diego, CA: Biovia Inc.

Accelrys (2015). *Discovery Studio. 4.0 Edn*. San Diego, CA: Biovia Inc.

Adams, C. M., Hu, C.-W., Jeng, A. Y., Karki, R., Ksander, G., Lasala, D., et al. (2010). The discovery of potent inhibitors of aldosterone synthase that exhibit selectivity over 11-β-hydroxylase. *Bioorg. Med. Chem. Lett.* 20, 4324–4327. doi: 10.1016/j.bmcl.2010.06.086

Akram, M., Kaserer, T., and Schuster, D. (2015). "Pharmacophore modeling and pharmacophore-based virtual screening," in *In Silico Drug Discovery and Design*, ed C. N. Cavasotto (Boca Raton, FL: CRC Press), 123–153.

Azizi, M., Amar, L., and Menard, J. (2013). Aldosterone synthase inhibition in humans. *Nephrol. Dial. Trans.* 28, 36–43. doi: 10.1093/ndt/gfs388

Baell, J. B., and Holloway, G. A. (2010). New substructure filters for removal of pan assay interference compounds (PAINS) from screening libraries and for their exclusion in bioassays. *J. Med. Chem.* 53, 2719–2740. doi: 10.1021/jm901137j

Belkina, N. V., Lisurek, M., Ivanov, A. S., and Bernhardt, R. (2001). Modelling of three-dimensional structures of cytochromes P450 11B1 and 11B2. *J. Inorg. Biochem.* 87, 197–207. doi: 10.1016/S0162-0134(01)00331-2

Berman, H. M., Westbrook, J., Feng, Z., Gilliland, G., Bhat, T. N., Weissig, H., et al. (2000). The protein data bank. *Nucleic Acids Res.* 28, 235–242. doi: 10.1093/nar/28.1.235

Blass, B. (2013a). Aldosterone synthase inhibitors. *ACS Med. Chem. Lett.* 4, 375–376. doi: 10.1021/ml4000589

Blass, B. (2013b). Selective Cyp11B1 inhibitors for the treatment of cortisol dependent diseases. *ACS Med. Chem. Lett.* 4, 377–378. doi: 10.1021/ml4000595

Briet, M., and Schiffrin, E. L. (2010). Aldosterone: effects on the kidney and cardiovascular system. *Nat. Rev. Nephrol.* 6, 261–273. doi: 10.1038/nrneph.2010.30

Brilla, C. G. (2000). Aldosterone and myocardial fibrosis in heart failure. *Herz* 25, 299–306. doi: 10.1007/s000590050024

Bureik, M., Hübel, K., Dragan, C.-A., Scher, J., Becker, H., Lenz, N., et al. (2004). Development of test systems for the discovery of selective human aldosterone synthase (CYP11B2) and 11β-hydroxylase (CYP11B1) inhibitors: discovery of a new lead compound for the therapy of congestive heart failure, myocardial fibrosis and hypertension. *Mol. Cell. Endocrinol.* 217, 249–254. doi: 10.1016/j.mce.2003.10.027

Cain, D. W., and Cidlowski, J. A. (2017). Immune regulation by glucocorticoids. *Nat. Rev. Immunol.* 17, 233–247. doi: 10.1038/nri.2017.1

Cambridgesoft (1986–2015). *ChemBioDraw Ultra. 14.0 Edn*. Waltham, MA: Perkin Elmer.

Cereto-Massagué, A., Guasch, L., Valls, C., Mulero, M., Pujadas, G., and Garcia-Vallvé, S. (2012). DecoyFinder: an easy-to-use python GUI application for building target-specific decoy sets. *Bioinformatics* 28, 1661–1662. doi: 10.1093/bioinformatics/bts249

Chen, Z., Li, H.-L., Zhang, Q.-J., Bao, X.-G., Yu, K.-Q., Luo, X.-M., et al. (2009). Pharmacophore-based virtual screening versus docking-based virtual screening: a benchmark comparison against eight targets. *Acta Pharmacol. Sin.* 30, 1694–1708. doi: 10.1038/aps.2009.159

Denner, K., Doehmer, J., and Bernhardt, R. (1995a). Cloning of CYP11B1 and CYP11B2 from normal human adrenal and their functional expression in COS-7 and V79 Chinese hamster cells. *Endocr. Res.* 21, 443–448. doi: 10.3109/07435809509030460

Denner, K., Vogel, R., Schmalix, W., Doehmer, J., and Bernhardt, R. (1995b). Cloning and stable expression of the human mitochondrial cytochrome P45011B1 cDNA in V79 Chinese hamster cells and their application for testing of potential inhibitors. *Pharmacogenetics* 5, 89–96. doi: 10.1097/00008571-199504000-00005

Devore, N. M., and Scott, E. E. (2012). Structures of cytochrome P450 17A1 with prostate cancer drugs abiraterone and TOK-001. *Nature* 482, 116–119. doi: 10.1038/nature10743

Dorr, H. G., Kuhnle, U., Holthausen, H., Bidlingmaier, F., and Knorr, D. (1984). Etomidate: a selective adrenocortical 11 beta-hydroxylase inhibitor. *Klin. Wochenschr.* 62, 1011–1013. doi: 10.1007/BF01711722

Ehmer, P. B., Bureik, M., Bernhardt, R., Müller, U., and Hartmann, R. W. (2002). Development of a test system for inhibitors of human aldosterone synthase (CYP11B2): screening in fission yeast and evaluation of selectivity in V79 cells. *J. Steroid Biochem. Mol. Biol.* 81, 173–179. doi: 10.1016/S0960-0760(02)00056-0

Ehmer, P. B., Jose, J., and Hartmann, R. W. (2000). Development of a simple and rapid assay for the evaluation of inhibitors of human 17alpha-hydroxylase-C(17,20)-lyase (P450cl7) by coexpression of P450cl7 with NADPH-cytochrome-P450-reductase in *Escherichia coli. J. Steroid Biochem. Mol. Biol.* 75, 57–63. doi: 10.1016/S0960-0760(00)00137-0

Emmerich, J., Hu, Q., Hanke, N., and Hartmann, R. W. (2013). Cushing's syndrome: development of highly potent and selective CYP11B1 inhibitors of the (pyridylmethyl)pyridine type. *J. Med. Chem.* 56, 6022–6032. doi: 10.1021/jm400240r

Faggiano, A., Pivonello, R., Melis, D., Filippella, M., Di Somma, C., Petretta, M., et al. (2003). Nephrolithiasis in Cushing's disease: prevalence, etiopathogenesis, and modification after disease cure. *J. Clin. Endocrinol. Metab.* 88, 2076–2080. doi: 10.1210/jc.2002-021494

Ferlin, M. G., Carta, D., Bortolozzi, R., Ghodsi, R., Chimento, A., Pezzi, V., et al. (2013). Design, synthesis, and structure–activity relationships of azolylmethylpyrroloquinolines as nonsteroidal aromatase inhibitors. *J. Med. Chem.* 56, 7536–7551. doi: 10.1021/jm400377z

Gobbi, S., Hu, Q., Negri, M., Zimmer, C., Belluti, F., Rampa, A., et al. (2013). Modulation of cytochromes P450 with xanthone-based molecules: from aromatase to aldosterone synthase and steroid 11β-hydroxylase inhibition. *J. Med. Chem.* 56, 1723–1729. doi: 10.1021/jm301844q

Gobbi, S., Hu, Q., Zimmer, C., Engel, M., Belluti, F., Rampa, A., et al. (2016). Exploiting the chromone scaffold for the development of inhibitors of corticosteroid biosynthesis. *J. Med. Chem.* 59, 2468–2477. doi: 10.1021/acs.jmedchem.5b01609

Guengerich, F. P. (2007). Mechanisms of cytochrome P450 substrate oxidation: minireview. *J. Biochem. Mol. Toxicol.* 21, 163–168. doi: 10.1002/jbt.20174

Hartmann, R. W., Müller, U., and Ehmer, P. B. (2003). Discovery of selective CYP11B2 (aldosterone synthase) inhibitors for the therapy of congestive heart failure and myocardial fibrosis. *Eur. J. Med. Chem.* 38, 363–366. doi: 10.1016/S0223-5234(03)00049-7

Hawkins, P. C. D., and Nicholls, A. (2012). Conformer generation with OMEGA: learning from the data set and the analysis of failures. *J. Chem. Inf. Model.* 52, 2919–2936. doi: 10.1021/ci300314k

Hawkins, P. C. D., Skillman, A. G., Warren, G. L., Ellingson, B. A., and Stahl, M. T. (2010). Conformer generation with OMEGA: algorithm and validation using high quality structures from the protein databank and cambridge structural database. *J. Chem. Inf. Model.* 50, 572–584. doi: 10.1021/ci100031x

Heim, R., Lucas, S., Grombein, C. M., Ries, C., Schewe, K. E., Negri, M., et al. (2008). Overcoming undesirable CYP1A2 inhibition of pyridylnaphthalene-type aldosterone synthase inhibitors: influence of heteroaryl derivatization on potency and selectivity. *J. Med. Chem.* 51, 5064–5074. doi: 10.1021/jm800377h

Hille, U. E., Zimmer, C., Haupenthal, J., and Hartmann, R. W. (2011a). Optimization of the first selective steroid-11β-hydroxylase (CYP11B1) inhibitors for the treatment of cortisol dependent diseases. *ACS Med. Chem. Lett.* 2, 559–564. doi: 10.1021/ml100283h

Hille, U. E., Zimmer, C., Vock, C. A., and Hartmann, R. W. (2011b). First selective CYP11B1 inhibitors for the treatment of cortisol-dependent diseases. *ACS Med. Chem. Lett.* 2, 2–6. doi: 10.1021/ml100071j

Hoyt, S. B., Petrilli, W., London, C., Liang, G.-B., Tata, J., Hu, Q., et al. (2015). Discovery of triazole CYP11B2 inhibitors with *in vivo* activity in rhesus monkeys. *ACS Med. Chem. Lett.* 6, 861–865. doi: 10.1021/acsmedchemlett.5b00048

Hu, Q., Yin, L., and Hartmann, R. W. (2012). Selective dual inhibitors of CYP19 and CYP11B2: targeting cardiovascular diseases hiding in the shadow of breast cancer. *J. Med. Chem.* 55, 7080–7089. doi: 10.1021/jm3004637

Irwin, J. J., and Shoichet, B. K. (2005). ZINC – a free database of commercially available compounds for virtual screening. *J. Chem. Inf. Model.* 45, 177–182. doi: 10.1021/ci049714+

Johnstone, R. W., Ruefli, A. A., and Smyth, M. J. (2000). Multiple physiological functions for multidrug transporter P-glycoprotein? *Trends Biochem. Sci.* 25, 1–6. doi: 10.1016/S0968-0004(99)01493-0

Jones, G., Willett, P., and Glen, R. C. (1995). Molecular recognition of receptor sites using a genetic algorithm with a description of desolvation. *J. Mol. Biol.* 245, 43–53. doi: 10.1016/S0022-2836(95)80037-9

Jones, G., Willett, P., Glen, R. C., Leach, A. R., and Taylor, R. (1997). Development and validation of a genetic algorithm for flexible docking1. *J. Mol. Biol.* 267, 727–748. doi: 10.1006/jmbi.1996.0897

Kaserer, T., Beck, K., Akram, M., Odermatt, A., and Schuster, D. (2015). Pharmacophore models and pharmacophore-based virtual screening: concepts and applications exemplified on hydroxysteroid dehydrogenases. *Molecules* 20:19880. doi: 10.3390/molecules201219880

Kawamoto, T., Mitsuuchi, Y., Toda, K., Yokoyama, Y., Miyahara, K., Miura, S., et al. (1992). Role of steroid 11 beta-hydroxylase and steroid 18-hydroxylase in the biosynthesis of glucocorticoids and mineralocorticoids in humans. *Proc. Natl. Acad. Sci. U.S.A.* 89, 1458–1462. doi: 10.1073/pnas.89.4.1458

Krautscheid, Y., Senning, C. J. Å., Sartori, S. B., Singewald, N., Schuster, D., and Stuppner, H. (2014). Pharmacophore modeling, virtual screening, and *in vitro* testing reveal haloperidol, eprazinone, and fenbutrazate as neurokinin receptors ligands. *J. Chem. Inf. Model.* 54, 1747–1757. doi: 10.1021/ci500106z

Lagorce, D., Sperandio, O., Baell, J. B., Miteva, M. A., and Villoutreix, B. O. (2015). FAF-Drugs3: a web server for compound property calculation and chemical library design. *Nucleic Acids Res.* 43, W200–W207. doi: 10.1093/nar/gkv353

Lifton, R. P., Gharavi, A. G., and Geller, D. S. (2001). Molecular mechanisms of human hypertension. *Cell* 104, 545–556. doi: 10.1016/S0092-8674(01)00241-0

Lijnen, P., and Petrov, V. (2000). Induction of cardiac fibrosis by aldosterone. *J. Mol. Cell. Cardiol.* 32, 865–879. doi: 10.1006/jmcc.2000.1129

Lucas, S., Heim, R., Negri, M., Antes, I., Ries, C., Schewe, K. E., et al. (2008a). Novel Aldosterone synthase inhibitors with extended carbocyclic skeleton by a combined ligand-based and structure-based drug design approach. *J. Med. Chem.* 51, 6138–6149. doi: 10.1021/jm800683c

Lucas, S., Heim, R., Ries, C., Schewe, K. E., Birk, B., and Hartmann, R. W. (2008b). *In vivo* active aldosterone synthase inhibitors with improved selectivity: lead optimization providing a series of pyridine substituted 3,4-dihydro-1H-quinolin-2-one derivatives. *J. Med. Chem.* 51, 8077–8087. doi: 10.1021/jm800888q

Lucas, S., Negri, M., Heim, R., Zimmer, C., and Hartmann, R. W. (2011). Fine-tuning the selectivity of aldosterone synthase inhibitors: structure–activity and structure–selectivity insights from studies of heteroaryl substituted 1,2,5,6-tetrahydropyrrolo[3,2,1-ij]quinolin-4-one derivatives. *J. Med. Chem.* 54, 2307–2319. doi: 10.1021/jm101470k

Martin, R. E., Aebi, J. D., Hornsperger, B., Krebs, H.-J., Kuhn, B., Kuglstatter, A., et al. (2015). Discovery of 4-Aryl-5,6,7,8-tetrahydroisoquinolines as potent, selective, and orally active aldosterone synthase (CYP11B2) inhibitors: *in vivo* evaluation in rodents and cynomolgus monkeys. *J. Med. Chem.* 58, 8054–8065. doi: 10.1021/acs.jmedchem.5b00851

Meredith, E. L., Ksander, G., Monovich, L. G., Papillon, J. P. N., Liu, Q., Miranda, K., et al. (2013). Discovery and *in vivo* evaluation of potent dual CYP11B2 (Aldosterone Synthase) and CYP11B1 inhibitors. *ACS Med. Chem. Lett.* 4, 1203–1207. doi: 10.1021/ml400324c

Newell-Price, J., Trainer, P., Besser, M., and Grossman, A. (1998). The diagnosis and differential diagnosis of Cushing's syndrome and pseudo-Cushing's states. *Endocr. Rev.* 19, 647–672.

Nieman, L. K. (2002). Medical therapy of Cushing's disease. *Pituitary* 5, 77–82. doi: 10.1023/A:1022308429992

Ogishima, T., Shibata, H., Shimada, H., Mitani, F., Suzuki, H., Saruta, T., et al. (1991). Aldosterone synthase cytochrome P-450 expressed in the adrenals of patients with primary aldosteronism. *J. Biol. Chem.* 266, 10731–10734.

Orth, D. N. (1978). MEtyrapone is useful only as adjunctive therapy in cushing's disease. *Ann. Intern. Med.* 89, 128–130. doi: 10.7326/0003-4819-89-1-128

Pecori Giraldi, F., Moro, M., and Cavagnini, F. (2003). Gender-related differences in the presentation and course of Cushing's disease. *J. Clin. Endocrinol. Metab.* 88, 1554–1558. doi: 10.1210/jc.2002-021518

Pinto-Bazurco Mendieta, M. A. E., Hu, Q., Engel, M., and Hartmann, R. W. (2013). Highly potent and selective nonsteroidal dual inhibitors of CYP17/CYP11B2 for the treatment of prostate cancer to reduce risks of Cardiovascular diseases. *J. Med. Chem.* 56, 6101–6107. doi: 10.1021/jm400484p

Pitt, B., Zannad, F., Remme, W. J., Cody, R., Castaigne, A., Perez, A., et al. (1999). The effect of spironolactone on morbidity and mortality in patients with severe heart failure. *N. Engl. J. Med.* 341, 709–717. doi: 10.1056/NEJM199909023411001

Ramires, F. J. A., Sun, Y., and Weber, K. T. (1998). Myocardial fibrosis associated with aldosterone or angiotensin II administration: attenuation by calcium channel blockade. *J. Mol. Cell. Cardiol.* 30, 475–483. doi: 10.1006/jmcc.1997.0612

Rogers, D., and Hahn, M. (2010). Extended-connectivity fingerprints. *J. Chem. Inf. Model.* 50, 742–754. doi: 10.1021/ci100050t

Roumen, L., Peeters, J. W., Emmen, J. M. A., Beugels, I. P. E., Custers, E. M. G., De Gooyer, M., et al. (2010). Synthesis, biological evaluation, and molecular modeling of 1-Benzyl-1H-imidazoles as selective inhibitors of aldosterone synthase (CYP11B2). *J. Med. Chem.* 53, 1712–1725. doi: 10.1021/jm901356d

Savage, M. O., Lienhardt, A., Lebrethon, M. C., Johnston, L. B., Huebner, A., Grossman, A. B., et al. (2001). Cushing's disease in childhood: presentation, investigation, treatment and long-term outcome. *Horm. Res.* 55, 24–30. doi: 10.1159/000063459

Sayers, G. (1950). The adrenal cortex and homeostasis. *Phy. Rev.* 30, 241–320.

Schuster, D., Waltenberger, B., Kirchmair, J., Distinto, S., Markt, P., Stuppner, H., et al. (2010). Predicting cyclooxygenase inhibition by three-dimensional pharmacophoric profiling. Part I: model generation, validation and applicability in ethnopharmacology. *Mol. Inform.* 29, 75–86. doi: 10.1002/minf.200900071

Scior, T., Bender, A., Tresadern, G., Medina-Franco, J. L., Martínez-Mayorga, K., Langer, T., et al. (2012). Recognizing pitfalls in virtual screening: a critical review. *J. Chem. Inf. Model.* 52, 867–881. doi: 10.1021/ci200528d

Sergejew, T., and Hartmann, R. W. (1994). Pyridyl substituted benzocycloalkenes: new inhibitors of 17α-Hydroxylase/ 17,20-Lyase (P450 17α). *J. Enzyme Inhib. Med. Chem.* 8, 113–122. doi: 10.3109/14756369409020194

Soberman, J. E., and Weber, K. T. (2000). Spironolactone in congestive heart failure. *Curr. Hypertens. Rep.* 2, 451–456. doi: 10.1007/s11906-000-0027-x

Stefanachi, A., Favia, A. D., Nicolotti, O., Leonetti, F., Pisani, L., Catto, M., et al. (2011). Design, synthesis, and biological evaluation of imidazolyl derivatives of 4,7-disubstituted coumarins as aromatase inhibitors selective over 17-α-Hydroxylase/C17-20 lyase. *J. Med. Chem.* 54, 1613–1625. doi: 10.1021/jm101120u

Strushkevich, N., Gilep, A. A., Shen, L., Arrowsmith, C. H., Edwards, A. M., Usanov, S. A., et al. (2013). Structural insights into aldosterone synthase substrate specificity and targeted inhibition. *Mol. Endocrinol.* 27, 315–324. doi: 10.1210/me.2012-1287

Taymans, S. E., Pack, S., Pak, E., Torpy, D. J., Zhuang, Z., and Stratakis, C. A. (1998). Human CYP11B2 (Aldosterone Synthase) maps to chromosome 8q24.3. *J. Clin. Endocrinol. Metab.* 83, 1033–1036. doi: 10.1210/jcem.83.3.4801

Tritos, N. A., Biller, B. M. K., and Swearingen, B. (2011). Management of Cushing disease. *Nat. Rev. Endocrinol.* 7, 279–289. doi: 10.1038/nrendo.2011.12

Ulmschneider, S., Müller-Vieira, U., Klein, C. D., Antes, I., Lengauer, T., and Hartmann, R. W. (2005a). Synthesis and evaluation of (Pyridylmethylene)tetrahydronaphthalenes/-indanes and structurally modified derivatives: potent and selective inhibitors of aldosterone synthase. *J. Med. Chem.* 48, 1563–1575. doi: 10.1021/jm0492397

Ulmschneider, S., Müller-Vieira, U., Mitrenga, M., Hartmann, R. W., Oberwinkler-Marchais, S., Klein, C. D., et al. (2005b). Synthesis and evaluation of imidazolylmethylenetetrahydronaphthalenes and imidazolylmethyleneindanes: potent inhibitors of aldosterone synthase. *J. Med. Chem.* 48, 1796–1805. doi: 10.1021/jm049600p

Ulmschneider, S., Negri, M., Voets, M., and Hartmann, R. W. (2006). Development and evaluation of a pharmacophore model for inhibitors of aldosterone synthase (CYP11B2). *Bioorg. Med. Chem. Lett.* 16, 25–30. doi: 10.1016/j.bmcl.2005.09.059

Voets, M., Antes, I., Scherer, C., Müller-Vieira, U., Biemel, K., Barassin, C., et al. (2005). Heteroaryl-substituted naphthalenes and structurally modified derivatives: selective inhibitors of CYP11B2 for the treatment of congestive heart failure and myocardial fibrosis. *J. Med. Chem.* 48, 6632–6642. doi: 10.1021/jm0503704

Voets, M., Antes, I., Scherer, C., Müller-Vieira, U., Biemel, K., Marchais-Oberwinkler, S., et al. (2006). Synthesis and evaluation of heteroaryl-substituted dihydronaphthalenes and indenes: potent and selective inhibitors of aldosterone synthase (CYP11B2) for the treatment of congestive heart failure and myocardial fibrosis. *J. Med. Chem.* 49, 2222–2231. doi: 10.1021/jm060055x

Vuorinen, A., Nashev, L. G., Odermatt, A., Rollinger, J. M., and Schuster, D. (2014). Pharmacophore model refinement for 11β-hydroxysteroid dehydrogenase inhibitors: search for modulators of intracellular glucocorticoid concentrations. *Mol. Inform.* 33, 15–25. doi: 10.1002/minf.201300063

Wolber, G., and Langer, T. (2005). LigandScout: 3-D pharmacophores derived from protein-bound ligands and their use as virtual screening filters. *J. Chem. Inf. Model.* 45, 160–169. doi: 10.1021/ci049885e

Yin, L., Hu, Q., Emmerich, J., Lo, M. M.-C., Metzger, E., Ali, A., et al. (2014). Novel pyridyl- or isoquinolinyl-substituted indolines and indoles as potent and selective aldosterone synthase inhibitors. *J. Med. Chem.* 57, 5179–5189. doi: 10.1021/jm500140c

Yin, L., Hu, Q., and Hartmann, R. W. (2013). Tetrahydropyrroloquinolinone type dual inhibitors of aromatase/aldosterone synthase as a novel strategy for breast cancer patients with elevated cardiovascular risks. *J. Med. Chem.* 56, 460–470. doi: 10.1021/jm301408t

Yin, L., Lucas, S., Maurer, F., Kazmaier, U., Hu, Q., and Hartmann, R. W. (2012). Novel imidazol-1-ylmethyl substituted 1,2,5,6-tetrahydropyrrolo[3,2,1-ij]quinolin-4-ones as potent and selective CYP11B1 inhibitors for the treatment of Cushing's syndrome. *J. Med. Chem.* 55, 6629–6633. doi: 10.1021/jm3003872

Young, M., and Funder, J. W. (2000). Aldosterone and the heart. *Trends Endocrinol. Metab.* 11, 224–226. doi: 10.1016/S1043-2760(00)00270-8

Zhu, W., Chen, Z., Li, Q., Tan, G., and Hu, G. (2016). Inhibitors of 11beta-Hydroxylase (CYP11B1) for treating diseases related to excess cortisol. *Curr. Med. Chem.* 23, 623–633. doi: 10.2174/0929867323666160122114947

Zimmer, C., Hafner, M., Zender, M., Ammann, D., Hartmann, R. W., and Vock, C. A. (2011). N-(Pyridin-3-yl)benzamides as selective inhibitors of human aldosterone synthase (CYP11B2). *Bioorg. Med. Chem. Lett.* 21, 186–190. doi: 10.1016/j.bmcl.2010.11.040

5

An Efficient Implementation of the Nwat-MMGBSA Method to Rescore Docking Results in Medium-Throughput Virtual Screenings

*Irene Maffucci, Xiao Hu, Valentina Fumagalli and Alessandro Contini**

Dipartimento di Scienze Farmaceutiche, Sezione di Chimica Generale e Organica "Alessandro Marchesini," Università degli Studi di Milano, Milan, Italy

***Correspondence:**
Alessandro Contini
alessandro.contini@unimi.it

Nwat-MMGBSA is a variant of MM-PB/GBSA based on the inclusion of a number of explicit water molecules that are the closest to the ligand in each frame of a molecular dynamics trajectory. This method demonstrated improved correlations between calculated and experimental binding energies in both protein-protein interactions and ligand-receptor complexes, in comparison to the standard MM-GBSA. A protocol optimization, aimed to maximize efficacy and efficiency, is discussed here considering penicillopepsin, HIV1-protease, and BCL-XL as test cases. Calculations were performed in triplicates on both classic HPC environments and on standard workstations equipped by a GPU card, evidencing no statistical differences in the results. No relevant differences in correlation to experiments were also observed when performing Nwat-MMGBSA calculations on 4 or 1 ns long trajectories. A fully automatic workflow for structure-based virtual screening, performing from library set-up to docking and Nwat-MMGBSA rescoring, has then been developed. The protocol has been tested against no rescoring or standard MM-GBSA rescoring within a retrospective virtual screening of inhibitors of AmpC β-lactamase and of the Rac1-Tiam1 protein-protein interaction. In both cases, Nwat-MMGBSA rescoring provided a statistically significant increase in the ROC AUCs of between 20 and 30%, compared to docking scoring or to standard MM-GBSA rescoring.

Keywords: MM-GBSA, explicit water, molecular dynamics, GPU, structure based virtual screening, protease, protein-protein interactions

INTRODUCTION

Structure based virtual screening (SBVS) methods are widely applied in drug discovery (Enyedy and Egan, 2008; Sousa et al., 2013). In most of the cases, SBVSs are done in the hit-to-lead development phase of the drug discovery process, with multiple successful outcomes (Enyedy et al., 2001a,b; Vangrevelinghe et al., 2003). In SBVS-related studies, scoring functions are mostly applied for potential hit selection. In general, the scoring functions are based on either empirical, knowledge-based, or molecular mechanics force field derived potentials (Wang et al., 2003; Raha et al., 2007). Additionally, to make the virtual screening process computational inexpensive, the scoring functions are most likely simplified. Thus, some important contributions known to influence the binding affinity are neglected (Sousa et al., 2006; Moitessier et al., 2008). Inevitably, applications of such simplified methods tend to fail in the hit optimization phase, where more meticulous selections are required about structurally similar compounds for better prediction of biological activity (Leach et al., 2006; Tirado-Rives and Jorgensen, 2006; Warren et al., 2006; Enyedy and Egan, 2008).

A better scoring can be achieved by considering energy evaluation averaged over an ensemble of conformations from a complex dynamic trajectory, as is the underlying concept of the molecular mechanics Poisson-Boltzmann / Generalized Born surface area (MM-PB/GBSA) analysis. Of course, the applications of MM-PB/GBSA methods are at the cost of increased computational expenses (Massova and Kollman, 2000). Nonetheless, the MM-PB/GBSA methods have been successfully applied to estimate binding energies (Kollman et al., 2000), or incorporated as a scoring method in SBVS applications (Lyne et al., 2006; Zhou et al., 2006; Ferrari et al., 2007; Xiong et al., 2007; Xu et al., 2010; Xu, 2012; Knight et al., 2014). The treatment of the solvent in MM-PB/GBSA calculations is implicit, providing an acceptable estimations of the energy contribution while bulk water is the only solvent-related concern (Wong and Lightstone, 2011; Yang et al., 2013). However, explicit water molecules might also be important in forming biomolecular complexes (Chong and Ham, 2017), particularly waters involved in bridging the ligand and the receptor (Wong et al., 2009; Abel et al., 2011; Ahmad et al., 2011; Wallnoefer et al., 2011; Maffucci and Contini, 2013; Mikulskis et al., 2014). Indeed, by analyzing several thousand of crystallographic complexes, it was recently observed that at least a water molecule mediates contacts between the partners in about two thirds of all the considered systems (Hendlich et al., 2003). Thus, several computational methods were proposed to aid the identification of important water molecules in crystal structures (Raymer et al., 1997; García-Sosa et al., 2003; Amadasi et al., 2006). Moreover, although replacing a water molecule in the binding site is a generally accepted strategy to increase drug potency, it has been shown that better pharmacodynamic properties might be obtained by keeping a tightly bound water as a bridge between the ligand and the receptor (García-Sosa, 2013). The effects of targeting or displacing binding site waters in drug design can be rigorously assessed by free energy calculations (García-Sosa and Mancera, 2010), that however are still too demanding when libraries of hundreds of molecules need to be evaluated. Therefore, some approaches have been attempted to consider the contribution of water-mediated interactions into the ligand docking score (Young et al., 2007; Ricchiuto et al., 2008; Forli and Olson, 2012; Ross et al., 2012; Kumar and Zhang, 2013; Murphy et al., 2016) or into the MM-PB/GBSA estimated binding energy (Checa et al., 1997; Wong et al., 2009; Genheden et al., 2011; Wallnoefer et al., 2011; Greenidge et al., 2013; Maffucci and Contini, 2013).

In this framework, we developed a MM-PB/GBSA variant, that we refer as Nwat-MMGBSA, which provided good-to-excellent results in ranking the binding energies of different protein-ligand or protein-protein complexes (Maffucci and Contini, 2013, 2016). Nwat-MMGBSA is based on the inclusion of a number of explicit water molecules, that are selected to be the closest to the ligand in each frame of the MD trajectory and are included as part of the receptor during the analysis. In addition to our work (Maffucci and Contini, 2013, 2016), Aldeghi and coworkers recently validated, by a thorough statistical analysis, the use of this approach on bromodomains (Aldeghi et al., 2017). Compared to other methods that include explicit water in MM-PB/GBSA calculations, Nwat-MMGBSA might have some advantages. For instance, relevant explicit water might be selected from the crystal structure (Wong et al., 2009; Wallnoefer et al., 2011). However, this imply that high resolution crystal structures are available, while Nwat-MMGBSA calculations can be performed on receptor models obtained by other techniques, such as homology modeling or NMR. Moreover, crystallographic water sites might derive from the average electron density of several molecules competing for the same position (Schiffer and Hermans, 2003). Indeed, we previously observed that a water-bridge between the ligand and the receptor found in the crystal structure of topoisomerase I in complex with topotecan (Staker et al., 2002) was described by the competition of three different waters in a 4 ns MD trajectory (Maffucci and Contini, 2013). It was also reported that explicit water for MM-GB/PBSA calculations might be selected from MD simulations accordingly to their distance from the ligand (Zhu et al., 2014). In this case, the distance from the ligand atoms is fixed, while the number of waters is different in each snapshot selected for MM-PB/GBSA analysis. However, by comparing this method to Nwat-MMGBSA, where the number of selected water is constant among all snapshots, we observed that Nwat-MMGBSA provided a better correlation with experiments and a better reproducibility among multiple repetitions of the same calculation (Maffucci and Contini, 2016). In this work, aiming to make Nwat-MMGBSA suitable for rescoring ligands in low- to medium-throughput SBVS experiments, we optimized the protocol to improve its efficiency, without losing in accuracy. We selected penicillopepsin (James et al., 1992; Ding et al., 1998; Hou et al., 2011a), HIV1-protease mutants (Shen et al., 2010; Olajuyigbe et al., 2011) and BCL-X_L (Lessene et al., 2013) as test systems with known experimental data, either binding free energy (ΔG), inhibition constant (k_i), or IC_{50}. Our studies have shown improvements in the coefficient of determination to experimental data (r^2) ranging from 10 to 60%, depending on the number of explicit water molecules considered in the energy evaluation. Moreover, we assessed the Nwat-MMGBSA approach for SBVS rescoring performance in a ligand-protein interaction and a protein-protein interaction (PPI) scenario (AmpC β-lactamase and Rac1-Tiam1, respectively). In both cases, improved outcomes were observed compared to either docking scoring or to standard MM-GBSA rescoring. Furthermore, the complete SBVS workflow applied in this

Abbreviations: SBVS, structure based virtual screening; VS, virtual screening; ROC, receiving operator characteristic; AUC, area under curve; MD, molecular dynamics; MM-GBSA, molecular mechanics Generalized Born surface area; PPI, protein-protein interaction; SD, steepest descendent; CG, conjugated gradient; NVT, constant number of particles, volume and temperature; NPT, constant number of particles, pressure and temperature.

work, including Nwat-MMGBSA rescoring, is provided in the Supplementary Information as a set of bash and tcsh scripts that, together with working tutorials, should make it readily applicable to other biomolecular systems of interest.

METHODS

Preparation of Complexes

Crystal structures of the penicillopepsin [PDB codes: 1APU, 1APV, 1APT, 1APW (James et al., 1992), 2WEA, 2WEB, and 2WEC (Ding et al., 1998)] and HIV1-protease [PDB codes: 3NU3, 3NU4, 3NU5, 3NU6, 3NUJ, 3NU9, 3NUO (Shen et al., 2010), 3NDW, and 3NDX (Olajuyigbe et al., 2011)] complexes (Table S1) were obtained from RCSB Protein Databank (Figures S1, S2). However, for the BCL-X_L system, (Figure S3) only 3ZK6, 3ZLN, 3ZLO, and 3ZLR complexes were available as crystal structures (Lessene et al., 2013). Therefore, the starting structures of the unavailable complexes were reconstructed using MOE software (Molecular Operating Environment, v2016.08, 2016) starting from the available ones. Ligand partial charges were derived with the AM1-BCC method using the *antechamber* (Wang et al., 2006) software of AmberTools15 package (Case et al., 2014). All waters, ions and stabilizing agents present in the crystal structures were removed. The protonation state of every titratable residue within the complexes were assigned at physiological conditions using the Protonate-3D module of MOE.

MD Simulations

MD simulations were performed with the *pmemd.MPI* or *pmemd.cuda* (Götz et al., 2012; Salomon-Ferrer et al., 2013) modules, depending on the hardware (classical HPC environment or GPU equipped workstations, respectively), included in the Amber14 package (Case et al., 2014). The ff14SB (Maier et al., 2015) and the gaff (Wang et al., 2004) force fields were adopted for the protein and the ligand in all simulations respectively. In each complex, the total charge was neutralized by adding Na+ or Cl- ions, and the systems were solvated by an octahedral box of TIP3P water (Jorgensen et al., 1983), with a box size of 10 Å from the solute.

The equilibration and production protocols were updated to optimize performance, in respect to previous studies (Maffucci and Contini, 2013, 2016). The systems were initially relaxed by optimizing the position of hydrogens (1,000 cycles of steepest descent (SD) and 5,000 cycles of conjugated gradient (CG), up to a gradient of 0.01 kcal $mol^{-1} \cdot$ Å; restraints of 100 kcal·$mol^{-1} \cdot$ Å^2 were applied on heavy atoms) and of ions and waters (2,000 cycles of SD and 5000 cycles of CG up to a gradient of 0.1 kcal·mol^{-1}·Å; restraints of 50 kcal·mol^{-1}·Å^2 were applied on atoms other than ions and water). The solvent box was then equilibrated at 300 K by 100 ps of NVT and 100 ps of NPT simulation using a Langevin thermostat with a collision frequency of 2.0 ps^{-1} (restraints of 50 and 25 kcal·mol^{-1}·Å^2 were applied on the solute for NVT and NPT simulations, respectively). Successively, two cycles of restrained minimization (2500 cycles of steepest descent and 5,000 cycles of conjugated gradient, up to a gradient of 0.1 kcal mol^{-1} Å, with restraints of 25 and 10 kcal mol^{-1} Å^2 on backbone atoms, respectively) were performed. The systems were then heated up to 300 K in 6 steps ($\Delta T = 50$ K) of 5 ps each, where backbone restraints were gradually reduced from 10.0 to 5.0 kcal mol^{-1} Å^2. An equilibration of 1.6 ns was then performed by initially using the NVT ensemble (100 ps, ligand and backbone restraints = 5.0 kcal mol^{-1} Å^2) followed by NPT (1 step of 200 ps with ligand and backbone restraints = 5 kcal mol^{-1} Å^2, then 3 steps of 100 ps each reducing the ligand and backbone restraints from 5.0 to 1.0 kcal mol^{-1} Å^2, and finally 1 step of 500 ns with ligand and backbone restraints of 1.0 kcal mol^{-1} Å^2). The last equilibration step consisted in 500 ps of unrestrained NVT simulation. Finally, production runs were conducted under the NVT condition at 300 K for 1 or 4 ns. An electrostatic cutoff of 8.0 Å, PME (Darden et al., 1993) for long electrostatic interactions, and the SHAKE (Ryckaert et al., 1977) algorithm were applied to all the calculations. Three independent simulations were performed for each hardware set-up (GPU workstation or CPU HPC cluster). For the simulations performed on GPUs, the default single precision/fixed precision (SPFP) version of *pmemd.cuda* (Le Grand et al., 2013) was applied in all steps, except for geometry minimizations where the double precision/fixed precision (DPFP) version was adopted.

All MD production trajectories were processed by *cpptraj* for backbone RMSD analyses (Figures S4–S11), solute-solvent hydrogen bond (donor-acceptor distance cutoff at 4.0 Å, angle cutoff at 150°) and water density (grid analysis over a cubic box 50 Å × 50 Å × 50 Å, mesh = 0.5 Å, centered on ligands) analyses. Images of water density plots were obtained by using UCSF Chimera (Pettersen et al., 2004).

Nwat-MMGBSA Analyses

MM-GBSA and Nwat-MMGBSA analyses were performed with the *MMPBSA.py* script (Miller et al., 2012) of the AmberTools15 package. The analyses were conducted on either the 1st or the 4th ns of the production runs by selecting 100 frames evenly spaced out. The GB-Neck2 implicit solvent model (Nguyen et al., 2013) was chosen for the GB calculations and the salt molar concentration in solution was set at 0.15 M. Entropy was neglected in all calculations, since the benefits of including its contribution still remain controversial (Weis et al., 2006; Hou et al., 2011a; Wallnoefer et al., 2011; Yang et al., 2011) and normal mode calculations are also extremely time consuming. It should be noted that neglecting entropy, although acceptable when comparing ligands of similar size and structure (Kollman et al., 2000; Wang et al., 2001; Wong et al., 2009), might lead to errors when the analysis involves ligands that are structurally rather different (Oehme et al., 2012).

The *Nwat-MMGBSA* script (**Figure 1**) uses the *cpptraj* module of AmberTools15 to process the solvated MD trajectory. When Nwat > 0, the water molecules closest to the ligand were preserved while the remaining were stripped from the selected frames by using the *cpptraj* command *closest*. The total number of water molecules to be kept in the trajectory is given by the *Nwat* flag in the script input section (in this work, we evaluated Nwat = 10, 20, 30, 40, 50, 60, 70, 80, 90, or 100). The number of frames that are going to be selected from the original MD trajectory is defined by the *r* flag in the script input section, that

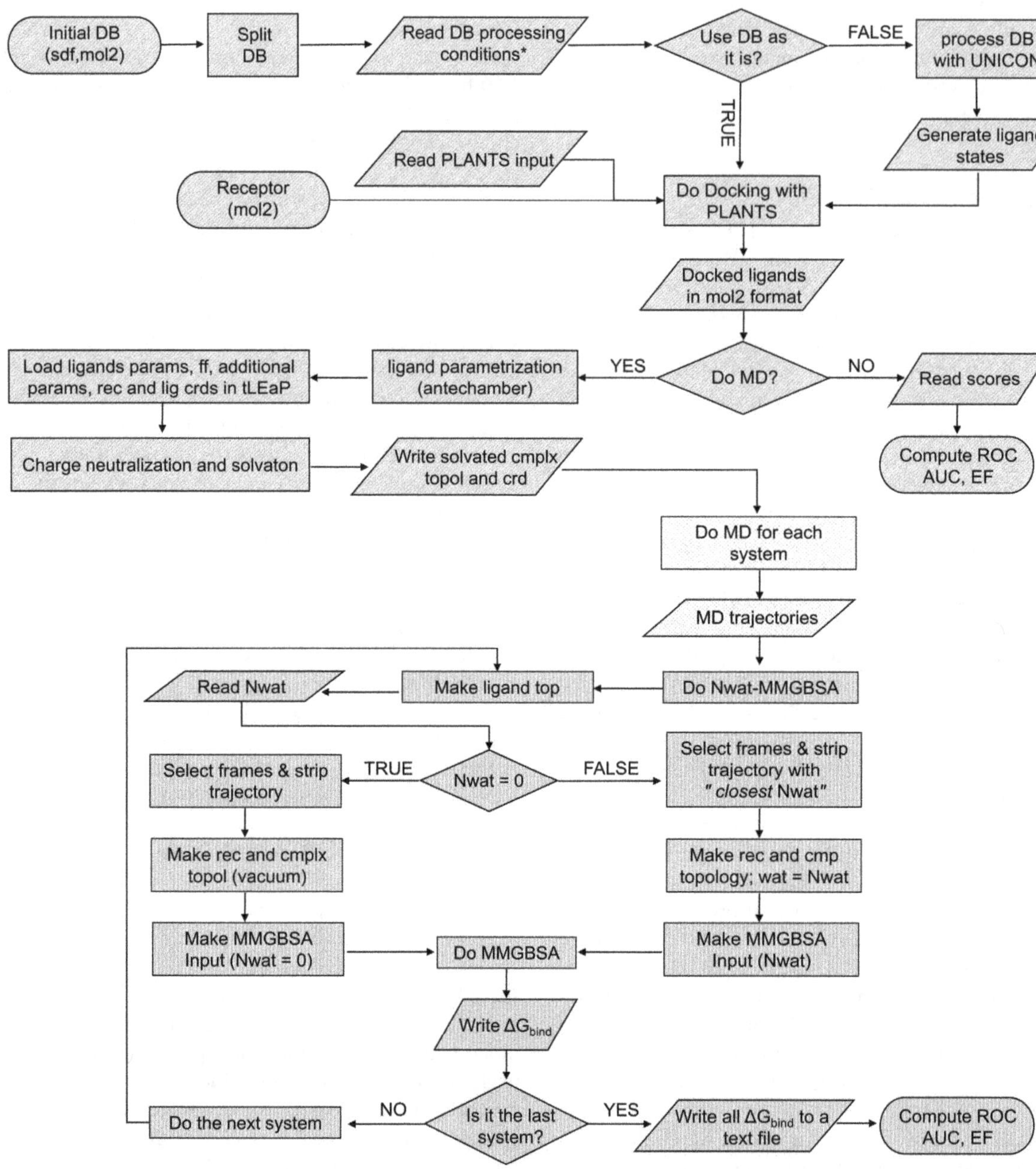

FIGURE 1 | Pseudocode of the complete screening and rescoring workflow. Each texture represents an independent script: VScreen (diagonal), autoMD (dots), and Nwat-MMGBSA (vertical).

corresponds to the *interval* keyword in the *MMPBSA.py* script (Miller et al., 2012). In this work, *r* was set at 10, meaning that one every 10 frames (i.e., 100 frames per nanosecond) was sampled. The preserved closest water molecules are considered as part of the receptor during the MM-GBSA analysis. In analogy with studies on the MM-PB/GBSA performance previously reported by us and by others (Hou et al., 2011b; Maffucci and Contini, 2013, 2016; Xu et al., 2013), the coefficient of determination (r^2) between experimental data and calculated binding energies was used as the evaluation metric.

Restrospective Virtual Screening

Preparation of the Receptor

The AmpC β-lactamase receptor was derived from the 2HDS PDB file (Babaoglu and Shoichet, 2006) according to what described on the DUD-E website (Mysinger et al., 2012). Starting from the crystal structure, only chain B was preserved, crystallographic water molecules were removed and the "Structure preparation" module of the MOE software was used to check the protein structure and correct eventual errors. The receptor was then capped by acetyl (ACE) and methylamino

(NME) groups at the N- and C-termini, respectively. Missing hydrogen atoms were added using the "Protonate 3D" function of the MOE package, considering a physiological pH. Partial charges were added accordingly to the AMBER10:EHT force field and solvation was treated with the Born model. The system geometry was then optimized up to a gradient of 0.1 kcal mol^{-1} Å, with protein backbone atoms restrained to the original position.

The Rac1 receptor, used in the VS simulation, was prepared as described elsewhere (Ferri et al., 2009, 2013a; Ruffoni et al., 2014).

AmpC β-Lactamase Testing Library

The DUD-E database provides 48 experimentally determined active ligands and 2850 decoy molecules for AmpC β-lactamase. However, considering the computational cost of rescoring by MD simulations followed by Nwat-MMGBSA analyses, we considered using a smaller library that decently represent the original database. Hence, fingerprint clustering methods included in MOE package were applied to reduce the size of the test set. Multiple fingerprint/similarity metric method combinations have been trial-and-error-ed. We found that the application of Typed Graph Triangle (TGT) fingerprint and Tanimoto Superset/Subset (tanimoto-ss) similarity metric method provides the closest reproduction of virtual screening results as the data provided by DUD-E. However, the combination applied here might not be directly transferred to other biomolecular systems. The clustering process reduced the original database to 20 active ligands and 378 decoys (Table S2) with a docking AUC at 74.82% and top 1% enrichment factor of 9.5, in comparison to the original 78.92% and 8.3 provided on DUD-E database. The smiles of the final database are reported in Table S2.

Rac1 Testing Library

By analyzing the literature and by using in-house data, we collected a set of 116 compounds, 10 of which were active and 106 inactive on the Rac1 protein (Table S3). The active compounds were selected among those able to inhibit at least the 50% of Rac1 activity, as assessed by G-LISA biochemical assays (Ferri et al., 2009, 2013a). Conversely, the decoys were chosen among molecules that were designed (or identified by computational screening) as Rac1 inhibitors, but turned out to be completely inactive on experimental evaluation (Ferri et al., 2009, 2013a; Hernández et al., 2010; Surviladze et al., 2010; Shang et al., 2012; Rahimi et al., 2015; Lu et al., 2017). The selected compounds were designed with MOE, minimized and subjected to a conformational search (MMFF94x force field, Born solvation, with the other parameters as default). The lowest energy conformation of each compound was selected to form the final test set.

Virtual Screening

The workflow included in the *VScreen* script (see Supplementary Information) allows the following combinations for library processing:

1) Use the library as it is
2) Generate tautomers
3) Generate stereoisomers and tautomers
4) Generate ring conformations and tautomers
5) Generate stereoisomers, ring conformations, and tautomers
6) Generate stereoisomers, ring conformations, tautomers, and protonation states.

The sixth library processing tandem was applied in this work. The UNICON software is used to generate tautomer and protonation states (Sommer et al., 2016). We chose the *topscoring* keyword to generate only the most favored tautomers and protomers, as in preliminary evaluation we observed that the generation of all tautomers and protomers (using the *ensemble* keyword) did not provide improved results and was significantly more time consuming. The SPORES software (ten Brink and Exner, 2009, 2010) is instead used to obtain stereoisomer and ring conformation, as well as for the final assignment of atom types, as requested by the PLANTS software (Korb et al., 2006, 2007, 2009, 2010) used for all dockings. Specific docking parameters, including search speed and scoring functions, can be set directly in the *VScreen* script. In the examples reported here, PLANTS was used in a low speed / high accuracy mode (search speed = *speed1*) and with the *CHEMPLP* scoring function (Korb et al., 2009). Additional PLANTS commands, such as H-bond or NMR constraints (Korb et al., 2010), can also be inserted in the input section of the *VScreen* script. Concerning the Rac1 example, we requested a H-bond constrain of 3 kcal/mol between any H-bond donor of the docking ligand and the carbonyl oxygen of Leu 70, since the literature evidence the importance of such ligand-receptor interaction for a proper activity (Montalvo-Ortiz et al., 2012; Ferri et al., 2013a; Ruffoni et al., 2014). Binding site radii were optimized to 16 Å for Rac1 and 7 Å for AmpC β-lactamase test sets, respectively. After the virtual screening process, the outcomes were ranked according to total $\text{PLANTS}_{\text{CHEMPLP}}$ score, using the top ranked pose of each ligand. Receiver operating characteristic (ROC) curves and corresponding area under curve (AUC) were then generated at the end of each docking run by using an R script integrated in the *VScreen* program.

Ligand Parameterization

Following the docking, automatized parametrization of ligands for later MD simulations can be enabled by setting the *doMD* keyword to 1. The user is allowed to choose a "top percentage" of the ranked ligands to be subjected to parametrization, by setting the *fract* keyword. We have chosen 100% (*fract* = 100), *i.e.*, the full test set, as we were interested in a full assessment of the Nwat-MMGBSA methods in terms of virtual screening rescoring. The *antechamber* software (Wang et al., 2006) of the AmberTools15 package is used for deriving AM1-BCC partial charges for each ligand and to assign atom types accordingly to the *gaff* force field (Jakalian et al., 2002; Wang et al., 2004). The quantum mechanical calculations necessary to perform the charge parameterization can be accomplished by using the default *sqm* software included in AmberTools15, or with MOPAC2016 (Stewart, 2016) by setting the *qm* keyword to 2 or 0, respectively. The topology and starting coordinate files of each complex are then generated by calling the *tleap* software, included in the AmberTools15 package. Each complex is neutralized and solvated by adding Na^+ or

Cl⁻ ions and a TIP3P water box of 10 Å from the solute. MD simulations and Nwat-MMGBSA analyses can then be performed as detailed in previous sections.

Nwat-MMGBSA analyses were performed on the obtained trajectories with number of closest water molecules set to 0, 30, 60, or 100. ROC curves and corresponding AUCs were evaluated by using the rankings derived from each Nwat-MMGBSA analysis.

All scripts applied in this work are available in the Supplement Materials. Eventual updates might also be requested to the authors.

RESULTS

Optimization of the Nwat-MMGBSA Protocol

To optimize the Nwat-MMGBSA protocol for low- or medium-throughput virtual screening procedures, such as those applied in the hit-to-lead optimization phase of a drug discovery process, we worked on a significant reduction of the overall simulation time in comparison to our previous implementations (Maffucci and Contini, 2013, 2016). Then, we integrated Nwat-MMGBSA in a continuous workflow that includes the library setup, docking and the preparation of complexes that is propaedeutic to MD, as shown in **Figure 1**. The following steps of the protocol were redesigned for an optimal ratio between accuracy and speed:

- The application of AM1-BBC charges to reduce the computational cost for ligand parameterizations. Indeed, it has been reported that AM1-BCC charges behaved fairly well in MM-PB/GBSA calculations, compared to more sophisticated methods (Xu et al., 2013; Sun et al., 2014).
- The use of the NVT ensemble instead of NPT for last equilibration step and production run. This allowed a 30% reduction on the overall MD simulation time, without a significant variation in the results.

Generalized Born (GB) implicit solvent model is used by default in Nwat-MMGBSA calculations. Indeed, several articles report that GB can provide outcomes comparable to the PB method, at a fraction of the computational cost, especially when relatively short MD trajectories are used for MM-PB/GBSA calculations (Hou et al., 2011a,b; Maffucci and Contini, 2013, 2015, 2016). However, the PB method can still be requested by the user by setting the *solv* keyword in the input section of the Nwat-MMGBSA script (see scripts and examples provided as Supplementary Information).

Moreover, the reproducibility between independent MD simulation repeats of the same system, especially when using GPU, was also improved. This required some protocol adjustments, including a longer equilibration of the solvent box, the use of geometric restraints instead of constraints, the use of the Langevin thermostat instead of the weak coupling algorithm, and a slightly extended final equilibration phase.

The protocol modifications allowed approximately 1.5 h per ligand on a standard workstation equipped with a single GeForce GTX TITAN Black card, including parameterization, minimization, equilibration, 1 ns of production run and Nwat-MMGBSA analysis. This is roughly the same time required for the simulation on a HPC architecture using 12 nodes equipped with two 2.40 GHz octa-core processors under similar simulation settings.

Considering our interest in using Nwat-MMGBSA calculations to rescore docking results in a reasonable time, the following tests were also designed to evidence any statistical difference in the correlation to experiment when the analysis is performed on 1 ns or 4 ns long MD trajectories. All the energies computed for the discussed examples are reported in Tables S4–S39. Correlations to experiments and statistical analyses are shown in Tables S40–S42 and Table S43, respectively.

Test on Penicillopepsin

This system was already evaluated, although with a different protocol, in a previous work where the bases of the Nwat-MMGBSA approach were described (Maffucci and Contini, 2013). The results of the Nwat-MMGBSA analysis obtained with the new protocol agreed with those reported in the

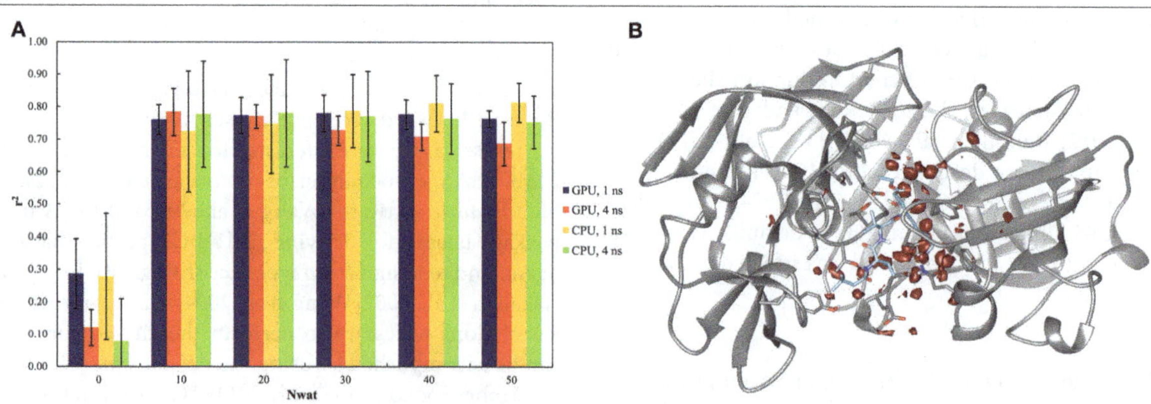

FIGURE 2 | Results of the penicillopepsin system regarding the application of Nwat-MMGBSA method. **(A)** Bar chart of r^2 in dependency at different Nwat and computational conditions. Nwat = 0 corresponds to a standard MM-GBSA calculation. **(B)** Water density plot obtained by grid analysis of penicillopepsin-1APT complex (visualization with Chimera, step = 1, level = 15).

previous work in terms of correlation between predicted and experimental binding energies (**Figure 2A** and Table S40). This confirms the robustness of the Nwat-MMGBSA method toward the modifications in the MD simulation conditions. However, the new protocol showed the beneficiary application of Nwat-MMGBSA method even when only 10 closest water molecules were considered (Nwat = 10), while in the previous evaluation no significant improvement was observed at this condition. Water density plot around the binding site (**Figure 2B**) confirm the role of water in mediating the ligand-receptor binding. Indeed, for this system, the use of the Nwat-MMGBSA methods allowed to increase the r^2 from about 0.3, obtained with the standard MM-GBSA approach (Nwat = 0), to about 0.8 (**Figure 2A**).

In addition, relatively low standard deviations, obtained when averaging the r^2 obtained by independent repetitions of the whole run, were observed when higher numbers of closest water molecules were considered (Table S40 and **Figure 2A**), thus suggesting that the inclusion of explicit waters is likely to improve the reproducibility of results from individual runs.

Moreover, the outcome obtained by running simulations on GPU and CPU hardware were statistically equivalent (Table S43), and the same was true for the analyses performed on either the 1st or the 4th ns of MD simulations (**Figure 2A**). This suggests that Nwat-MMGBSA analysis is suitable for the analysis of short MD simulations run on GPU cards, with a great improvement in speed and no impairments in accuracy.

Test on HIV1-Protease

Similarly to other aspartic proteases (Brik and Wong, 2003). HIV1-protease exhibits a close relationship with water-mediated bridging effects in the crystal structure (Shen et al., 2010). Consequently, the effects of explicit waters were also reflected by the Nwat-MMGBSA workflow (**Figure 3A**). The high water-density around a wide area at the binding site also confirms the likelihood of the involvement of explicit water during binding process (**Figure 3B**).

When considering the correlation between the experimental k_i and the predicted binding energies, a significant improvement in r^2 was obtained with the inclusion of a hydration shell of 30–70 water molecules (**Figure 3A** and Table S41). Although, results with a lower Nwat value showed no significant difference from standard MM-GBSA analyses, suggesting that smaller hydration shells around the ligand might have excluded certain solute-solvent interactions important for binding free energy estimations. However, water-mediated H-bond analyses showed that only one or two stable (occupancy > 20%) water-mediated interactions did involve the ligand, while majority of the bridging water molecules were found between protein residues (Tables S44, S45). Furthermore, crystallographic data provides that only 10–15 water molecules are generally present within 4 Å from the ligand molecules (Olajuyigbe et al., 2011). These imply potential conflicts between the lower numbers of the observed "stable" bridging water molecules to the evidently better binding free energy estimations when higher amount of closest explicit solvent (up to 70) is included. Such conflicts can only be explained when transient water bridges are considered. The averaged free energy contribution of these transient interactions is more likely been captured by Nwat-MMGBSA calculations, whereas not necessarily detectable through population distribution or electron density analyses. Indeed, for example, the inclusion of crystallographic water molecules up to 3.5 Å from the ligand did not provide a clear benefit over standard MM-PB/GBSA approach (Greenidge et al., 2013).

Similar to the penicillopepsin system, the outcomes did not show statistically significant differences between the 1st and 4th ns of MD simulations and were independent from the hardware. Apparently, 4 ns MD simulations performed using CPU averagely provided higher correlation to experiments for Nwat $\leq$ 20, although the high standard deviations make this result not statistically significant (**Figure 3A** and Table S41).

Test on BCL-X_L

The Nwat-MMGBSA trails up to 50 closest water molecules have no statistical difference from standard MM-GBSA calculations, despite of different hardware environment (**Figure 4A**). A lower water density was indeed observed around the ligand for BCL-X_L system (**Figure 4B**). This implies that explicit water molecules are playing a less important role in ligand binding,

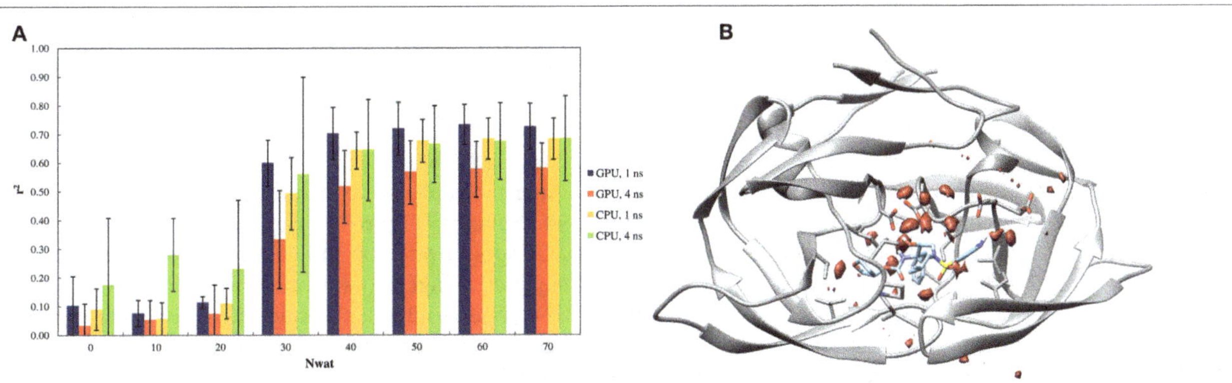

FIGURE 3 | (A) Trend of r^2 in dependency of Nwat for HIV1-protease. Nwat = 0 corresponds to a standard MM-GBSA calculation. **(B)** Water density plot obtained by grid analysis of HIV1-protease-3NUO complex (visualization with Chimera, step = 1, level = 15).

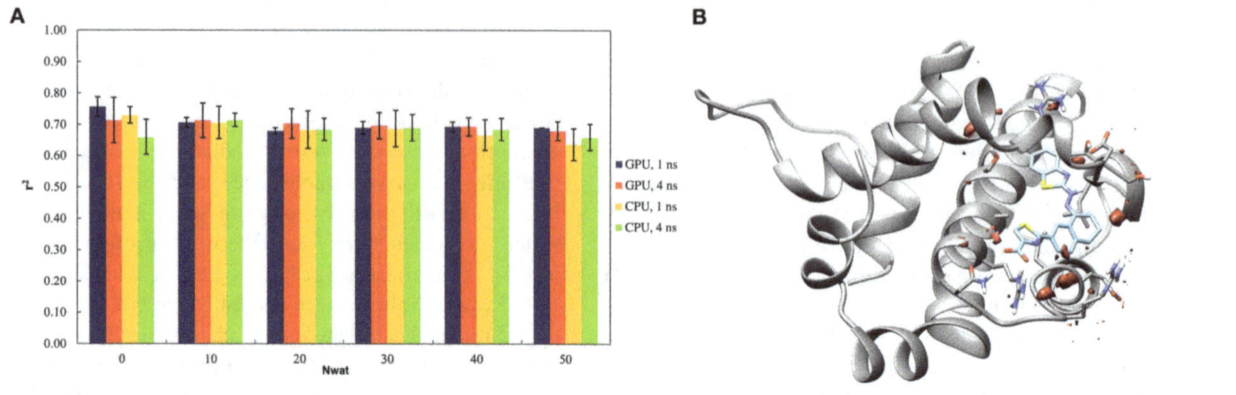

FIGURE 4 | (A) Trend of r^2 in dependency of Nwat for BCL-X_L. **(B)** Water density plot obtained by grid analysis of BCL-X_L-3ZC4 complex (visualization with Chimera, step = 1, level = 15).

as reflected by the relatively deluding performance of Nwat-MMGBSA compared to MM-GBSA. A relatively high r^2 (~0.7) was indeed consistent throughout the multiple trials for all of the conditions evaluated. These apparently non-effective results, however, positively suggest that the Nwat-MMGBSA method does not impair the statistical outcomes of the estimations for systems where explicit water molecules are deemed less important. Thus, it can be concluded that, even if system-specific tuning is necessary for optimal performance, Nwat-MMGBSA can be safe for binding free energy estimation even without an *a priori* knowledge of the bridging water in the system of interest.

Retrospective Virtual Screening Test

To assess the performance of the Nwat-MMGBSA method in rescoring virtual screening results, we have chosen two case studies for protein-ligand (PLI) and protein-protein (PPI) interactions, respectively. The first system, AmpC β-lactamase (Usher et al., 1998), was selected from the Dud-E database to provide an example were water plays an active role in the target catalytic cycle. Indeed, the inclusion of an explicit water molecule was found beneficial in previously reported virtual screenings (Powers et al., 2002). Conversely, the second system, the Rac1 protein targeted at the Tiam1 binding site (Worthylake et al., 2000), was chosen because of the availability of reliable in-house activity data, including those of several inactive compounds that were however selected as potential hits by virtual screening studies previously conducted (Ferri et al., 2009, 2013a).

The AUC of the ROC curves was chosen as the main metric of comparison, since enrichment values are not indicated for databases of limited sizes (Enyedy and Egan, 2008). For the AmpC system, the full virtual screening workflow, followed by MD simulation and Nwat-MMGBSA (Nwat = 0, 30, 60 and, for Rac1 only, 100) rescoring, was repeated twice, while for Rac1 a third repetition was added due to a higher variance among the obtained correlations. Docking scores and Nwat-MMGBSA binding energies for AmpC and Rac1 screenings are reported in Tables S46, S47 and Tables S48–S50, respectively.

TABLE 1 | ROC AUC values obtained at different scoring conditions for AmpC β-lactamase.

	Docking	Nwat0[a]	Nwat30	Nwat60
r^2 [b]	0.72 ± 0.00	0.76 ± 0.01	0.88 ± 0.01	0.88 ± 0.00
$P_{docking}$		0.019	0.002	<0.001[c]
P_{MMGBSA}			0.004	0.002
$\Delta\%_{docking}$		4.9	22.7	21.7
$\Delta\%_{MMGBSA}$			17.0	16.0

Percentage of variation ($\Delta\%_{docking}$ and $\Delta\%_{MMGBSA}$) and P values respect to ChemPLP scoring ($P_{docking}$) and to standard MM-GBSA rescoring (P_{MMGBSA}) are also reported.
[a]Corresponding to a standard MM-GBSA calculation, with no explicit waters included.
[b]Average of two full repetitions.
[c]0.00001.

AmpC β-Lactamase

The receptor in Dud-E include an explicit water molecule. We did preliminary docking evaluations by including the water, using the "water_molecule" function implemented in PLANTS, but comparable results were obtained (see Figure S12). For this reason, to simplify and standardize the procedure, we decided not to include any explicit water in the docking part of the virtual screening workflow.

We initially noticed that virtual screening has already provided a decent discrimination of active from decoys with a ROC AUC that averaged at 72.0% (**Table 1**). The application of the standard MM-GBSA method (Nwat = 0) only provided a barely significant increase of ROC AUC value, respect to docking (**Table 1**), while improvements appeared once explicit water molecules were included, as shown by the Nwat = 30 and 60 scenarios (**Figure 5**, Figure S15). Considering that the ROC AUCs for Nwat = 30 and 60 were fully converged, no additional analyses at higher Nwat values were done. Additionally, ligand-to-ligand correlations in calculated free energies were evaluated between the two repeated runs. The standard MM-GBSA run provides a r^2 of 0.66 when correlating the energies obtained by the two repetitions, while Nwat-MMGBSA with Nwat = 30 and 60 resulted in r^2 of 0.84 and 0.91, respectively (**Figure 6**). This implies that Nwat-MMGBSA rescoring is likely to provide

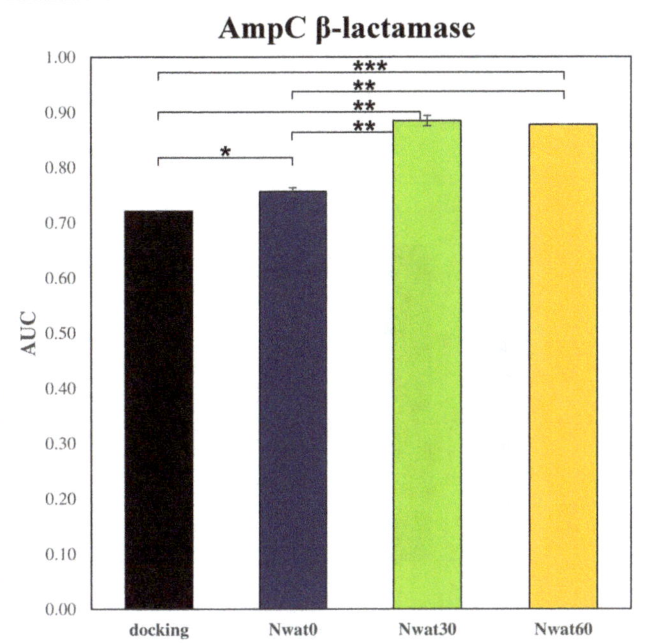

FIGURE 5 | Average ROC AUC values for AmpC β-lactamase. Statistical significance was calculated by *t*-test and is graphically reported only when a significant variation was observed (*$P < 0.05$; **$P < 0.01$; ***$P < 0.001$).

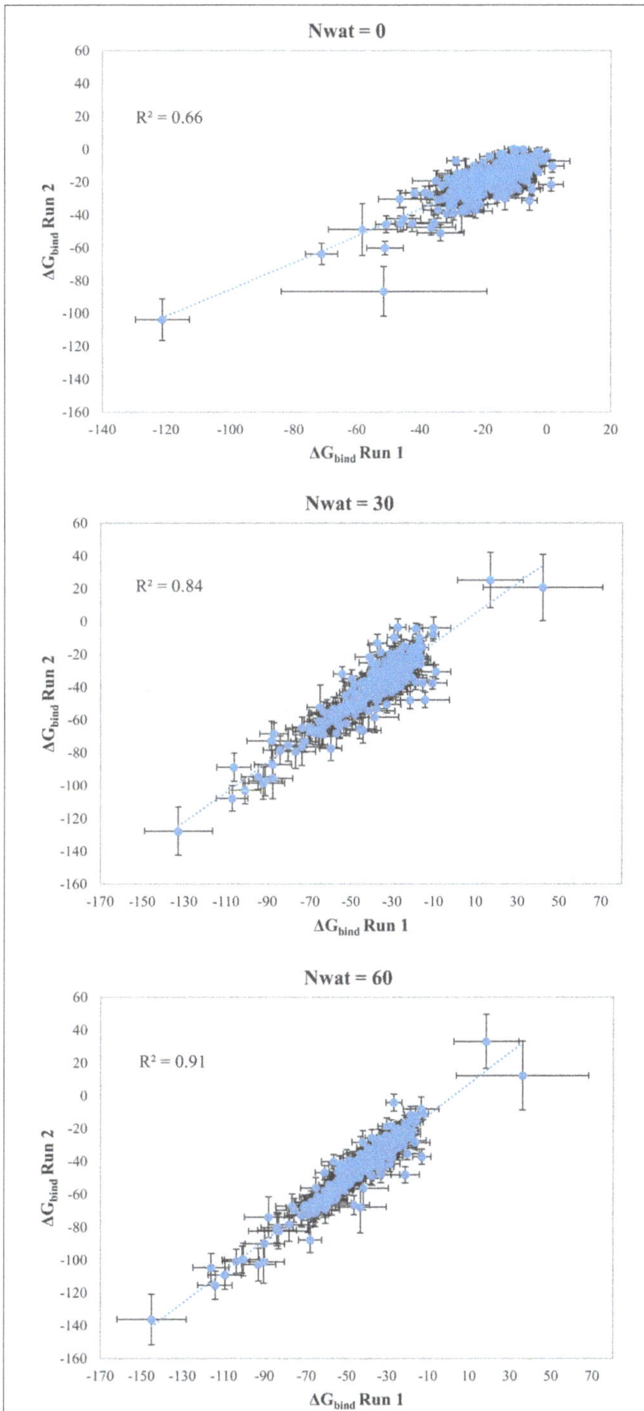

FIGURE 6 | Correlations between the binding energies computed in two independent repetitions (Run 1 and Run 2) for AmpC β-lactamase by standard MM-GBSA (Nwat = 0) or by Nwat-MMGBSA *with* Nwat = 30 or Nwat = 60.

better reproducibility between separate runs. Moreover, the good ligand-to-ligand inter-method correlation between Nwat = 60 and 30 (r^2 = 0.95 and 0.94 for runs 1 and 2, respectively; Figure S13) further confirmed the improvements in reproducibility. Interestingly, a positive binding energy was computed for two ligands by Nwat-MMGBSA calculations, but not by docking or standard MM-GBSA rescoring. The two ligands belong to the decoy set (ligands 088 and 179, Tables S46, S47) and are thus supposed to be poorly ranked. Indeed, by analyzing the binding modes of the decoy 088 (Figure S17), it can be observed that an isopropyl group overlaps with the position occupied by a water molecule present in the crystal structure (Babaoglu and Shoichet, 2006), but not explicitly considered during docking (see Methods). Conversely, decoy 179 does not overlap with the crystallographic water site (Figure S18). However, it can be observed that a solvent-exposed chloropropyl group overlaps to a position occupied by a hydrophilic amino acidic moiety of the crystallographic ligand. In both cases, it appears that Nwat-MMGBSA rescoring can correctly penalize compounds that do not offer an optimal orientation of hydrophobic groups.

Tiam1-Rac1 PPI Interface as the PPI Test Set

Virtual screening targeting PPIs has been suggested as a challenging task, especially when only traditional docking and scoring procedures are used (Bienstock, 2012; Scott et al., 2016). In the past, we have applied standard computational methods to identify and design inhibitors of the Rac1-Tiam1 PPI, thus collecting data on compounds identified as potential hits, but that turned out to be inactive upon experiments (Ferri et al., 2009, 2013a,b; Ruffoni et al., 2014). In addition, we searched the literature to identify compounds that were tested against Rac1 inhibition, but turned out to be inactive (Hernández et al., 2010; Surviladze et al., 2010; Shang et al., 2012; Rahimi et al., 2015; Lu et al., 2017). By this way, the resulting ligand test set

TABLE 2 | ROC AUC values obtained at different scoring conditions for the Rac1-Tiam1 system.

	Docking	Nwat0	Nwat30	Nwat60	Nwat100
$r^{2\,a}$	0.59 ± 0.00	0.56 ± 0.06	0.53 ± 0.04	0.71 ± 0.07	0.76 ± 0.06
$P_{docking}$		0.536	0.077	0.029	0.007
P_{MMGBSA}			0.520	0.045	0.016
$\Delta\%_{docking}$		−4.1	−9.2	21.4	29.1
$\Delta\%_{MMGBSA}$			−5.3	26.7	34.7

Percentage of variation ($\Delta\%_{docking}$ and $\Delta\%_{MMGBSA}$) and P-values respect to ChemPLP scoring ($P_{docking}$) and to standard MM-GBSA rescoring (P_{MMGBSA}) are also reported.
[a]Average of three full repetitions.

shared similar physico-chemical and structural features between the actives and the inactives, thus making this virtual screening a difficult discrimination process to tackle.

The docking protocol was optimized to maximize AUC by evaluating the effect of the different scoring functions available in PLANTS, by variating the binding site radius, the search speed and by using hydrogen bond constraints with residues known to be essential for activity (i.e., Leu70 or Ser71) (Gao et al., 2004). The docking poses were visually inspected to check their consistency with the poses obtained in previous studies (Ferri et al., 2013a). With the optimized protocol and for each library processing condition, all the active compounds showed a similar binding pose, except for ligand109 (Figure S14).

The ROC computed on the scores obtained by docking showed a moderate ability of this procedure in discriminating active from inactive compounds, with AUCs of about 0.6 (**Table 2**, **Figure 7**). Considering the strained characteristic of both the target and database, this result is acceptable, if compared to the ROC AUCs obtained in other benchmarks reported by literature (Brozell et al., 2012; Liebeschuetz et al., 2012; McGann, 2012; Neves et al., 2012; Novikov et al., 2012; Repasky et al., 2012; Schneider et al., 2012; Lavecchia and Di Giovanni, 2013; Yuriev et al., 2015).

This time, the application of the standard MM-GBSA (Nwat = 0) rescoring did not provide any significant improvement in the AUC compared to docking (**Table 2**). Unexpectedly, Nwat-MMGBSA performed with 30 water molecules (Nwat = 30) behaved similarly. Conversely, the ROC AUCs improved of about 20 and 30% after rescoring with Nwat = 60 or 100, respectively (**Table 2**, **Figure 7**, and Figure S16). Since the difference in AUC between the two last scenarios was not statistically significant, no additional simulations were conducted at higher Nwat. An improvement in the ROC AUC of about 20–30%, although reproducible and significant (Zhang et al., 2014), might be questionable against the increased computational effort of rescoring with either MM-GBSA or Nwat-MMGBSA. However, in the framework of a lead optimization study, the payback of a simulation that can be easily run on relatively inexpensive hardware can be an increased chance of synthesizing a good molecule. Considering the costs associated with the synthesis of new molecules, having even only a 20% higher probability of preparing an active compound can be considered a rather good result.

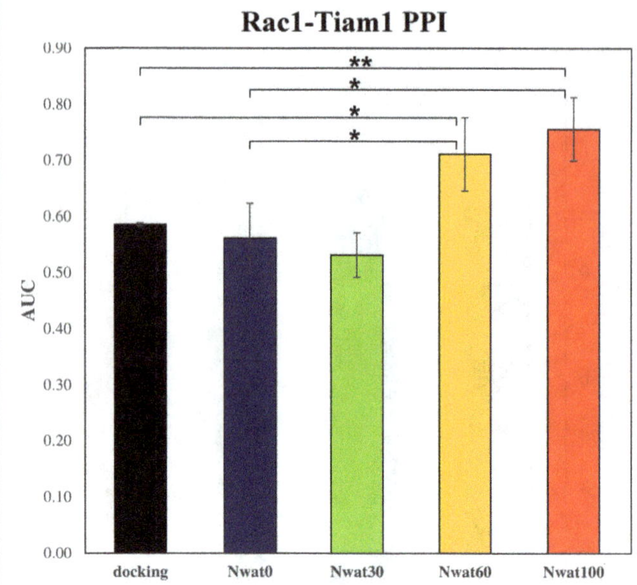

FIGURE 7 | Average ROC AUC values for Rac1-Tiam1 virtual screenings. Statistical significance was calculated by *t*-test and is graphically reported only when a significant variation was observed (*$P < 0.05$; **$P < 0.01$).

DISCUSSION

When developing new drugs, computational calculation can help in identifying new hits in either the hit-to-lead or lead optimization phases. While the first task is generally performed by using very fast computational methods to screen large databases, the lead optimization phase is generally done by applying more accurate, although more computationally demanding, methods. Indeed, starting from a lead, a virtual library of hundreds-to-thousands congeneric molecules can be generated and evaluated computationally. However, the prioritization of the synthesis of a few derivatives by computational methods might still be quite challenging. In this framework, we optimized a variant on the well-known MM-GBSA method, referred as Nwat-MMGBSA (Maffucci and Contini, 2013, 2016). This approach consists in the inclusion, during the MM-GBSA analysis, of a fixed number of water molecules, which in each frame of the MD simulation are the closest to the ligand, or to a binding interface, and are therefore potentially mediating interactions between the receptor and the ligand. We demonstrated that this approach might improve the correlation between predicted and experimental binding energies up to 50%, compared to the standard MM/GBSA method (corresponding to Nwat = 0), with only a modest increase in computation time (Maffucci and Contini, 2016). Of course, the potential improvement in correlation depends on the role played by water in facilitating the ligand-receptor binding. However, we also found that when water does not play a specific role in mediating this interaction, the application of Nwat-MMGBSA is not detrimental on the quality of correlation, compared to the default approach. In the light of this, we automatized the process and optimized the MD protocol for running simulations on standard workstations equipped with a GPU, on which a full calculation can be completed in about 1–2 h per complex, depending on system size. Indeed, the results obtained by using a single GPU card are comparable, in both quality and duration, with those obtained by running MDs on a relatively large HPC environment (12 nodes with 2 octa core processors per node). Moreover, we also observed that Nwat-MMGBSA analyses provided comparable results when applied on 1 or on 4 ns MD trajectories, thus making this simulation attractive for medium-throughput virtual screenings.

In the second part of this article, we described the integration of Nwat-MMGBSA as a method to rescore docking results in SBVS studies. By applying Nwat-MMGBSA rescoring (Nwat = 60 or 100) we obtained, in both the examples, an increase in the ROC AUCs of between 20 and 30%, compared to the docking scorings or default MM/GBSA (Nwat = 0), depending on the system. In the adopted conditions, we were able to process more than 20 compounds per day using a standard octa core workstation equipped by a single GPU. Although this might appear a quite long time, compared to the thousands of compounds that can be screened per day by docking, the investment becomes reasonable when considering the time and resources required for the synthesis of new molecules. Moreover, we can expect that the fast development of GPU hardware will make MD-based rescoring even faster in short time. Indeed, in 2010 we could run a MD simulation on a Rac1 complex at a speed of 8.7 ns/day on a Tesla C1060 card, while a few years later, the same simulation was run at a speed of 59.3 ns/day on a GeForce GTX TITAN Black card.

Unfortunately, we were not able to find an ideal number of water that need to be included during Nwat-MMGBSA rescoring. Indeed, while Nwat = 30 appeared to be reasonable in most of the examples, including those reported previously (Maffucci and Contini, 2013, 2016), it failed in the Rac1 VS example. Indeed, in this case, at least 60 waters were necessary to observe a significant improvement over docking and standard MM-GBSA, possibly due to the large and solvent-exposed nature of the Rac1 binding site. Conversely, it was recently reported that MM-PBSA calculations on a set of Mnk1 and Mnk2 inhibitors provided improved correlations to experiments only when including up to 10 water molecules (Kannan et al., 2017). This quite low number, compared to other examples, was justified by the rather small interface between Mnk1/Mnk2 kinases and the respective ligands.

AUTHOR CONTRIBUTIONS

AC coordinated the team, designed the scripts and performed the calculations on Rac1. IM performed the calculations on penicillopepsin, HIV1 and BCL-X_L. XH provided important updates to the VScreen script. VF performed the calculations on AmpC β-lactamase. IM, XH, and AC wrote the article.

FUNDING

This work was partially supported by the Italian Ministry of Education, University and Research (MIUR) through the FIRB—Programma 'Futuro in Ricerca' (grant No. RBFR087YAY), by the European Union's Horizon 2020 research and innovation programme under the Marie Skłodowska-Curie ITN-European Joint Doctorate grant agreement No. 675527 MOGLYNET-programme in Drug Discovery and Development, and by NVIDIA through the GPU Grant Program.

ACKNOWLEDGMENTS

We acknowledge the CINECA for high performance computer service and the MIUR for the Ph.D. scholarship that supported IM. We also acknowledge João Cavalheiro for having run calculations on the BCL-X_L example during his Erasmus Programme. Daniela Albo and Cecilia Carvoli are also acknowledged for their work during their BS theses.

REFERENCES

Abel, R., Salam, N. K., Shelley, J., Farid, R., Friesner, R. A., and Sherman, W. (2011). Contribution of explicit solvent effects to the binding affinity of small-molecule inhibitors in blood coagulation factor serine proteases. *ChemMedChem.* 6, 1049–1066. doi: 10.1002/cmdc.201000533

Ahmad, M., Gu, W., Geyer, T., and Helms, V. (2011). Adhesive water networks facilitate binding of protein interfaces. *Nat. Commun.* 2, 261–267. doi: 10.1038/ncomms1258

Aldeghi, M., Bodkin, M. J., Knapp, S., and Biggin, P. C. (2017). A statistical analysis on the performance of MMPBSA versus absolute binding free energy calculations: bromodomains as a case study. *J. Chem. Inf. Model.* 57, 2203–2221. doi: 10.1021/acs.jcim.7b00347

Amadasi, A., Spyrakis, F., Cozzini, P., Abraham, D. J., Kellogg, G. E., and Mozzarelli, A. (2006). Mapping the Energetics of Water–Protein and Water–Ligand Interactions with the "Natural" HINT Forcefield: Predictive Tools for Characterizing the Roles of Water in Biomolecules. *J. Mol. Biol.* 358, 289–309. doi: 10.1016/j.jmb.2006.01.053

Babaoglu, K., and Shoichet, B. K. (2006). Deconstructing fragment-based inhibitor discovery. *Nat. Chem. Biol.* 2, 720–723. doi: 10.1038/nchembio831

Bienstock, R. J. (2012). Computational drug design targeting protein-protein interactions. *Curr. Pharm. Des.* 18, 1240–1254. doi: 10.2174/138161212799436449

Brik, A., and Wong, C.-H. (2003). HIV-1 protease: mechanism and drug discovery. *Org. Biomol. Chem.* 1, 5–14. doi: 10.1039/b208248a

Brozell, S. R., Mukherjee, S., Balius, T. E., Roe, D. R., Case, D. A., and Rizzo, R. C. (2012). Evaluation of DOCK 6 as a pose generation and database enrichment tool. *J. Comput. Aided Mol. Des.* 26, 749–773. doi: 10.1007/s10822-012-9565-y

Case, D. A., Babin, V., Berryman, J. T., Betz, R. M., Cai, Q., Cerutti, D. S., et al. (2014). *AMBER 14.* University of California, (San Francisco, CA).

Checa, A., Ortiz, A. R., de Pascual-Teresa, B., and Gago, F. (1997). Assessment of solvation effects on calculated binding affinity differences: trypsin inhibition by flavonoids as a model system for congeneric series. *J. Med. Chem.* 40, 4136–4145. doi: 10.1021/jm970245v

Chong, S.-H., and Ham, S. (2017). Dynamics of hydration water plays a key role in determining the binding thermodynamics of protein complexes. *Sci. Rep.* 7, 8744–8753. doi: 10.1038/s41598-017-09466-w

Darden, T., York, D., and Pedersen, L. (1993). Particle mesh ewald: an N·log(N) method for ewald sums in large systems. *J. Chem. Phys.* 98, 10089–10092. doi: 10.1063/1.464397

Ding, J., Fraser, M. E., Meyer, J. H., Bartlett, P. A., and James, M. N. G. (1998). Macrocyclic inhibitors of penicillopepsin. II. X-ray crystallographic analyses of penicillopepsin complexed with a P3-P1 macrocyclic peptidyl inhibitor and with its two acyclic analogues. *J. Am. Chem. Soc.* 120, 4610–4621. doi: 10.1021/ja973714r

Enyedy, I. J., and Egan, W. J. (2008). Can we use docking and scoring for hit-to-lead optimization? *J. Comput. Aided Mol. Des.* 22, 161–168. doi: 10.1007/s10822-007-9165-4

Enyedy, I. J., Lee, S.-L., Kuo, A. H., Dickson, R. B., Lin, C.-Y., and Wang, S. (2001a). Structure-based approach for the discovery of bis-benzamidines as novel inhibitors of matriptase. *J. Med. Chem.* 44, 1349–1355. doi: 10.1021/jm000395x

Enyedy, I. J., Ling, Y., Nacro, K., Tomita, Y., Wu, X., Cao, Y., et al. (2001b). Discovery of small-molecule inhibitors of Bcl-2 through structure-based computer screening. *J. Med. Chem.* 44, 4313–4324. doi: 10.1021/jm010016f

Ferrari, A. M., Degliesposti, G., Sgobba, M., and Rastelli, G. (2007). Validation of an automated procedure for the prediction of relative free energies of binding on a set of aldose reductase inhibitors. *Bioorg. Med. Chem.* 15, 7865–7877. doi: 10.1016/j.bmc.2007.08.019

Ferri, N., Bernini, S. K., Corsini, A., Clerici, F., Erba, E., Stragliotto, S., et al. (2013a). 3-Aryl-N-aminoylsulfonylphenyl-1H-pyrazole-5-carboxamides: a new class of selective Rac inhibitors. *MedChemComm.* 4, 537–541. doi: 10.1039/C2MD20328F

Ferri, N., Contini, A., Bernini, S. K., and Corsini, A. (2013b). Role of small GTPase protein Rac1 in Cardiovascular diseases: development of new selective pharmacological inhibitors. *J. Cardiovasc. Pharmacol.* 62, 425–435. doi: 10.1097/FJC.0b013e3182a18bcc

Ferri, N., Corsini, A., Bottino, P., Clerici, F., and Contini, A. (2009). Virtual screening approach for the identification of new Rac1 inhibitors. *J. Med. Chem.* 52, 4087–4090. doi: 10.1021/jm8015987

Forli, S., and Olson, A. J. (2012). A force field with discrete displaceable waters and desolvation entropy for hydrated ligand docking. *J. Med. Chem.* 55, 623–638. doi: 10.1021/jm2005145

Gao, Y., Dickerson, J. B., Guo, F., Zheng, J., and Zheng, Y. (2004). Rational design and characterization of a Rac GTPase-specific small molecule inhibitor. *Proc. Natl. Acad. Sci. U.S.A.* 101, 7618–7623. doi: 10.1073/pnas.0307512101

García-Sosa, A. T. (2013). Hydration properties of ligands and drugs in protein binding sites: tightly-bound, bridging water molecules and their effects and consequences on molecular design strategies. *J. Chem. Inf. Model.* 53, 1388–1405. doi: 10.1021/ci3005786

García-Sosa, A. T., and Mancera, R. L. (2010). Free energy calculations of mutations involving a tightly bound water molecule and ligand substitutions in a ligand-protein complex. *Mol. Inform.* 29, 589–600. doi: 10.1002/minf.201000007

García-Sosa, A. T., Mancera, R. L., and Dean, P. M. (2003). WaterScore: a novel method for distinguishing between bound and displaceable water molecules in the crystal structure of the binding site of protein-ligand complexes. *J. Mol. Model.* 9, 172–182. doi: 10.1007/s00894-003-0129-x

Genheden, S., Mikulskis, P., Hu, L., Kongsted, J., Söderhjelm, P., and Ryde, U. (2011). Accurate predictions of nonpolar solvation free energies require explicit consideration of binding-site hydration. *J. Am. Chem. Soc.* 133, 13081–13092. doi: 10.1021/ja202972m

Götz, A. W., Williamson, M. J., Xu, D., Poole, D., Le Grand, S., and Walker, R. C. (2012). Routine microsecond molecular dynamics simulations with AMBER on GPUs. 1. generalized born. *J. Chem. Theory Comput.* 8, 1542–1555. doi: 10.1021/ct200909j

Greenidge, P. A., Kramer, C., Mozziconacci, J.-C., and Wolf, R. M. (2013). MM/GBSA binding energy prediction on the PDBbind data set: successes, failures, and directions for further improvement. *J. Chem. Inf. Model.* 53, 201–209. doi: 10.1021/ci300425v

Hendlich, M., Bergner, A., Günther, J., and Klebe, G. (2003). Relibase: Design and development of a database for comprehensive analysis of protein-ligand interactions. *J. Mol. Biol.* 326, 607–620. doi: 10.1016/S0022-2836(02)01408-0

Hernández, E., Dharmawardhane, S., De La Mota-Peynado, A., and Vlaar, C. (2010). Novel inhibitors of Rac1 in metastatic breast cancer. *P. R. Health Sci. J.* 29, 348–356. Available online at: http://prhsj.rcm.upr.edu/index.php/prhsj/article/view/451

Hou, T., Wang, J., Li, Y., and Wang, W. (2011a). Assessing the performance of the MM/PBSA and MM/GBSA methods. 1. The accuracy of binding free energy calculations based on molecular dynamics simulations. *J. Chem. Inf. Model.* 51, 69–82. doi: 10.1021/ci100275a

Hou, T., Wang, J., Li, Y., and Wang, W. (2011b). Assessing the performance of the molecular mechanics/Poisson Boltzmann surface area and molecular mechanics/generalized Born surface area methods. II. The accuracy of ranking poses generated from docking. *J. Comput. Chem.* 32, 866–877. doi: 10.1002/jcc.21666

Jakalian, A., Jack, D. B., and Bayly, C. I. (2002). Fast, efficient generation of high-quality atomic charges. AM1-BCC model: II. Parameterization and validation. *J. Comput. Chem.* 23, 1623–1641. doi: 10.1002/jcc.10128

James, M. N. G., Sielecki, A. R., and Moult, J. (1992). Crystallographic analysis of transition state mimics bound to penicillopepsin: difluorostatine- and difluorostatone-containing peptides. *Biochemistry* 31, 3872–3886. doi: 10.1021/bi00130a019

Jorgensen, W. L., Chandrasekhar, J., Madura, J. D., Impey, R. W., and Klein, M. L. (1983). Comparison of simple potential functions for simulating liquid water. *J. Chem. Phys.* 79, 926–935. doi: 10.1063/1.445869

Kannan, S., Pradhan, M. R., Cherian, J., Joseph, T. L., Poh, Z. Y., Hai Yan, Y., et al. (2017). Small Molecules Targeting the Inactive Form of the Mnk1/2 Kinases. *ACS Omega* 2, 7881–7891. doi: 10.1021/acsomega.7b01403

Knight, J. L., Krilov, G., Borrelli, K. W., Williams, J., Gunn, J. R., Clowes, A., et al. (2014). Leveraging data fusion strategies in multireceptor lead optimization MM/GBSA End-point methods. *J. Chem. Theory Comput.* 10, 3207–3220. doi: 10.1021/ct500189s

Kollman, P. A., Massova, I., Reyes, C., Kuhn, B., Huo, S., Chong, L., et al. (2000). Calculating structures and free energies of complex molecules: combining molecular mechanics and continuum models. *Acc. Chem. Res.* 33, 889–897. doi: 10.1021/ar000033j

Korb, O., Möller, H. M., and Exner, T. E. (2010). NMR-guided molecular docking of a protein-peptide complex based on ant colony optimization. *ChemMedChem* 5, 1001–1006. doi: 10.1002/cmdc.201000090

Korb, O., Stützle, T., and Exner, T. E. (2006). "PLANTS: application of ant colony optimization to structure-based drug design," in *Ant Colony Optimization and Swarm Intelligence. ANTS 2006. Lecture Notes in Computer Science,* Vol. 4150, eds M. Dorigo, L. M. Gambardella, M. Birattari, A. Martinoli, R. Poli, and T. Stützle (Berlin; Heidelberg: Springer), 247–258.

Korb, O., Stützle, T., and Exner, T. E. (2007). An ant colony optimization approach to flexible protein–ligand docking. *Swarm Intell.* 1, 115–134. doi: 10.1007/s11721-007-0006-9

Korb, O., Stützle, T., and Exner, T. E. (2009). Empirical scoring functions for advanced protein-ligand docking with PLANTS. *J. Chem. Inf. Model.* 49, 84–96. doi: 10.1021/ci800298z

Kumar, A., and Zhang, K. Y. J. (2013). Investigation on the effect of key water molecules on docking performance in CSARdock exercise. *J. Chem. Inf. Model.* 53, 1880–1892. doi: 10.1021/ci400052w

Lavecchia, A., and Di Giovanni, C. (2013). Virtual screening strategies in drug discovery: a critical review. *Curr. Med. Chem.* 20, 2839–2860. doi: 10.2174/09298673113209990001

Leach, A. R., Shoichet, B. K., and Peishoff, C. E. (2006). Prediction of protein-ligand interactions. Docking and scoring: successes and gaps. *J. Med. Chem.* 49, 5851–5855. doi: 10.1021/jm060999m

Le Grand, S., Götz, A. W., and Walker, R. C. (2013). SPFP: speed without compromise—A mixed precision model for GPU accelerated molecular dynamics simulations. *Comput. Phys. Commun.* 184, 374–380. doi: 10.1016/j.cpc.2012.09.022

Lessene, G., Czabotar, P. E., Sleebs, B. E., Zobel, K., Lowes, K. N., Adams, J. M., et al. (2013). Structure-guided design of a selective BCL-XL inhibitor. *Nat. Chem. Biol.* 9, 390–397. doi: 10.1038/nchembio.1246

Liebeschuetz, J. W., Cole, J. C., and Korb, O. (2012). Pose prediction and virtual screening performance of GOLD scoring functions in a standardized test. *J. Comput. Aided Mol. Des.* 26, 737–748. doi: 10.1007/s10822-012-9551-4

Lu, Q., Zhou, H., Chen, Y., and Friesland, A. (2017). *Cdc42 Inhibitor and Uses Thereof.* US9725417 B2.

Lyne, P. D., Lamb, M. L., and Saeh, J. C. (2006). Accurate prediction of the relative potencies of members of a series of kinase inhibitors using molecular docking and MM-GBSA scoring. *J. Med. Chem.* 49, 4805–4808. doi: 10.1021/jm060522a

Maffucci, I., and Contini, A. (2013). Explicit ligand hydration shells improve the correlation between MM-PB/GBSA binding energies and experimental activities. *J. Chem. Theory Comput.* 9, 2706–2717. doi: 10.1021/ct400045d

Maffucci, I., and Contini, A. (2015). "Tuning the solvation term in the MM-PBSA/GBSA binding affinity predictions," in *Frontiers in Computational Chemistry*, eds J. D. Madura and Z. Ul-Haq (Elsevier Inc.), 82–120.

Maffucci, I., and Contini, A. (2016). Improved computation of protein–protein relative binding energies with the Nwat-MMGBSA method. *J. Chem. Inf. Model.* 56, 1692–1704. doi: 10.1021/acs.jcim.6b00196

Maier, J. A., Martinez, C., Kasavajhala, K., Wickstrom, L., Hauser, K. E., and Simmerling, C. (2015). ff14SB: improving the accuracy of protein side chain and backbone parameters from ff99SB. *J. Chem. Theory Comput.* 11, 3696–3713. doi: 10.1021/acs.jctc.5b00255

Massova, I., and Kollman, P. A. (2000). Combined molecular mechanical and continuum solvent approach (MM-PBSA/GBSA) to predict ligand binding. *Perspect. Drug Discov. Des.* 18, 113–135. doi: 10.1023/A:1008763014207

McGann, M. (2012). FRED and HYBRID docking performance on standardized datasets. *J. Comput. Aided Mol. Des.* 26, 897–906. doi: 10.1007/s10822-012-9584-8

Mikulskis, P., Genheden, S., and Ryde, U. (2014). Effect of explicit water molecules on ligand-binding affinities calculated with the MM/GBSA approach. *J. Mol. Model.* 20:2273. doi: 10.1007/s00894-014-2273-x

Miller, B. R. I., Mcgee, T. D., Swails, J. M., Homeyer, N., Gohlke, H., and Roitberg, A. E. (2012). MMPBSA. py: an efficient program for end-state free energy calculations. *J. Chem. Theory Comput.* 8, 3314–3321. doi: 10.1021/ct300418h

Moitessier, N., Englebienne, P., Lee, D., Lawandi, J., and Corbeil, C. R. (2008). Towards the development of universal, fast and highly accurate docking/scoring methods: a long way to go. *Br. J. Pharmacol.* 153(Suppl.), S7–S26. doi: 10.1038/sj.bjp.0707515

Molecular Operating Environment, v2016.08 (2016). *Chemical Computing Group Inc.,* Montreal, QC, Canada, H3A 2R7.

Montalvo-Ortiz, B. L., Castillo-Pichardo, L., Hernández, E., Humphries-Bickley, T., De la Mota-Peynado, A., Cubano, L. A., et al. (2012). Characterization of EHop-016, novel small molecule inhibitor of Rac GTPase. *J. Biol. Chem.* 287, 13228–13238. doi: 10.1074/jbc.M111.334524

Murphy, R. B., Repasky, M. P., Greenwood, J. R., Tubert-Brohman, I., Jerome, S., Annabhimoju, R., et al. (2016). WScore: a flexible and accurate treatment of explicit water molecules in ligand–receptor docking. *J. Med. Chem.* 59, 4364–4384. doi: 10.1021/acs.jmedchem.6b00131

Mysinger, M. M., Carchia, M., Irwin, J. J., and Shoichet, B. K. (2012). Directory of useful decoys, enhanced (DUD-E): better ligands and decoys for better benchmarking. *J. Med. Chem.* 55, 6582–6594. doi: 10.1021/jm300687e

Neves, M. A. C., Totrov, M., and Abagyan, R. (2012). Docking and scoring with ICM: the benchmarking results and strategies for improvement. *J. Comput. Aided Mol. Des.* 26, 675–686. doi: 10.1007/s10822-012-9547-0

Nguyen, H., Roe, D. R., and Simmerling, C. (2013). Improved generalized born solvent model parameters for protein simulations. *J. Chem. Theory Comput.* 9, 2020–2034. doi: 10.1021/ct3010485

Novikov, F. N., Stroylov, V. S., Zeifman, A. A., Stroganov, O. V., Kulkov, V., and Chilov, G. G. (2012). Lead Finder docking and virtual screening evaluation with Astex and DUD test sets. *J. Comput. Aided Mol. Des.* 26, 725–735. doi: 10.1007/s10822-012-9549-y

Oehme, D. P., Brownlee, R. T. C., and Wilson, D. J. D. (2012). Effect of atomic charge, solvation, entropy, and ligand protonation state on MM-PB(GB)SA binding energies of HIV protease. *J. Comput. Chem.* 33, 2566–2580. doi: 10.1002/jcc.23095

Olajuyigbe, F. M., Demitri, N., and Geremia, S. (2011). Investigation of 2-fold disorder of inhibitors and relative potency by crystallizations of HIV-1 protease in ritonavir and saquinavir mixtures. *Cryst. Growth Des.* 11, 4378–4385. doi: 10.1021/cg200514z

Pettersen, E. F., Goddard, T. D., Huang, C. C., Couch, G. S., Greenblatt, D. M., Meng, E. C., et al. (2004). UCSF Chimera—A visualization system for exploratory research and analysis. *J. Comput. Chem.* 25, 1605–1612. doi: 10.1002/jcc.20084

Powers, R. A., Morandi, F., and Shoichet, B. K. (2002). Structure-Based Discovery of a Novel, Noncovalent Inhibitor of AmpC β-Lactamase. *Structure* 10, 1013–1023. doi: 10.1016/S0969-2126(02)00799-2

Raha, K., Peters, M. B., Wang, B., Yu, N., Wollacott, A. M., Westerhoff, L. M., et al. (2007). The role of quantum mechanics in structure-based drug design. *Drug Discov. Today* 12, 725–731. doi: 10.1016/j.drudis.2007.07.006

Rahimi, R., Mahdavi, M., Pejman, S., Zare, P., and Balalaei, S. (2015). Inhibition of cell proliferation and induction of apoptosis in K562 human leukemia cells by the derivative (3-NpC) from dihydro-pyranochromenes family. *Acta Biochim. Pol.* 62, 83–88. doi: 10.18388/abp.2014_825

Raymer, M. L., Sanschagrin, P. C., Punch, W. F., Venkataraman, S., Goodman, E. D., and Kuhn, L. A. (1997). Predicting conserved water-mediated and polar ligand interactions in proteins using a K-nearest-neighbors genetic algorithm. *J. Mol. Biol.* 265, 445–464. doi: 10.1006/jmbi.1996.0746

Repasky, M. P., Murphy, R. B., Banks, J. L., Greenwood, J. R., Tubert-Brohman, I., Bhat, S., et al. (2012). Docking performance of the glide program as evaluated on the Astex and DUD datasets: a complete set of glide SP results and selected results for a new scoring function integrating WaterMap and glide. *J. Comput. Aided Mol. Des.* 26, 787–799. doi: 10.1007/s10822-012-9575-9

Ricchiuto, P., Rocco, A. G., Gianazza, E., Corrada, D., Beringhelli, T., and Eberini, I. (2008). Structural and dynamic roles of permanent water molecules in ligand molecular recognition by chicken liver bile acid binding protein. *J. Mol. Recognit.* 21, 348–354. doi: 10.1002/jmr.908

Ross, G. A., Morris, G. M., and Biggin, P. C. (2012). Rapid and accurate prediction and scoring of water molecules in protein binding sites. *PLoS ONE* 7:e32036. doi: 10.1371/journal.pone.0032036

Ruffoni, A., Ferri, N., Bernini, S. K., Ricci, C., Corsini, A., Maffucci, I., et al. (2014). 2-Amino-3-(phenylsulfanyl)norbornane-2-carboxylate: an appealing scaffold for the Design of Rac1–Tiam1 protein–protein interaction inhibitors. *J. Med. Chem.* 57, 2953–2962. doi: 10.1021/jm401924s

Ryckaert, J.-P., Ciccotti, G., and Berendsen, H. J. C. (1977). Numerical integration of the cartesian equations of motion of a system with constraints: molecular dynamics of n-alkanes. *J. Comput. Phys.* 23, 327–341. doi: 10.1016/0021-9991(77)90098-5

Salomon-Ferrer, R., Götz, A. W., Poole, D., Le Grand, S., and Walker, R. C. (2013). Routine microsecond molecular dynamics simulations with AMBER on GPUs. 2. Explicit solvent particle mesh ewald. *J. Chem. Theory Comput.* 9, 3878–3888. doi: 10.1021/ct400314y

Schiffer, C., and Hermans, J. (2003). "Promise of advances in simulation methods for protein crystallography: implicit solvent models, time- averaging refinement, and quantum mechanical modeling," in *Methods in Enzymology*, eds C. W. Carter Jr, and R. M. Sweet (New York, NY: Elsevier Inc), 412–461.

Schneider, N., Hindle, S., Lange, G., Klein, R., Albrecht, J., Briem, H., et al. (2012). Substantial improvements in large-scale redocking and screening using the novel HYDE scoring function. *J. Comput. Aided Mol. Des.* 26, 701–723. doi: 10.1007/s10822-011-9531-0

Scott, D. E., Bayly, A. R., Abell, C., and Skidmore, J. (2016). Small molecules, big targets: drug discovery faces the protein–protein interaction challenge. *Nat. Rev. Drug Discov.* 15, 533–550. doi: 10.1038/nrd.2016.29

Shang, X., Marchioni, F., Sipes, N., Evelyn, C. R., Jerabek-Willemsen, M., Duhr, S., et al. (2012). Rational design of small molecule inhibitors targeting RhoA subfamily Rho GTPases. *Chem. Biol.* 19, 699–710. doi: 10.1016/j.chembiol.2012.05.009

Shen, C. H., Wang, Y. F., Kovalevsky, A. Y., Harrison, R. W., and Weber, I. T. (2010). Amprenavir complexes with HIV-1 protease and its drug-resistant mutants altering hydrophobic clusters. *FEBS J.* 277, 3699–3714. doi: 10.1111/j.1742-4658.2010.07771.x

Sommer, K., Friedrich, N.-O., Bietz, S., Hilbig, M., Inhester, T., and Rarey, M. (2016). UNICON: a powerful and easy-to-use compound library converter. *J. Chem. Inf. Model.* 56, 1105–1111. doi: 10.1021/acs.jcim.6b00069

Sousa, S. F., Fernandes, P. A., and Ramos, M. J. (2006). Protein-ligand docking: current status and future challenges. *Proteins* 65, 15–26. doi: 10.1002/prot.21082

Sousa, S. F., Ribeiro, A. J. M., Coimbra, J. T. S., Neves, R. P., Martins, S. A., Moorthy, N. S. H. N., et al. (2013). Protein-ligand docking in the new millennium–a retrospective of 10 years in the field. *Curr. Med. Chem.* 20, 2296–2314. doi: 10.2174/0929867311320180002

Staker, B. L., Hjerrild, K., Feese, M. D., Behnke, C. A., Burgin, A. B., and Stewart, L. (2002). The mechanism of topoisomerase I poisoning by a camptothecin analog. *Proc. Natl. Acad. Sci. U.S.A.* 99, 15387–15392. doi: 10.1073/pnas.242259599

Stewart, J. J. P. (2016). *Stewart Computational Chemistry, MOPAC2016*. Colorado Springs. Available online at: http://OpenMOPAC.net

Sun, H., Li, Y., Tian, S., Xu, L., and Hou, T. (2014). Assessing the performance of MM/PBSA and MM/GBSA methods. 4. Accuracies of MM/PBSA and MM/GBSA methodologies evaluated by various simulation protocols using PDBbind data set. *Phys. Chem. Chem. Phys.* 16, 16719–16729. doi: 10.1039/C4CP01388C

Surviladze, Z., Waller, A., Strouse, J. J., Bologa, C., Ursu, O., Salas, V., et al. (2010). "A potent and selective inhibitor of Cdc42 GTPase," in *Probe Reports from the NIH Molecular Libraries Program [Internet]* (Bethesda, MD: National Center for Biotechnology Information US), Available online at: https://www.ncbi.nlm.nih.gov/books/NBK51965/

ten Brink, T., and Exner, T. E. (2009). Influence of protonation, tautomeric, and stereoisomeric states on protein-ligand docking results. *J. Chem. Inf. Model.* 49, 1535–1546. doi: 10.1021/ci800420z

ten Brink, T., and Exner, T. E. (2010). pK(a) based protonation states and microspecies for protein-ligand docking. *J. Comput. Aided Mol. Des.* 24, 935–942. doi: 10.1007/s10822-010-9385-x

Tirado-Rives, J., and Jorgensen, W. L. (2006). Contribution of conformer focusing to the uncertainty in predicting free energies for protein-ligand binding. *J. Med. Chem.* 49, 5880–5884. doi: 10.1021/jm060763i

Usher, K. C., Blaszczak, L. C., Weston, G. S., Shoichet, B. K., and Remington, S. J. (1998). Three-dimensional structure of AmpC β-lactamase from *Escherichia coli* bound to a transition-state analogue: possible implications for the oxyanion hypothesis and for inhibitor design. *Biochemistry* 37, 16082–16092. doi: 10.1021/bi981210f

Vangrevelinghe, E., Zimmermann, K., Schoepfer, J., Portmann, R., Fabbro, D., and Furet, P. (2003). Discovery of a potent and selective protein kinase CK2 inhibitor by high-throughput docking. *J. Med. Chem.* 46, 2656–2662. doi: 10.1021/jm030827e

Wallnoefer, H. G., Liedl, K. R., and Fox, T. (2011). A challenging system: free energy prediction for factor Xa. *J. Comput. Chem.* 32, 1743–1752. doi: 10.1002/jcc.21758

Wang, J., Morin, P., Wang, W., and Kollman, P. A. (2001). Use of MM-PBSA in reproducing the binding free energies to HIV-1 RT of TIBO derivatives and predicting the binding mode to HIV-1 RT of efavirenz by docking and MM-PBSA. *J. Am. Chem. Soc.* 123, 5221–5230. doi: 10.1021/ja003834q

Wang, J., Wang, W., Kollman, P. A., and Case, D. A. (2006). Automatic atom type and bond type perception in molecular mechanical calculations. *J. Mol. Graph. Model.* 25, 247–260. doi: 10.1016/j.jmgm.2005.12.005

Wang, J., Wolf, R. M., Caldwell, J. W., Kollman, P. A., and Case, D. A. (2004). Development and testing of a general amber force field. *J. Comput. Chem.* 25, 1157–1174. doi: 10.1002/jcc.20035

Wang, R., Lu, Y., and Wang, S. (2003). Comparative evaluation of 11 scoring functions for molecular docking. *J. Med. Chem.* 46, 2287–2303. doi: 10.1021/jm0203783

Warren, G. L., Andrews, C. V., Capelli, A.-M., Clarke, B., LaLonde, J., Lambert, M. H., et al. (2006). A critical assessment of docking programs and scoring functions. *J. Med. Chem.* 49, 5912–5931. doi: 10.1021/jm050362n

Weis, A., Katebzadeh, K., Söderhjelm, P., Nilsson, I., and Ryde, U. (2006). Ligand affinities predicted with the MM/PBSA method: dependence on the simulation method and the force field. *J. Med. Chem.* 49, 6596–6606. doi: 10.1021/jm0608210

Wong, S., Amaro, R. E., and McCammon, J. A. (2009). MM-PBSA captures key role of intercalating water molecules at a protein-protein interface. *J. Chem. Theory Comput.* 5, 422–429. doi: 10.1021/ct8003707

Wong, S. E., and Lightstone, F. C. (2011). Accounting for water molecules in drug design. *Expert Opin. Drug Discov.* 6, 65–74. doi: 10.1517/17460441.2011.534452

Worthylake, D. K., Rossman, K. L., and Sondek, J. (2000). Crystal structure of Rac1 in complex with the guanine nucleotide exchange region of Tiam1. *Nature* 408, 682–688. doi: 10.1038/35047014

Xiong, Y., Li, Y., He, H., and Zhan, C.-G. (2007). Theoretical calculation of the binding free energies for pyruvate dehydrogenase E1 binding with ligands. *Bioorg. Med. Chem. Lett.* 17, 5186–5190. doi: 10.1016/j.bmcl.2007.06.095

Xu, D. (2012). *Autodock2MMGBSA, A Multi-Level Virtual Screening Rescoring and Refinement Scheme that Combines Consensus Scoring, Simulated Annealing and MM-GBSA Binding Free Energy Methods*. American Chemical Society (Washington, DC), NORM-153.

Xu, D., Sawaya, N., McCammon, J. A., and Li, W. W. (2010). *Autodock2MMGBSA, A Multi-Level Virtual Screening Rescoring and Refinement Scheme that Combines Consensus Scoring and MM-GBSA Binding Free Energy Methods*. American Chemical Society (Washington, DC), COMP-78.

Xu, L., Sun, H., Li, Y., Wang, J., and Hou, T. (2013). Assessing the performance of MM/PBSA and MM/GBSA methods. 3. The impact of force fields and ligand charge models. *J. Phys. Chem. B* 117, 8408–8421. doi: 10.1021/jp404160y

Yang, T., Wu, J. C., Yan, C., Wang, Y., Luo, R., Gonzales, M. B., et al. (2011). Virtual screening using molecular simulations. *Proteins* 79, 1940–1951. doi: 10.1002/prot.23018

Yang, Y., Lightstone, F. C., and Wong, S. E. (2013). Approaches to efficiently estimate solvation and explicit water energetics in ligand binding: the use of WaterMap. *Expert Opin. Drug Discov.* 8, 277–287. doi: 10.1517/17460441.2013.749853

Young, T., Abel, R., Kim, B., Berne, B. J., and Friesner, R. A. (2007). Motifs for molecular recognition exploiting hydrophobic enclosure in protein-ligand binding. *Proc. Natl. Acad. Sci. U.S.A.* 104, 808–813. doi: 10.1073/pnas.0610202104

Yuriev, E., Holien, J., and Ramsland, P. A. (2015). Improvements, trends, and new ideas in molecular docking: 2012-2013 in review. *J. Mol. Recognit.* 28, 581–604. doi: 10.1002/jmr.2471

Zhang, X., Wong, S. E., and Lightstone, F. C. (2014). Toward fully automated high performance computing drug discovery: a massively parallel virtual screening pipeline for docking and molecular mechanics/generalized born surface area rescoring to improve enrichment. *J. Chem. Inf. Model.* 54, 324–337. doi: 10.1021/ci4005145

Zhou, Z., Bates, M., and Madura, J. D. (2006). Structure modeling, ligand binding, and binding affinity calculation (LR-MM-PBSA) of human heparanase for inhibition and drug design. *Proteins* 65, 580–592. doi: 10.1002/prot.21065

Zhu, Y.-L., Beroza, P., and Artis, D. R. (2014). Including explicit water molecules as part of the protein structure in MM/PBSA calculations. *J. Chem. Inf. Model.* 54, 462–469. doi: 10.1021/ci4001794

6

Discovery of Novel Bovine Viral Diarrhea Inhibitors Using Structure-Based Virtual Screening on the Envelope Protein E2

Mariela Bollini[1], Emilse S. Leal[1], Natalia S. Adler[2], María G. Aucar[2], Gabriela A. Fernández[1], María J. Pascual[3], Fernando Merwaiss[3], Diego E. Alvarez[3] and Claudio N. Cavasotto[2*]*

[1] Laboratorio de Química Medicinal, Centro de Investigaciones en Bionanociencias, Consejo Nacional de Investigaciones Científicas y Técnicas, Ciudad de Buenos Aires, Argentina, [2] Laboratory of Computational Chemistry and Drug Design, Instituto de Investigación en Biomedicina de Buenos Aires, Consejo Nacional de Investigaciones Científicas y Técnicas, Partner Institute of the Max Planck Society, Ciudad de Buenos Aires, Argentina, [3] Instituto de Investigaciones Biotecnológicas, Universidad Nacional de San Martín, Consejo Nacional de Investigaciones Científicas y Técnicas, San Martín, Argentina

***Correspondence:**
Mariela Bollini
mariela.bollini@cibion.conicet.gov.ar
Claudio N. Cavasotto
cnc@cavasotto-lab.net;
ccavasotto@ibioba-mpsp-conicet.gov.ar

orcid.org/0000-0002-1372-0379

Bovine viral diarrhea virus (BVDV) is a member of the genus Pestivirus within the family Flaviviridae. BVDV causes both acute and persistent infections in cattle, leading to substantial financial losses to the livestock industry each year. The global prevalence of persistent BVDV infection and the lack of a highly effective antiviral therapy have spurred intensive efforts to discover and develop novel anti-BVDV therapies in the pharmaceutical industry. Antiviral targeting of virus envelope proteins is an effective strategy for therapeutic intervention of viral infections. We performed prospective small-molecule high-throughput docking to identify molecules that likely bind to the region delimited by domains I and II of the envelope protein E2 of BVDV. Several structurally different compounds were purchased or synthesized, and assayed for antiviral activity against BVDV. Five of the selected compounds were active displaying IC_{50} values in the low- to mid-micromolar range. For these compounds, their possible binding determinants were characterized by molecular dynamics simulations. A common pattern of interactions between active molecules and aminoacid residues in the binding site in E2 was observed. These findings could offer a better understanding of the interaction of BVDV E2 with these inhibitors, as well as benefit the discovery of novel and more potent BVDV antivirals.

Keywords: BVDV entry inhibitors, structure-based virtual screening, molecular dynamics simulation, envelope protein, molecular docking

INTRODUCTION

Bovine viral diarrhea virus (BVDV) is a worldwide distributed pathogen of cattle. Together with classical swine fever virus (CSFV) and border disease virus (BDV) of sheep, BVDV belongs to the genus Pestivirus of the Flaviviridae family. The pestiviral genome is a positive, single-stranded RNA molecule of about 12.3 kb in length encoding a single polyprotein that is processed into individual viral proteins: Npro -C-Erns -E1-E2-p7-NS2-NS3-NS4A-NS4B-NS5A-NS5B (Collett et al., 1988). Pestivirus particles consist of a lipid bilayer with envelope glycoproteins Erns, E1, and E2 surrounding the nucleocapsid, composed by the capsid protein C and the RNA genome (Callens et al., 2016). BVDV infection is distributed worldwide resulting in major economic losses to the livestock industry. The virus is primarily a pathogen of cattle and the clinical manifestations are presented as acute infection, fetal infection, or mucosal disease (Lanyon et al., 2014). Based on genetic and antigenic differences, BVDV is segregated into genotypes 1 and 2. For each of these genotypes, cytopathic and non-cytopathic biotypes are distinguished according to the capacity of virus infection to induce cell death in culture (Ridpath, 2003). Non cytopathic (ncp) BVDV biotypes cause acute infections in adult animals and can be transmitted across the placenta to the fetus. Fetal infection is particularly relevant and it can lead to congenital malformations and abortion, or to the birth of persistently infected (PI) calves that spread and maintain the disease in cattle populations (Lanyon et al., 2014). Cytopathic (cp) BVDV biotypes arise in PI cattle from recombination events in the infecting ncpBVDV genome, and are associated with the development of fatal mucosal disease (Becher and Tautz, 2011).

Control and prevention of BVDV infection should combine systematic vaccination with detection and culling of persistently infected cattle from herds (Newcomer and Givens, 2013). However, immunization is complicated due to the wide antigenic diversity of the virus, and fails to target the emergence of persistently infected animals (Fulton et al., 2003; Newcomer et al., 2017). Previous studies showed that antivirals directed against the pestivirus polymerase NS5B provide immediate protection from viral challenge (Newcomer et al., 2012), thus prophylactic treatment with antivirals represents an alternative for therapeutic intervention in outbreaks of BVDV.

Computer-aided drug design has become an integral part of drug discovery and development in the pharmaceutical and biotechnology industry, and is nowadays extensively used in lead identification and optimization (Cavasotto and Orry, 2007; Jorgensen, 2009; Spyrakis and Cavasotto, 2015). Virus envelope proteins are attractive targets for the development of antiviral agents, and structure-based drug design has been successfully used to identify small molecule ligands of envelope proteins that block entry of flaviviruses (Zhou et al., 2008; Kampmann et al., 2009; Leal et al., 2017). With the aim of finding novel targets for pestivirus drug design, we focused on the *in silico* identification of antivirals directed against the envelope protein E2 of BVDV. E2 mediates receptor recognition on the cell surface and is required for fusion of virus and cell membranes after the endocytic uptake of the virus during entry (Ronecker et al., 2008; Wang et al., 2009). In this work, we expand on a structure-based approach to seek hit small-molecules that dock into the druggable pocket at the interface between domains I and II of the envelope protein E2 of BVDV (Pascual et al., 2018). Around a million compounds from different chemical libraries were screened in a high-throughput docking (HTD) fashion. This led to the selection of nineteen lead candidates that were either purchased or synthesized, and evaluated in a reporter-based assay for antiviral activity. The likely interaction of active compounds with the protein E2 was further characterized by molecular dynamics (MD) simulations. The approach presented here led to the identification of five of novel compounds with anti-BVDV activity displaying IC_{50} values in the low to mid-micromolar range.

MATERIALS AND METHODS

Computational Chemistry

Molecular System Preparation

All simulations were based on the crystal structure of the pestivirus of the envelope glycoprotein E2 from BVDV (PDB 2YQ2) (El Omari et al., 2013). Protein domains were designated from the N- to the C-terminus of E2 as I, II and III according to the nomenclature used by Li et al. (2013). The molecular system was described in terms of torsional coordinates using the ECEPP/3 force field (Nemethy et al., 1992) as implemented in the ICM program (version 3.7-2c, MolSoft LLC, La Jolla, CA; Abagyan et al., 1994), and prepared in a similar fashion as earlier works (He et al., 2012; Brand et al., 2013; Leal et al., 2017; Pascual et al., 2018). Hydrogen atoms were added to the receptor structure followed by local energy minimization. All Asp and Glu residues were assigned a −1 charge, and all Arg and Lys residues were assigned a +1 charge. Histidine tautomers were assigned according to the hydrogen bonding pattern.

High-Throughput Docking

As in an earlier work (Pascual et al., 2018), docking was performed within Site I located at the interface of domains I and II of E2. All water molecules and co-factors were deleted. A flexible-ligand:rigid-receptor docking methodology as implemented in ICM was used. The receptor was represented by six potential energy maps, while the docked molecule was considered flexible and subjected to global energy minimization within the field of the receptor using a Monte Carlo protocol (Abagyan et al., 1994; Cavasotto et al., 2006); thus, the intra- and inter-molecular energy of the molecule are minimized. Each molecule was assigned an empirical docking score according to its fit within the binding site (Totrov et al., 2001). Two independent runs of HTD were performed to improve convergence of the global optimization energy, while the best score per molecule was kept.

Small-Molecule Libraries and Filtering

The ZINC (Irwin and Shoichet, 2005) (accessed Nov. 2014), Maybridge (http://www.maybridge.com/), and in house databases were chosen for HTD. They were first filtered to remove the compounds containing inorganic atoms, PAINS (Filtering Pan-assay interfering substances) structures, and other reactive groups. Then the complete virtual library was pre-filtered for properties based on Lipinski's rules (Lipinski et al., 1997). Finally about a total of one million small-molecules were used. The PAINS filter was implemented through the online server FAF-Drugs3 (Lagorce et al., 2015).

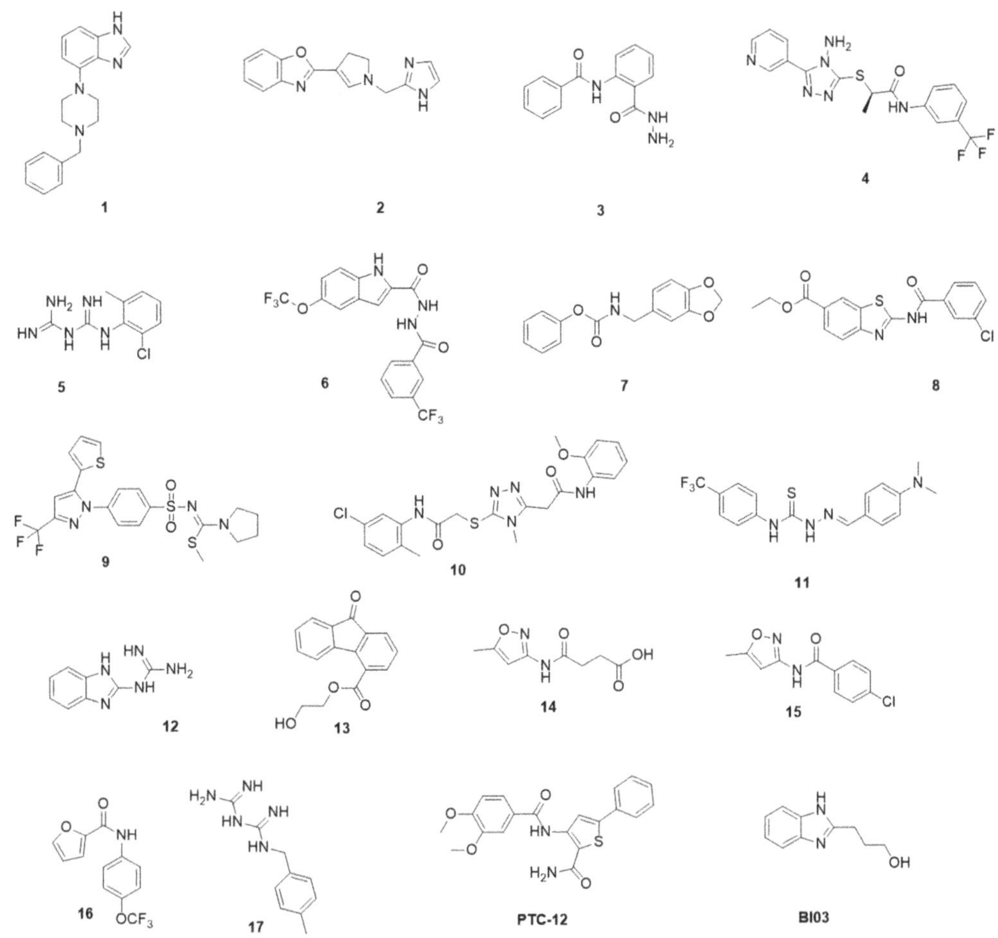

FIGURE 1 | Chemical structures of the **19** hits from docking-based virtual screening.

Molecular Dynamics

MD simulations were performed using GROMACS v5.1 package (Abraham et al., 2015) using the Amber99SB force field (Hornak et al., 2006). The system was solvated with the SPCE water model in a triclinic box, extending 10 Å from the protein, and neutralized adding sufficient NaCl counter ions to reach 0.15 M concentration. Bond lengths were constrained using the LINCS algorithm allowing a 2 fs time-step. Long-range electrostatics interactions were taken into account using the particle-mesh Ewald (PME) approach. The non-bonded cut-off for Coulomb and Van der Waals interactions were both 10 Å, and the non-bonded pair list was updated every 25 fs. Energy minimization was conducted through the steepest-descent algorithm, until the maximum force decayed to 1,000 [kJ mol^{-1} nm^{-1}]. Then an equilibration of the whole system was performed by 500 of NVT simulation followed by 500 ps of NPT simulation. Temperature was kept constant at 300 K using a modified Berendsen thermostat (Berendsen et al., 1984) with a coupling constant of 0.1 ps. Constant pressure of 1 bar was applied in all directions with a coupling constant of 2.0 ps and a compressibility of 4.5 10^{-5} bar^{-1}.

Biological Evaluation

Cell Culture

MDBK cells (Bos taurus kidney, ATCC CCL-22) were purchased from ATCC and grown in Dulbecso's modified Eagle medium (DMEM) supplemented with 10% fetal bovine serum and antibiotics under 5% CO2 at 37°C. For infections, cells were cultivated in DMEM supplemented with 2% Horse serum and antibiotics under 5% CO2 at 37°C.

Cytotoxicity Assay

Cell viability assays were performed on confluent cell cultures in 96 well plates (~15,000 cells per well). For each compound, cells were treated with serial dilutions of the compound in quadruplicates and incubated at 37°C for 3 days. Then, cell viability was measured using crystal violet staining. Briefly, cells were fixed with 10% formaldehyde, stained with crystal violet solution (20% Ethanol, 0.1% Crystal Violet), and after washing, the absorbance at 595 nm was recorded for each well in a spectrophotometer. Assays were conducted at least in duplicates, and the cytotoxic concentration 50 (CC_{50}) was estimated by a nonlinear regression fitting of five data points as the compound

TABLE 1 | Antiviral activity against BVDV.

Compound	$IC_{50}(\mu M)^a$ BVDV	CC_{50} $(\mu M)^b$
1	NA	>50
2	44.3 ± 10.3	>50
3	NA	>50
4	30.1 ± 2.9	>50
5	NA	>50
6	ND	7.2 ± 1.3
7	NA	>50
8	20.2 ± 3.6	>50
9	NA	>50
10	NA	>50
11	23.9 ± 7.9	>50
12	44.4 ± 11.5	>50
13	NA	61.5±1.4
14	NA	>50
15	NA	>50
16	NA	49.8 ± 1.5
17	NA	>50
BI03[c]	17.6 ± 6.4	>200
PTC12[c]	0.30 ± 0.10	89.5 ± 1.1

[a]*IC_{50}: inhibitory concentration 50%. Data represent the mean and standard deviation of at least two independent experiments.*

[b]*CC_{50}: cytotoxic concentration 50%. Data represent the mean and standard deviation of at least two independent experiments.*

[c]*Pascual et al. (2018).*

NA indicates assayed but not active compounds; ND Not determined.

concentration necessary to reduce cell viability by 50% compared to control non-treated cells.

Reporter-Based Assay for Antiviral Activity

Antiviral activity was evaluated in a reporter-based assay using a recombinant virus expressing GFP, cpBVDV/Npro GFP (Pascual et al., 2018). MDBK cells were seeded onto 24 well plates, infected with cpBVDV/Npro GFP at a multiplicity of infection of 0.1 in the presence of increasing concentrations of compounds. At 48 h post-infection cells were thoroughly washed, lifted with trypsin 0.05% and fixed using 4% paraformaldehyde in PBS. The fluorescence signal was measured using a flow cytometer (CyFlow® Space, Partec) at a detection spectrum of 488 nm. Data were analyzed in the FlowJo 7.6.2 software package. The inhibitory concentrations 50 (IC50s) for the compounds tested in the assay were calculated from curves constructed by plotting the percentage of infected cells versus the concentration of compound as the compound concentration necessary to reduce the number of infected cells by 50% compared to control non-treated cells.

Chemistry

General Information

NMR spectra were recorded on Bruker Biospin 600 MHz AVIII600, Bruker advance II 500 MHZ and Bruker 300 MHZ spectrometers at room temperature. Chemical shifts (δ) are reported in ppm and coupling constants (J) in Hertz. Column chromatography was carried out employing Merck silica gel (Kieselgel 60, 63–200 μm). Precoated silica gel plates F-254 were used for thin-layer analytical chromatography. The mass spectrometer utilized was a Xevo G2S QTOF (Waters Corporation, Manchester, UK) with an electrospray ionization (ESI) source. The mass spectrometer was operated in positive and negative ion modes with probe capillary voltages of 2.5 and 2.3 kV, respectively. The purity (≥95%) of all final synthesized compounds was determined by reverse phase HPLC, using a Waters 2487 dual λ absorbance detector with a Waters 1,525 binary pump and a Phenomenex Luna 5 μ C18(2) 250 × 4.6 mm column. Samples were run at 1 mL/min using gradient mixtures of 5–100% of water with 0.1% trifluoroacetic acid (TFA) (A) and 10:1 acetonitrile:water with 0.1% TFA (B) for 22 min followed by 3 min at 100% B. UV spectra were measured with a Shimadzu 3600 UV/vis/NIR spectrophotometer.

Synthetic Procedures of New Compounds From Our in House Library

Synthesis of (E)-2-(4-(dimethylamino)benzylidene)-N-(4-(trifluoromethyl)phenyl)hydrazinecarbothioamide (11)

Synthesis of N-(4-trifluoromethoxyphenyl)hydrazinecarbothioamide (**19**) Sodium hydroxide (0.14 g, 3.4 mmol) and carbon disulphide (0.2 mL, 2.8 mmol) were added to a solution of 4-(trifluoromethoxy)aniline **18** (0.50 g, 2.8 mmol) in DMF (5 mL). The mixture was stirred at room temperature for 1 h. Then, hydrazine hydrate (0.5 mL, 8.5 mmol) was added and stirring continued at 70°C for 1 h. After water addition compound **19** precipitate and the solid was filtrated off. The crude was recristallized from ethanol:water (0.28 g, 39.1 %). ^{1}H NMR (500 MHz, $CDCl_3$) δ 9.30 (s, 1H), 7.82 (s, 1H), 7.68 (d, J = 7.1 Hz, 2H), 7.24 (d, J = 8.7 Hz, 2H), 4.01 (s, 2H). To a solution of **19** (0.10 g; 0.40 mmol) in ethanol (3 mL) was added 4-dimethylaminobenzaldehyde (0. 65 g, 0.44 mmol). The mixture was stirred under reflux for 1 h. The reaction was then cooled to room temperature, and precipitate solid was filtered and washed with cyclohexane to give **11**, which was recristallized from ethanol. (0.07 g, 43.5 %). ^{1}H NMR (600 MHz, $CDCl_3$) δ 9.37 (s, 1H), 9.20 (s, 1H), 7.79 (s, 1H), 7.76 (dd, J = 8.9, 2.1 Hz, 2H), 7.57 (dd, J = 8.9, 2.1 Hz, 2H), 7.27 (d, J = 8.5 Hz, 2H), 6.72 (dd, J = 8.9, 1.9 Hz, 2H), 3.07 (s, 6H). ^{13}C NMR (151 MHz, $CDCl_3$) δ 175.2, 152.2, 146.5, 144.2, 144.1, 136.75, 129.0, 125.4, 125.3, 121.3, 121.2, 121.2, 120.1, 119.6, 111.8, 111.7, 40.1, 40.09. HR-MS (ES) calcd for $C_{17}H_{18}F_3N_4OS$ $[M+H]^+$ 383.1153, found 383.1141.

4-((5-methylisoxazol-3-yl)amino)-4-oxobutanoic acid. (14)

To a solution of isoxazol-5-amine (0.20 g, 2.0 mmol) **20** in dioxane (5 mL) was added succinic anhydride (0.20 g, 2.0 mmol). The mixture was stirred at 80–90°C overnight. The solvent was evaporated and the obtained yellowish solid was suspended in water, collected by filtration, and crystallized from ethanol to give the pure product as a white solid (0.088 g, 0.44 mmol, 22%). ^{1}H NMR (600 MHz, dmso-d_6) δ 12.14 (s, 1H), 10.87 (s, 1H), 6.58 (s, 1H), 2.55 (t, J = 6.5 Hz, 2H), 2.34 (s, 3H). The other methylene group was determined by HSQC, due to the

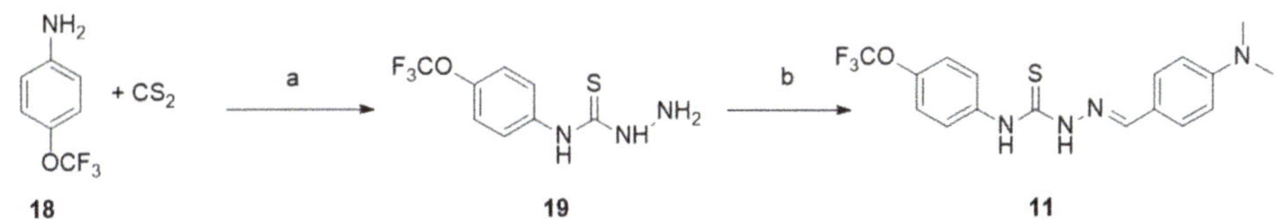

SCHEME 1 | Synthesis of compound **11**. Reagents and conditions. (a) CS_2, NaOH, DMF, 25°C, 1 h. NH_2NH_2, 70°C, 1 h. (b) 4-dimethylaminobenzaldehyde, EtOH, Reflux, 1 h.

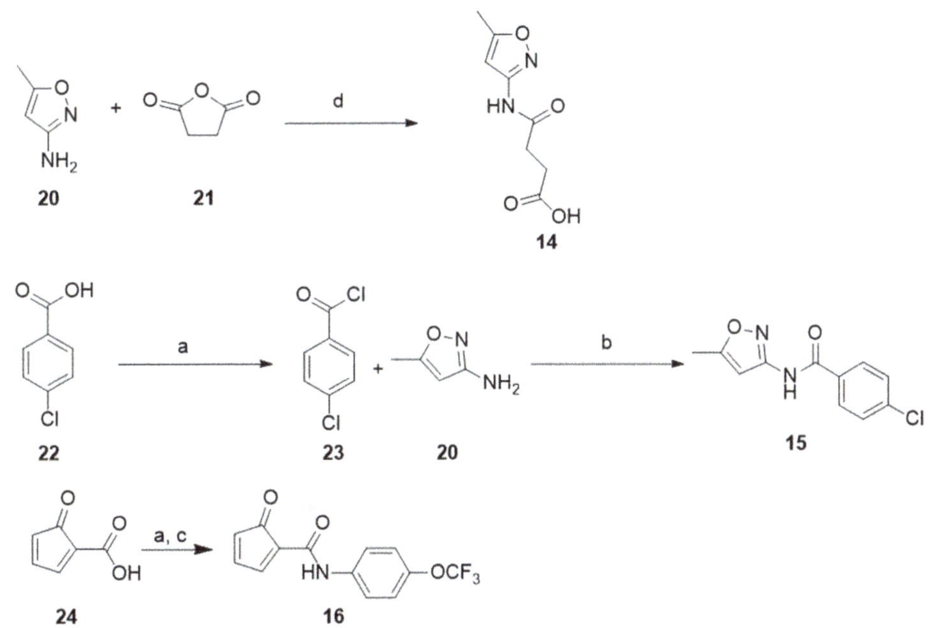

SCHEME 2 | Synthesis of compound **15** and **16**. Reagents and conditions. (a) $SOCl_2$, TEA, DCM, N_2, rt, 5 h; (b) Cs_2CO_3, ACN, rt, overnight; (c) 4-(trifluoromethoxy)aniline, TEA, DCM, rt, overnight; (d) dioxane 80–90°C, 5 h.

overlapping with solvent signal (SI). ^{13}C NMR (151 MHz, dmso-d_6): δ 173.4, 170.3, 169.2, 158.1, 96.2, 30.4, 28.4, 12.1. HRMS (ES) *m/z* calc. for $C_8H_{10}N_2O_4Na$ $[M+Na]^+$: 221.0538; found: 221.0533, $C_8H_{11}N_2O_4$ $[M+H]^+$: 119.0719; found: 199.0714.

4-chloro-N-(isoxazol-5-yl)benzamide (15)

A mixture of *p*-chloro benzoic acid (1.0 g, 6.4 mmol), and an excess of thionyl chloride (4.92 g, 3 mL, 41.7 mmol) was refluxed for 2 h. The excess of thionyl chloride was distilled in vacuo and the acyl chloride was used without further purification. To a solution of *p*-chlorobenzoyl chloride **23** in MeCN (10 mL) was added Cs_2CO_3 (3.7 g, 19 mmol) and isoxazol-5-amine **20** (0.63 g, 6.4 mmol) at 0°C and the obtained suspension was stirred at r.t. overnight. Then, the reaction mixture was concentrated under vacuo and the obtained residue was treated with water and extracted with EtOAc (4 × 20 mL). The organic layers were dried over Na_2SO_4, filtered-off and concentrated under vacuo to give a residue that was purified by silica gel column chromatography eluting with cHex/EtOAc (95:5–70:30). The product was obtained as a white solid (0.146 g, 0.63 mmol, 10%).

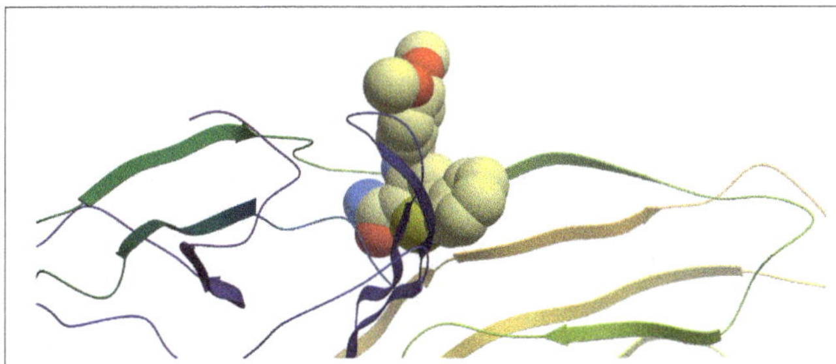

FIGURE 2 | Ribbon representation of protein E2 with PTC12 ligand within the binding site. Figure prepared with ICM (MolSoft LLC, La Jolla, CA).

^{1}H NMR (600 MHz, dmso-d_6) δ 11.39 (s, 1H), 8.02 (d, $J = 8.6$ Hz, 2H), 7.60 (d, $J = 8.6$ Hz, 2H), 6.74 (s, 1H), 2.41 (s, 3H). ^{13}C NMR (151 MHz, dmso-d_6) δ 169.4, 164.2, 158.5, 137.1, 131.9, 129.9, 128.5, 96.9, 12.1. HRMS (ES) *m/z* calc. for $C_{11}H_9ClN_2O_2Na$ $[M+Na]^+$: 259.0250; found: 259.0247, $C_{11}H_{10}ClN_2O_2$ $[M+H]^+$ 237.0431; found: 237.0428.

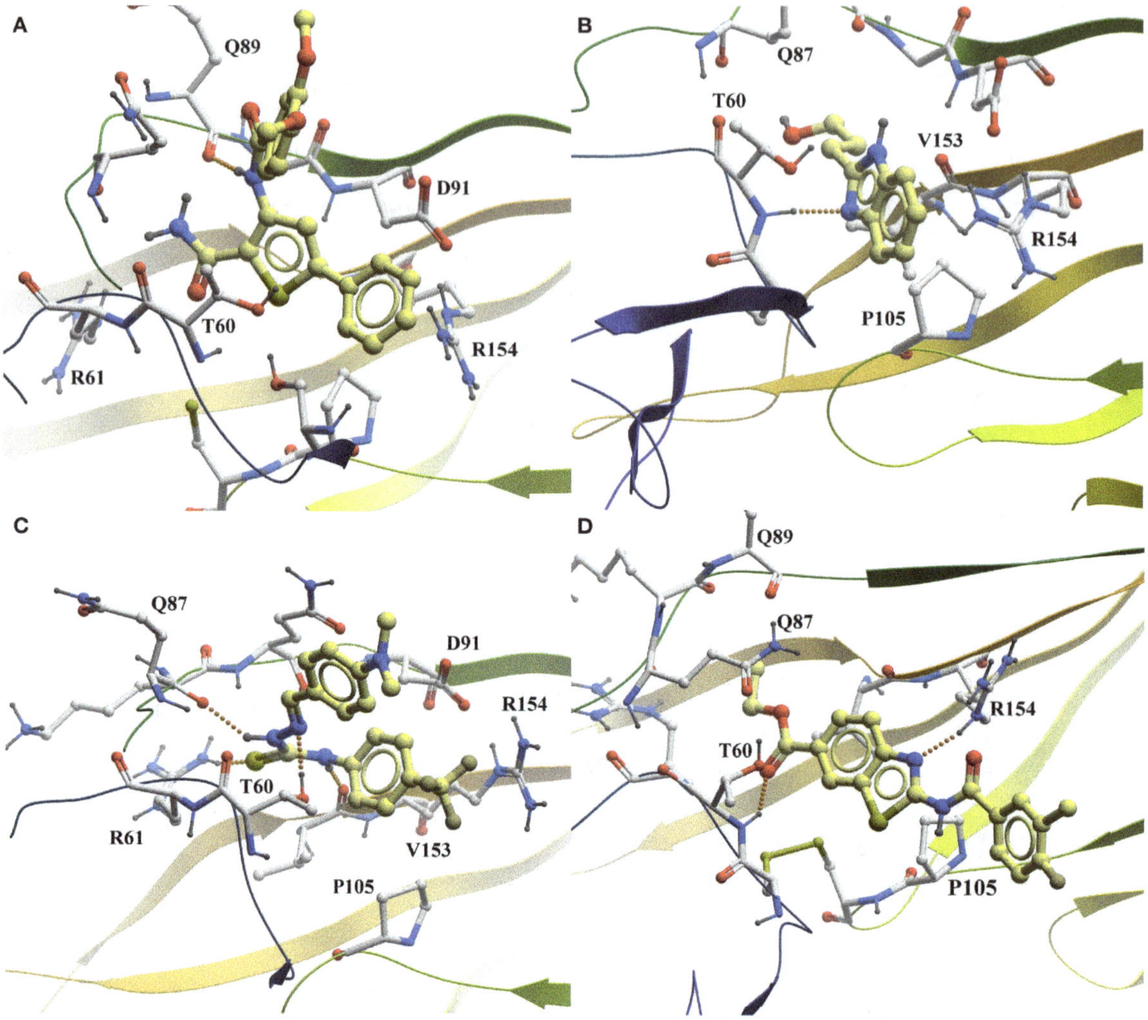

FIGURE 3 | Predicted interaction of active compounds PTC12 **(A)**, BI03 **(B)**, **11 (C)**, and **8 (D)** within the E2 protein binding site, extracted from the molecular dynamics simulations. For simplicity, only aminoacids within 4 Å of the ligand and polar hydrogens are shown. Hydrogen bonds are shown as a line of orange colored spheres. Color code: ligand carbons, yellow; E2 protein carbons, white; oxygens, red; nitrogens, blue; sulfur, dark yellow; polar hydrogens, dark gray. Figure prepared with ICM (MolSoft LLC, La Jolla, CA).

N-(4-(trifluoromethoxy)phenyl)furan-2-carboxamide (16)

Thionyl chloride (0.1 mL, 1.34 mmol) was added dropwise to a mixture of 2-furoic acid **20** (0.15 g, 1.34 mmol) and triethylamine (0.26 mL, 1.82 mmol) in DCM (5 mL) under N_2 atmosphere. The reaction mixture was stirred at room temperature for 5 h. The crude was added to another flask containing 4-(trifluoromethoxy)aniline (0.16 mL, 1.22 mmol) and triethylamine (0.34 mL, 2.43 mmol) in DCM (5 mL). The reaction mixture was stirred at room temperature overnight. After complete reaction, the solvent was the removed under reduced pressure, water added and extracted with dichloromethane. The organic layer was sequentially washed with brine, dried over anhydrous Na_2SO_4 and concentrated in vacuo. The crude was purified by column chromatography (SiO_2, dichloromethane) to give a white solid **16** (0.25 g, 75.6 %). ^{1}H NMR (600 MHz, DMSO-d_6) δ 10.38 (s, 1H), 7.96 (d, J = 0.9 Hz, 1H), 7.88 (dd, J = 9.1, 2.0Hz, 2H), 7.40–7.32 (m, 3H), 6.72 (dd, J = 3.4, 1.7 Hz, 1H). ^{13}C NMR (126 MHz, $CDCl_3$) δ 156.0, 147.4, 145.4, 144.3, 136.0, 121.8, 121.5, 121.0, 119.4, 115.6, 112.7. HR-MS (ES) calcd for $C_{12}H_8F_3NO_3Na$ $[M+Na]^+$ 294.0354, found 294.0345. Synthetic procedure of compounds **5, 12, 13** and **17** from the ZINC library are described in Supporting information (Scheme S1 and S2).

RESULTS AND DISCUSSION

Computer-Aided Indentification, Chemical Synthesis, and Biological Evaluation of Novel Inhibitors

We employed a multistep HTD screening framework to efficiently identify novel inhibitors of the E2 protein using commercially available (ZINC and Maybridge chemical libraries) and synthetic druglike compounds (from our in house library)

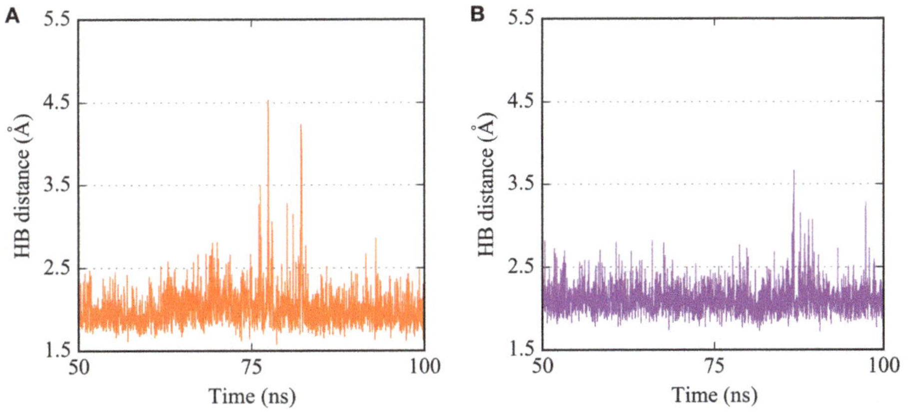

FIGURE 4 | Time dependence of hydrogen bond (HB) distances between **(A)** the carbonyl O of Gln89 and the benzamide H of PTC12 ligand, and **(B)** the backbone amide H of Thr60 and the N2 atom of BI03 ligand.

using the available structural data of the BVDV virus envelope protein E2. Initially, several chemical filters were applied on the chemical libraries to remove pan assay interference compounds (PAINS) (Baell and Holloway, 2010), compounds containing inorganic atoms, unwanted functionalities, reactive groups, and compounds having (i) MW <500 Dalton; (ii) more than one violation or the Lipinsky rules (Lipinski et al., 1997), or (iii) more than two violation of the rule of three, or more than six #STARS using the program QikProp (Jorgensen, 2005). The #stars parameter indicates the number of property descriptors computed by QikProp that fall outside the optimum range of values for 95% of known drugs.

The selected molecules were subjected to independent parallel HTD cycles and the top 1,000 scoring compounds were further analyzed. To ensure diversity, these highly ranked compounds were clustered based on chemical similarity using ICM. For each cluster, several compounds were selected manually based on commercial availability, synthetic tractability for potential modifications, interaction with binding site amino acids and adequate pharmacological characteristics for drug candidates. Finally, 19 compounds were purchased from vendors (**1–10**) or synthesized (**11–16**), and then evaluated in a reporter-based assay for antiviral activity (**Figure 1**, **Table 1**). Compounds **5** and **17** were obtained via reaction of the corresponding amine and dicyandiamide under acidic conditions to give the required phenylbiguanide (**5**, **17**) in high yields. 2-Guanidinobenzimidazole (**12**) was prepared by the cyclocondensation of o-phenylendiamine with cyanoguanidine (Scheme S1 of Supplementary Material) according to the method reported by King et al. (1948). Synthesis of new compounds is shown in **Scheme 1**. Compound (**11**) was obtained by ccondensation of thiosemicarbazide with 4-(dimethylamino)benzaldehyde. Compounds **14–16** were prepared by acylation of the corresponding amine with the adequate carboxilic acid chloride (**15**, **16**) or by reaction with succinic anhydride (**14**) (see **Scheme 2**).

First, we assayed selected compounds for cytotoxicity in cultured cells. Only compound **6** displayed high toxicity and was discarded from further analysis (**Table 1**). The remainder of the compounds were evaluated for antiviral activity in a reporter-based assay using a recombinant BVDV virus carrying GFP on its genome to infect MDBK cells (Pascual et al., 2018). Expression of GFP induced by BVDV infection was measured 2 days after infection using flow cytometry. Inhibition of BVDV infection was assessed by comparing the number of GFP positive cells in non-treated control cells and in cells treated with increasing amounts of compound. Structurally different compounds **4**, **8**, **11**, **BI03**, and **PTC12** showed activity with IC_{50} values of 30.1, 20.2, 23.9, 17.6, 0.30 μM, respectively, and no cytotoxicity was detected at 50 μM. In accordance with targeting of envelope protein function, we have previously shown that compounds BI03 and PTC12 specifically block BVDV cell entry (Pascual et al., 2018).

Analysis of Binding Determinants Using Molecular Dynamics

To further characterize the likely interaction between the new molecules and protein E2, we performed 100 ns MD simulation on the most active compounds listed on **Table 1**. The docked poses of the ligands within the binding site between domains I and II were used as the initial conformations. For compound **8** two conformationally different poses with very similar docking scores were used as starting conformations, and the most probable pose was assigned based on the molecular dynamics simulation results and the analysis of interactions (Liu and Kokubo, 2017). The protein and ligands remained stable in every simulation (Figure S1), displaying the ligands the following RMSF values: **PCT12**, 0.4 Å; **BI03**, 0.4 Å; **8**, 0.3 Å; **11**, 0.2 Å. The analysis of the binding determinants of the most active compounds is described in the following paragraphs.

The predicted binding mode of **PTC12** within the E2 protein is shown in **Figures 2**, **3**. The 3,4-dimethoxybenzamide group remained exposed to the solvent, whereas the thiophene ring made contacts with Asp91, Thr60, and Arg61. The system also presented a strong hydrogen bond between the benzamide group of the ligand and the carbonyl O of Gln89, exhibiting an interatomic distance of ~2 Å and an angle of 160° during the last 50 ns simulation (**Figure 4**). A moderate hydrogen bond between the NH of the thiophencarboxamide and the carbonyl O Gln89 was detected, with interatomic distances and angles closer to 2.5 Å and 140°, respectively. This group was also intermittently exposed to the solvent through a narrow channel. A stable cation-π interaction between the aromatic ring of the 3, 4 dimethoxyphenyl group and Arg154 was observed throughout the simulation, with a N^+-ring centroid distance below 6 Å at all times and a favorable θ angle below 40° during half of the last 50 ns simulation (Marshall et al., 2009).

The predicted interaction of **BI03** is shown in **Figure 3**. This ligand also presented a strong hydrogen bond between N2 and the backbone amide H of Thr60, with an average interatomic distance of 2.1 Å (**Figure 4**) and an angle of ~165° during the final half of the simulation. A stable cation-π interaction was also found in this case between the ligand ring and Arg154, showing again distances and θ angles below 6 Å and 40°, respectively for most of the final 50 ns of the simulation. A moderate hydrogen bond was also formed between the ring and the HO atom of Thr60. The system was further stabilized by close contacts with Thr60, Gln87, Arg154, Val153, and Pro105, while the ligand ring, NH and OH groups were mainly exposed to the solvent.

Compound **11** is shown within its predicted binding site in **Figure 3** Two stable hydrogen bond occurred between the HN atoms of the ligand and the carbonyl O atom in Val153 and Gln87. In both cases interatomic distances and angles were very favorable with average values of 2 Å and 155° respectively. The cation-π interaction between Arg154 and the aromatic ring of 4-trifluoromethylphenyl group was less favorable than for the other compounds showing higher N^+-ring centroid distances and θ angles, probably due to a moderate interaction between the CF_3 group and the charged portion of Arg154. The ligand made contacts with Asp91, Arg61, Arg154, Gln87, Val153, Pro105, and Thr60 while the CF_3 and NMe_2 groups were mostly exposed to the solvent.

The predicted binding mode of compound **8** is shown in **Figure 3**. This pose was selected as the most probable one based on the analysis of the interactions and binding free energy estimations. In the last half of the simulation, a moderate hydrogen bond between N1 (N with no H) and the side chain of Arg154 was observed, with average interactomic distances of 2.5 Å and angles of ~140°. No cation-π interaction was detected, and the charged portion of Arg154 seemed to interact strongly with the amide group of the ligand. The 3-chloro-4-fluorobenzamide remained exposed to the solvent and there were close contacts of the ligand with Ser57, Thr60, Gln87, Gln89, Pro105, and Arg154.

Overall, molecular dynamics simulations reveal a common pattern of interactions with the binding site in E2. Taken together with previous studies on the mode of action (Pascual et al., 2018), our data support binding of active compounds to E2. Further studies including *in vitro* binding to the recombinant protein are still required to confirm the interaction of active compounds with E2.

CONCLUSIONS

We have undertaken a structure-based virtual screening approach to identify small-molecules that dock into the druggable binding site at the interface between domains I and II of the E2 of BVDV, a virus responsible of both acute and persistent infections in cattle, with the consequent financial losses to the livestock industry each year. Around a million compounds were screened, and after chemical clustering, the top nineteen lead candidates were selected, and either purchased or synthesized, and evaluated in a reporter-based assay for antiviral activity. Five of these compounds exhibited IC_{50} values in the low micromolar range. The likely binding determinants of these compounds is supported by molecular dynamics simulations, where a common pattern of interaction with the binding site in E2 could be identified. These findings should benefit the design of novel and improved BVDV antivirals.

AUTHOR CONTRIBUTIONS

MB and CNC: Designed and supervised the study; NSA, MGA, and CNC: Performed the computational simulations; MB and CNC: The virtual screening; ESL, GAF, and MB: Conducted chemical synthesis; MJP and FM: Performed biological experiments under the supervision of DEA; MB, DEA, and CNC: Analyzed data. All authors were involved in the preparation of the manuscript and approved the final version.

ACKNOWLEDGMENTS

This work has been supported by the Agencia Nacional de Promoción Científica y Tecnológica, Argentina (PICT 2013-0778 and PICT 2014-1884 to MB; PICT 2011-2778 to CNC; PICT 2014-3599 to CNC and MB), CONICET (PIP 2014 11220130100721 to MB, CNC, and DEA), and FOCEM-Mercosur (COF 03/11). MB thanks William Jorgensen for providing an academic license for QikProp software. CNC thanks Molsoft LLC for providing an academic license for the ICM program. The authors thank the National System of High Performance Computing (Sistemas Nacionales de Computación de Alto Rendimiento, SNCAD) and the Computational Centre of High Performance Computing (Centro de Computación de Alto Rendimiento, CeCAR) for granting use of their computational resources.

REFERENCES

Abagyan, R., Totrov, M., and Kuznetsov, D. (1994). ICM - a new method for protein modeling and design - applications to docking and structure prediction from the distorted native conformation. *J. Comput. Chem.* 15, 488–506. doi: 10.1002/jcc.540150503

Abraham, M. J., Murtola, T., Schulz, R., Páll, S., Smith, J. C., Hess, B., et al. (2015). GROMACS: high performance molecular simulations through multi-level parallelism from laptops to supercomputers. *SoftwareX* 1, 19–25. doi: 10.1016/j.softx.2015.06.001

Baell, J. B., and Holloway, G. A. (2010). New substructure filters for removal of pan assay interference compounds (PAINS) from screening libraries and for their exclusion in bioassays. *J. Med. Chem.* 53, 2719–2740. doi: 10.1021/jm901137j

Becher, P., and Tautz, N. (2011). RNA recombination in pestiviruses: cellular RNA sequences in viral genomes highlight the role of host factors for viral persistence and lethal disease. *RNA Biol.* 8, 216–224. doi: 10.4161/rna.8.2.14514

Berendsen, H. J. C., Postma, J. P. M., Gunsteren, W. F., van, DiNola, A., and Haak, J. R. (1984). Molecular dynamics with coupling to an external bath. *J. Chem. Phys.* 81, 3684–3690. doi: 10.1063/1.448118

Brand, C. S., Hocker, H. J., Gorfe, A. A., Cavasotto, C. N., and Dessauer, C. W. (2013). Isoform selectivity of adenylyl cyclase inhibitors: characterization of known and novel compounds. *J. Pharmacol. Exp. Ther.* 347, 265–275. doi: 10.1124/jpet.113.208157

Callens, N., Brügger, B., Bonnafous, P., Drobecq, H., Gerl, M. J., Krey, T., et al. (2016). Morphology and molecular composition of purified bovine viral diarrhea virus envelope. *PLoS Pathog.* 12:e1005476. doi: 10.1371/journal.ppat.1005476

Cavasotto, C. N., and Orry, A. J. W. (2007). Ligand docking and structure-based virtual screening in drug discovery. *Curr. Top. Med. Chem.* 7, 1006–1014. doi: 10.2174/156802607780906753

Cavasotto, C. N., Ortiz, M. A., Abagyan, R. A., and Piedrafita, F. J. (2006). *In silico* identification of novel EGFR inhibitors with antiproliferative activity against cancer cells. *Bioorg. Med. Chem. Lett.* 16, 1969–1974. doi: 10.1016/j.bmcl.2005.12.067

Collett, M. S., Larson, R., Belzer, S. K., and Retzelt, E. (1988). Proteins encoded by bovine viral diarrhea virus : the genomic organization of a pestivirus. *Virology* 165, 200–208. doi: 10.1016/0042-6822(88)90673-3

El Omari, K., Iourin, O., Harlos, K., Grimes, J. M., and Stuart, D. I. (2013). Structure of a pestivirus envelope glycoprotein E2 clarifies its role in cell entry. *Cell Rep.* 3, 30–35. doi: 10.1016/j.celrep.2012.12.001

Fulton, R. W., Ridpath, J. F., Confer, A. W., Saliki, J. T., Burge, L. J., and Payton, M. E. (2003). Bovine viral diarrhoea virus antigenic diversity: impact on disease and vaccination programmes. *Biologicals* 31, 89–95. doi: 10.1016/S1045-1056(03)00021-6

He, W., Elizondo-Riojas, M. A., Li, X., Lokesh, G. L., Somasunderam, A., Thiviyanathan, V., et al. (2012). X-aptamers: a bead-based selection method for random incorporation of druglike moieties onto next-generation aptamers for enhanced binding. *Biochemistry* 51, 8321–8323. doi: 10.1021/bi300471d

Hornak, V., Abel, R., Okur, A., Strockbine, B., Roitberg, A., and Simmerling, C. (2006). Comparison of multiple Amber force fields and development of improved protein backbone parameters. *Proteins* 65, 712–725. doi: 10.1002/prot.21123

Irwin, J. J., and Shoichet, B. K. (2005). ZINC–a free database of commercially available compounds for virtual screening. *J. Chem. Inf. Model.* 45, 177–182. doi: 10.1021/ci049714+

Jorgensen, W. L. (2009). Efficient drug lead discovery and optimization. *Acc. Chem. Res.* 42, 724–733. doi: 10.1021/ar800236t

Jorgensen, W. L. (2005). *QikProp, v 3.0.* New York, NY: Schrödinger, LLC.

Kampmann, T., Yennamalli, R., Campbell, P., Stoermer, M. J., Fairlie, D. P., Kobe, B., et al. (2009). *In silico* screening of small molecule libraries using the dengue virus envelope E protein has identified compounds with antiviral activity against multiple flaviviruses. *Antiviral Res.* 84, 234–241. doi: 10.1016/j.antiviral.2009.09.007

King, F. E., Acheson, R. M., and Spensley, P. C. (1948). 275. Benziminazole analogues of paludrine. *J. Chem. Soc.* 1948, 1366–1371. doi: 10.1039/jr9480001366

Lagorce, D., Sperandio, O., Baell, J. B., Miteva, M. A., and Villoutreix, B. O. (2015). FAF-Drugs3: a web server for compound property calculation and chemical library design. *Nucleic Acids Res.* 43, W200–W207. doi: 10.1093/nar/gkv353

Lanyon, S. R., Hill, F. I., Reichel, M. P., and Brownlie, J. (2014). Bovine viral diarrhoea : pathogenesis and diagnosis. *Vet. J.* 199, 201–209. doi: 10.1016/j.tvjl.2013.07.024

Leal, E. S., Aucar, M. G., Gebhard, L. G., Iglesias, N. G., Pascual, M. J., Casal, J. J., et al. (2017). Discovery of novel dengue virus entry inhibitors via a structure-based approach. *Bioorg. Med. Chem. Lett.* 27, 3851–3855. doi: 10.1016/j.bmcl.2017.06.049

Li, Y., Wang, J., Kanai, R., and Modis, Y. (2013). Crystal structure of glycoprotein E2 from bovine viral diarrhea virus. *Proc. Natl. Acad. Sci. U. S. A.* 110, 6805–6810. doi: 10.1073/pnas.1300524110

Lipinski, C. A., Lombardo, F., Dominy, B. W., and Feeney, P. J. (1997). Experimental and computational approaches to estimate solubility and permeability in drug discovery and development settings. *Adv. Drug Deliv. Rev.* 46, 3–26. doi: 10.1016/S0169-409X(96)00423-1

Liu, K., and Kokubo, H. (2017). Exploring the stability of ligand binding modes to proteins by molecular dynamics simulations: a cross-docking study. *J. Chem. Inf. Model.* 57, 2514–2522. doi: 10.1021/acs.jcim.7b00412

Marshall, M. S., Steele, R. P., Thanthiriwatte, K. S., and Sherrill, C. D. (2009). Potential energy curves for cation-π interactions: off-axis configurations are also attractive. *J. Phys. Chem. A* 113, 13628–13632. doi: 10.1021/jp906086x

Nemethy, G., Gibson, K. D., Palmer, K. A., Yoon, C. N., Paterlini, M. G., Zagari, A., et al. (1992). Energy parameters in polypeptides. 10. Improved geometrical parameters and nonbonded interactions for use in the ECEPP/3 algorithm, with application to proline-containing peptides. *J. Phys. Chem.* 96, 6472–6484. doi: 10.1021/j100194a068

Newcomer, B. W., Chamorro, M. F., and Walz, P. H. (2017). Vaccination of cattle against bovine viral diarrhea virus. *Vet. Microbiol.* 206, 78–83. doi: 10.1016/j.vetmic.2017.04.003

Newcomer, B. W., and Givens, M. D. (2013). Approved and experimental countermeasures against pestiviral diseases : bovine viral diarrhea, classical swine fever and border disease. *Antiviral Res.* 100, 133–150. doi: 10.1016/j.antiviral.2013.07.015

Newcomer, B. W., Marley, M. S., Galik, P. K., Walz, P. H., Zhang, Y., Riddell, K. P., et al. (2012). Antiviral treatment of calves persistently infected with bovine viral diarrhoea virus. *Antivirus Chem. Chemother.* 22, 171–179. doi: 10.3851/IMP1903

Pascual, M. J., Merwaiss, F., Leal, E., Quintana, M. E., Capozzo, A. V., Cavasotto, C. N., et al. (2018). Structure-based drug design for envelope protein E2 uncovers a new class of bovine viral diarrhea inhibitors that block virus entry. *Antiviral Res.* 149, 179–190. doi: 10.1016/j.antiviral.2017.10.010

Ridpath, J. F. (2003). BVDV genotypes and biotypes: practical implications for diagnosis and control. *Biologicals* 31, 127–131. doi: 10.1016/S1045-1056(03)00028-9

Ronecker, S., Zimmer, G., Herrler, G., Greiser-wilke, I., and Grummer, B. (2008). Formation of bovine viral diarrhea virus E1 – E2 heterodimers is essential for virus entry and depends on charged residues in the transmembrane domains. *J. Gen. Virol.* 89, 2114–2121. doi: 10.1099/vir.0.2008/001792-0

Spyrakis, F., and Cavasotto, C. N. (2015). Open challenges in structure-based virtual screening: receptor modeling, target flexibility consideration and active site water molecules description. *Arch. Biochem. Biophys.* 583, 105–119. doi: 10.1016/j.abb.2015.08.002

Totrov, M., Abagyan, R., and Raffa, R. B. (2001). "Protein-ligand docking as an energy optimization problem," in *Drug-receptor Thermodynamics: Introduction and Experimental Applications*, ed R. B. Raffa (New York, NY: John Wiley and Sons), 603–624.

Wang, Q. Y., Patel, S. J., Vangrevelinghe, E., Hao, Y. X., Rao, R., Jaber, D., et al. (2009). A small-molecule dengue virus entry inhibitor. *Antimicrob. Agents Chemother.* 53, 1823–1831. doi: 10.1128/AAC.01148-08

Zhou, Z., Khaliq, M., Suk, J. E., Patkar, C., Li, L., Kuhn, R. J., et al. (2008). Antiviral compounds discovered by virtual screening of small-molecule libraries against dengue virus E protein. *ACS Chem. Biol.* 3, 765–775. doi: 10.1021/cb800176t

7

Insights into the Bifunctional Aphidicolan-16-ß-ol Synthase through Rapid Biomolecular Modeling Approaches

Max Hirte, Nicolas Meese, Michael Mertz, Monika Fuchs and Thomas B. Brück**

Werner Siemens Chair of Synthetic Biotechnology, Department of Chemistry, Technical University of Munich, Munich, Germany

Correspondence:
Monika Fuchs
monika.fuchs@tum.de
Thomas B. Brück
brueck@tum.de

Diterpene synthases catalyze complex, multi-step C-C coupling reactions thereby converting the universal, aliphatic precursor geranylgeranyl diphosphate into diverse olefinic macrocylces that form the basis for the structural diversity of the diterpene natural product family. Since catalytically relevant crystal structures of diterpene synthases are scarce, homology based biomolecular modeling techniques offer an alternative route to study the enzyme's reaction mechanism. However, precise identification of catalytically relevant amino acids is challenging since these models require careful preparation and refinement techniques prior to substrate docking studies. Targeted amino acid substitutions in this protein class can initiate premature quenching of the carbocation centered reaction cascade. The structural characterization of those alternative cyclization products allows for elucidation of the cyclization reaction cascade and provides a new source for complex macrocyclic synthons. In this study, new insights into structure and function of the fungal, bifunctional Aphidicolan-16-ß-ol synthase were achieved using a simplified biomolecular modeling strategy. The applied refinement methodologies could rapidly generate a reliable protein-ligand complex, which provides for an accurate *in silico* identification of catalytically relevant amino acids. Guided by our modeling data, ACS mutations lead to the identification of the catalytically relevant ACS amino acid network I626, T657, Y658, A786, F789, and Y923. Moreover, the ACS amino acid substitutions Y658L and D661A resulted in a premature termination of the cyclization reaction cascade *en-route* from syn-copalyl diphosphate to Aphidicolan-16-ß-ol. Both ACS mutants generated the diterpene macrocycle syn-copalol and a minor, non-hydroxylated labdane related diterpene, respectively. Our biomolecular modeling and mutational studies suggest that the ACS substrate cyclization occurs in a spatially restricted location of the enzyme's active site and that the geranylgeranyl diphosphate derived pyrophosphate moiety remains in the ACS active site thereby directing the cyclization process. Our cumulative data confirm that amino acids constituting the G-loop of diterpene synthases are involved in the open to the closed, catalytically active enzyme conformation. This study demonstrates that a simple and rapid biomolecular modeling procedure can predict catalytically relevant amino acids. The approach reduces computational and experimental screening efforts for diterpene synthase structure-function analyses.

Keywords: homology modeling, aphidicolin, diterpene, diterpene synthase, homology model refinement

INTRODUCTION

With more than 50,000 different molecules known to date terpenes are the greatest natural occurring product family found in organisms from bacteria to fungi, mammals, and plants. They are all derived from the isoprene units' dimethylallyl diphosphate and isopentenyl diphosphate. Condensation reactions of this molecules lead to the formation of different length phosphorylated linear terpenes, serving as substrate for terpene synthases. This enzyme family carry out highly stereo complex C-C coupling reactions, resulting in structurally complex macrocycles that contribute to the structural and functional diversity of terpenes (Christianson, 2017). Diterpenes are derived from the linear aliphatic precursor geranylgeranyl diphosphate (GGDP) being cyclized by diterpene synthases. More specifically, diterpene synthases are classified into class I and class II enzymes based on the structural presence of the conserved motifs DDXD or DDXXD/E and NSE/DTE, respectively. While class II reactions perform a protonation initiated cyclization reaction to generate phosphorylated bicyclic structures, class I reactions are initiated by hydrolyses of the GGDP pyrophosphate moiety that is coordinated by a Mg^{2+}-triad thereby generating mono- or poly-cyclic structures.

The natural product Aphidicolin, initially isolated from the fungus *Cephalosporium aphidicola,* is a hydroxylated, tetracyclic diterpenoid that exhibits a broad range of biological activities and applications (Brundret et al., 1972; Dalziel et al., 1973). More specifically, it is a potent inhibitor of the eukaryotic DNA α-polymerase with a commercial application as a cell synchronization agent. The compound is in pharmaceutical development due anti-tumor, anti-viral, and anti-leishmanial activity (Ikegami et al., 1978; Pedrali-Noy et al., 1980; Kayser et al., 2001; Edwards et al., 2013; Starczewska et al., 2016). Recently, other organisms including the fungus *Nigrospora sphaerica* and the pathogenic fungus *Phoma betae* have been identified as natural Aphidicolin producers. Current data suggests that Aphidicolin biosynthesis is exclusive to fungal metabolism and that natural sources for Aphidicolin are limited (Starratt and Loschiavo, 1974; Fujii et al., 2011; Lopes and Pupo, 2011). Nevertheless, elucidation of the responsible Aphidicolin biosynthetic gene cluster in *P. betae* allowed for the identification of a bifunctional diterpene synthase that contains both a functional class I and class II domain (Oikawa et al., 2001). The Aphidicolan-16-ß-ol synthase (ACS) generates the stereo-chemically demanding Aphidicolan-16-ß-ol (AD)—core structure of Aphidicolin—structure via a two-step reaction as depicted in **Figure 1** (Oikawa et al., 2002).

Initially, GGDP is rearranged in the class II active site cleft by protonation to the bicyclic syn-copalyl diphosphate (syn-CDP). Subsequently, syn-CDP is elaborated to AD in the class I active site (Adams and Bu'Lock, 1975; Oikawa et al., 2002). As depicted in **Figure 2** the cyclization mechanism in the class I active site, initiated by the hydrolysis of the pyrophosphate group, results

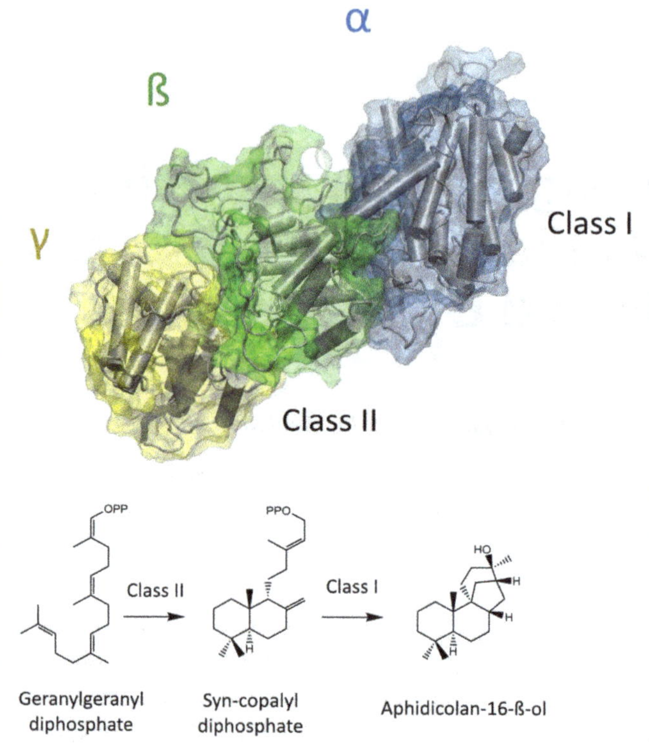

FIGURE 1 | Model of a bifunctional diterpene synthase. In the case of ACS GGDP is initially converted to syn-CDP in the class II active site (located between ß and γ domain). Syn-CDP is further cyclizied to AD in class I active site (α-domain).

in 8-ß-pimaradienyl carbocation formation. A subsequent attack of the vinyl group, bridging the C ring, directly undergoes a Wagner-Meerwein rearrangement and results in the formation of the aphidicolenyl carbocation. Eventually, this cation is quenched by water thereby generating AD.

Terpene cyclization mechanisms are conventionally elucidated by radio labeling of protons and carbons (Dickschat, 2017). This substrate specific labeling provides for identification of unusual hydride shifts and rearrangements. Alternatively, the enzyme's cyclization mechanisms can be probed by altering amino acids, trying to terminate the reaction cascade at a specific transition state (Morrone et al., 2008; Janke et al., 2014; Schrepfer et al., 2016; Jia et al., 2017). Therefore, random mutagenesis can be performed but the screening effort for this methodology is elaborate without an efficient high throughput screening options (Lauchli et al., 2013). Biomolecular modeling allows for the rational identification and *in silico* modulation of amino acid networks that are involved in complex reaction cascades (Pemberton et al., 2015; Schrepfer et al., 2016; Christianson, 2017; Escorcia et al., 2018). This methodology provides for a knowledge based approach of enzyme mutagenesis and screening. Nevertheless, a particular challenge for this strategy is based on the missing structural information for most terpene synthases. However, as their structural elements and domains are highly conserved (Christianson, 2017), homology

Abbreviations: ACS, Aphidicolan-16-β-ol synthase; AD, Aphidicolan-16-β-ol; GGDP, geranylgeranyl diphosphate; LRS, labdane related diterpene synthase; syn-CDP, syn-copalyl diphosphate.

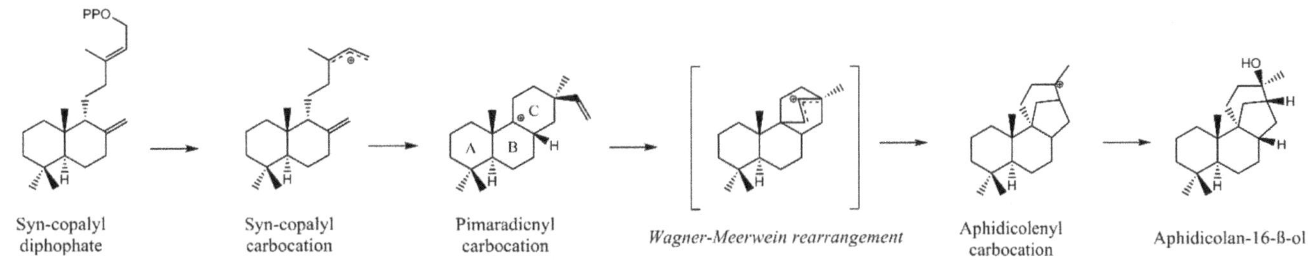

FIGURE 2 | Proposed cyclization mechanism of the ACS class I reaction (Oikawa et al., 2002).

modeling is a potential route to identify catalytically relevant amino acids despite the low primary sequence identities in this enzyme family (Xu and Li, 2003). Unfortunately, most available crystal structures of terpene synthase are deposited in the open apo-enzyme configuration that is catalytically inactive. This open enzyme conformation presents an additional obstacle when catalytically relevant amino acids have to be identified *in silico*. At present, only two diterpene synthase structures have been reported in the closed, catalytically active form (Liu et al., 2014; Serrano-Posada et al., 2015). Therefore, automated homology modeling approaches will almost always result in catalytically non-relevant open enzyme configuration. Moreover, while prediction tools can place large cofactors (i.e., FAD, NADH, Heme) correctly in the apo-protein framework, ligand-metal interactions are difficult to predict because of the multiple coordination geometries and the lack of sufficiently accurate force field parameters (Khandelwal et al., 2005). Hence, structure function predictions that depend on the interplay between the amino acids of the protein framework with small metal ions cannot be conducted solely by application of automated software tools. In this context, a rational combination of structural information by superposition and extraction of cofactors is performed to prepare the protein structure for docking studies. Nevertheless, this approach often neglects reliable positioning of the cofactor coordinating amino acids. Additionally, falsely predicted positioning of amino acid side chains in the active site cleft can lead to invalid interpretation of a homology model based protein-ligand complex. To improve this situation, this study elucidated rapid and simple methodologies to refine diterpene homology models for docking studies thereby allowing for reliable structure-function predictions. In this context, an ACS class I homology model of the α-domain was predicted from the primary sequence. Subsequently, these models were compared to catalytically relevant closed terpene synthases structures. The location of metals was refined and fitted against specifically selected structural templates and multiple docking studies were carried out and validated. Our *in silico* results were experimentally evaluated by ACS mutagenesis studies. This lead to an identification of essential amino acid residue sidechains that are necessary for retaining the enzymes activity. Additionally, we detected amino acid substitutions that abort the catalytic reaction cascade *en- route* from syn-CDP to AD. Structural analyses and elucidation of these compounds revealed the formation of syn-copalol and a labdane related, non-hydroxylated diterpene by the ACS mutants Y658L and D661A. Our approach of a protein homology model based structure function analysis can be easily adapted for other terpene synthases. This methodology allows for rapid and simple analysis of the catalytically relevant amino acid network that help studying complex reaction cascades and developing new biocatalysts.

MATERIALS AND METHODS

Materials and Chemicals

All genes used were synthesized by Life technologies GmbH and the codon usage was optimized for *E. coli* if not stated otherwise. Primers were obtained from Eurofins Genomics GmbH. Strains and plasmids were obtained from Merck KGaA. All chemicals used were obtained at highest purity from Roth chemicals or Applichem GmbH. Enzymes were purchased from Thermo Fisher Scientific.

Software and Web-Tools

RaptorX was applied for homology modeling studies (http://raptorx.uchicago.edu; Källberg et al., 2012). The initial predicted structure was analyzed and further modified in the environment of UCSF Chimera software package (Pettersen et al., 2004; http://www.cgl.ucsf.edu/chimera). Comparative modeling by spatial restraints was performed by MODELLER (Eswar et al., 2006), and all substrate docking studies performed by AutoDock Vina (Trott and Olson, 2010; http://vina.scripps.edu). Chemical structures were drawn by PerkinElmer ChemBioDraw Ultra (http://www.cambridgesoft.com). For ligand preparation the Avogadro (Hanwell et al., 2012; https://avogadro.cc/) software package was used. A syn-CDP toppar stream file was generated by CHARMM General Force Field program version 1.0.0 for use with CGenFF version 3.0.1 (https://cgenff.paramchem.org; Vanommeslaeghe et al., 2010, 2012; Vanommeslaeghe and MacKerell, 2012). Two ns molecular dynamic studies of the docked ACS model B in a water sphere have been performed under CHARMM general force field by NAMD (Phillips et al., 2005; http://www.ks.uiuc.edu/Research/namd/). NAMD was developed by the Theoretical and Computational Biophysics Group in the Beckman Institute for Advanced Science and Technology at the University of Illinois at Urbana-Champaign. For high resolution pictures the protein was prepared by Visual Molecular Dynamics (http://www.ks.

uiuc.edu/Research/vmd/; Humphrey et al., 1996) and rendered by Tachyon implemented in the VMD software package (Stone, 1998).

Docking

Ligand structures were downloaded from https://pubchem.ncbi.nlm.nih.gov/ available and geometrically optimized by 500 steps of steepest descent under MMFF94 force field parameters included in Avogadro. Protein structures were prepared by Dock Prep, which is part of the Chimera software environment. The AMBER force field (AMBERff14SB) was applied to the receptor while Gasteiger charges were added to the ligand and co-factors. As recently reported, docking can be improved by assigning partial charges to metal ions (Hu and Shelver, 2003). In this context, Mg-ion charges were set to +1. Syn-CDP charge was set to −3. Docking was performed by AutoDock Vina using standard parameters. Docking poses were chosen based on a structural comparison to the pyrophosphate group that is co-crystallized in pdb 5A0J (see Figure S1B). The chosen pose was furthermore validated by re-dock approaches. Therefore, the predicted syn-CDP pose was *de novo* geometrically optimized by 500 steps of steepest descent under MMFF94 force field parameters included in Avogadro software environment prior to docking repetition (see Figure S1A).

Model Generation

An initial homology model of the ACS α-domain was predicted by RaptorX starting from the amino acid 565. A model based on the pdb crystal structure 5A0J, referring to a labdane related diterpene synthase, was manually selected for further structure function analyses. In order to prepare the model for docking studies, the coordinating Mg^{2+}-ion triad and water molecules were implemented in the structure by different methods. Model A was generated by structural alignment to 5A0J. Cofactor positions were transferred from the structure template to Model A without any further adjustment prior to docking studies. Model B was created by MODELLER implemented in the Chimera software environment using the 5A0J as template structure. In this model hetero atoms and water molecules in the structure environment were computationally implemented. The pyrophosphate group was removed prior to docking with syn-CDP. Model C was prepared analogously to Model B but prior to refinement by MODELLER, syn-CDP was docked into the template structure 5A0J.

Model Validation

The protein ligand complex of Model B was validated by molecular dynamics studies. Therefore, syn-CDP was initially extracted from Model B and parameterized by CHARMM General Force Field program version 1.0.0 for use with CGenFF version 3.0.1. VMD was used to parameterize the protein and for merging ligand and protein. Subsequently, a water sphere was added around the protein-ligand complex. Two nanoseconds of molecular dynamic studies under CHARMM General Force Field was applied to the protein complex by NAMD. The calculated rmsd of the generated frames was plotted over time (Figure S2). A constant rmsd value was chosen as the criteria for an equilibrated protein-ligand complex. The last frame obtained was compared to the initial model B (Figure S3).

Plasmids for Diterpene Production

For all cloning procedures *E. coli* HMS 174 (DE3) was used. Clones were cultivated at 37°C in Luria-Bertani (LB) medium. Chloramphenicol (34 μg/L) and Kanamycin (50 μg/L) were added as required. For efficient production of the diterpene AD, *E. coli's* internal 1-deoxy-xylulose-5 phosphate pathway flux was increased by overexpression of deoxy-xylulose 5 phosphate synthase (dxs: GenBank: YP001461602.1), isopentenyl-diphosphate delta isomerase (idi: GenBank: AAC32208.1), and further extended by expressing geranylgeranyl diphosphate synthase (crtE: GenBank: KPA04564.1) and Aphidicolan-16-ß-ol synthase (acs: GenBank: AB049075.1). Therefore, dxs and acs were amplified from original sources by PCR. Polycistronic operons (**Table 1**) were constructed by BioBrick cloning standard (Shetty et al., 2008).

Site directed mutations of acs were generated by PCR. Forward primers were designed exhibiting the respective mutation at the 5′ end while the corresponding reverse primers were phosphorylated at 5′ end (Table S1). PCR products were ligated by T4 Ligase prior to transformation. All amino acid exchanges were confirmed by sequencing.

Production of Diterpenes

All diterpene production experiments were performed in *E. coli* BL 21 (DE3). To investigate the product outcome of ACS mutants, pACYC acs plasmids were co-transformed with pAX dic. Cultivation was performed in minimal media supplemented with 6 g/L yeast extract and 30 g/L glycerol at 25°C. After 60 h the culture was extracted with a mixture of hexane, ethanol and ethyl acetate (1:1:1) (v/v/v) for 1 h. The extract was centrifuged at 10,000 g for 2 min. The upper, organic phase was directly analyzed for diterpene products via GC-MS.

Diterpene Analytics

GC-MS analyses of diterpenes was performed by a Trace GC Ultra with DSQII (Thermo Fisher Scientific). Therefore, 1 μL sample was loaded (Split 1/10) by TriPlus AS onto a SGE BPX5 column (30 m, I.D 0.25 mm, Film 0.25 μm). The initial column temperature was set to 160°C and maintained for 5 min before a temperature gradient at 8°C/min up to 320°C was applied. The final temperature was kept for additional 3 min. MS data were recorded at 70 eV (EI) and m/z (rel. intensity in %) as total ion current (TIC). The recorded m/z range was in between 50 to 650.

NMR spectra were recorded in $CDCl_3$ with an Avance III 500 MHz (Bruker) at 300 K. ^1H NMR chemical shifts are given in ppm relative to $CDCl_3$ (δ = 7.26 ppm). The 2D experiments

TABLE 1 | Plasmids used for AD production in *E. coli*.

Name	Promotor strength	Genes	Resistance	vector
pAX dic	Weak	dxs, idi, crtE	Kanamycin	pBR322
pACYC acs	Strong	acs	Chloramphenicol	pACYC duet

(HSQC) were performed using standard Bruker pulse sequences and parameters.

RESULTS AND DISCUSSION

Homology Model Refinement

The steady increase in published protein crystal structures provides for an accelerated improvement of computational homology prediction. Especially due to the high structurally conservation of the terpene synthase enzyme families, biomolecular tools can predict structures solely based on the amino acid sequence. In this context, structure prediction of the bifunctional ACS was performed to analyze the highly complex conversion of GGDP via syn-CDP to the tetracyclic AD which is the core structure of the cytostatic compound Aphidicolin. ACS belongs to the diterpene synthase family and we identified three highly structurally conserved domains. The initial conversion from the universal diterpene precursor GGDP to syn-CDP occurs in class II active site, located between the ACS ß- and γ-domain. The subsequent syn-CDP cyclization to AD is then conducted in the class I active site that is positioned in the middle of an α-helical bundle forming the ACS α-domain. Notably, the fungal ACS is structurally highly similar to the previously crystallized plant diterpene synthases Abietadiene (pdb: 3S9V) and Taxadiene synthase (pdb: 3P5R), respectively. Homology prediction based on the full ACS sequence took those two structures into account, but for both, crystals could only be achieved in N-terminal truncated forms. Furthermore, these crystal structures have only been solved in an open conformation that is catalytically inactive. In order to circumvent the consideration of these catalytically inactive templates, only the ACS α-domain sequence was used for homology prediction. A model based on the labdane related diterpene synthases (LRS) (pdb: 5A0J), which is provided in a catalytically active holo-complex (Serrano-Posada et al., 2015), was selected for ACS homology refinement. The structural superposition of Abietadiene (pdb: 3S9V), LRS (pdb: 5A0J), and the ACS model, as depicted in **Figure 3**, explicitly demonstrates that there is a better fit between the ACS model and the LRS crystal structure. While the structural fit between LRS and the ACS model is visually well apparent, we have not calculated an rmsd value qualifier as structural domains that do not constitute the active site region are highly variable.

Co-crystallized cofactors (Mg^{2+}-ion triad) and waters, both provided in the LRS structure, are also involved in the ACS reaction *en-route* from syn-CDP to AD. Therefore, we differentially adapted both, the positions of the Mg^{2+} ions and waters into the ACS models that resulted in the generation of three ACS models (A–C). Model A was prepared by adaptation of cofactor positions from the template structure LRS after structural alignment. Initial evaluation of this model indicated that this un-refined modeling method results in clashes of cofactors positions with amino acids side chains. Generally, in homology prediction the active site's cavity is not reserved for the substrate or cofactors specifically. Therefore, we presume that amino acid sidechains occupy this free space due to applied energy minimization optimizations. This is demonstrated in

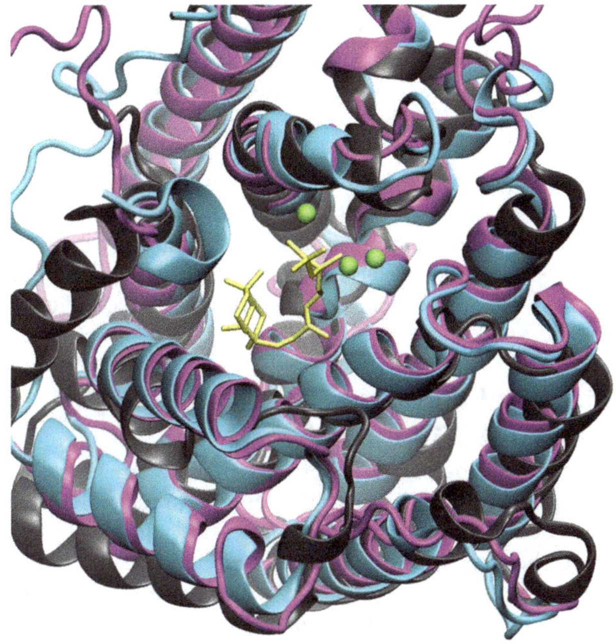

FIGURE 3 | Structural alignment of Abietadiene synthase (gray), LRS (blue), and ACS (purple) in complex with Mg^{2+}-ions and syn-CDP.

our docking studies of model A, where ACS amino acid Y658 is preventing syn-CDP to completely access the active site cavity. With the MODELLER package, which is based on comparative protein structure modeling by spatial restraints, a protein structure can be refined based on a template structure. Additionally, hetero-atoms and water molecules can be included directly in the model refinement. This refinement methodology applied to our initial model structure lead to the generation of ACS model B. This model B computationally included the three Mg^{2+}-ions, a pyrophosphate group (conventionally derived by Mg^{2+} based hydrolysis of the phosphorylated substrate [syn-CDP] substrate) and water molecules directly as they are all present in the LRS template structure. Model B provides reliable positioning of the conserved amino acids that constitute the class I diterpene synthase signature DDXXD/E and NSE/DTE motifs in relation to the adapted Mg^{2+}- ions, water and pyrophosphate moieties, respectively. Subsequently, we removed the pyrophosphate group from the model B structure to enable docking with the native syn-CDP substrate. Our docking data indicated that in Model B syn-CDP can completely access the active site's cavity. A specific syn-CDP conformation was selected pointing toward the ACS G-Helix, as this flexible helix is proposed to be involved in terpene cyclization reactions (Yoshikuni et al., 2006; Baer et al., 2014; Jia et al., 2017). This docking pose was validated by multiple re-docking approaches (Figure S1A). Additionally, we validated the pose while the position of the pyrophosphate moiety was compared to the pyrophosphate group co-crystallized in LRS (Figure S1B). Finally, a third approach for structure-function analyses was performed by docking syn-CDP into LRS prior to ACS refinement with MODELLER. Again, a syn-CDP conformation was chosen with close proximity toward the G-Helix. On the basis of this LRS holo-protein complex, an ACS holo-complex model C was generated. This method provided for a protein model that was refined around the substrate and cofactors. This methodology also provided for a precise specification of amino acids involved in the AD cyclization reaction. For all three models amino acids located within a five Å vicinity to the docked substrate syn-CDP (thereby neglecting the pyrophosphate moiety) were analyzed by mutational studies to elucidate their catalytic relevance (see **Figure 4**, Table S2).

Mutational Validation of Catalytically Relevant ACS Amino Acids

Due to their stereo-chemical diversity, natural diterpene scaffolds are attractive research leads. The enormous stereo-chemical demand of diterpene macrocycles renders them difficult to access via total chemical synthesis approaches. Therefore, biosynthetic routes to generate these complex structures are currently an intense research focus (Dickschat, 2016; Bian et al., 2017; Jones, 2017). The ability to access new diterpene macrocycles via selective alteration of amino acids in diterpene synthases provides for a highly varied accessible chemical space. For the class I cyclooctat-9-en-7-ol synthase, which naturally generates a tricyclic fusicoccin type diterpene, amino acid mutations in the vicinity of the active site lead to intermittent abortion of the reaction cascade. Hence, alternative macrocyclic structures, such as the bicyclic dolabellane and the monocyclic cembrane, could be generated thereby elucidating the reaction cascade (Görner et al., 2013; Janke et al., 2014). In this study, insights into the class I reaction of the ACS were achieved by mutational studies. In that respect, we intended to quench the reaction from syn-CDP to AD at previously proposed transitional states (Adams and Bu'Lock, 1975; Oikawa et al., 2002). Based on the proposed ACS transitional states we presume that syn-labdatriene and syn-copalol (termination product of the syn-copalyl carbocation), stereoisomers of syn-pimaradiene (termination products of the pimaradienyl carbocation), or aphidicolene and stemodene (termination products of the aphidicolenyl carbocation) are potential abortion products (see **Figure 5**).

For an intermittent abortion of the reaction cascade from syn-CDP to AD, we have selected amino acids within a range of five Å to the docked ligands as prime targets for mutagenesis (see **Figure 4**). Preliminary studies revealed that sidechain substitutions encompassing amino acids exchanges that inherently change physico-chemical properties frequently resulted in inactive enzyme variants (Janke et al., 2014; Schrepfer et al., 2016). In this context, we focused on changing the size of the respective amino acid sidechain thereby trying to preserve physico-chemical characteristics. Alternatively, we chose amino acid side chain substitutions that would replace polar groups with similar size amino acids (Table S2).

ACS syn-CDP docking results pointed toward a strong interaction between the decalin core and surrounding hydrophobic sidechains. However, as the decalin structure of syn-CDP remains untouched in further cyclization steps most of the implemented mutations near this particular moiety resulted in inactive (I626A, Y923L, F789L) or wildtype activity variants (F629L, Y658F, C831G, C831T, T920G, Y923F). Based on our modeling results, we also identified specific amino acids located in the ACS G-helix that in other studies have been proposed to be of catalytic relevance (Baer et al., 2014;

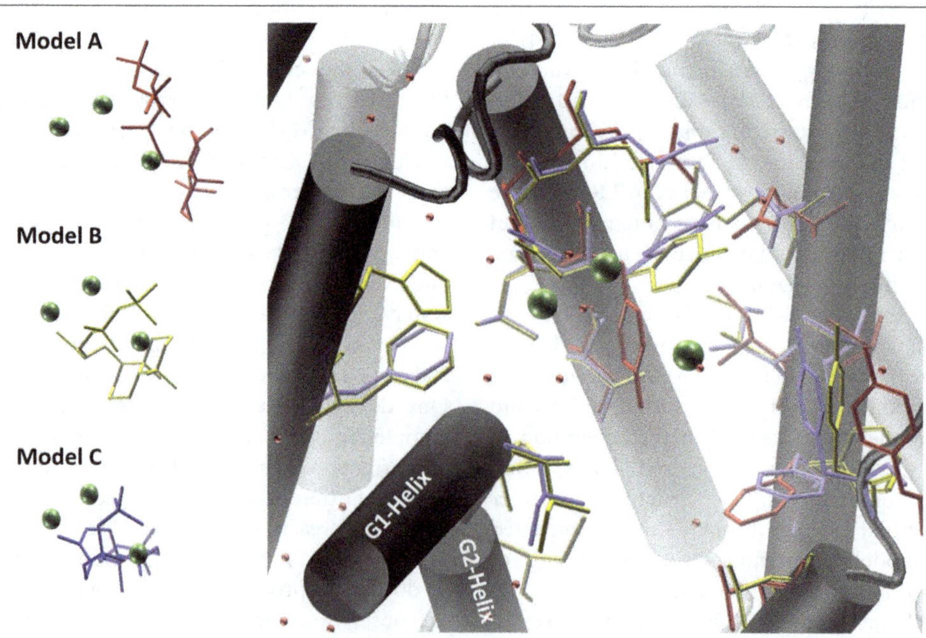

FIGURE 4 | Homology models of ACS synthase refined and prepared for docking of the substrate syn-CDP. Model A results are colored red, Model B results yellow, and Model C results blue.

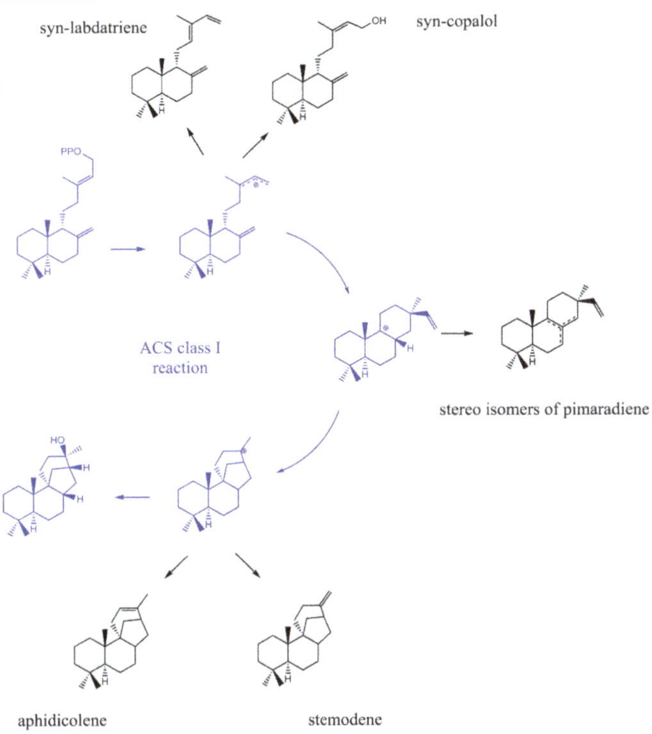

FIGURE 5 | Expected products generated by ACS if the reaction cascade *en-route* from syn-CDP to AD is prematurely terminated.

Jia et al., 2017). While mutational changes in the G-Helix of Kaurene synthase like diterpene synthases resulted in alternative product profiles (Jia et al., 2017), our analogous approaches with ACS only provided inactive (A786L, F789L) or wildtype active (A786G, F789Y) variants. Nevertheless, our results support previous findings that propose the G-Helix as an essential flexible motif which is involved in the catalytically relevant structural change from the open to the closed enzyme configuration (Baer et al., 2014).

Only the substitution of ACS Y658L and D661A provided for a varied product outcome. In addition to amino acids that constitute the DXXDD/E and NSE/DTE signature motifs that are responsible for Mg^{2+}-ion coordination, our combined *in silico* and experimental study identified only a few amino acids (see **Figure 6**, colored in pink) capable to terminate activity. Our successful mutations (D661A, Y658L) indicated that the unusual cyclization from syn-CDP to AD proceeds in a spatially restricted area of the active site's cleft. Additionally, our data suggests that the pyrophosphate group remains in the active site and coordinates the reaction cascade. This is in accordance to the recently postulated Taxadiene synthase reaction mechanism (Schrepfer et al., 2016).

ACS Mutants D661A and Y658L

GC-MS analyses of the ACS mutants Y658L and D661A revealed that this mutations lead to the formation of two unknown diterpene products (see **Figure 7**). In contrast to the native AD, which had a GC retention time of 17.67 min, these new diterpenes had a retention time of 12.79 and 13.46 min, respectively. The latter product with a retention time of 13.46 min, showed a total mass of 290 m/z. Comparison of the MS spectral data suggests that this was a hydroxylated diterpene with a similar structure to syn-copalol (Hoshino et al., 2011). Subsequently, this compound was isolated and structural characterized by NMR (Figures S4, S5). The results are in accordance to previous spectral data for syn-copalol (Yee and Coates, 1992). One plausible explanation for syn-copalol formation is the quenching of the syn-copalyl carbocation intermediate by water in the active site of the enzyme. The other diterpene product with a retention time of 12.79 min had a total mass of 272 m/z indicating that this structure was not-hydroxylated. While we expected the formation of syn-labda-8(17),12E,14-triene, comparison with published MS-spectra revealed significant differences (Morrone et al., 2011). Unfortunately, due to the low amounts produced and purification issues for this highly hydrophobic compound, we could not conduct NMR analysis. However, we presume that this compound is also originated from the syn-copalyl carbocation and that a labdane related diterpene with high structural similarity to syn-labda-8(17),12E,14-triene was generated by the ACS mutants. The newly generated diterpenes are of great interest as copalol derivatives display various biological activities analogous to aphidicolin (Hanson, 2015).

The structural changes (D661A and Y658L) still allowed syn-CDP binding in the active site with subsequent hydrolyses of the pyrophosphate group. The syn-copalyl carbocation was then quenched either by water (release of syn-copalol) or an amino acid side chain (release of non-hydroxylated diterpene). Furthermore, as we did not find other substitution that stopped cyclization at the proposed transitional states and as we could not even detect changes in the byproduct formation of the active mutants, we presume that the ACS cyclization occurs in a spatially restricted area and that the pyrophosphate group remains in the active site, which is in accordance to recent reports (Schrepfer et al., 2016).

Former diterpene centered production processes were limited by low target compound yields. However, optimization of recombinant diterpene production hosts has extensively progressed to provide gram per liter yields (Ajikumar et al., 2010; Schalk et al., 2012). Today, access to novel diterpene lead structures is limited by the effective identification of relevant enzyme systems from large scale genome sequencing projects. Therefore, rational alteration of known terpene synthase product profiles by using a combination of *in silico* prediction and knowledge based mutagenesis studies can allow for a more rapid and targeted expansion of the desired chemical space.

CONCLUSION

A model of ACS synthase was computed that required the application of various methods for model refinement to improve the quality of *in silico* structure function analysis. A model of the

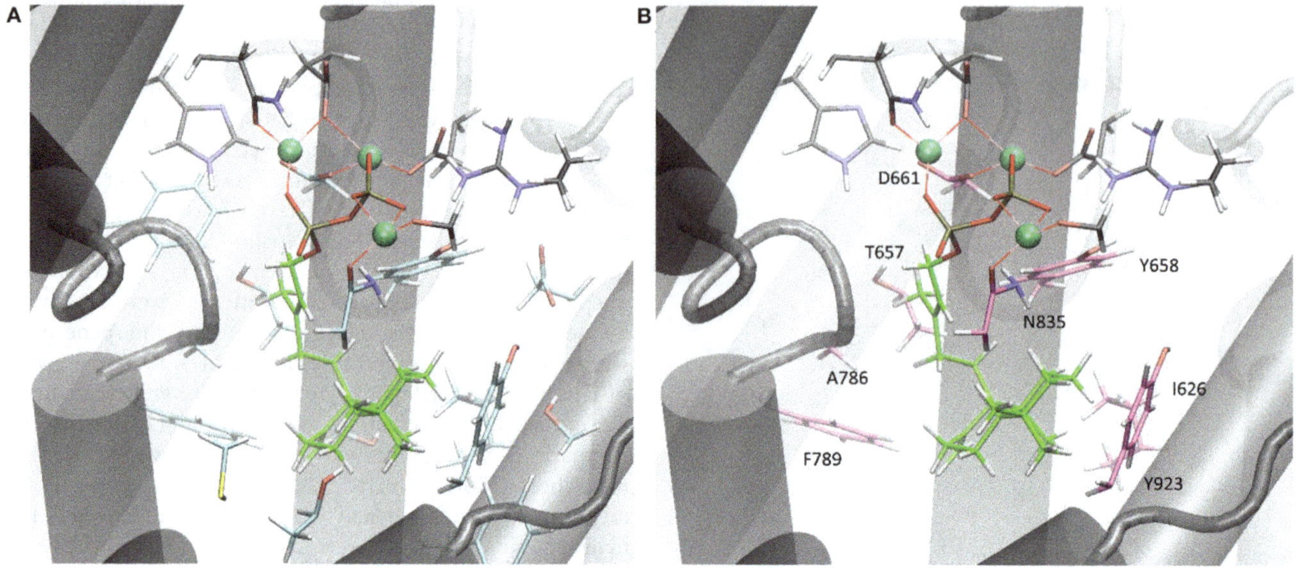

FIGURE 6 | (A) ACS active sites cleft in complex with Mg^{2+} and syn-CDP. Amino acid network within five Å to syn-CDP are displayed. **(B)** ACS active sites cleft in complex with Mg^{2+} and syn-CDP. Substitution of labeled amino acid (displayed in pink) resulted in inactive enzyme versions or mutants with altered product outcome.

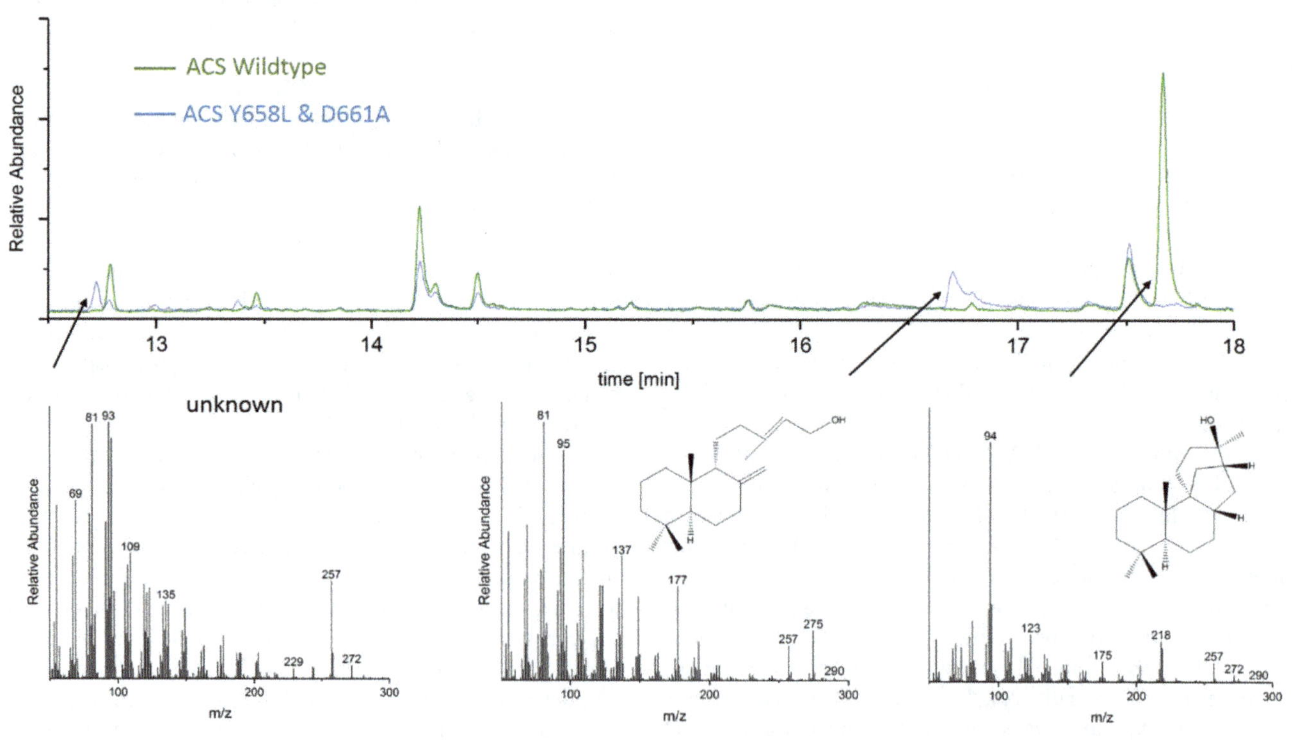

FIGURE 7 | Analysis of ACS wildtype and ACS D661A mutant product outcome by GC. The MS-patterns for syn-labdatriene, syn-copalol and AD (from right to left) are presented below.

catalytically active, closed ACS α-domain complex was generated. Examination of this model provided for the identification of catalytically active amino acid sidechains. The *in silico* results were confirmed by mutational studies of the ACS. The amino acid substitutions Y658L and D661A in the vicinity of the ACS active site lead to formation of the alternative cyclization products syn-copalol and a minor labdane related diterpene. Formation of these products were delineated by quenching of the syn-copalyl carbocation *en-route* to AD. Additional mutants leading to inactive enzyme variants (A786L, F789L) provided insights into catalytically relevant amino acid residues within the G-Helix. The cumulative *in-silico* and experimental data suggests that amino acids constituting the G-loop motif of class I terpene cyclases are involved in the transformation of the open to the closed, catalytically active enzyme conformation. Moreover, as we only obtained a limited number of alternative cyclization products in our mutational screens, we presume that AD formation occurs in a rather confined location of the ACS active site. With respect to our biomolecular modeling approaches, we demonstrated that application of simple and rapid computational methodologies can be employed for prediction and structure function analyses of class I diterpene synthases.

AUTHOR CONTRIBUTIONS

TB and MF supervised this study. MH initiated this study and performed virtual modeling and docking studies. NM and MM conducted mutagenesis experiments and screening under supervision of MH and MF. Data was analyzed by MH, MF, NM, MM, and TB. All figures were created by MH. All authors verified the data, contributed to the manuscript, and approved the final version.

ACKNOWLEDGMENTS

MH, MF, and TB would like to acknowledge the financial support of the German ministry for Education and Research (BMBF) with the grant number 031A305A. TB gratefully acknowledges funding by the Werner Siemens foundation for establishing the field of Synthetic Biotechnology at the Technical University of Munich (TUM).

REFERENCES

Adams, M. R., and Bu'Lock, J. D. (1975). Biosynthesis of the diterpene antibiotic, aphidicolin, by radioisotope and ^{13}C nuclear magnetic resonance methods. *J. Chem. Soc. Chem. Commun.* 389–391. doi: 10.1039/c39750000389

Ajikumar, P. K., Xiao, W.-H., Tyo, K. E., Wang, Y., Simeon, F., Leonard, E., et al. (2010). Isoprenoid pathway optimization for Taxol precursor overproduction in *Escherichia coli*. *Science* 330, 70–74. doi: 10.1126/science.1191652

Baer, P., Rabe, P., Fischer, K., Citron, C. A., Klapschinski, T. A., Groll, M., et al. (2014). Induced-fit mechanism in class I terpene cyclases. *Angew. Chem. Int. Edn.* 53, 7652–7656. doi: 10.1002/anie.201403648

Bian, G., Deng, Z., and Liu, T. (2017). Strategies for terpenoid overproduction and new terpenoid discovery. *Curr. Opin. Biotechnol.* 48, 234–241. doi: 10.1016/j.copbio.2017.07.002

Brundret, K. M., Dalziel, W., Hesp, B., Jarvis, J. A. J., and Neidle, S. (1972). X-Ray crystallographic determination of the structure of the antibiotic aphidicolin: a tetracyclic diterpenoid containing a new ring system. *J. Chem. Soc. Chem. Commun.* 1027–1028. doi: 10.1039/c39720001027

Christianson, D. W. (2017). Structural and chemical biology of terpenoid cyclases. *Chem. Rev.* 117, 11570–11648. doi: 10.1021/acs.chemrev.7b00287

Dalziel, W., Hesp, B., Stevenson, K. M., and Jarvis, J. A. J. (1973). The structure and absolute configuration of the antibiotic aphidicolin: a tetracyclic diterpenoid containing a new ring system. *J. Chem. Soc. Perkin Trans.* 1, 2841–2851. doi: 10.1039/p19730002841

Dickschat, J. S. (2016). Bacterial terpene cyclases. *Nat. Prod. Rep.* 33, 87–110. doi: 10.1039/C5NP00102A

Dickschat, J. S. (2017). Modern aspects of isotopic labellings in terpene biosynthesis. *Eur. J. Org. Chem.* 2017, 4872–4882. doi: 10.1002/ejoc.201700482

Edwards, T. G., Helmus, M. J., Koeller, K., Bashkin, J. K., and Fisher, C. (2013). Human papillomavirus episome stability is reduced by aphidicolin and controlled by DNA Damage response pathways. *J. Virol.* 87, 3979–3989. doi: 10.1128/JVI.03473-12

Escorcia, A. M., van Rijn, J. P. M., Cheng, G.-J., Schrepfer, P., Brück, T. B., and Thiel, W. (2018). Molecular dynamics study of taxadiene synthase catalysis. *J. Comput. Chem.* doi: 10.1002/jcc.25184. [Epub ahead of print].

Eswar, N., Webb, B., Marti-Renom, M. A., Madhusudhan, M. S., Eramian, D., Shen, M.-Y., et al. (2006). Comparative protein structure modeling using modeller. *Curr. Protoc. Bioinformatics* Chapter 5, Unit-5.6. doi: 10.1002/0471250953.bi0506s15

Fujii, R., Minami, A., Tsukagoshi, T., Sato, N., Sahara, T., Ohgiya, S., et al. (2011). Total biosynthesis of diterpene aphidicolin, a specific inhibitor of DNA polymerase α: heterologous expression of four biosynthetic genes in *Aspergillus oryzae*. *Biosci. Biotechnol. Biochem.* 75, 1813–1817. doi: 10.1271/bbb.110366

Görner, C., Häuslein, I., Schrepfer, P., Eisenreich, W., and Brück, T. (2013). Targeted engineering of cyclooctat-9-en-7-ol synthase: a stereospecific access to two new non-natural fusicoccane-type diterpenes. *ChemCatChem* 5, 3289–3298. doi: 10.1002/cctc.201300285

Hanson, J. R. (2015). Diterpenoids of terrestrial origin. *Nat. Prod. Rep.* 32, 76–87. doi: 10.1039/C4NP00108G

Hanwell, M. D., Curtis, D. E., Lonie, D. C., Vandermeersch, T., Zurek, E., and Hutchison, G. R. (2012). Avogadro: an advanced semantic chemical editor, visualization, and analysis platform. *J. Cheminform.* 4:17. doi: 10.1186/1758-2946-4-17

Hoshino, T., Nakano, C., Ootsuka, T., Shinohara, Y., and Hara, T. (2011). Substrate specificity of Rv3378c, an enzyme from *Mycobacterium tuberculosis*, and the inhibitory activity of the bicyclic diterpenoids against macrophage phagocytosis. *Org. Biomol. Chem.* 9, 2156–2165. doi: 10.1039/C0OB00884B

Hu, X., and Shelver, W. H. (2003). Docking studies of matrix metalloproteinase inhibitors: zinc parameter optimization to improve the binding free energy prediction. *J. Mol. Graph. Modell.* 22, 115–126. doi: 10.1016/S1093-3263(03)00153-0

Humphrey, W., Dalke, A., and Schulten, K. (1996). VMD: Visual molecular dynamics. *J. Mol. Graph.* 14, 33–38. doi: 10.1016/0263-7855(96)00018-5

Ikegami, S., Taguchi, T., Ohashi, M., Oguro, M., Nagano, H., and Mano, Y. (1978). Aphidicolin prevents mitotic cell division by interfering with the activity of DNA polymerase-α. *Nature* 275:458. doi: 10.1038/275458a0

Janke, R., Görner, C., Hirte, M., Brueck, T., and Loll, B. (2014). The first structure of a bacterial diterpene cyclase: CotB2. *Acta Crystallogr. D Biol. Crystallogr.* 70, (Pt 6), 1528–1537. doi: 10.1107/S1399004714005513

Jia, M., Zhou, K., Tufts, S., Schulte, S., and Peters, R. J. (2017). A pair of residues that interactively affect diterpene synthase product outcome. *ACS Chem. Biol.* 12, 862–867. doi: 10.1021/acschembio.6b01075

Jones, B. (2017). *Diterpenoids: Types, Functions and Research*. New York, NY: Nova Science Publishers, Incorporated.

Källberg, M., Wang, H., Wang, S., Peng, J., Wang, Z., Lu, H., et al. (2012). Template-based protein structure modeling using the RaptorX web server. *Nat. Protoc.* 7, 1511–1522. doi: 10.1038/nprot.2012.085

Kayser, O., Kiderlen, A. F., Bertels, S., and Siems, K. (2001). Antileishmanial activities of aphidicolin and its semisynthetic derivatives. *Antimicrob. Agents Chemother.* 45, 288–292. doi: 10.1128/AAC.45.1.288-292.2001

Khandelwal, A., Lukacova, V., Comez, D., Kroll, D. M., Raha, S., and Balaz, S. (2005). A Combination of docking, QM/MM methods, and MD simulation for binding affinity estimation of metalloprotein ligands. *J. Med. Chem.* 48, 5437–5447. doi: 10.1021/jm049050v

Lauchli, R., Rabe, K. S., Kalbarczyk, K. Z., Tata, A., Heel, T., Kitto, R. Z., et al. (2013). High-throughput screening and directed evolution of terpene synthase-catalyzed cylization(). *Angew. Chem. Int. Ed. Engl.* 52, 5571–5574. doi: 10.1002/anie.201301362

Liu, W., Feng, X., Zheng, Y., Huang, C.-H., Nakano, C., Hoshino, T., et al. (2014). Structure, function and inhibition of ent-kaurene synthase from *Bradyrhizobium japonicum*. *Sci. Rep.* 4:6214. doi: 10.1038/srep06214

Lopes, A. A., and Pupo, M. T. (2011). Biosynthesis of aphidicolin proceeds via the mevalonate pathway in the endophytic fungus *Nigrospora sphaerica*. *J. Braz. Chem. Soc.* 22, 80–85. doi: 10.1590/S0103-50532011000100010

Morrone, D., Hillwig, M. L., Mead, M. E., Lowry, L., Fulton, D. B., and Peters, R. J. (2011). Evident and latent plasticity across the rice diterpene synthase family with potential implications for the evolution of diterpenoid metabolism in the cereals. *Biochem. J.* 435, 589–595. doi: 10.1042/BJ20101429

Morrone, D., Xu, M., Fulton, D. B., Determan, M. K., and Peters, R. J. (2008). Increasing complexity of a diterpene synthase reaction with a single residue switch. *J. Am. Chem. Soc.* 130, 5400–5401. doi: 10.1021/ja710524w

Oikawa, H., Nakamura, K., Toshima, H., Toyomasu, T., and Sassa, T. (2002). Proposed mechanism for the reaction catalyzed by a diterpene cyclase, aphidicolan-16β-ol synthase: experimental results on biomimetic cyclization and examination of the cyclization pathway by ab initio calculations. *J. Am. Chem. Soc.* 124, 9145–9153. doi: 10.1021/ja025830m

Oikawa, H., Toyomasu, T., Toshima, H., Ohashi, S., Kawaide, H., Kamiya, Y., et al. (2001). Cloning and functional expression of cDNA encoding aphidicolan-16β-ol synthase: a key enzyme responsible for formation of an unusual diterpene skeleton in biosynthesis of aphidicolin. *J. Am. Chem. Soc.* 123, 5154–5155. doi: 10.1021/ja015747j

Pedrali-Noy, G., Spadari, S., Miller-Faurès, A., Miller, A. O., Kruppa, J., and Koch, G. (1980). Synchronization of HeLa cell cultures by inhibition of DNA polymerase alpha with aphidicolin. *Nucleic Acids Res.* 8, 377–387. doi: 10.1093/nar/8.2.377

Pemberton, R. P., Ho, K. C., and Tantillo, D. J. (2015). Modulation of inherent dynamical tendencies of the bisabolyl cation via preorganization in epi-isozizaene synthase. *Chem. Sci.* 6, 2347–2353. doi: 10.1039/C4SC03782K

Pettersen, E. F., Goddard, T. D., Huang, C. C., Couch, G. S., Greenblatt, D. M., Meng, E. C., et al. (2004). UCSF Chimera—A visualization system for exploratory research and analysis. *J. Comput. Chem.* 25, 1605–1612. doi: 10.1002/jcc.20084

Phillips, J. C., Braun, R., Wang, W., Gumbart, J., Tajkhorshid, E., Villa, E., et al. (2005). Scalable molecular dynamics with NAMD. *J. Comput. Chem.* 26, 1781–1802. doi: 10.1002/jcc.20289

Schalk, M., Pastore, L., Mirata, M. A., Khim, S., Schouwey, M., Deguerry, F., et al. (2012). Toward a biosynthetic route to sclareol and amber odorants. *J. Am. Chem. Soc.* 134, 18900–18903. doi: 10.1021/ja307404u

Schrepfer, P., Buettner, A., Goerner, C., Hertel, M., van Rijn, J., Wallrapp, F., et al. (2016). Identification of amino acid networks governing catalysis in the closed complex of class I terpene synthases. *Proc. Natl. Acad. Sci. U.S.A.* 113, E958–E967. doi: 10.1073/pnas.1519680113

Serrano-Posada, H., Centeno-Leija, S., Rojas-Trejo, S., Stojanoff, V., Rodriguez-Sanoja, R., Rudino-Pinera, E., et al. (2015). Crystallization and X-ray diffraction analysis of a putative bacterial class I labdane-related diterpene synthase. *Acta Crystallogr. Sect. F* 71, 1194–1199. doi: 10.1107/S2053230X15014363

Shetty, R. P., Endy, D., and Knight, T. F. (2008). Engineering BioBrick vectors from BioBrick parts. *J. Biol. Eng.* 2:5. doi: 10.1186/1754-1611-2-5

Starczewska, E., Beyaert, M., Michaux, L., Vekemans, M.-C., Saussoy, P., Bol, V., et al. (2016). Targeting DNA repair with aphidicolin sensitizes primary chronic lymphocytic leukemia cells to purine analogs. *Oncotarget* 7, 38367–38379. doi: 10.18632/oncotarget.9525

Starratt, A. N., and Loschiavo, S. R. (1974). The production of aphidicolin by *Nigrospora sphaerica*. *Can. J. Microbiol.* 20, 416–417. doi: 10.1139/m74-063

Stone, J. E. (1998). *An Efficient Library for Parallel Ray Tracing and Animation: A Thesis Presented to the Faculty of the Graduate School of the University of Missouri-Rolla in Partial Fulfillment of Requirements for the Degree of Master of Science in Computer Science.* Master thesis, University of Missouri-Rolla, Rolla, MO.

Trott, O., and Olson, A. J. (2010). AutoDock Vina: improving the speed and accuracy of docking with a new scoring function, efficient optimization, and multithreading. *J. Comput. Chem.* 31, 455–461. doi: 10.1002/jcc.21334

Vanommeslaeghe, K., Hatcher, E., Acharya, C., Kundu, S., Zhong, S., Shim, J., et al. (2010). CHARMM General Force Field (CGenFF): a force field for drug-like molecules compatible with the CHARMM all-atom additive biological force fields. *J. Comput. Chem.* 31, 671–690. doi: 10.1002/jcc.21367

Vanommeslaeghe, K., and MacKerell, A. D. (2012). Automation of the CHARMM General Force Field (CGenFF) I: bond perception and atom typing. *J. Chem. Inf. Model.* 52, 3144–3154. doi: 10.1021/ci300363c

Vanommeslaeghe, K., Raman, E. P., and MacKerell, A. D. (2012). Automation of the CHARMM General Force Field (CGenFF) II: assignment of bonded parameters and partial atomic charges. *J. Chem. Inf. Model.* 52, 3155–3168. doi: 10.1021/ci3003649

Xu, J., and Li, M. (2003). Assessment of RAPTOR's linear programming approach in CAFASP3. *Proteins* 53, 579–584. doi: 10.1002/prot.10531

Yee, N. K. N., and Coates, R. M. (1992). Total synthesis of (+)-9,10-syn- and (+)-9,10-anti-copalol via epoxy trienylsilane cyclizations. *J. Org. Chem.* 57, 4598–4608. doi: 10.1021/jo00043a014

Yoshikuni, Y., Martin, V. J. J., Ferrin, T. E., and Keasling, J. D. (2006). Engineering cotton (+)-δ-cadinene synthase to an altered function: germacrene D-4-ol synthase. *Chem. Biol.* 13, 91–98. doi: 10.1016/j.chembiol.2005.10.016

8

Structure-Based Design, Synthesis, Biological Evaluation and Molecular Docking of Novel PDE10 Inhibitors with Antioxidant Activities

Jinxuan Li†, Jing-Yi Chen†, Ya-Lin Deng, Qian Zhou, Yinuo Wu, Deyan Wu* and Hai-Bin Luo*

School of Pharmaceutical Sciences, Sun Yat-sen University, Guangzhou, China

***Correspondence:**
Yinuo Wu
wyinuo3@mail.sysu.edu.cn
Deyan Wu
wudeyan3@mail.sysu.edu.cn

†These authors have contributed equally to this work.

Phosphodiesterase 10 is a promising target for the treatment of a series of central nervous system (CNS) diseases. Imbalance between oxidative stress and antioxidant defense systems as a universal condition in neurodegenerative disorders is widely studied as a potential therapy for CNS diseases, such as Alzheimer's disease (AD), Parkinson's disease (PD) and amyotrophic lateral sclerosis (ALS). To discover multifunctional pharmaceuticals as a treatment for neurodegenerative diseases, a series of quinazoline-based derivatives with PDE10 inhibitory activities and antioxidant activities were designed and synthesized. Nine out of 13 designed compounds showed good PDE10 inhibition at the concentration of 1.0 μM. Among these compounds, eight exhibited moderate to excellent antioxidant activity with ORAC (oxygen radical absorbance capacity) value above 1.0. Molecular docking was performed for better understanding of the binding patterns of these compounds with PDE10. Compound **11e**, which showed remarkable inhibitory activity against PDE10 and antioxidant activity may serve as a lead for the further modification.

Keywords: Phosphodiesterase-10A, papaverine, antioxidant activity, Alzheimer's disease, molecular docking

INTRODUCTION

Phosphodiesterases (PDEs) are a super enzyme family in charge of hydrolyzing the intracellular second messenger molecules 3′,5′-cyclic adenosine monophosphate (cAMP) and 3′,5′-cyclic guanosine monophosphate (cGMP) by degrading their phosphodiester bonds (Liu et al., 2001; Mehats et al., 2002; Castro et al., 2005; Bender and Beavo, 2006; Conti and Beavo, 2007; Houslay, 2010). As both cAMP and cGMP are involved in various extracellular signals and biological processes, the inhibition of PDEs can improve abnormal physiological processes caused by the low concentration of cAMP and/or cGMP by inhibiting their degradation (Lugnier, 2006; Francis et al., 2011). Thus, PDEs have been considered as promising targets for various diseases. Currently, up to 12 PDEs inhibitors have been approved, including PDE5 inhibitor sildenafil for erectile dysfunction and pulmonary arterial hypertension, PDE4 inhibitor roflumilast for chronic obstructive pulmonary disease (Sung et al., 2003; Christie, 2005). PDEs are classified into 11 distinct families (PDE1-11) based on the amino acid sequences, substrate specificities, and pharmacological properties (Bender and Beavo, 2006). The different expression of each subfamily on the organs and tissues makes specific PDE inhibitors have different therapeutic effects.

Phosphodiesterase 10 (PDE10) is a dual-specificity superfamily responsible for hydrolyzing both cAMP (K_m = 0.05 µM) and cGMP (K_m = 3 µM) (Soderling et al., 1999), which is highly expressed in the brain and has been considered as a potential target for the treatment of several central nervous system (CNS) disorders such as Schizophrenia and Huntington's disease (Hebb et al., 2004). Recent work has shown that blockade of PDE10A with selective inhibitors increases striatal cGMP and phosphorylated cAMP-response element binding protein (CREB), a downstream marker of cAMP production (Siuciak et al., 2006b). PDE10 inhibitors regulate the levels of cAMP and cGMP and activate the downstream dopaminergic pathways and glutamatergic pathways, which may avoid side effects of extrapyramidal system (EPS) caused by current anti-Schizophrenia drugs. In conditioned avoidance responding (CAR), an animal model predictive of drug antipsychotic activity, PDE10A inhibitors exhibited a dose-dependent inhibition. (Jones et al., 2015; Suzuki et al., 2015). Great efforts have been devoted in the development of PDE10 inhibitors in the last decade. Up to 7 candidates such as **MP-10** and **TAK-063** have entered the preclinical or clinical trials (Kehler, 2013; Gentzel et al., 2015; Wilson et al., 2015). However, there is still no PDE10 inhibitor approved on the market as a drug.

Oxidative stress (OS) has been suggested as a possible element in the pathogenesis of neurodegenerative disorders (Ceballos et al., 1990; Islam, 2017). Researches showed that neurodegenerative disorders are qualified by different levels of oxidative stress biomarkers and antioxidant defense biomarkers in the brain and peripheral tissues. Recently, some pharmaceuticals on the market with anti-oxidant activities have been demonstrated to decelerate neurodegenerative processes and enhance comprehension ability of the Oxidative stress (OS) characteristics in the pathobiology of these stubborn conditions (Mecocci and Polidori, 2012; Danta and Piplani, 2014). Moreover, experimental studies have proved the presence of elevated levels of Oxidative stress (OS) biomarkers accompanied with the impairments to antioxidant defenses in central and peripheral tissues in pathological process of Parkinson's disease (PD), Alzheimer's disease (AD), and amyotrophic lateral sclerosis (ALS). Pharmaceuticals with antioxidant activity enable biomarkers of the oxidant/antioxidant to rebalance in animal models, thus are widely studied as possible anti-neurodegenerative agents (Zhang et al., 2006; Niedzielska et al., 2016). Vinpocetine, a moderate PDE1 inhibitor with antioxidant activity, can significantly improve the learning and memory in the streptozotocin infused AD rat models. Vinpocetine acts as a neuroprotective agent, which is widely applied to the treatment of CNS disorders with good antioxidant activity and the observed cognitive effects and memory improvement of vinpocetine is believed to be bound up with the antioxidant mechanism and elevations of cGMP levels (Hindmarch et al., 1991; Bönöczk et al., 2000). As noted above, PDE inhibitors with antioxidant activities have potential possibility to apply in the treatment of several CNS disorders.

Till now, compounds with both PDE10A inhibitory activities and antioxidant activities have seldom been reported. Taking all these into consideration, a strategy to design lead compounds combining the pharmacophore of PDE10A inhibitors and antioxidants seems to be attractive and challenging. In this study, a series of compounds expected to exhibit both PDE10A inhibition and antioxidant activity were designed and synthesized based on the chemical structure of a natural derivative papaverine. Five compounds showed moderate to good PDE10A inhibitory activities. Compound **11e** showed good antioxidant activity as well as PDE10A inhibitory activity.

MATERIALS AND METHODS

All starting materials and reagents were purchased from commercial suppliers (Adamas, Energy, Bide, Sigma-Aldrich, ShuYa, J&K, and Meryer) and used directly without further purification. Chemical HG/T2354-92 silica gel (200–300 mesh, Haiyang®) was used for chromatography, and silica gel plates with fluorescence F254 (0.25 mm, Huanghai®) were used for thin-layer chromatography (TLC) analysis. Reactions requiring anhydrous conditions were performed under argon or a calcium chloride tube. ^{1}H NMR and ^{13}C NMR spectra were recorded at room temperature on a Bruker AVANCE III 400 instrument with tetramethylsilane (TMS) as an internal standard (**Presentation 1**). The following abbreviations are used: s (singlet), d (doublet), t (triplet), m (multiplet), dd (doublet of doublets), dt (doublet of triplets), td (triplet of doublets), and br (broad signal). Coupling constants were reported in Hz. Low- and high-resolution mass spectra (LRMS and HRMS) were recorded on a MAT-95 spectrometer. The purity of compounds was determined by reverse-phase high-performance liquid chromatography (HPLC) analysis confirming to be over 95%. HPLC instrument: SHIMADZU LC-20AT (column: Hypersil BDS C_{18}, 5.0 µm, 4.6 × 150 mm (Elite); Detector: SPD-20A UV/VIS detector, UV detection at 254 nm; Elution, MeOH in water (60–80%, v/v); T = 25°C; and flow rate = 0.8–1.0 mL/min.

7-methoxy-4-oxo-3,4-dihydroquinazolin-6-yl Acetate (4)

Pyridine (4 mL) was added dropwise to the solution of 6-hydroxy-7-methoxyquinazolin-4(3H)-one **3** (1.92 g, 10.0 mmol) in acetic anhydrate (20 mL). The reaction mixture was heated at 100°C for 2 h and then cooled to room temperature. After the mixture was poured into ice water, a white solid was precipitated. The precipitate was collected, washed with water and dried to give the compound **4** (2.32 g, 99%) as a white solid. ^{1}H NMR (400 MHz, DMSO – d_6) δ 8.09 (s, 1H), 7.76 (s, 1H), 7.28 (s, 1H), 3.92 (s, 3H), 2.30 (s, 3H).

4-chloro-7-methoxyquinazolin-6-yl acetate (5)

To a solution of **4** (2.34 g, 10.0 mmol) in $SOCl_2$ (20 mL) was added DMF (0.1 mL) dropwise. The mixture was stirred at 80°C for 2.5 h and then concentrated under vacuum, providing compound **5** (2.22 g, 88%) which could be used in the next step without further purification. ^{1}H NMR (400 MHz, DMSO – d_6) δ 9.02 (s, 1H), 8.02 (s, 1H), 7.65 (s, 1H), 4.03 (s, 4H), 2.36 (s, 3H).

7-methoxy-4-morpholinoquinazolin-6-ol (7)

A solution of compound **5** (2.52 g, 10.0 mmol) and morpholine (1.04 g, 12.0 mmol) in DMF (20 mL) was stirred at 80°C for 6 h. The mixture was then poured into the ice water and a white solid was precipitated, which was collected and washed with ice water to afford compound **6**. The compound **6** was dissolved in methanol (20 mL). Ammonia (2.5 mL) was added to the mixture and the mixture was then stirred under reflux for 2 h. The solvents were evaporated under vacuum. The crude product was recrystallized using methanol to afford compound **7** (1.87 g, 72%). ^{1}H NMR (400 MHz, DMSO – d_6) δ 8.52 (s, 1H), 7.24 (s, 1H), 7.21 (s, 1H), 3.93 (s, 3H), 3.83 – 3.75 (m, 4H), 3.54 – 3.47 (m, 4H).

4-(6-(2-(1H-indol-3-yl)ethoxy)-7-methoxyquinazolin-4-yl) morpholine (8a)

To a solution of compound **7** (522 mg, 2.0 mmol) in DMF (20 mL) was added 3-(2-bromoethyl)-1H-indole (538 mg, 2.4 mmol) and potassium carbonate (690 mg, 5.0 mmol). The reaction mixture was refluxed for 3 h. After cooling to room temperature, adding water to quench the mixture, and then the residue was diluted with CH_2Cl_2 (30 mL) and washed with saturated aqueous sodium bicarbonate and water. The organic layer was dried over anhydrous sodium sulfate, and purified by silica gel column chromatography (petroleum ether/EtOAc, 3:1–1:1) to afford the title compound as a yellow solid. Purity: 97%; yield: 20%; ^{1}H NMR (400 MHz, $CDCl_3$) δ 8.67 (s, 1H), 8.29 (s, 1H), 7.69 (d, J = 7.8 Hz, 1H), 7.38 (d, J = 8.0 Hz, 1H), 7.22 (t, J = 7.5 Hz, 1H), 7.17 (s, 1H), 7.15 (t, J = 7.4 Hz, 1H), 7.08 (s, 1H), 4.37 (t, J = 7.0 Hz, 2H), 4.02 (s, 3H), 3.82 (s, 4H), 3.60 (s, 4H), 3.39 (t, J = 7.0 Hz, 2H); ^{13}C NMR (101 MHz, $CDCl_3$) δ 163.76, 155.11, 152.96, 149.17, 148.04, 136.26, 127.46, 122.49, 122.22, 119.51, 118.76, 111.85, 111.42, 111.28, 107.65, 104.44, 69.48, 66.63 × 2, 56.19, 50.21×2, 25.19; LRMS (ESI) m/z $[M+H]^+$ 405.2; HRMS (ESI) m/z calcd $C_{23}H_{24}N_4O_3$ $[M+H]^+$ 405.1927, found 405.1922.

General Procedure for Synthesis of Compounds 8b-8c

To a solution of compound **7** (522 mg, 2.0 mmol) in DMF (20 mL) was added the EDCI (575 mg, 3.0 mmol) and DMAP (12 mg, 0.1 mmol). The reaction mixture was stirred at room temperature for 0.5 h, and then the corresponding acid (2.4 mmol) was added, the reaction mixture was refluxed overnight. After cooling to room temperature, adding water to quench the mixture, and then the residue was diluted with CH_2Cl_2 (30 mL) and washed with saturated aqueous sodium bicarbonate and water. The organic layer was dried over anhydrous sodium sulfate, and purified by silica gel column chromatography (petroleum ether/EtOAc, 3:1 to 1:1) to afford the title compound as a white solid.

7-methoxy-4-morpholinoquinazolin-6-yl 3-(4-hydroxyphenyl)Acrylate (8b)

White solid; purity: 97%; yield: 10%; ^{1}H NMR (400 MHz, $CDCl_3$) δ 8.70 (s,1H), 7.86 (d, J = 16.0 Hz, 1H), 7.61 (s, 1H), 7.52 (d, J = 7.5 Hz, 2H), 7.35 (s, 1H), 6.90 (d, J = 7.5 Hz, 2H), 6.54 (d, J = 15.7 Hz, 1H), 5.35 (br, 1H), 3.96 (s, 3H), 3.91–3.85 (m, 4H), 3.78–3.73 (m, 4H); ^{13}C NMR (101 MHz, $CDCl_3$) δ 177.80, 164.07, 155.98, 154.20, 151.68, 147.48, 139.24, 138.32, 130.45 × 2, 117.87, 116.23 × 2, 113.08, 110.55, 108.16, 94.86, 66.76 × 2, 56.28, 50.18 × 2; HRMS (ESI) m/z calcd $C_{22}H_{21}N_3O_5$ $[M+H]^+$ 408.1559, found 408.1554.

7-methoxy-4-morpholinoquinazolin-6-yl 5-(1,2-dithiolan-3-yl)pentanoate (8c)

White solid; purity: 97%; yield: 16%; ^{1}H NMR (400 MHz, $CDCl_3$) δ 8.66 (s, 1H), 7.48 (s, 1H), 7.31 (s, 1H), 3.93 (s, 3H), 3.90–3.78 (m, 4H), 3.75–3.64 (m, 4H), 3.59 (dt, J = 12.9, 6.4 Hz, 1H), 3.14 (dtd, J = 17.9, 11.4, 6.8 Hz, 2H), 2.63 (t, J = 7.3 Hz, 2H), 2.46 (td, J = 12.4, 6.4 Hz, 1H), 1.91 (td, J = 13.7, 7.0 Hz, 1H), 1.76 (ddd, J = 29.4, 14.5, 8.2 Hz, 4H), 1.58 (ddd, J = 22.9, 14.4, 8.1 Hz, 2H); ^{13}C NMR (101 MHz, $CDCl_3$) δ 177.02, 155.73, 153.99, 151.77, 145.91, 139.05, 117.65, 111.54, 106.70, 66.68 × 2, 56.36, 50.08 × 2, 40.19, 38.45, 34.62, 34.29, 33.71, 28.81, 24.78; HRMS (ESI) m/z calcd $C_{21}H_{27}N_3O_4S_2$ $[M+H]^+$ 450.1521, found 450.1534.

4-chloro-6,7-dimethoxyquinazoline (10)

To a solution of **9** (10.0 mmol) in $SOCl_2$ (20 mL) was added DMF (0.1 mL) dropwise. The mixture was stirred at 80°C for 2.5 h and then concentrated under vacuum, providing compound **10** (2.22 g, 90%) which could be used in the next step without further purification. ^{1}H NMR (400 MHz, DMSO – d_6) δ 8.88 (s, 1H), 7.46 (s, 1H), 7.40 (s, 1H), 4.01 (d, J = 6.0 Hz, 6H).

General Procedure for Synthesis of Compounds 11a-11h, 12 and 13

To a solution of **10** (2.0 mmol), the corresponding amine (3.0 mmol) in isopropanol (20 mL) was added triethylamine (6.0 mmol) dropwise. The reaction mixture was refluxed for 4 h and then concentrated under vacuum, providing crude product. The crude product was purified by silica gel column chromatography (CH_2Cl_2/MeOH, 100:1–40:1) to afford the title compound as a white solid.

N-(2-(1H-indol-3-yl)ethyl)-6,7-dimethoxyquinazolin-4-amine (11a)

White solid; purity: 97%; yield: 60%; ^{1}H NMR (400 MHz, DMSO-d_6) δ 10.92 (s, 1H), 10.27 (br, 1H), 8.80 (s, 1H), 8.06 (s, 1H), 7.63 (d, J = 7.8 Hz, 1H), 7.35 (d, J = 8.1 Hz, 1H), 7.26 (d, J = 11.6 Hz, 2H), 7.07 (t, J = 7.5 Hz, 1H), 6.98 (t, J = 7.4 Hz, 1H), 3.97 (s, 1H), 3.95 (s, 7H), 3.93–3.91 (m, 1H), 3.13 (t, J = 7.4 Hz, 2H); ^{13}C NMR (101 MHz, DMSO-d_6) δ 159.44, 156.13, 150.20, 149.28, 136.72, 134.53, 127.62, 123.40, 121.49, 118.80, 114.08, 111.92, 111.57, 107.09, 104.42, 99.94, 57.29, 56.77, 42.80, 24.94; HRMS (ESI) m/z calcd $C_{20}H_{20}N_4O_2$ $[M+H]^+$ 349.1665, found 349.1670.

N-(1-(1H-indol-3-yl)propan-2-yl)-6,7-dimethoxyquinazolin-4-amine (11b)

White solid; purity: 96%; yield: 55%; ^{1}H NMR (400 MHz, $CDCl_3$) δ 8.59 (s, 1H), 8.37 (br, 1H), 7.70 (d, *J* = 7.8 Hz, 1H), 7.41 (d, *J* = 8.1 Hz, 1H), 7.28 (s, 1H), 7.21 (t, *J* = 7.5 Hz, 1H), 7.12 (t, *J* = 7.2 Hz, 2H), 6.56 (s, 1H), 5.74 (br, 1H), 4.96–4.85 (m, 1H), 3.97 (s, 3H), 3.75 (s, 3H), 3.24 (dd, *J* = 14.5, 5.9 Hz, 1H), 3.13 (dd, *J* = 14.4, 4.6 Hz, 1H), 1.40 (d, *J* = 6.4 Hz, 3H); ^{13}C NMR (101 MHz, $CDCl_3$) δ 157.73, 154.22, 154.00, 148.80, 146.09, 136.30, 128.25, 123.26, 122.12, 119.79, 118.90, 111.41, 111.28, 108.60, 107.39, 99.58, 56.13, 56.08, 46.72, 31.11, 20.06; HRMS (ESI) m/z calcd $C_{21}H_{22}N_4O_2$ $[M+H]^+$ 363.1821, found 363.1806.

6,7-dimethoxy-N-(2-(5-methoxy-1H-indol-3-yl)ethyl)quinazolin-4-amine (11c)

White solid; purity: 97%; yield: 62%; ^{1}H NMR (400 MHz, DMSO-d_6) δ 10.67 (br, 1H), 8.41 (s, 1H), 8.10 (t, *J* = 5.5 Hz, 1H), 7.59 (s, 1H), 7.24 (d, *J* = 8.7 Hz, 1H), 7.17 (d, *J* = 2.3 Hz, 1H), 7.13 (d, *J* = 2.4 Hz, 1H), 7.11 (s, 1H), 6.72 (dd, *J* = 8.7, 2.4 Hz, 1H), 3.89 (d, *J* = 9.2 Hz, 6H), 3.88 (s, 3H), 3.81 (dd, *J* = 14.3, 6.3 Hz, 2H), 3.71 (s, 3H), 3.10–3.00 (m, 2H); ^{13}C NMR (101 MHz, DMSO-d_6) δ 158.27, 153.68, 153.60, 152.96, 148.25, 145.80, 131.37, 127.70, 123.27, 112.00, 111.86, 111.10, 108.56, 106.91, 101.99, 100.20, 55.97, 55.62, 55.17, 41.43, 24.85; HRMS (ESI) m/z calcd $C_{21}H_{22}N_4O_3$ $[M+H]^+$ 379.1770, found 379.1766.

6,7-dimethoxy-N-(1-(5-methoxy-1H-indol-3-yl)propan-2-yl)quinazolin-4-amine (11d)

White solid; purity: 98%; yield: 51%; ^{1}H NMR (400 MHz, $CDCl_3$) δ 8.61 (s, 1H), 8.23 (br, 1H), 7.31 (d, *J* = 8.8 Hz, 1H), 7.20 (s, 1H), 7.14 (d, *J* = 1.9 Hz, 1H), 7.10 (s, 1H), 6.87 (dd, *J* = 8.8, 2.1 Hz, 1H), 6.47 (s, 1H), 5.41 (br, 1H), 4.91 (dt, *J* = 12.5, 6.4 Hz, 1H), 3.99 (s, 3H), 3.73 (s, 3H), 3.70 (s, 3H), 3.69–3.64 (m, 1H), 3.22 (dd, *J* = 14.5, 6.0 Hz, 1H), 3.08 (dd, *J* = 14.4, 4.1 Hz, 1H), 1.38 (d, *J* = 6.5 Hz, 3H); ^{13}C NMR (101 MHz, $CDCl_3$) δ 157.73, 154.25, 154.02, 148.91, 146.18, 131.36, 128.62, 124.05, 112.49, 112.18, 110.96, 108.61, 107.43, 100.45, 99.50, 56.14, 55.92, 55.52, 46.61, 31.10, 19.92; HRMS (ESI) m/z calcd $C_{22}H_{24}N_4O_3$ $[M+H]^+$ 393.1927, found 393.1916.

3-(2-((6,7-dimethoxyquinazolin-4-yl)amino)ethyl)-1H-indol-5-ol (11e)

White solid; purity: 97%; yield: 62%; ^{1}H NMR (400 MHz, DMSO-d_6) δ 10.58 (s, 1H), 10.23 (t, *J* = 5.0 Hz, 1H), 8.79 (s, 1H), 8.71 (s, 1H), 8.09 (s, 1H), 7.30 (s, 1H), 7.14 (d, *J* = 8.5 Hz, 2H), 6.98 (d, *J* = 2.0 Hz, 1H), 6.62 (dd, *J* = 8.6, 2.2 Hz, 1H), 3.95 (d, *J* = 4.5 Hz, 6H), 3.90 (dd, *J* = 14.5, 6.7 Hz, 2H), 3.06–3.02 (m, 2H); ^{13}C NMR (101 MHz, DMSO-d_6) δ 159.03, 154.98, 152.15, 151.72, 150.69, 149.35, 131.28, 128.41, 123.65, 112.17, 111.80, 111.13, 108.23, 104.32, 103.27, 102.82, 56.79, 56.41, 42.20, 25.32; HRMS (ESI) m/z calcd $C_{20}H_{20}N_4O_3$ $[M+H]^+$ 365.1614, found 365.1611.

N-(2-(6-fluoro-1H-indol-3-Yl)ethyl)-6,7-dimethoxyquinazolin-4-amine (11f)

White solid; purity: 97%; yield: 44%; ^{1}H NMR (400 MHz, DMSO-d_6) δ 10.90 (br, 1H), 8.39 (s, 1H), 8.09 (t, *J* = 5.5 Hz, 1H), 7.62 (dd, *J* = 8.6, 5.5 Hz, 1H), 7.59 (s, 1H), 7.21 (d, *J* = 2.1 Hz, 1H), 7.12 (dd, *J* = 11.1, 3.2 Hz, 2H), 6.85 (ddd, *J* = 9.8, 8.8, 2.3 Hz, 1H), 3.90 (s, 3H), 3.88 (s, 3H), 3.79 (dd, *J* = 14.3, 6.3 Hz, 2H), 3.08–3.02 (m, 2H); ^{13}C NMR (101 MHz, DMSO-d_6) δ 158.75, 154.27, 153.81, 148.81, 145.57, 136.57, 124.68, 123.73, 119.88, 112.71, 108.88, 107.32, 107.08, 102.48, 97.92, 97.67, 56.50, 56.17, 41.87, 25.22; HRMS (ESI) m/z calcd $C_{20}H_{19}FN_4O_2$ $[M+H]^+$ 367.1570, found 367.1766.

6,7-dimethoxy-N-(2-(5-methyl-1H-indol-3-Yl)ethyl)quinazolin-4-amine (11g)

White solid; purity: 97%; yield: 68%; ^{1}H NMR (400 MHz, DMSO-d_6) δ 10.67 (br, 1H), 8.39 (s, 1H), 8.05 (t, *J* = 5.4Hz, 1H), 7.58 (s, 1H), 7.38 (s, 1H), 7.23 (d, *J* = 8.2 Hz, 1H), 7.15 (s, 1H), 7.10 (s, 1H), 6.90 (d, *J* = 8.2 Hz, 1H), 3.90 (s, 3H), 3.88 (s, 3H), 3.79 (dd, *J* = 13.5, 6.7 Hz, 2H), 3.04 (t, *J* = 7.5 Hz, 2H), 2.35 (s, 3H); ^{13}C NMR (101 MHz, DMSO-d_6) δ 158.70, 154.14, 148.70, 146.49, 135.13, 128.07, 127.01, 123.19, 122.95, 118.54, 112.04, 111.54, 109.07, 107.54, 102.47, 99.99, 56.47, 56.12, 42.00, 25.38, 21.74; HRMS (ESI) m/z calcd $C_{21}H_{22}N_4O_2$ $[M+H]^+$ 363.1821, found 363.1816.

N-(2-(5-bromo-1H-indol-3-yl)ethyl)-6,7-dimethoxyquinazolin-4-amine (11h)

White solid; purity: 97%; yield: 72%; ^{1}H NMR (400 MHz, DMSO-d_6) δ 11.04 (br, 1H), 8.40 (s, 1H), 8.13 (t, *J* = 5.6 Hz, 1H), 7.82 (d, *J* = 1.7 Hz, 1H), 7.57 (s, 1H), 7.32 (d, *J* = 8.6 Hz, 1H), 7.27 (d, *J* = 2.1 Hz, 1H), 7.18 (dd, *J* = 8.6, 1.9 Hz, 1H), 7.10 (s, 1H), 3.90 (d, *J* = 6.6 Hz, 6H), 3.78 (dd, *J* = 13.5, 6.8 Hz, 2H), 3.05 (t, *J* = 7.3 Hz, 2H); ^{13}C NMR (101 MHz, DMSO − d_6) δ 158.85, 154.49, 153.24, 149.00, 144.50, 135.41, 129.75, 125.00, 123.79, 121.34, 113.87, 112.42, 111.43, 108.78, 106.27, 102.90, 56.67, 56.23, 42.06, 25.07; HRMS (ESI) m/z calcd $C_{20}H_{20}BrN_4O_2$ $[M+H]^+$ 427.0770, found 427.0759.

N-(4-(1H-indol-2-yl)butan-2-yl)-6,7-dimethoxyquinazolin-4-amine (12)

White solid; purity: 97%; yield: 60%; ^{1}H NMR (400 MHz, DMSO − d_6) δ 10.71 (s, 1H), 8.32 (s, 1H), 7.67 (s, 1H), 7.58 (d, *J* = 7.6 Hz, 1H), 7.49 (d, *J* = 7.6 Hz, 1H), 7.32 (d, *J* = 8.0 Hz, 1H), 7.09 (t, *J* = 7.1 Hz, 2H), 7.04 (d, *J* = 7.7 Hz, 1H), 6.94 (t, *J* = 7.2 Hz, 1H), 4.58 − 4.48 (m, 1H), 3.90 (dd, *J* = 9.9, 4.6 Hz, 6H), 2.77 (t, *J* = 6.6 Hz, 2H), 2.02 − 1.88 (m, 2H), 1.31 (d, *J* = 6.3 Hz, 3H); ^{13}C NMR (101 MHz, $CDCl_3$) δ 157.79, 154.22, 154.19, 148.79, 146.52 136.45, 127.22, 122.06, 121.39, 119.24, 118.75, 115.83, 111.19, 108.52, 107.79, 99.31, 56.22, 56.15, 47.07, 36.86, 22.15, 21.13; HRMS (ESI) m/z calcd $C_{22}H_{24}N_4O_2$ $[M+H]^+$ 377.1978, found 377.1972.

N-(2-(1H-benzo[d]imidazol-2-yl)ethyl)-6,7-dimethoxyquinazolin-4-amine (13)

White solid; purity: 98%; yield: 68%; ^{1}H NMR (400 MHz, DMSO - d_6) δ 9.31(br, 1H), 8.56 (s, 1H), 7.84 (s, 1H), 7.52 (dd, J = 5.9, 3.2 Hz, 2H), 7.19 (s, 2H), 7.18 (d, J = 3.2 Hz, 1H), 4.17–4.01 (m, 2H), 3.92 (s, 3H), 3.89 (s, 3H), 3.34–3.26 (m, 2H); ^{13}C NMR (101 MHz, DMSO-d_6) δ 159.33, 155.46, 152.92, 150.99, 150.93, 149.68, 149.66, 137.57, 137.46, 122.67×2, 114.82, 107.93, 103.66, 102.90, 56.97, 56.55, 31.18, 28.19; HRMS (ESI) m/z calcd $C_{19}H_{19}N_5O_2$ $[M+H]^+$ 350.1617, found 350.1616.

Protein Expression and Purification

The recombinant pET15b-PDE10A plasmid coding the catalytic domain (residues 446-789) was subcloned and purified according to the following protocols previously reported (Li et al., 2015). Then it was transferred into *E. coli strain* BL21 (Codonplus, Stratagene). The *E. coli* cells carrying the recombinant plasmid were cultured in an 2XYT medium (containing 100 μg/mL ampicillin and 30 μg/mL chloramphenicol) at 37°C until OD_{600} = 0.6-0.8. And then, 1 mM isopropyl-β-D-thiogalactopyranoside was added in to induce the PDE10A protein expression at 20°C for 24 h. The nickel nitriloacetic acid (Ni-NTA) column (Qiagen) was used for purifying PDE10A proteins. The concentration of the PDE10 fractions was estimated based on the absorbance at 280 nm (calculated by the ProtParam software). A typical batch of purification yielded 100-200 mg PDE10A protein from a 1.0 L cell culture.

PDE10A Enzymatic Assays

The enzymatic activities of the catalytic domains of PDE10A were performed using ^{3}H-cGMP solution in the assay buffer of 50 mM Tris pH = 7.5, 4 mM $MgCl_2$, 1 mM DTT, and ^{3}H-cGMP giving 20,000–30,000 cpm after the reaction terminated per assay. To a solution (DMSO) of test compounds in different concentration, the PDE10A enzyme in the assay buffer was added to perform the enzymatic reaction and then incubated at room temperature for 15 min. The assay was then terminated by addition of 0.2 M $ZnSO_4$, Subsequently, 0.2 N $Ba(OH)_2$ was added to precipitate the reaction product ^{3}H-GMP, whereas unreacted ^{3}H-cGMP remained in the supernatant. The radioactivity in the supernatant was measured in 2.5 mL Ultima Gold liquid scintillation cocktails (PerkinElmer) by a liquid scintillation counter (PerkinElmer 2910). The IC_{50} values of test compounds at PDE10A enzymes were measured by repeating of three independent experiments using the nonlinear regression method. Papaverine with an IC_{50} of 0.1 μM was used as the reference compound for enzymatic assay.

Antioxidant Assay

The modified oxygen radical absorbance capacity fluorescein (ORAC-FL) method was performed to determine the antioxidant activity (Ou et al., 2001; Dávalos et al., 2004). The reaction was diluted with 75 mM phosphate buffer (pH = 7.4), and the volume of the final reaction mixture was 200 μL in well. Test compound (20 μL) and fluorescein (120 μL, 150 nM final concentration) were placed in the well of a black 96 well optical bottom plates. After the mixture was incubated at 37°C for 15 min, AAPH solution (60 μL, 12 mM final concentration) was added rapidly. The plate was placed in a Spectrafluor Plus plate reader (Tecan, Crailsheim, Germany) and the fluorescence was recorded every minute for 4 h with an excitation wavelength at 485 nm and emission wavelength at 535 nM. Trolox was used as standard (1–8 μM, final concentration). A blank (fluorescein + AAPH) with phosphate buffer instead of test compounds and trolox calibration were performed for the assays of antioxidants. The samples were measured at different concentration (1–10 μM). All the reaction mixtures were prepared fourfold, and at least three independent assays were performed for each sample. Fluorescence in time course was normalized on basis of the blank (without antioxidants). The ORAC-FL values were calculated as the reported method. Final ORAC-FL values were expressed in μM of trolox equivalents. Ferulic acid was used as the positive reference compound, showing an ORAC-FL value of 1.6 trolox equivalents.

Molecular Docking Studies

The starting conformation of synthesized compounds was generated using Accelrys Discovery Studio 2.5.5. The crystal structure of PDE10A protein with a bound inhibitor possessing the same quinazoline core (PDB code: 3QPN) was used as the reference (Helal et al., 2011). The binding site was defined by the co-crystallized PDE10A inhibitor in PDB entry 3QPN. The Surflex-dock in the software Tripos Sybyl 1.2 (Jain, 2003) was used to obtain the dominant docking conformations in this study.

RESULTS AND DISCUSSION

Rational Design of PDE10 Inhibitors

Papaverine, a natural drug used for the prevention of vasospasm in the clinic, has been proved to have good inhibitory activity toward PDE10A (IC_{50} = 10–300 nM) (Siuciak et al., 2006a). Based on the structure of papaverine, several quinazoline compounds have been developed as PDE10A inhibitors such as compound **1** and compound **2** (**Figure 1**; Chappie et al., 2007; Helal et al., 2011). Observed from the crystal structure of **1** and PDE10A complex, following information for further structural modification were obtained. Firstly, the quinazoline ring located in a hydrophobic clamp comprised of Phe719 and Phe686 in the PDE10A protein, forming π-π interaction with Phe719. Secondly, the 6,7-dimethoxy group in the quinazoline ring formed a bidentate interaction with Gln716 in the pocket. As Gln716 has been regarded as a conserved amino acid residue in PDE10A, the interaction with Gln716 is the main reason for the high affinity of compounds with PDE10A protein. Thus, in our designed compounds, the quinazoline ring was kept as core. Last but not least, the piperazine ring of **1** located outside of the catalytic site in PDE10 protein, providing room for introducing a fragment with antioxidant activity. Furthermore, compound **2**, a PDE10 inhibitor developed from **1**, had a quinoline ring attached on the quinazoline core in order to completely fill the selectivity pocket mainly composed of Tyr683, Met703 and Gly715 in the PDE10A protein. Occupying this unique pocket in PDE10A may significantly enhance the selectivity of the inhibitors over other PDEs. In addition, 6-position at the quinazoline core also provides space and synthetic possibilities for conveniently introducing a fragment. Based on these evidences, the strategy combining PDE10A inhibitory activity and antioxidant activity might improve the druggability of hits. Different fragment from antioxidants (such as melatonin, ferulic acid and lipolic acid) were attached on the 6-position or 4-position of quinazoline ring to form the designed compounds and went into the following synthetic work.

Chemistry

The synthetic route of compounds **8a-8c** is outlined in the **Scheme 1** (Chandregowda et al., 2009). 6-hydroxy-7-methoxyquinazolin-4(3H)-one was reacted with acetic anhydride in pyridine to protect the phenolic hydroxyl group, providing the intermediated **4**. Chlorination of **4** was accomplished with $SOCl_2$ to give 4-chloro-7-methoxyquinazolin-6-yl acetate **5**, which could be used in the reaction with the morpholine directly without further purification, providing 7-methoxy-4-morpholinoquinazolin-6-yl acetate **6**. Hydrolysis of the acetyl group of **6** was performed with concentrated ammonia in MeOH to give **7**. The final products **8a-8c** were obtained by the S_N2 displacement with corresponding bromides or condensation reaction with corresponding acids in moderate yields.

The series of compound **11a-11h**, **12**, and **13** were synthesized in three steps (**Scheme 2**). With 6, 7-dimethoxyquinazolinone as the starting material, a following chlorination led to intermediate **10**, which reacted with different melatonin derivatives to acquire compounds **11a-11h**, **12**, and **13** in high yields (Garofalo et al., 2012; Min et al., 2016).

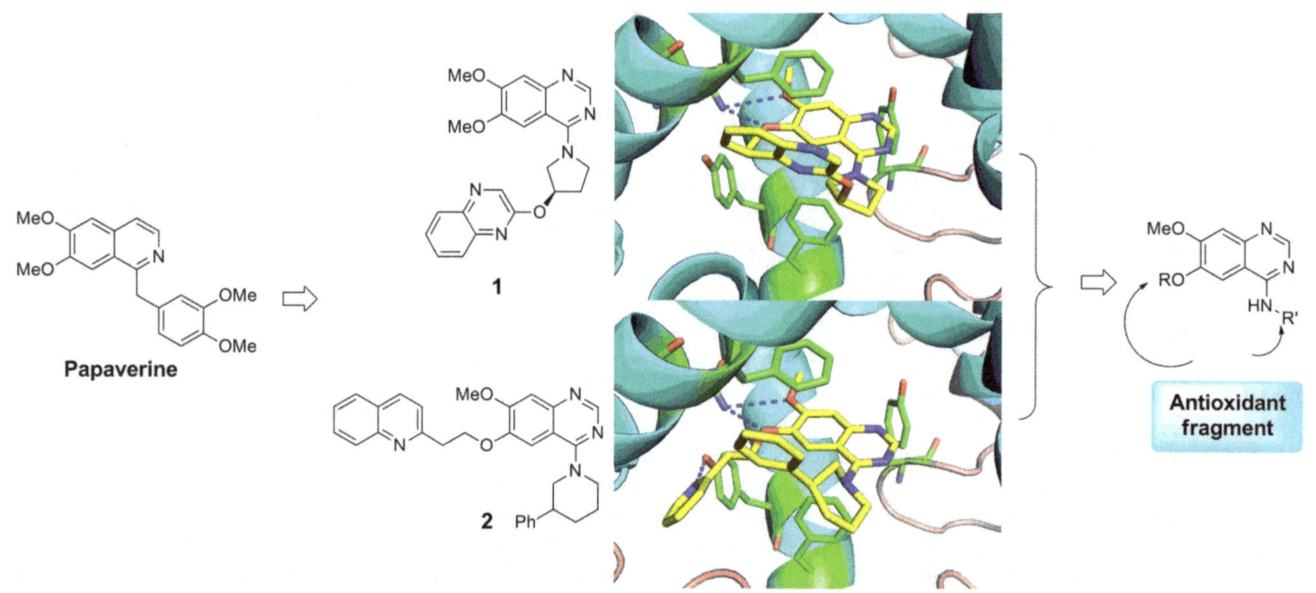

FIGURE 1 | Rational design of novel PDE10 inhibitors with antioxidant activity.

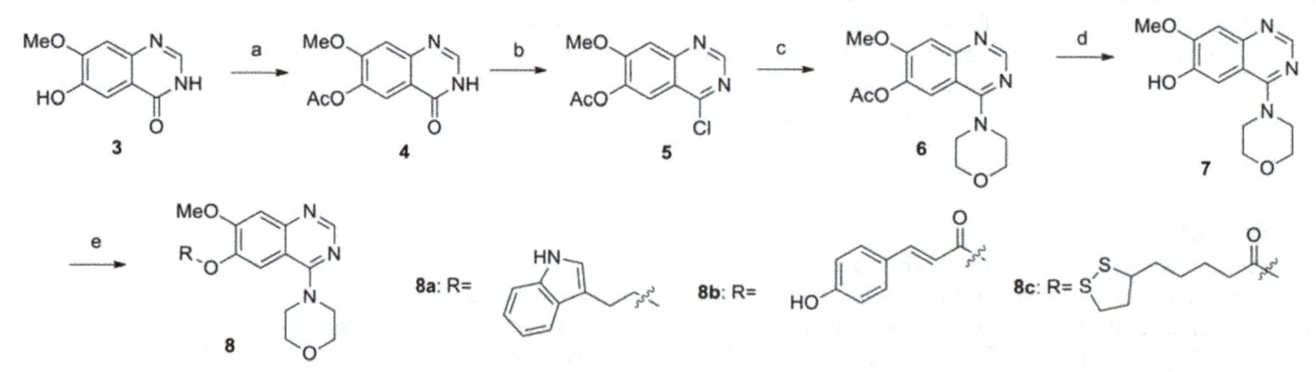

SCHEME 1 | The synthesis route of compounds **8a–8c**. Reagents and conditions: (a) Aceticanhydride, pyridine, 100°C, 2 h; (b)$SOCl_2$, DMF, 80°C, 2.5 h; (c) Morpholine, DMF, 80°C, 6 h; (d) Ammonia, methanol, reflux, 2 h; (e) The corresponding bromide, K_2CO_3, DMF, reflux for 3 h; or the corresponding acid, EDCI, DMAP, DMF, reflux overnight.

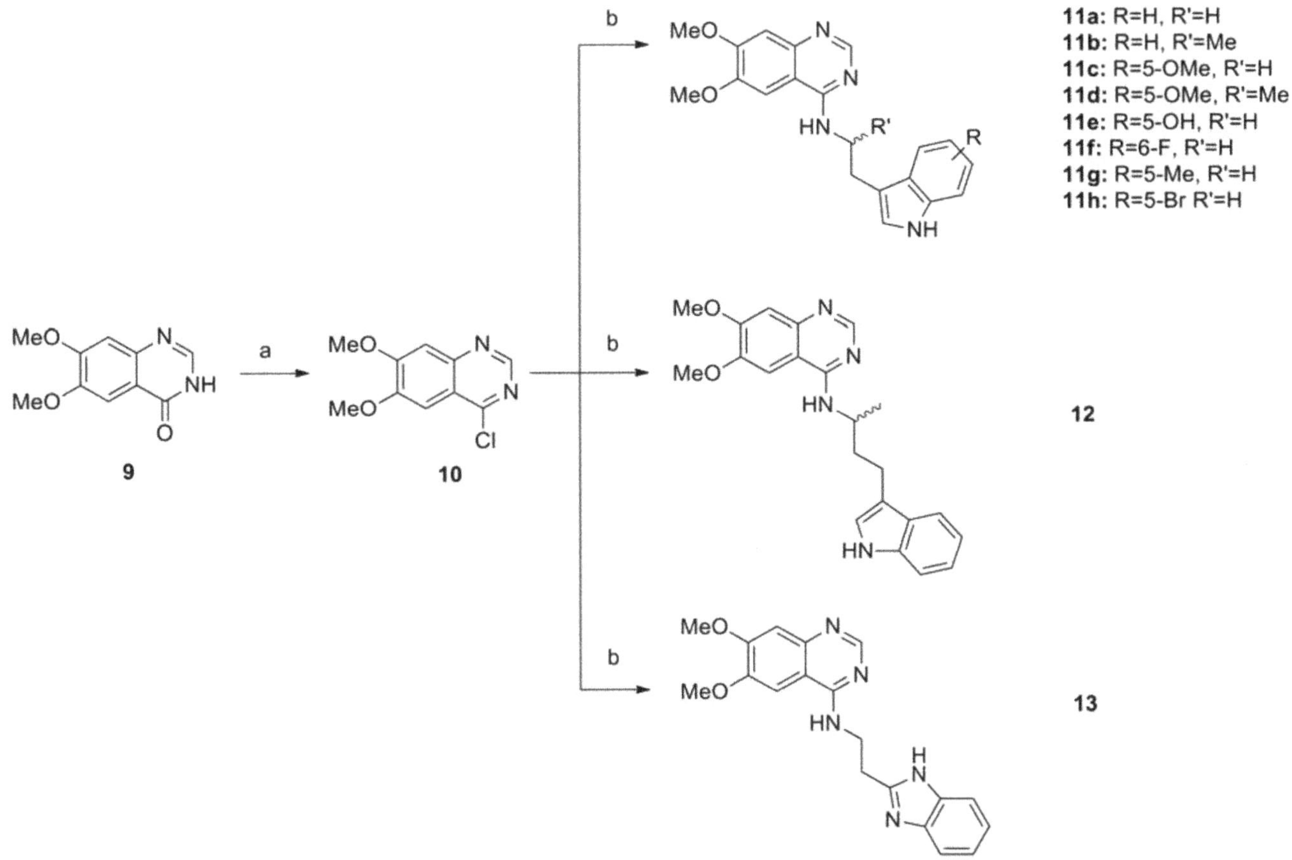

SCHEME 2 | The synthesis route of compounds **11a–11h**, **12**, and **13**. Reagents and conditions: (a) $SOCl_2$, DMF, 80°C, 2.5 h; (b) the corresponding amine, isopropanol, triethylamine, reflux.

Structure-Activity Relationships

Two series of compounds with antioxidant fragments on 4- or 6-position at the quinazoline core were synthesized. The inhibitory activities of these compounds toward PDE10A were evaluated with papaverine as the positive control. LogP (Octanol-Water Partition Coefficient) were calculated as the measure of lipophilicity, mostly drug candidates have LogP value below 5 based on Lipinski's Rule of Five. For our study, all synthetic and designed compounds have good LogP value. TPSA (Topological Polar Surface Area) provided a good estimate of proportion of compounds passed through BBB (blood-brain barrier), high penetration is necessary for drug candidates that targeted central nervous system (CNS) diseases. We were pleased to find that compound **8a**, with a fragment "2-(1H-indol-3-yl)ethyl" substituted on the 6-position, showed good inhibitory activity in the series of compounds **8a-8c**, although not as good as the papaverine and **1**, which also gave ORAC value of 1.0. Compound **8b** and **8c** only showed 26 and 24% inhibition on PDE10A at the concentration of 1 μM, respectively, despite that **8b** showed good TPSA value and antioxidant activity with ORAC value of 3.3 (**Table 1**). We concluded that the ester group in the linker caused steric hindrance in PDE10A pocket, resulting the low inhibitory activities.

According to the structures of reported PDE10/inhibitor complexes, Gln716 and Tyr683 in the PDE10 catalytic domain are two key amino residues for the interaction between inhibitors and PDE10 protein. From this point, we hypothesized that introducing a long chain at the 6-position of our hit compounds to form an interaction with the residue Tyr683 may be useful for the improvement of inhibitory activity toward PDE10. In the other series of compounds **11a-11h, 12 and 13**, different groups were placed on the 4-position of the quinazoline core and the methoxy group on the 6-position remain unchanged. The results were encouraging. Compound **11a**, **11e**, **11f**, **12**, and **13** showed good PDE10A inhibitory activities with IC_{50} below 1 μM. As depicted in **Figure 2**, compound **11f** and **12** exhibited the best PDE10A inhibitory activities with the IC_{50} of 0.33 and 0.24 μM. However, they showed moderate antioxidant activities with ORAC (oxygen radical absorbance capacity) 1.0 and 1.3. Compound **11e**, giving the third best IC_{50} of 0.64 μM on PDE10A and good ORAC (oxygen radical absorbance capacity) value of 2.3, reached a compromise between the PDE10A inhibitory activity and antioxidant activity. From

TABLE 1 | The Inhibitory activities against PDE10A, TPSA, LogP, and oxygen radical absorbance capacity of compounds **8a**-**8c**, **11a**-**11h**, **12**, and **13**.

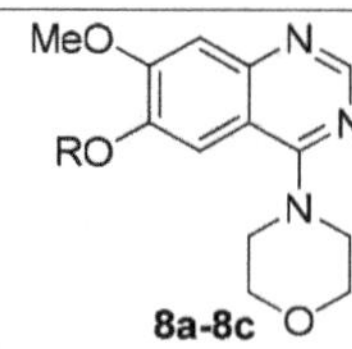

8a-8c

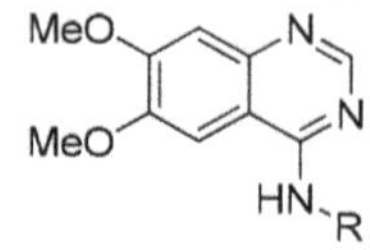

11a-11h

Compound	R	PDE10 inhibitory assay		TPSA[b]	LogP[b]	ORAC[c]
		Inhibition ratio (1 μM) (%)	IC_{50} (μM)[a]			
8a	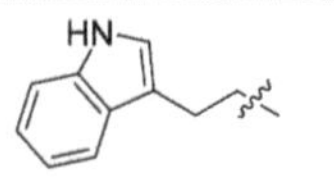	57	–	67.719	3.942	1.0 ± 0.1
8b	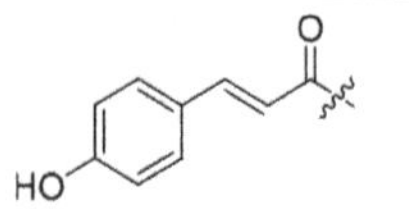	26	–	90.781	3.418	3.3 ± 0.1
8c	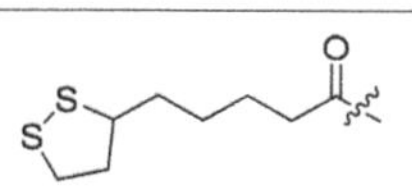	24	–	69.965	3.991	0.3 ± 0.01
11a	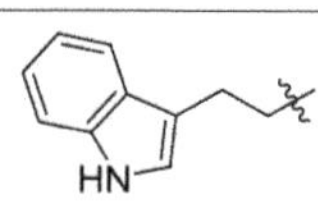	72	0.76 ± 0.09	68.247	3.901	1.3 ± 0.1
11b	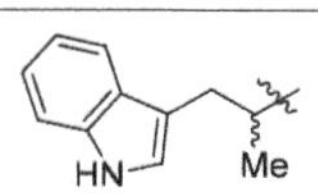	66	–	68.247	4.278	1.5 ± 0.1
11c	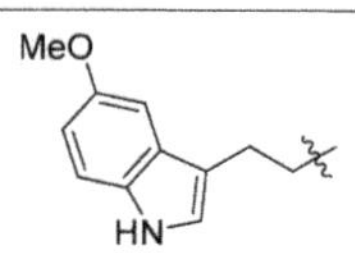	49	–	77.177	3.885	2.2 ± 0.03
11d	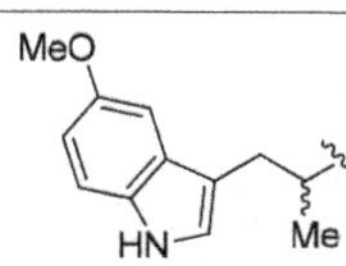	56	–	77.177	4.262	1.3 ± 0.1
11e	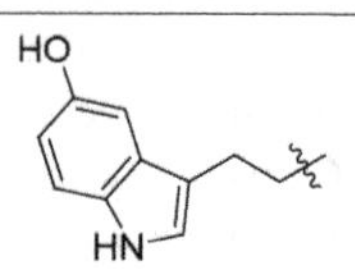	76	0.64 ± 0.05	89.063	3.659	2.3 ± 0.2
11f	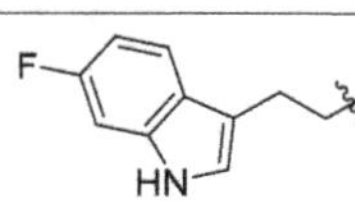	78	0.33 ± 0.04	68.247	4.106	1.0 ± 0.1
11g	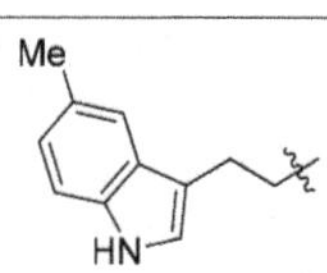	64	–	68.247	4.387	1.0 ± 0.2
11h	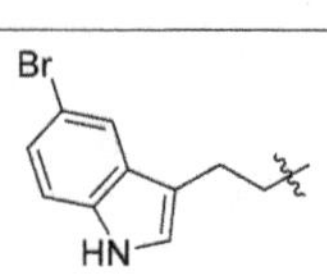	66	–	68.247	4.649	1.9 ± 0.1

(Continued)

TABLE 1 | Continued

Compound	R	PDE10 inhibitory assay		$TPSA^b$	$LogP^b$	$ORAC^c$
		Inhibition ratio (1 μM) (%)	IC_{50} (μM)[a]			
12	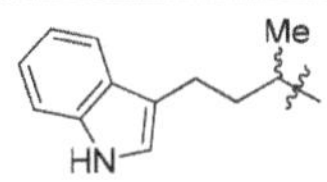	84	0.24 ± 0.02	68.247	4.735	1.3 ± 0.2
13	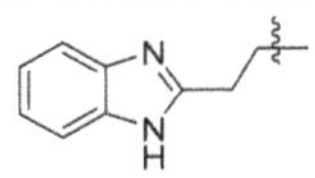	80	0.68 ± 0.09	79.5	3.243	0.15 ± 0.02
Papaverine	–	–	0.1	–	–	–
Ferulic acid	–	–	–	–	–	1.6 ± 0.1

[a] *IC_{50} values are given as the mean of three independent determinations.*
[b] *PSA and LogP values are calculated by Accelrys Discovery Studio 2.5.5.*
[c] *ORAC results are expressed as trolox equivalents.*

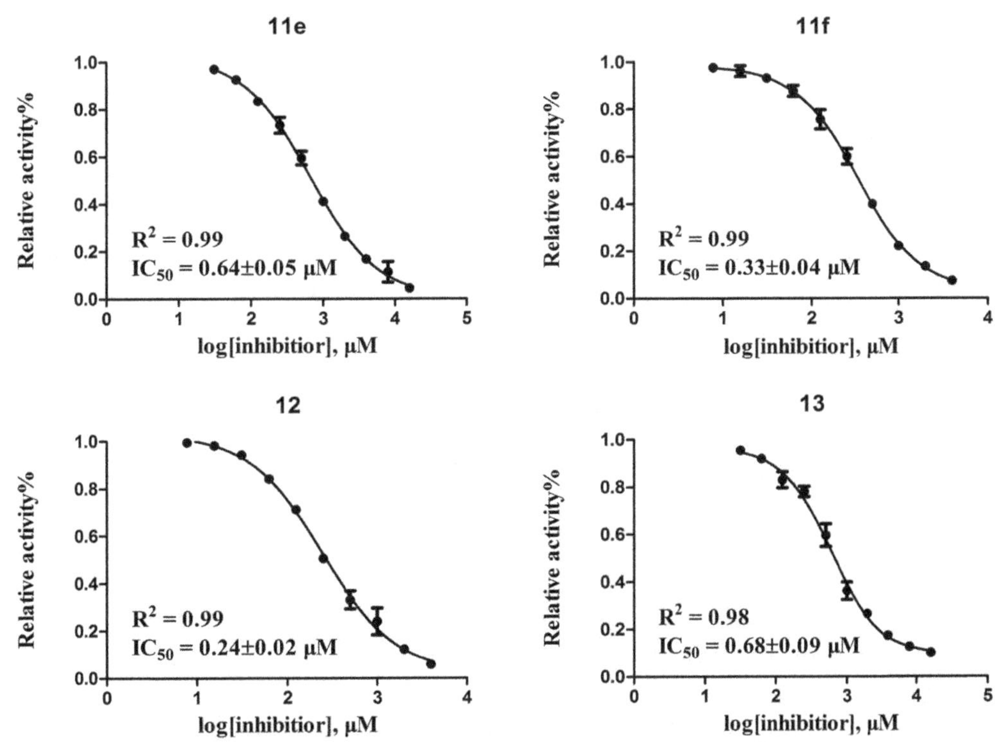

FIGURE 2 | Inhibitory curves of four of the most potent compounds toward PDE10A.

11a to **11b** and **12**, it can be observed that the inhibition on PDE10 was affected by introducing extra carbon atom and methyl group in the linker, while the antioxidant activity was not much affected. In contrast, the antioxidant activities were weakened from **11c** to **11d**, with the ORAC (oxygen radical absorbance capacity) of 2.2–1.3, we concluded that the slight change of introducing a methyl group may cause the steric hindrance (**11b**, **11d** and **12** compared to **11a**, **11c** and **11d**) and leading to impropriate occupation in PDE10 protein, thus responsible for the decreased inhibition on PDE10A. The predict TPSA value of **8b** and **11e** seems good for the BBB penetration. Taking all into consideration, compound **11e**, which showed good PDE10 inhibitory activity and antioxidant activity was good lead for the further modification.

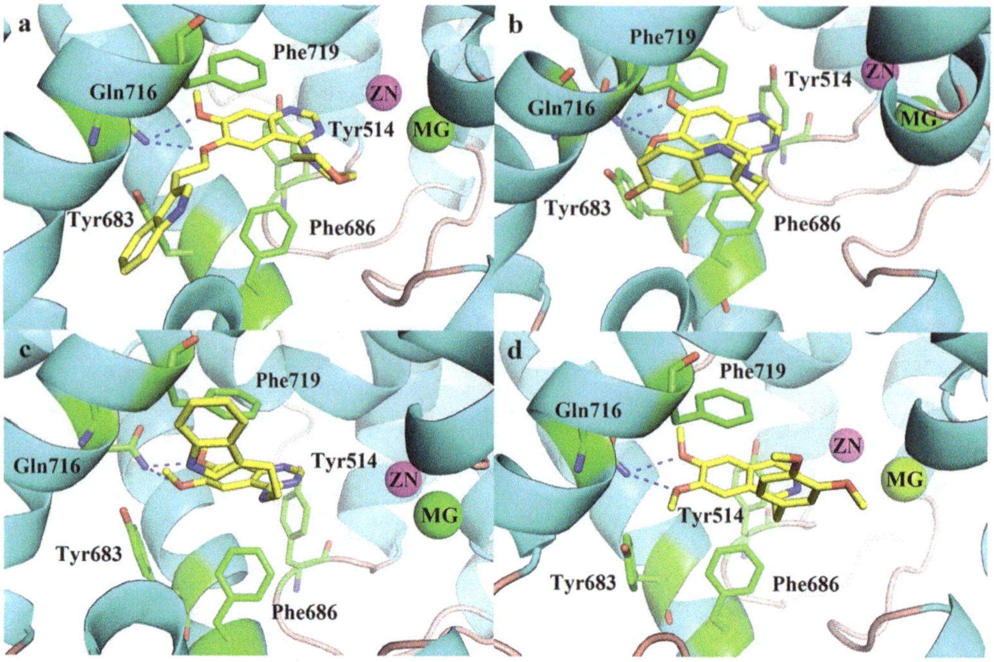

FIGURE 3 | Docked conformation of **(a)** compound **8a**, **(b)** compound **11e**, **(c)** compound **11a** in complex with PDE10A and crystal structure of **(d)** papaverine in complex with PDE10A.

Molecular Docking

The molecular docking was performed to better understand the binding modes between the inhibitors and the PDE10 protein. The structure of PDE10 complex with papaverine has been reported in 2009 (PDB code: 2WEY), which clarified the interaction between papaverine and PDE10 (Andersen et al., 2009). All compounds of **8a-8c**, **11a-11h**, **12**, and **13** were docked into the PDE10 catalytic domain by the Surflex-dock in the software Tripos Sybyl 1.2 (Jain, 2003). From the docking results (**Figure 3**), we found that the quinazoline core of this series compounds occupied the same position as papaverine, and the oxygen of the quinazoline core formed a hydrogen bond interaction with the residue of Gln716. Besides, the quinazoline ring has the hydrophobic interactions with the residues of Phe719 and Phe686. These interactions have been reported to be the critical forces to determine the binding capacity of PDE10 inhibitors. In the series of compounds **8a-8c**, introducing groups at the 6-position of the quinazoline core could fill in the selective pocket of PDE10. However, no hydrogen bond was observed between compounds and Tyr683. The substituted groups of **8b** and **8c** might be too large in terms of volume size for the PDE10 selective pocket. Thus, the PDE10 inhibitory activities of them were weaker than that of **8a**. Compounds **11a-11h** had similar docking patterns since they structurally resemble each other. Besides, compound **8a** and **11a** have the same 2-(1H-indol-3-yl)ethyl group. By observing the docked conformations of **8a** and **11a** in complex with PDE10A, we found that the side chains stretch in different directions, respectively. The side chain of **8a** resides in the selective pocket of PDE10A, however, no hydrogen bond is formed with Tyr683. On the contrary, the side chain of **11a** stretches out of the catalytic site, possessing the same pattern as papaverine (**Figure 3d**).

CONCLUSION

In summary, a series of novel PDE10A inhibitors with antioxidant activities were successfully designed and synthesized using a structure-based discovery strategy, which are potential pharmaceuticals as anti-neurodegenerative PD, AD, or ALS therapies. On the basis of the lead compound papaverine, 13 new quinazoline-based derivatives have been synthesized and evaluated by the inhibitory assays. Nine out of 13 compounds showed good PDE10A inhibitory activities at the concentration of 1 μM. Among these compounds, eight exhibited moderate to good antioxidant activity with the ORAC above 1.0. Especially worthy to mention is that compound **11e**, gave an IC_{50} value of 0.64 μM on PDE10A and good ORAC value of 2.3. In conclusion, this work has described a structure-based discovery strategy and the synthesized quinazoline-based derivatives with both PDE10A inhibitory activity and antioxidant activity, and might provide a new perspective for the development of novel PDE10A inhibitors.

AUTHOR CONTRIBUTION

All authors listed have made a substantial, direct and intellectual contribution to the work, and approved it for publication.

ACKNOWLEDGMENTS

This work was supported by the Natural Science Foundation of China (81602955, 81522041, 21572279, and 81373258), Science Foundation of Guangdong Province (2016A030310144), the Fundamental Research Funds for the Central Universities (Sun Yat-Sen University) (17ykpy20), and Medical Scientific Research Foundation of Guangdong Province (A2016104). We cordially thank Prof. Hengming Ke from Department of Biochemistry and Biophysics at the University of North Carolina, Chapel Hill, for his help with molecular cloning, expression, purification, crystal structure, and bioassay of PDEs.

REFERENCES

Andersen, O., Schönfeld, D., Toogood-Johnson, I., Felicetti, B., Albrecht, C., Fryatt, T., et al. (2009). Cross-linking of protein crystals as an aid in the generation of binary protein-ligand crystal complexes, exemplified by the human PDE10a-papaverine structure. *Acta Crystallogr. D Biol. Crystallogr.* 65, 872–874. doi: 10.1107/S0907444909017855

Bender, A. T., and Beavo, J. A. (2006). Cyclic nucleotide phosphodiesterases: molecular regulation to clinical use. *Pharmacol. Rev.* 58, 488–520. doi: 10.1124/pr.58.3.5

Bönöczk, P., Gulyas, B., Adam-Vizi, V., Nemes, A., Karpati, E., Kiss, B., et al. (2000). Role of sodium channel inhibition in neuroprotection: effect of vinpocetine. *Brain Res. Bull.* 53, 245–254. doi: 10.1016/S0361-9230(00)00354-3

Castro, A., Jerez, M. J., Gil, C., and Martinez, A. (2005). Cyclic nucleotide phosphodiesterases and their role in immunomodulatory responses: advances in the development of specific phosphodiesterase inhibitors. *Med. Res. Rev.* 25, 229–244. doi: 10.1002/med.20020

Ceballos, I., Javoy-Agid, F., Delacourte, A., Defossez, A., Nicole, A., and Sinet, P. M. (1990). Parkinson's disease and Alzheimer's disease: neurodegenerative disorders due to brain antioxidant system deficiency? *Adv. Exp. Med. Biol.* 264, 493–498.

Chandregowda, V., Kush, A. K., and Chandrasekara Reddy, G. (2009). Synthesis and *in vitro* antitumor activities of novel 4-anilinoquinazoline derivatives. *Eur. J. Med. Chem.* 44, 3046–3055. doi: 10.1016/j.ejmech.2008.07.023

Chappie, T. A., Humphrey, J. M., Allen, M. P., Estep, K. G., Fox, C. B., Lebel, L. A., et al. (2007). Discovery of a series of 6,7-dimethoxy-4-pyrrolidylquinazoline PDE10A inhibitors. *J. Med. Chem.* 50, 182–185. doi: 10.1021/jm060653b

Christie, P. (2005). Roflumilast: a selective phosphodiesterase 4 inhibitor. *Drugs Today* 41, 667–675. doi: 10.1358/dot.2005.41.10.920428

Conti, M., and Beavo, J. (2007). Biochemistry and physiology of cyclic nucleotide phosphodiesterases: essential components in cyclic nucleotide signaling. *Annu. Rev. Biochem.* 76, 481–511. doi: 10.1146/annurev.biochem.76.060305.150444

Danta, C. C., and Piplani, P. (2014). The discovery and development of new potential antioxidant agents for the treatment of neurodegenerative diseases. *Expert Opin. Drug Discov.* 9, 1205–1222. doi: 10.1517/17460441.2014.942218

Dávalos, A., Gomez-Cordoves, C., and Bartolome, B. (2004). Extending applicability of the oxygen radical absorbance capacity (ORAC-fluorescein) assay. *J. Agric. Food Chem.* 52, 48–54. doi: 10.1021/jf0305231

Francis, S. H., Blount, M. A., and Corbin, J. D. (2011). Mammalian cyclic nucleotide phosphodiesterases: molecular mechanisms and physiological functions. *Physiol. Rev.* 91, 651–690. doi: 10.1152/physrev.00030.2010

Garofalo, A., Farce, A., Ravez, S., Lemoine, A., Six, P., Chavatte, P., et al. (2012). Synthesis and structure-activity relationships of (aryloxy)quinazoline ureas as novel, potent, and selective vascular endothelial growth factor receptor-2 inhibitors. *J. Med. Chem.* 55, 1189–1204. doi: 10.1021/jm2013453

Gentzel, R. C., Toolan, D., Roberts, R., Koser, A. J., Kandebo, M., Hershey, J., et al. (2015). The PDE10A inhibitor MP-10 and haloperidol produce distinct gene expression profiles in the striatum and influence cataleptic behavior in rodents. *Neuropharmacology* 99, 256–263. doi: 10.1016/j.neuropharm.2015.05.024

Hebb, A. L., Robertson, H. A., and Denovan-Wright, E. M. (2004). Striatal phosphodiesterase mRNA and protein levels are reduced in Huntington's disease transgenic mice prior to the onset of motor symptoms. *Neuroscience* 123, 967–981. doi: 10.1016/j.neuroscience.2003.11.009

Helal, C. J., Kang, Z., Hou, X., Pandit, J., Chappie, T. A., Humphrey, J. M., et al. (2011). Use of structure-based design to discover a potent, selective, *in vivo* active phosphodiesterase 10A inhibitor lead series for the treatment of schizophrenia. *J. Med. Chem.* 54, 4536–4547. doi: 10.1021/jm2001508

Hindmarch, I., Fuchs, H. H., and Erzigkeit, H. (1991). Efficacy and tolerance of vinpocetine in ambulant patients suffering from mild to moderate organic psychosyndromes. *Int. Clin. Psychopharmacol.* 6, 31–43.

Houslay, M. D. (2010). Underpinning compartmentalised cAMP signalling through targeted cAMP breakdown. *Trends Biochem. Sci.* 35, 91–100. doi: 10.1016/j.tibs.2009.09.007

Islam, M. T. (2017). Oxidative stress and mitochondrial dysfunction-linked neurodegenerative disorders. *Neurol. Res.* 39, 73–82. doi: 10.1080/01616412.2016.1251711

Jain, A. N. (2003). Surflex: fully automatic flexible molecular docking using a molecular similarity-based search engine. *J. Med. Chem.* 46, 499–511. doi: 10.1021/jm020406h

Jones, P. G., Hewitt, M. C., Campbell, J. E., Quinton, M. S., Engel, S., Lew, R., et al. (2015). Pharmacological evaluation of a novel phosphodiesterase 10A inhibitor in models of antipsychotic activity and cognition. *Pharmacol. Biochem. Behav.* 135, 46–52. doi: 10.1016/j.pbb.2015.04.017

Kehler, J. (2013). Phosphodiesterase 10A inhibitors: a 2009 - 2012 patent update. *Expert Opin. Ther. Pat.* 23, 31–45. doi: 10.1517/13543776.2012.739157

Li, Z., Lu, X., Feng, L. J., Gu, Y., Li, X., Wu, Y., et al. (2015). Molecular dynamics-based discovery of novel phosphodiesterase-9A inhibitors with non-pyrazolopyrimidinone scaffolds. *Mol. Biosyst.* 11, 115–125. doi: 10.1039/c4mb00389f

Liu, Y., Shakur, Y., Yoshitake, M., and Kambayashi Ji, J. (2001). Cilostazol (pletal): a dual inhibitor of cyclic nucleotide phosphodiesterase type 3 and adenosine uptake. *Cardiovasc. Drug Rev.* 19, 369–386. doi: 10.1111/j.1527-3466.2001.tb00076.x

Lugnier, C. (2006). Cyclic nucleotide phosphodiesterase (PDE) superfamily: a new target for the development of specific therapeutic agents. *Pharmacol. Ther.* 109, 366–398. doi: 10.1016/j.pharmthera.2005.07.003

Mecocci, P., and Polidori, M. C. (2012). Antioxidant clinical trials in mild cognitive impairment and Alzheimer's disease. *Biochim. Biophys. Acta* 1822, 631–638. doi: 10.1016/j.bbadis.2011.10.006

Mehats, C., Andersen, C. B., Filopanti, M., Jin, S. L., and Conti, M. (2002). Cyclic nucleotide phosphodiesterases and their role in endocrine cell signaling. *Trends Endocrinol. Metab.* 13, 29–35. doi: 10.1016/S1043-2760(01)00523-9

Min, J., Guo, K., Suryadevara, P. K., Zhu, F., Holbrook, G., Chen, Y., et al. (2016). Optimization of a novel series of ataxia-telangiectasia mutated kinase inhibitors as potential radiosensitizing agents. *J. Med. Chem.* 59, 559–577. doi: 10.1021/acs.jmedchem.5b01092

Niedzielska, E., Smaga, I., Gawlik, M., Moniczewski, A., Stankowicz, P., Pera, J., et al. (2016). Oxidative stress in neurodegenerative diseases. *Mol. Neurobiol.* 53, 4094–4125. doi: 10.1007/s12035-015-9337-5

Ou, B., Hampsch-Woodill, M., and Prior, R. L. (2001). Development and validation of an improved oxygen radical absorbance capacity assay using fluorescein as the fluorescent probe. *J. Agric. Food Chem.* 49, 4619–4626. doi: 10.1021/jf010586o

Siuciak, J. A., Chapin, D. S., Harms, J. F., Lebel, L. A., McCarthy, S. A., Chambers, L., et al. (2006a). Inhibition of the striatum-enriched phosphodiesterase PDE10A: a novel approach to the treatment of psychosis. *Neuropharmacology* 51, 386–396. doi: 10.1016/j.neuropharm.2006.04.013

Siuciak, J. A., McCarthy, S. A., Chapin, D. S., Fujiwara, R. A., James, L. C., Williams, R. D., et al. (2006b). Genetic deletion of the striatum-enriched phosphodiesterase PDE10A: evidence for altered striatal function. *Neuropharmacology* 51, 374–385. doi: 10.1016/j.neuropharm.2006.01.012

Soderling, S. H., Bayuga, S. J., and Beavo, J. A. (1999). Isolation and characterization of a dual-substrate phosphodiesterase gene family: PDE10A. *Proc. Natl. Acad. Sci. U.S.A.* 96, 7071–7076.

Sung, B. J., Hwang, K. Y., Jeon, Y. H., Lee, J. I., Heo, Y. S., Kim, J. H., et al. (2003). Structure of the catalytic domain of human phosphodiesterase 5 with bound drug molecules. *Nature* 425, 98–102. doi: 10.1038/nature01914

Suzuki, K., Harada, A., Shiraishi, E., and Kimura, H. (2015). *In vivo* pharmacological characterization of TAK-063, a potent and selective phosphodiesterase 10A inhibitor with antipsychotic-like activity in rodents. *J. Pharmacol. Exp. Ther.* 352, 471–479. doi: 10.1124/jpet.114.218552

Wilson, J. M., Ogden, A. M., Loomis, S., Gilmour, G., Baucum, A. J. II, Belecky-Adams, T. L., et al. (2015). Phosphodiesterase 10A inhibitor, MP-10 (PF-2545920), produces greater induction of c-Fos in dopamine D2 neurons than in D1 neurons in the neostriatum. *Neuropharmacology* 99, 379–386. doi: 10.1016/j.neuropharm.2015.08.008

Zhang, H. Y., Yang, D. P., and Tang, G. Y. (2006). Multipotent antioxidants: from screening to design. *Drug Discov. Today* 11, 749–754. doi: 10.1016/j.drudis.2006.06.007

9

Design, Synthesis and Evaluation of Ribose-Modified Anilinopyrimidine Derivatives as EGFR Tyrosine Kinase Inhibitors

Xiuqin Hu[1], Disha Wang[1], Yi Tong[1], Linjiang Tong[2], Xia Wang[1], Lili Zhu[1], Hua Xie[2], Shiliang Li[1], You Yang[1] and Yufang Xu[1*]*

[1] *Shanghai Key Laboratory of New Drug Design, School of Pharmacy, East China University of Science and Technology, Shanghai, China,* [2] *Division of Anti-tumor Pharmacology, State Key Laboratory of Drug Research, Shanghai Institute of Materia Medica, Chinese Academy of Sciences, Shanghai, China*

***Correspondence:**
You Yang
yangyou@ecust.edu.cn
Yufang Xu
yfxu@ecust.edu.cn

The synthesis of a series of ribose-modified anilinopyrimidine derivatives was efficiently achieved by utilizing DBU or *t*BuOLi-promoted coupling of ribosyl alcohols with 2,4,5-trichloropyrimidine as key step. Preliminary biological evaluation of this type of compounds as new EGFR tyrosine kinase inhibitors for combating EGFR L858R/T790M mutant associated with drug resistance in the treatment of non-small cell lung cancer revealed that 3-*N*-acryloyl-5-*O*-anilinopyrimidine ribose derivative **1a** possessed potent and specific inhibitory activity against EGFR L858R/T790M over WT EGFR. Based upon molecular docking studies of the binding mode between compound **1a** and EGFR, the distance between the Michael receptor and the pyrimidine scaffold is considered as an important factor for the inhibitory potency and future design of selective EGFR tyrosine kinase inhibitors against EGFR L858R/T790M mutants.

Keywords: EGFR, tyrosine kinase inhibitors, anilinopyrimidine, glycosides, carbohydrate-based drugs

INTRODUCTION

Epidermal growth factor receptor (EGFR), a transmembrane protein with tyrosine kinase activity, is essential for cell growth, differentiation, migration, adhesion, and proliferation under normal physiological conditions (Gschwind et al., 2004). However, overexpression of EGFR has been associated with tumor growth and progression in a variety of cancers including non-small cell lung cancer (NSCLC), head and neck squamous cell carcinoma, and pancreatic cancer (Huang and Harari, 1999; Kris et al., 2003; Moore et al., 2007; Harrington et al., 2009). Therefore, regulation of EGFR has been deemed as an important strategy for the development of cancer therapy (Huang and Harari, 1999; Gschwind et al., 2004; Steuer et al., 2015).

First-generation EGFR tyrosine kinase inhibitors (TKIs) such as gefitinib and erlotinib that possess a 4-anilinoquinazoline scaffold, reversibly inhibit EGFR mutants (L858R and delE746_A750) as well as wild-type (WT) EGFR, resulting in significant disease control of patients with NSCLC (**Figure 1**) (Cohen et al., 2005; Cheng et al., 2016). However, drug resistance driven by activating mutation of the gatekeeper T790M residue in which the threonine group is replaced with the methionine moiety, greatly counteracted the clinical efficiency of first-generation TKIs against NSCLC (Ozvegy-Laczka et al., 2005; Balak et al., 2006; De Luca et al., 2008; Pao and Chmielecki, 2010). To address this issue, the irreversible EGFR TKIs (afatinib, osimertinib, WZ4002, and CO-1686) which contain a Michael acceptor moiety for binding covalently to the thiol group of

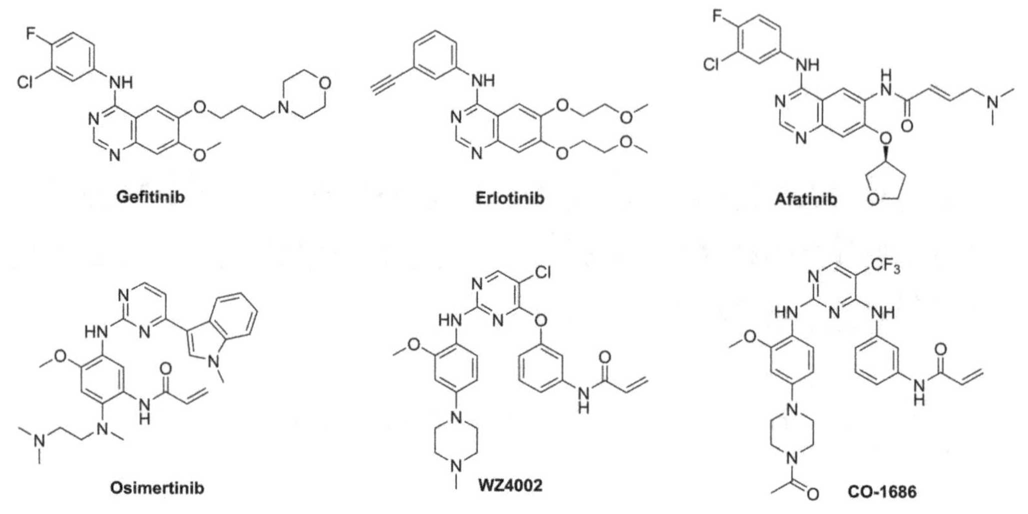

FIGURE 1 | Structures of three generations of EGFR tyrosine kinase inhibitors.

Cys797 in the ATP binding domain of EGFR, were developed to treat NSCLC via the efficient inhibition of EGFR mutants (**Figure 1**; Castellanos and Horn, 2015). Among them, second-generation TKIs such as afatinib potently inhibited both EGFR mutants (L858R/T790M) and WT-EGFR without mutant selectivity, thereby leading to side effects such as rash and diarrhea (Dungo and Keating, 2013). In contrast, third-generation TKIs such as osimertinib, WZ4002, and CO-1686 bearing an anilinopyrimidine core, showed high potency and selectivity for EGFR L858R/T790M over WT EGFR, therefore serving as mutant-selective TKIs targeting EGFR mutants involved in NSCLC (Zhou et al., 2009; Walter et al., 2013; Cross et al., 2014; Finlay et al., 2014; Gray and Haura, 2014).

Considering the drug resistance is rapidly emerging for third-generation TKIs (Eberlein et al., 2015; Niederst et al., 2015; Piotrowska et al., 2015; Thress et al., 2015), design of EGFR inhibitors with new structural skeletons could lead to the discovery of novel types of TKIs against EGFR mutants such as the triple mutant L858R/T790M/C797S (Günther et al., 2016, 2017; Jia et al., 2016; Juchum et al., 2017; Park et al., 2017). Based on the fact that most commercially available TKIs are ATP-competitive inhibitors for binding at the catalytic domain of the EGFR tyrosine kinase (Traxler and Furet, 1999; Grünwald and Hidalgo, 2003; Normanno et al., 2003), we envisioned that replacement of the phenyl ring on the right side of WZ4002 with a chiral ribosyl moiety would provide compound **1** as a novel type of carbohydrate-based EGFR TKI against the drug resistance involved in NSCLC (**Figure 2**). Here we report the synthesis, preliminary biological evaluation and molecular docking studies of ribose-containing anilinopyrimidine derivatives as EGFR TKIs against EGFR L858R/T790M.

MATERIALS AND METHODS

Commercial reagents were used without further purification except where noted. Solvents were dried and redistilled prior to use in the usual way. All reactions were performed in oven-dried glassware with magnetic stirring under an inert atmosphere unless noted otherwise. Analytical thin layer chromatography (TLC) was performed on precoated plates of Silica Gel (0.25–0.3 mm, Shanghai, China). The TLC plates were visualized with UV light and by staining with sulfuric acid-ethanol solution. Silica gel column chromatography was performed on Silica Gel AR (100–200 mesh, Shanghai, China). NMR spectra were measured with a Bruker Avance III 400 or Bruker Avance III 500 spectrometer. The ^{1}H and ^{13}C NMR spectra were calibrated against the residual proton and carbon signals of the solvents as internal references ($CDCl_3$: $\delta_H = 7.26$ ppm and $\delta_C = 77.2$ ppm; CD_3OD: $\delta_H = 3.31$ ppm and $\delta_C = 49.0$ ppm). Multiplicities are quoted as singlet (s), broad singlet (br s), doublet (d), doublet of doublets (dd), triplet (t), or multiplet (m). All NMR chemical shifts (δ) were recorded in ppm and coupling constants (*J*) were reported in Hz. Mass spectra were recorded on an Agilent Technologies 6120 or LCT Premier XE FTMS instrument.

1,2-*O*-Isopropylidene-3-*N*-acryloyl-3-deoxy-5-*O*-(2,5-dichloropyrimidin-4-yl)-α-D-ribofuranoside 7

To a solution of compound **5** (0.60 g, 2.47 mmol) in anhydrous CH_2Cl_2 (30 mL) at room temperature, was added DBU (1.48 mL, 5.94 mmol) and 2,4,5-trichloropyrimidine **6** (0.57 mL, 4.94 mmol). After stirring at room temperature for 2 h, the reaction mixture was diluted with saturated aqueous NH_4Cl, and extracted with CH_2Cl_2. The organic layer was washed with brine, dried over Na_2SO_4, and concentrated *in vacuo*. The residue was purified by silica gel chromatography (petroleum ether/EtOAc: 80/1) to give **7** (0.88 g, 92%) as a pale yellow syrup: ^{1}H NMR (400 MHz, $CDCl_3$) δ 8.30 (s, 1 H), 6.29 (dd, *J* = 1.2, 17.2 Hz, 1 H), 6.12 (dd, *J* = 10.4, 17.2 Hz, 1 H), 6.07 (d, *J* = 8.8 Hz, 1 H, NH), 5.90 (d, *J* = 3.6 Hz, 1 H, H-1), 5.69 (dd, *J* = 1.2, 10.4 Hz, 1 H), 4.73 (dd, *J* = 2.4, 12.0 Hz, 1 H), 4.66 (t, *J* = 4.0 Hz, 1 H), 4.61–4.55 (m, 2 H),

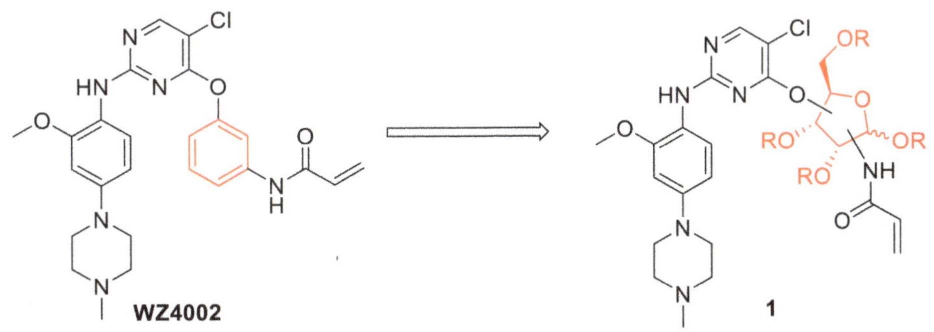

FIGURE 2 | Design of novel EGFR tyrosine kinase inhibitors.

4.16 (m, 1 H), 1.57 (s, 3 H), 1.35 (s, 3 H); ^{13}C NMR (100 MHz, $CDCl_3$) δ 165.4, 165.3, 157.4, 157.2, 130.1, 128.0, 117.0, 113.0, 104.7, 79.1, 78.2, 67.3, 52.1, 26.8, 26.5; ESI-MS (ESI) m/z calcd for $C_{15}H_{17}O_5N_3Cl_2Na$ $[M + Na]^+$ 412.0, found 412.0.

1,2-*O*-Isopropylidene-3-*N*-acryloyl-3-deoxy-5-*O*-[5-chloro-2-*N*-(2-methoxy-4-(4-methylpiperazin-1-yl)phenyl)pyrimidin-4-yl]-α-D-ribofuranoside 1a

To a solution of compound **7** (80 mg, 0.21 mmol) and aniline derivative **8** (91 mg, 0.41 mmol) in isobutanol (3 mL), was added TFA (0.12 mL, 1.55 mmol). The mixture was heated to 100°C and stirred for 5 h. After cooling down to room temperature, the mixture was quenched with Et_3N (3 mL) and concentrated *in vacuo* to give a residue, which was purified by silica gel column chromatography (CH_2Cl_2/MeOH: 30/1) to give **1a** (82 mg, 69%) as a pale yellow powder: ^{1}H NMR (400 MHz, $CDCl_3$) δ 8.10 (d, J = 8.8 Hz, 1 H), 8.08 (s, 1 H), 7.35 (br s, 1 H), 6.56 (dd, J = 2.4, 8.8 Hz, 1 H), 6.52 (d-like, J = 2.4 Hz, 1 H), 6.30 (dd, J = 1.2, 17.2 Hz, 1 H), 6.11 (m, 2 H), 5.91 (d, J = 3.6 Hz, 1 H, H-1), 5.67 (dd, J = 1.2, 10.4 Hz, 1 H), 4.66 (m, 2 H), 4.59–4.49 (m, 3 H), 4.22 (m, 1 H), 3.86 (s, 3 H), 3.16 (t-like, J = 5.2 Hz, 4 H), 2.58 (t-like, J = 5.2 Hz, 4 H), 2.34 (s, 3 H), 1.58 (s, 3 H), 1.35 (s, 3 H); ^{13}C NMR (100 MHz, $CDCl_3$) δ 165.4, 164.1, 157.9, 156.5, 149.2, 147.5, 130.2, 127.8, 122.0, 120.0, 112.9, 108.3, 106.2, 104.8, 100.6, 79.1, 78.2, 66.6, 55.8, 55.3, 52.7, 50.2, 46.2, 26.8, 26.5; HRMS (ESI) m/z calcd for $C_{27}H_{36}O_6N_6ClNa$ $[M + H]^+$ 575.2385, found 575.2385.

3-*N*-Acryloyl-3-deoxy-5-*O*-[5-chloro-2-*N*-(2-methoxy-4-(4-methylpiperazin-1-yl)phenyl)pyrimidin-4-yl]-D-ribofuranose 1b

A solution of compound **1a** (58 mg, 0.10 mmol) in TFA/acetic acid/water (1/15/4, v/v/v, 5 mL) was stirred at 70°C for 7 h. Concentration *in vacuo* and elution through reverse phase C-18 column (H_2O/MeOH: 2/3) provided **1b** (44 mg, 83%) as a pale yellow syrup: ^{1}H NMR (400 MHz, CD_3OD) δ 8.07 (s, 1 H), 8.05 (s, 2.4 H), 7.92 (m, 3.4 H), 6.67 (d-like, J = 2.4 Hz, 3.4 H), 6.58 (dd, J = 2.8, 8.8 Hz, 3.4 H), 6.35 (m, 3.4 H), 6.21 (m, 3.4 H), 5.67 (m, 3.4 H), 5.38 (d, J = 4.0 Hz, 1 H), 5.22 (s, 2.4 H), 4.67 (m, 2.4 H), 4.58 (m, 3.4 H), 4.49 (m, 4.4 H), 4.34–4.24 (m, 4.4 H), 4.00 (d-like, J = 4.4 Hz, 2.4 H), 3.87 (s, 10.2 H), 3.78 (m, 6.8 H), 3.58 (m, 6.8 H), 3.26 (m, 6.8 H), 3.03 (m, 6.8 H), 2.96 (s, 10.2 H); HRMS (ESI) m/z calcd for $C_{24}H_{32}O_6N_6ClNa$ $[M + H]^+$ 535.2072, found 535.2079.

2,3-*O*-Isopropylidene-5-*O*-(2,5-dichloropyrimidin-4-yl)-α-D-ribofuranosyl acrylamide 14

To a solution of compound **13** (147 mg, 0.60 mmol) in anhydrous CH_2Cl_2 (25 mL) at room temperature, was added DBU (0.21 mL, 1.42 mmol) and 2,4,5-trichloropyrimidine **6** (0.12 mL, 1.07 mmol). After stirring at room temperature for 2 h, the reaction mixture was diluted with saturated aqueous NH_4Cl, and extracted with CH_2Cl_2. The organic layer was washed with brine, dried over Na_2SO_4, and concentrated *in vacuo*. The residue was purified by silica gel chromatography (petroleum ether/EtOAc: 5/1) to give **14** (217 mg, 93%) as a colorless syrup: ^{1}H NMR (400 MHz, $CDCl_3$) δ 8.36 (s, 1 H), 6.58 (d, J = 9.2 Hz, 1 H, NH), 6.32 (dd, J = 1.2, 17.2 Hz, 1 H), 6.15 (dd, J = 10.4, 17.2 Hz, 1 H), 6.08 (dd, J = 4.0, 9.2 Hz, 1 H, H-1), 5.72 (dd, J = 1.2, 10.4 Hz, 1 H), 4.86 (d-like, J = 6.0 Hz, 1 H), 4.82 (dd, J = 4.4, 6.0 Hz, 1 H), 4.55 (m, 2 H), 4.45 (t, J = 2.8 Hz, 1 H), 1.57 (s, 3 H), 1.38 (s, 3 H); ^{13}C NMR (100 MHz, $CDCl_3$) δ 165.1, 165.0, 157.7, 157.4, 130.6, 128.2, 116.8, 113.4, 82.3, 81.6, 79.7, 79.4, 70.4, 26.4, 24.8; HRMS (ESI) m/z calcd for $C_{15}H_{17}O_5N_3Cl_2Na$ $[M + Na]^+$ 412.0443, found 412.0448.

5-*O*-[5-Chloro-2-*N*-(2-methoxy-4-(4-methylpiperazin-1-yl)phenyl)pyrimidin-4-yl]-D-ribofuranosyl acrylamide 1c

To a solution of compound **14** (58 mg, 0.15 mmol) and aniline derivative **8** (66 mg, 0.30 mmol) in isobutanol (3 mL), was added TFA (0.084 mL, 1.13 mmol). The mixture was heated to 100°C and stirred for 5 h. After cooling down to room temperature, the mixture was quenched with Et_3N (3 mL) and concentrated *in vacuo* to give a residue, which was purified by silica gel column chromatography (CH_2Cl_2/MeOH: 30/1) to give **15** (60 mg, 70%) as a pale yellow oil: HRMS (ESI) m/z calcd for $C_{27}H_{36}O_6N_6Cl$ $[M + H]^+$ 575.2385, found 575.2383. A solution of compound

15 (85 mg, 0.15 mmol) in TFA/acetic acid/water (1/20/4, v/v/v, 4 mL) was stirred at 50°C for 5 h. Concentration *in vacuo* and elution through reverse phase C-18 column (H_2O/MeOH: 2/3) provided **1c** (64 mg, 80%) as a pale yellow syrup. **1c** (α): ^{1}H NMR (400 MHz, CD_3OD) δ 8.06 (s, 1 H), 7.88 (d, J = 8.8 Hz, 1 H), 6.63 (d-like, J = 2.4 Hz, 1 H), 6.53 (dd, J = 2.8, 8.8 Hz, 1 H), 6.34 (dd, J = 10.0, 17.2 Hz, 1 H), 6.27 (dd, J = 2.0, 17.2 Hz, 1 H), 5.83 (d, J = 4.4 Hz, 1 H, H-1), 5.70 (dd, J = 2.0, 10.0 Hz, 1 H), 4.57 (dd, J = 3.2, 12.0 Hz, 1 H), 4.40 (dd, J = 4.0, 11.6 Hz, 1 H), 4.25 (m, 3 H), 3.85 (s, 3 H), 3.16 (t, J = 4.8 Hz, 4 H), 2.61 (t, J = 4.8 Hz, 4 H), 2.34 (s, 3 H); ^{13}C NMR (100 MHz, CD_3OD) δ 168.0, 165.6, 159.5, 157.3, 151.6, 148.8, 132.1, 128.1, 123.0, 122.3, 109.3, 106.7, 101.9, 81.9 (C-1), 81.5, 73.3, 71.8, 68.2, 56.4, 55.8, 50.2, 45.6; **1c** (β): ^{1}H NMR (400 MHz, CD_3OD) δ 8.05 (s, 1 H), 7.87 (d, J = 8.4 Hz, 1 H), 6.65 (d-like, J = 2.4 Hz, 1 H), 6.54 (dd, J = 2.4, 8.8 Hz, 1 H), 6.23 (m, 2 H), 5.67 (dd, J = 4.8, 6.8 Hz, 1 H), 5.48 (d, J = 4.4 Hz, 1 H, H-1), 4.58 (dd, J = 3.6, 12.0 Hz, 1 H), 4.41 (dd, J = 4.8, 12.0 Hz, 1 H), 4.24–4.14 (m, 2 H), 4.03 (t, J = 4.8 Hz, 1 H), 3.84 (s, 3 H), 3.76 (m, 2 H), 3.57 (m, 2 H), 3.23 (m, 2 H), 3.00 (m, 2 H), 2.93 (s, 3 H); HRMS (ESI) m/z calcd for $C_{24}H_{32}O_6N_6Cl$ [M + H]$^+$ 535.2072, found 535.2087.

5-*O*-*tert*-Butyldiphenylsilyl-3-*O*-(2,5-dichloropyrimidin-4-yl)-2-*O*-*tert*-butyldimethylsilyl-β-D-ribofuranosyl azide 21

To a solution of compound **19** (0.86 g, 1.63 mmol) in anhydrous CH_2Cl_2 (25 mL) at room temperature, was added *t*BuOLi (1.83 g, 22.82 mmol) and 2,4,5-trichloropyrimidine **6** (0.37 mL, 3.26 mmol). After stirring under reflux for 36 h, the reaction mixture was diluted with saturated aqueous NH_4Cl, and extracted with CH_2Cl_2. The organic layer was washed with brine, dried over Na_2SO_4, and concentrated *in vacuo*. The residue was purified by silica gel chromatography (petroleum ether/EtOAc: 80/1) to give **21** (0.88 g, 80%) as a pale yellow syrup: ^{1}H NMR (400 MHz, $CDCl_3$) δ 8.34 (s, 1 H), 7.71–7.67 (m, 4 H), 7.45–7.34 (m, 6 H), 5.66 (t, J = 4.8 Hz, 1 H, H-3), 5.25 (d, J = 3.6 Hz, 1 H, H-1), 4.40 (dd, J = 3.6, 7.6 Hz, 1 H), 4.33 (t, J = 4.4 Hz, 1 H), 3.91 (dd, J = 4.0, 11.6 Hz, 1 H), 3.84 (dd, J = 3.6, 11.6 Hz, 1 H), 1.09 (s, 9 H), 0.75 (s, 9 H), 0.05 (s, 3 H), −0.15 (s, 3 H); HRMS (ESI) m/z calcd for $C_{31}H_{42}O_4N_5Cl_2Si_2$ [M + H]$^+$ 674.2152, found 674.2155.

5-*O*-*tert*-Butyldiphenylsilyl-3-*O*-[5-chloro-2-*N*-(2-methoxy-4-(4-methylpiperazin-1-yl)phenyl)pyrimidin-4-yl]-2-*O*-*tert*-butyldimethylsilyl-β-D-ribofuranosyl azide 22

To a solution of compound **21** (0.53 g, 0.79 mmol) and aniline derivative **8** (0.70 g, 3.16 mmol) in isobutanol (12 mL), was added TFA (1.47 mL, 19.75 mmol). The mixture was heated to 100°C and stirred for 5 h. After cooling down to room temperature, the mixture was quenched with Et_3N (8 mL) and concentrated *in vacuo* to give a residue, which was purified by silica gel column chromatography (CH_2Cl_2/MeOH: 30/1) to give **22** (0.47 g, 69%) as a white powder: ^{1}H NMR (400 MHz, $CDCl_3$) δ 8.12 (s, 1 H), 8.08 (d, J = 9.2 Hz, 1 H), 7.69 (dd, J = 1.6, 7.6 Hz, 2 H), 7.63 (dd, J = 1.6, 8.0 Hz, 2 H), 7.43–7.25 (m, 6 H), 6.54 (m, 2 H), 5.58 (dd, J = 4.4, 7.2 Hz, 1 H, H-3), 5.29 (d, J = 1.6 Hz, 1 H, H-1), 4.47 (m, 1 H), 4.38 (dd, J = 2.0, 4.4 Hz, 1 H), 4.02 (dd, J = 2.8, 11.6 Hz, 1 H), 3.88 (s, 3 H), 3.83 (dd, J = 3.6, 12.0 Hz, 1 H), 3.17 (t, J = 5.2 Hz, 4 H), 2.61 (t, J = 4.8 Hz, 4 H), 2.37 (s, 3 H), 1.06 (s, 9 H), 0.78 (s, 9 H), −0.07 (s, 3 H), −0.25 (s, 3 H); ^{13}C NMR (100 MHz, $CDCl_3$) δ 163.6, 157.9, 156.9, 149.3, 147.6, 135.8, 135.7, 133.1, 133.0, 129.9, 127.9, 127.8, 121.8, 120.1, 108.4, 106.1, 100.6, 95.8, 81.6, 74.7, 74.2, 62.8, 55.8, 55.3, 50.1, 46.3, 26.9, 25.6, 19.3, 18.0, −4.9, −5.4; HRMS (ESI) m/z calcd for $C_{43}H_{60}O_5N_8ClSi_2$ [M + H]$^+$ 859.3914, found 859.3920.

5-*O*-*tert*-Butyldiphenylsilyl-3-*O*-[5-chloro-2-*N*-(2-methoxy-4-(4-methylpiperazin-1-yl)phenyl)pyrimidin-4-yl]-2-*O*-*tert*-butyldimethylsilyl-α-D-ribofuranosyl acrylamide 23

A mixture of compound **22** (190 mg, 0.22 mmol) and Pd/C (50 mg, 10%) in EtOH (7 mL) was stirred under an atmosphere of H_2 at room temperature for overnight. The mixture was filtered through celite, washed with EtOH and concentrated *in vacuo* to afford the corresponding amine for the next step without further purification. To a solution of the resulting amine in CH_2Cl_2 (7 mL) at room temperature, was added DCC (69 mg, 0.33 mmol), DMAP (41 mg, 0.33 mmol), and acrylic acid (0.061 mL, 0.89 mmol). After stirring at room temperature for 4 h, the mixture was concentrated *in vacuo* to give a residue, which was purified by silica gel column chromatography (CH_2Cl_2/MeOH: 30/1) to afford **23** (76 mg, 39% over two steps) as a pale yellow syrup: ^{1}H NMR (400 MHz, $CDCl_3$) δ 8.17 (s, 1 H), 8.09 (d, J = 8.8 Hz, 1 H), 7.71 (m, 4 H), 7.43–7.36 (m, 6 H), 7.12 (d, J = 9.2 Hz, 1 H), 6.53 (d, J = 2.4 Hz, 1 H), 6.42 (m, 1 H), 6.36 (dd, J = 1.2, 16.8 Hz, 1 H), 6.14 (dd, J = 10.4, 17.2 Hz, 1 H), 6.02 (d-like, J = 4.8 Hz, 1 H), 5.98 (dd, J = 6.0, 9.2 Hz, 1 H), 5.70 (dd, J = 1.2, 10.4 Hz, 1 H), 4.72 (dd, J = 5.2 Hz, 1 H), 4.36 (br s, 1 H), 3.86 (m, 5 H), 3.07 (br s, 4 H), 2.54 (br s, 4 H), 2.35 (s, 3 H), 1.11 (s, 9 H), 0.68 (s, 9 H), −0.02 (s, 3 H), −0.09 (s, 3 H); ^{13}C NMR (100 MHz, $CDCl_3$) δ 165.9, 164.0, 157.8, 157.0, 149.3, 147.6, 135.8, 135.5, 133.4, 132.5, 131.0, 130.1, 130.0, 128.9, 128.0, 127.4, 121.5, 120.0, 108.1, 105.8, 100.4, 82.2, 80.4, 77.4, 71.0, 64.2, 55.7, 55.2, 49.9, 46.2, 27.0, 25.4, 19.5, 17.7, −5.1, −5.3; HRMS (ESI) m/z calcd for $C_{46}H_{64}O_6N_6ClSi_2$ [M + H]$^+$ 887.4114, found 887.4116.

3-*O*-[5-Chloro-2-*N*-(2-methoxy-4-(4-methylpiperazin-1-yl)phenyl)pyrimidin-4-yl]-2-*O*-*tert*-butyldimethylsilyl-α-D-ribofuranosyl acrylamide 1d

To a solution of compound **23** (91 mg, 0.11 mmol) in pyridine (3 mL) at room temperature, was added HF·pyridine (0.19 mL). After stirring at room temperature for overnight, the mixture was poured into saturated aqueous $NaHCO_3$ and extracted with CH_2Cl_2. The combined organic layers were washed with brine, dried over Na_2SO_4, and concentrated *in vacuo*. The residue was purified by silica gel column chromatography (CH_2Cl_2/MeOH:

20/1) to afford **1d** (40 mg, 68%) as a pale yellow syrup: ^{1}H NMR (400 MHz, $CDCl_3$) δ 8.15 (s, 1 H), 8.02 (d, J = 8.4 Hz, 1 H), 7.71 (m, 4 H), 7.30 (br s, 1 H), 7.06 (d, J = 8.4 Hz, 1 H), 6.54 (m, 2 H), 6.33 (d-like, J = 17.2 Hz, 1 H), 6.12 (dd, J = 10.0, 16.8 Hz, 1 H), 5.90 (dd, J = 6.0, 8.4 Hz, 1 H), 5.73 (m, 2 H), 4.51 (t, J = 5.6 Hz, 1 H), 4.30 (br s, 1 H), 3.87 (s, 3 H), 3.82 (d-like, J = 12.4 Hz, 1 H), 3.71 (d-like, J = 11.2 Hz, 1 H), 3.18 (br s, 4 H), 2.61 (br s, 4 H), 2.37 (s, 3 H), 0.72 (s, 9 H), −0.02 (s, 3 H), −0.10 (s, 3 H); ^{13}C NMR (100 MHz, $CDCl_3$) δ 166.1, 163.8, 157.9, 157.0, 149.6, 147.5, 130.9, 127.7, 121.9, 120.5, 108.6, 106.1, 100.8, 82.1, 80.6, 76.3, 70.9, 62.5, 55.8, 55.0, 49.6, 45.7, 25.5, 17.9, −5.0, −5.2; HRMS (ESI) m/z calcd for $C_{30}H_{46}O_6N_6ClSi$ $[M + H]^+$ 649.2937, found 649.2940.

Kinase Assay

Kinases domain of EGFR WT and EGFR L858R/T790M were expressed using the Bac-to-Bac™ baculo virus expression system (Invitrogen, Carlsbad, CA, USA) and purified in Ni-NTA columns (QIAGEN Inc., Valencia, CA, USA). The kinase activity was evaluated with enzyme-linked immunosorbent assay (ELISA). Briefly, 20 μg/mL Poly (Glu, Tyr) 4:1 (Sigma, St. Louis, MO) was precoated in 96-well ELISA plates as substrate. After adding 50 μL of 10 μmol/L ATP solution which was diluted in kinase reaction buffer (50 mM HEPES pH 7.4, 20 mM $MgCl_2$, 0.1 mM $MnCl_2$, 0.2 mM Na_3VO_4, 1 mM DTT), the plate was treated with 1 μL of indicated concentrations of compounds (dissolved in DMSO) per well. Experiments at each concentration were performed in duplicate. Reaction was initiated by adding tyrosine kinase diluted in kinase reaction buffer. After incubation at 37°C for 1 h, the wells were washed three times with phosphate buffered saline (PBS) containing 0.1% Tween 20 (T-PBS). One hundred microliters of anti-phosphotyrosine (PY99) antibody (1:1,000, Santa Cruz Biotechnology, Santa Cruz, CA) diluted in T-PBS containing 5 mg/mL BSA was added and the plate was incubated at 37°C for 30 min. After the plate was washed three times, 100 μL horseradish peroxidase-conjugated goat anti-mouse IgG (1:2,000, Calbiochem, SanDiego, CA) was added and the plate was incubated at 37°C for 30 min. The plate was washed, added with 100 μL citrate buffer (0.1 M, pH 5.5) containing 0.03% H_2O_2. Then 2 mg/mL *o*-phenylenediamine was added, and samples were incubated at room temperature until color emerged. The reaction was terminated immediately by adding 50 μL of 2 M H_2SO_4. Plate was read using a multiwell spectrophotometer (VERSAmax™, Molecular Devices, Sunnyvale, CA, USA) at 492 nm. The inhibitory rate (%) was calculated with the formula: [1 − (A492 treated/A492 control)] × 100%. IC_{50} values were calculated from the inhibitory curves.

Molecular Docking

EGFR$^{T790M/L858R}$ structure (PDB: 3IKA) was retrieved from the Protein Data Bank and covalent docking was performed with maestro (Schrödinger, Inc., version 10.2). Compound **1a** was docked into the EGFR protein as an irreversible inhibitor using Covalent Docking module. The docking procedure was validated by re-docking the co-crystallized ligand WZ4002 into the ATP binding site of EGFR$^{T790M/L858R}$ structure. The details of the docking workflow are listed below:

(1) Protein was prepared using the "Protein Preparation Wizard" workflow. All water molecules were removed from the structure of the complex. Hydrogen atoms and charges were added during a brief relaxation. After optimizing the hydrogen bond network, the crystal structure was minimized using the OPLS_2005 force field with the maximum root mean square deviation (RMSD) value of 0.3 Å.
(2) The ligand was prepared with LigPrep module in Maestro, including adding hydrogen atoms, ionizing at a pH range from 5.0 to 9.0, and producing the corresponding low-energy 3D structure.
(3) Pose prediction mode of Covalent Docking module was adopted to dock the molecules into the ATP-binding site with the default parameters. The center of the grid box was defined with the intrinsic ligand and Michael addition reaction type was chosen. The top-ranking poses of molecule **1a** were retained.

RESULT AND DISCUSSION

The synthesis of 3-*N*-acryloyl-5-*O*-anilinopyrimidine ribose derivatives **1a** and **1b** commenced with 3-amino ribose derivative **3** that can be readily prepared from D-xylose **2** in 41% yield over six steps (**Scheme 1**; Shie et al., 2007). Protection of the primary hydroxyl group in **3** with TBDPSCl followed by condensation with acryloyl chloride using Et_3N as base gave ribose derivative **4** in 92% yield (two steps). Treatment of **4** with HF·pyridine afforded alcohol **5** in 71% yield. When **5** was reacted with 2,4,5-trichloropyrimidine **6** in the presence of K_2CO_3 or DIPEA, almost no desired product was observed. Exhilaratingly, nucleophilic reaction of **5** with **6** employing stronger base (DBU) as promoter proceeded smoothly to provide ribose derivative **7** in excellent yield (92%). Subjection of **7** to the known aniline derivative **8** (Han et al., 2014) under the promotion of TFA in isobutanol at 100°C delivered **1a** in 69% yield. Removal of the 1,2-*O*-isopropylidene group in **1a** with TFA in acetic acid and water at 70°C produced **1b** in 83% yield.

For the synthesis of 1-*N*-acryloyl-5-*O*-anilinopyrimidine ribose derivative **1c**, β-ribosyl azide **10** was conveniently prepared from D-ribose **9** in three steps and 53% yield according to the procedures described in the literature (**Scheme 2**; Bonache et al., 2009). The acetyl group in **10** was then replaced with TBS group to give compound **11** in 85% yield. Hydrogenolysis of the azide group in **11** over Pd/C followed by condensation with acrylic acid in the presence of DCC and DMAP afforded a mixture of ribose derivative **12** in 43% yield (α/β = 1:1; α-anomer: δ_H = 6.00 ppm, δ_C = 81.4 ppm; β-anomer: δ_H = 5.95 ppm, δ_C = 87.2 ppm), which were easily separated by silica gel column chromatography (Numao et al., 1981; Bonache et al., 2009). After removal of the TBS group in **12α**, the resulting alcohol **13** reacted with **6** in the presence of DBU to produce ribose derivative **14** in an excellent 93% yield. TFA-promoted reaction of **14** with aniline **8** led to **15** in 70% yield as a mixture of α/β anomers probably arising from the anomerization of the 1-*N*-acryloyl ribose derivative under

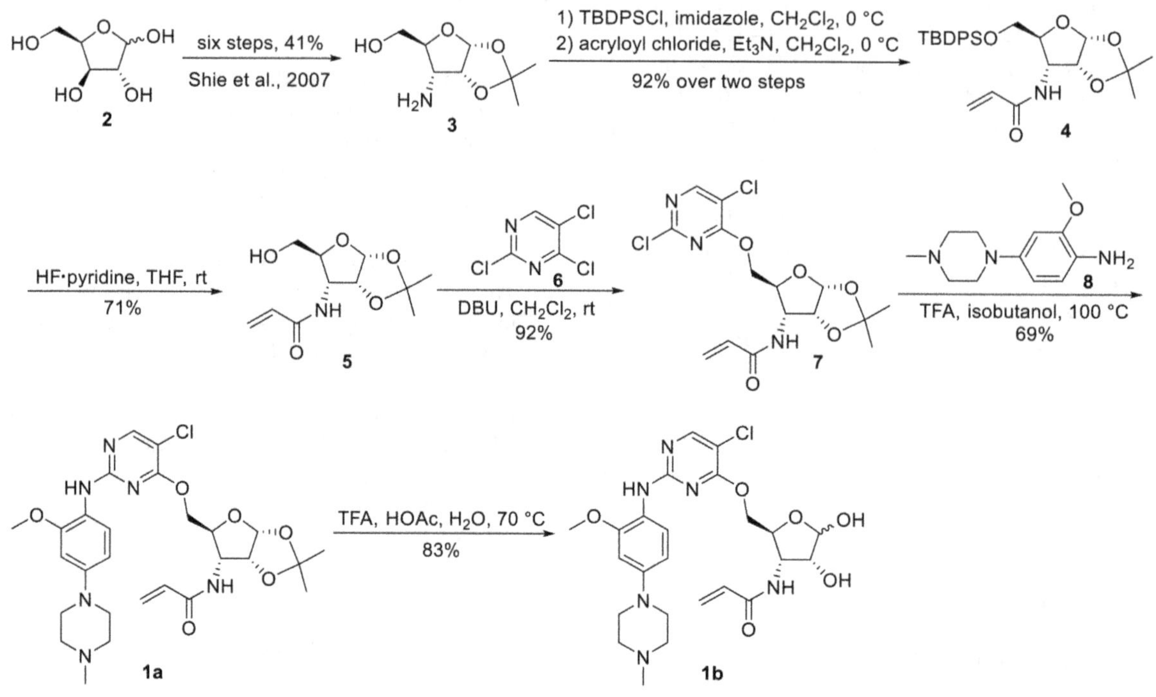

SCHEME 1 | Synthesis of 3-*N*-acryloyl-5-*O*-anilinopyrimidine ribose derivatives **1a** and **1b**.

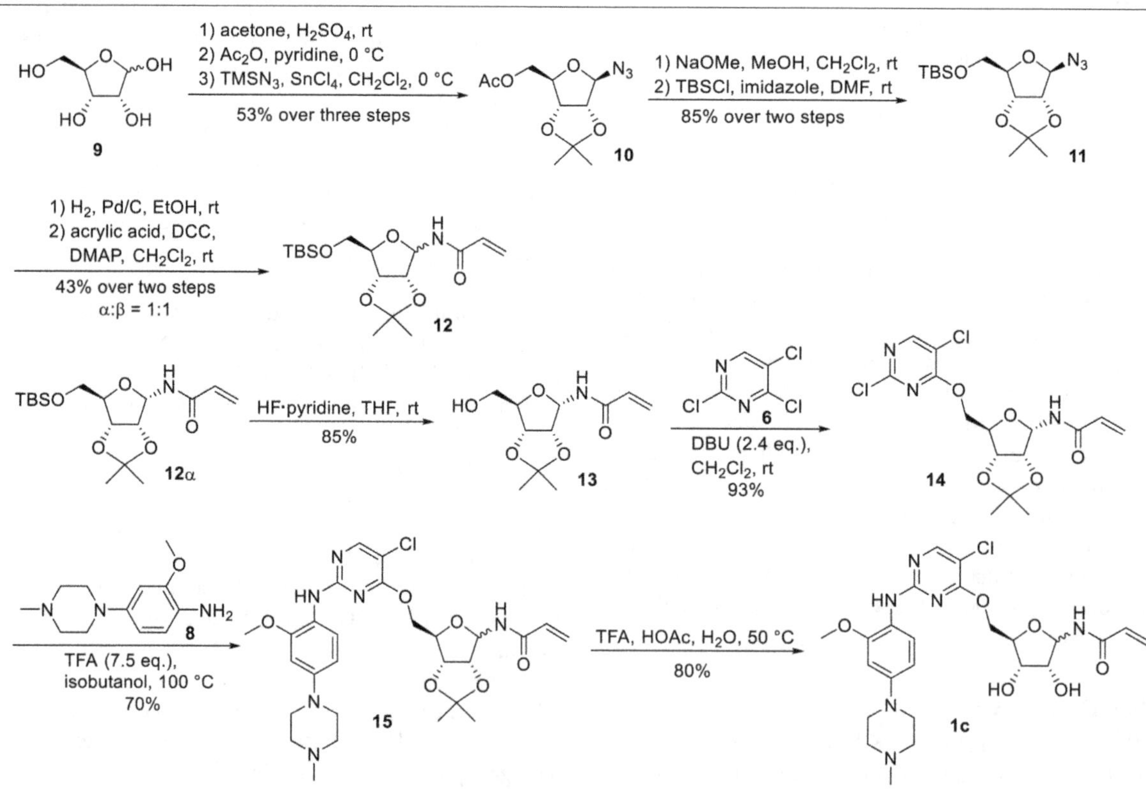

SCHEME 2 | Synthesis of 1-*N*-acryloyl-5-*O*-anilinopyrimidine ribose derivative **1c**.

strong acidic conditions (Boschelli et al., 1989). Finally, acidic cleavage of the isopropylidene group of **15** in the mixture of TFA/HOAc/water provided **1c** in 80% yield.

Synthetic work toward 1-*N*-acryloyl-3-*O*-anilinopyrimidine ribose derivative **1d** started from replacement of the 2,3-isopropylidene group of azide **10** with 2,3-orthoester group by treatment with TFA and subsequent protection with triethyl orthoacetate under the catalysis of $TsOH{\cdot}H_2O$, affording azide **16** in 76% yield over two steps (**Scheme 3**). Substitution of the acetyl group in **16** with TBDPS group and subsequent acidic cleavage of the orthoester group led to an inseparable mixture of 2-acetyl and 3-acetyl ribose derivatives **17** and **18** (77% yield over three steps). Treatment of the mixture of **17** and **18** with TBSCl followed by removal of the acetyl groups gave alcohols **19** and **20** in 83% yield, allowing for the separation of 3-hydroxyl ribose derivative **19** from 2-hydroxyl ribose derivative **20** (**19**:**20** = 3:2). Nucleophilic

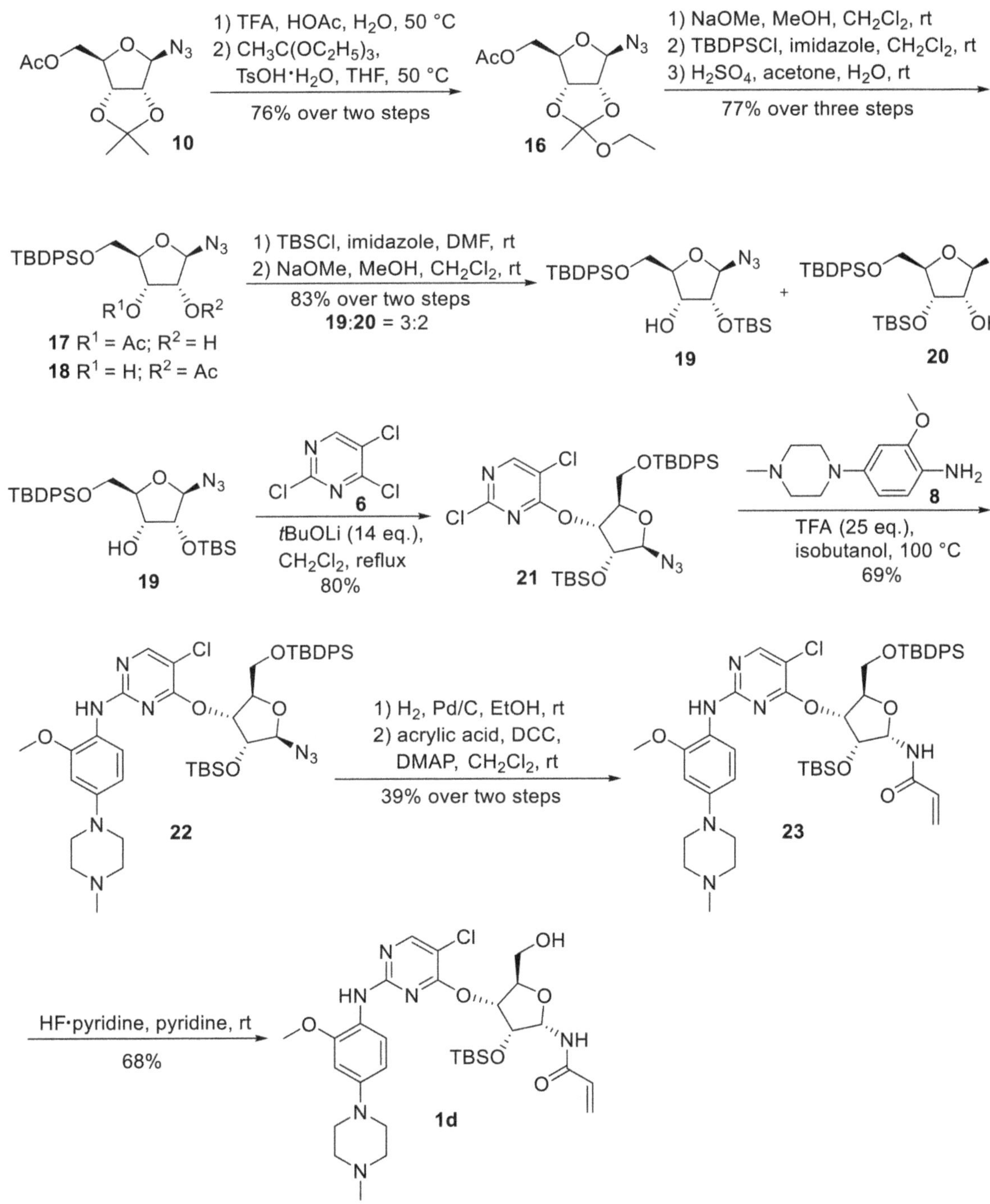

SCHEME 3 | Synthesis of 1-*N*-acryloyl-3-*O*-anilinopyrimidine ribose derivative **1d**.

attack of **19** on **6** required stronger basic conditions to promote the reaction due to the steric hindrance of the silyl groups on **19**. As such, excess *t*BuOLi in dichloromethane under reflux was employed for this conversion, providing ribose derivative **21** in 80% yield. TFA-promoted coupling of **21** with aniline **8** generated ribose derivative **22** (69%), which was then subjected to hydrogenolysis over Pd/C and subsequent condensation with acrylic acid to afford ribose derivative **23** as single anomer in moderate yield (39% over two steps). Exposure of **23** to HF·pyridine in pyridine resulted in cleavage of the TBDPS group without affecting the TBS group, providing **1d** in 68% yield.

To determine whether the Michael acceptor played a significant role in the inhibitory activity of ribose-modified pyrimidine derivatives against EGFR tyrosine kinase, 1-azide-5-*O*-anilinopyrimidine ribose derivative **24**, 1-azide-3-*O*-anilinopyrimidine ribose derivative **25**, and 5-*O*-anilinopyrimidine ribose derivative **26** were readily synthesized following the similar procedures described for **1a-1d** (**Table 1**; see Supplementary Material for details).

As shown in **Table 1**, compounds **1a** and **1b** containing 3-*N*-acryloyl-5-*O*-anilinopyrimidine ribosyl moiety potently inhibited EGFR L858R/T790M mutant with IC_{50} values of 0.62 and 2.64 μM, revealing specific inhibitory activity for EGFR L858R/T790M over WT EGFR, although they are not comparable to the positive controls osimertinib (IC_{50} = 1.5 nM for EGFR L858R/T790M) and afatinib (IC_{50} = 3.7 nM for EGFR L858R/T790M). In contrast, other compounds (**1c**, **1d**, and **24–26**) bearing 5-*O*-anilinopyrimidine ribosyl moiety, 1-*N*-acryloyl-5-*O*-anilinopyrimidine ribosyl moiety, 1-*N*-acryloyl-3-*O*-anilinopyrimidine ribosyl moiety, or their 1-azide counterparts, showed no inhibitory activities against EGFR tyrosine kinases.

In order to better understand the mechanism of this type of compounds binding to EGFR T790M, molecular docking was adopted to predict the binding mode of the representative compound **1a**. The docking procedure was validated in advance by re-docking the co-crystallized ligand WZ4002 (Zhou et al., 2009) into the ATP binding site of EGFR L858R/T790M structure (PDB ID: 3IKA). The root mean square deviation (RMSD) between the crystallographic and docked conformation of WZ4002 is 0.57 Å (Figure S1), demonstrating that the present docking procedure was feasible in generating the binding conformation accurately. As expected based upon co-crystal structure of the anilinopyrimidine-derived inhibitor WZ4002, the anilinopyrimidine core of compound **1a** forms a bidentate hydrogen bonding interaction with the "hinge" residue Met793 (**Figure 3**). The chlorine substituent on the pyrimidine ring could form hydrophobic contact with the mutant gatekeeper residue, Met790. The aniline ring is oriented to form hydrophobic interactions with Leu792 and Pro794 in the hinge region. Moreover, the acrylamide group attached to the sugar ring of compound **1a** could form a covalent bond with Cys797 to achieve irreversible binding. The sugar ring acts like a linker to tune the orientation of the electrophilic acrylamide moiety that can covalently alkylate the conserved cysteine residue Cys797. For the 1,2-*O*-isopropylidene moiety in compound **1a**, it could form favorable vdW interactions with residues ARG841, ASN842,

TABLE 1 | *In vitro* inhibitory activities of ribose-modified pyrimidine derivatives **1a–1d** and **24–26** against EGFR tyrosine kinase.

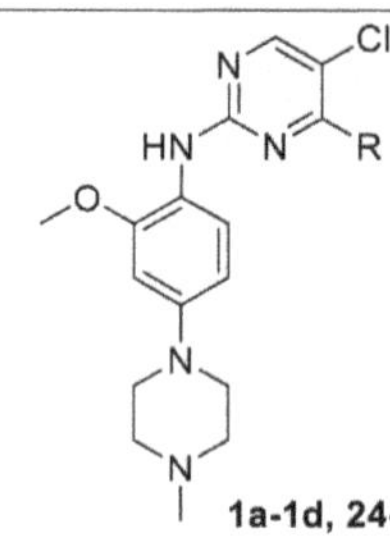

1a-1d, 24-26

Compound	R	EGFR tyrosine kinase IC_{50} (μM)[a]	
		EGFR	$EGFR^{T790M/L858R}$
1a	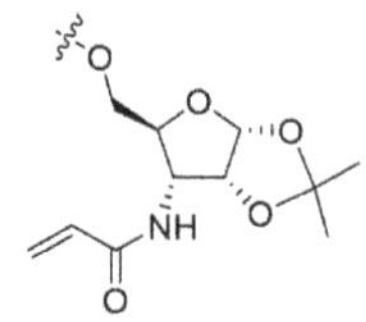	>10	0.6204 ± 0.1729
1b	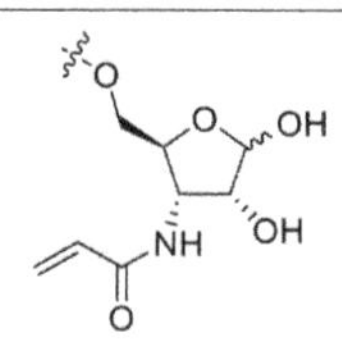	>10	2.6435 ± 1.8606
1c	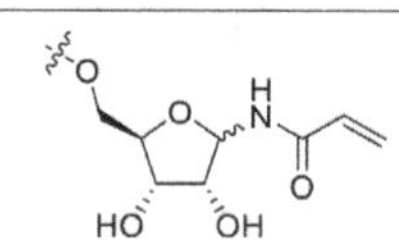	>10	>10
1d	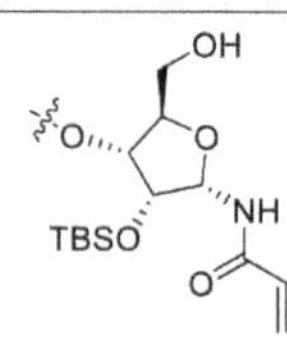	>10	>10
24	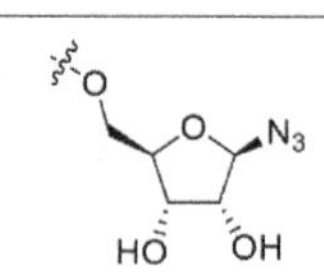	>10	>10
25	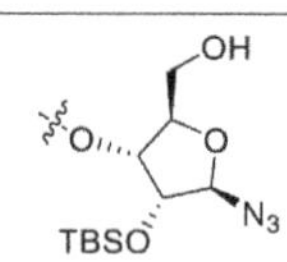	>10	>10
26	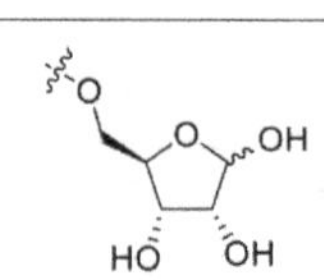	>10	>10
Osimertinib[b]		0.1586 ± 0.0428	0.0015 ± 0.0001
Afatinib[b]		0.00697 ± 0.00052	0.00374 ± 0.00035

[a] *Kinase activity assays were examined by using the ELISA-based EGFR-TK assay. Data are averages of at least two independent determinations and reported as the mean ± SD (standard deviation).*

[b] *Reported data.*

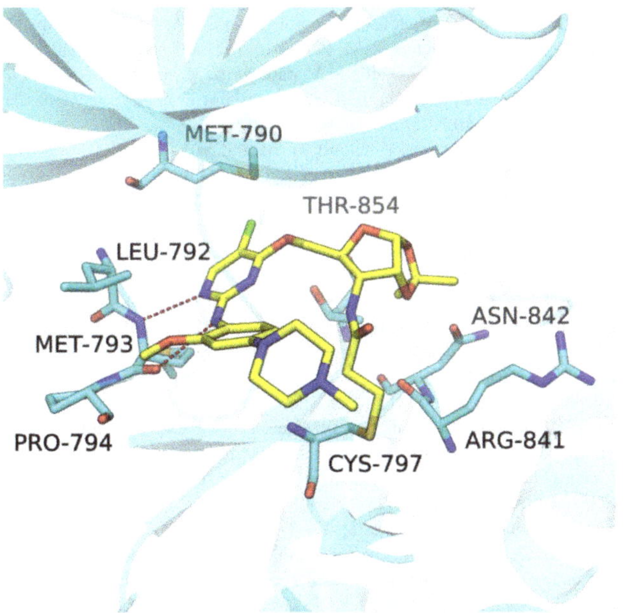

FIGURE 3 | Docking pose of compound **1a** in complex with the $EGFR^{T790M/L858R}$ (PDB ID 3IKA). The EGFR kinase is shown as cartoon (cyan) with the bound inhibitor in a stick representation (yellow). Key residues are represented as cyan sticks. The expected hydrogen bonds are indicated by red dashes.

and Thr854. Therefore, compound **1b** without that protecting group on the sugar ring, displayed less potent bioactivity against EGFR T790M/L858R compared with compound **1a**. Lacking of the Michael receptor, compounds **24–26** are unable to form covalent bond with Cys797 and thus displayed sharply decreased inhibitory activity against EGFR T790M/L858R. Compound **1c** displayed no inhibitory activity of EGFR probably because of the long distance between the Michael receptor and Cys797. Although compound **1d** also has an acrylamide group attached to the sugar ring, it showed no inhibitory activity probably due to the conformational alteration of compound **1d** caused by the TBS protecting group. Briefly, it could be concluded that the distance between the Michael receptor and the pyrimidine scaffold has a significant effect on the inhibitory potency of this type of compounds. Employing the ribosyl moiety as a chiral building block for modulating the distance between the Michael receptor and the pyrimidine scaffold could pave a new avenue for future design of EGFR inhibitors against EGFR mutants.

CONCLUSION

In summary, we have described a DBU- or *t*BuOLi-promoted coupling of ribosyl alcohols with 2,4,5-trichloropyrimidine as key step for the synthesis of a series of ribose-modified anilinopyrimidine derivatives as EGFR TKIs. Preliminary biological evaluation indicated that compound **1a** displayed potent inhibitory activity against EGFR L858R/T790M with an IC_{50} value of $0.62\,\mu M$, and good selectivity for EGFR L858R/T790M over WT EGFR. Molecular docking studies revealed that the inhibitory activities of this type of compounds are largely influenced by the distance between the Michael receptor and the pyrimidine scaffold. As a novel type of EGFR inhibitor, the ribose-modified anilinopyrimidine derivative **1a** might be used as a promising lead compound for further development of selective EGFR inhibitors to overcome EGFR L858R/T790M resistance mutation.

AUTHOR CONTRIBUTIONS

YY and YX designed and guided this study. XH conducted the chemical synthesis. YT, LT, LZ, and HX performed the kinase activity assays. DW, XW, and SL performed the molecular docking studies. XH, YY, and YX analyzed the data and wrote the manuscript with input from all authors.

ACKNOWLEDGMENTS

Financial support from the National Thousand Young Talents Program (YC0130518, YC0140103), the Shanghai Committee of Science and Technology (14431902100), and the Shanghai Pujiang Program (15PJ1401500), is gratefully acknowledged.

REFERENCES

Balak, M. N., Gong, Y., Riely, G. J., Somwar, R., Li, A. R., Zakowski, M. F., et al. (2006). Novel D761Y and common secondary T790M mutations in epidermal growth factor receptor-mutant lung adenocarcinomas with acquired resistance to kinase inhibitors. *Clin. Cancer Res.* 12, 6494–6501. doi: 10.1158/1078-0432.CCR-06-1570

Bonache, M. A., Nuti, F., Le Chevalier Isaad, A., Real-Fernandez, F., Chelli, M., Rovero, P., et al. (2009). Synthesis of new ribosylated Asn building blocks as useful tools for glycopeptide and glycoprotein synthesis. *Tetrahedron Lett.* 50, 4151–4153. doi: 10.1016/j.tetlet.2009.04.124

Boschelli, D. H., Powell, D., Sharky, V., and Semmelhack, M. F. (1989). An improved synthesis of glycinamide ribonucleotide. *Tetrahedron Lett.* 30, 1599–1600. doi: 10.1016/S0040-4039(00)99530-3

Castellanos, E. H., and Horn, L. (2015). Generations of epidermal growth factor receptor tyrosine kinase inhibitors: perils and progress. *Curr. Treat. Options Oncol.* 16, 51. doi: 10.1007/s11864-015-0365-1

Cheng, H., Nair, S. K., and Murray, B. W. (2016). Recent progress on third generation covalent EGFR inhibitors. *Bioorg. Med. Chem. Lett.* 26, 1861–1868. doi: 10.1016/j.bmcl.2016.02.067

Cohen, M. H., Johnson, J. R., Chen, Y. F., Sridhara, R., and Pazdur, R. (2005). FDA drug approval summary: erlotinib (Tarceva®) tablets. *Oncologist* 10, 461–466. doi: 10.1634/theoncologist.10-7-461

Cross, D. A., Ashton, S. E., Ghiorghiu, S., Eberlein, C., Nebhan, C. A., Spitzler, P. J., et al. (2014). AZD9291, an irreversible EGFR TKI, overcomes T790M-mediated resistance to EGFR inhibitors in lung cancer. *Cancer Discov.* 4, 1046–1061. doi: 10.1158/2159-8290.CD-14-0337

De Luca, A., Carotenuto, A., Rachiglio, A., Gallo, M., Maiello, M. R., Aldinucci, D., et al. (2008). The role of the EGFR signaling in tumor microenvironment. *J. Cell. Physiol.* 214, 559–567. doi: 10.1002/jcp.21260

Dungo, R. T., and Keating, G. M. (2013). Afatinib: first global approval. *Drugs* 73, 1503–1515. doi: 10.1007/s40265-013-0111-6

Eberlein, C. A., Stetson, D., Markovets, A. A., Al-Kadhimi, K. J., Lai, Z., Fisher, P. R., et al. (2015). Acquired resistance to the mutant-selective EGFR inhibitor AZD9291 is associated with increased dependence on RAS signaling in preclinical models. *Cancer Res.* 75, 2489–2500. doi: 10.1158/0008-5472.CAN-14-3167

Finlay, M. R., Anderton, M., Ashton, S., Ballard, P., Bethel, P. A., Box, M. R., et al. (2014). Discovery of a potent and selective EGFR inhibitor (AZD9291) of both sensitizing and T790M resistance mutations that spares the wild type form of the receptor. *J. Med. Chem.* 57, 8249–8267. doi: 10.1021/jm500973a

Gray, J., and Haura, E. (2014). Update on third-generation EGFR tyrosine kinase inhibitors. *Transl. Lung Cancer Res.* 3, 360–362. doi: 10.3978/j.issn.2218-6751.2014.09.08

Grünwald, V., and Hidalgo, M. (2003). Developing inhibitors of the epidermal growth factor receptor for cancer treatment. *J. Natl. Cancer Inst.* 95, 851–867. doi: 10.1093/jnci/95.12.851

Gschwind, A., Fischer, O. M., and Ullrich, A. (2004). The discovery of receptor tyrosine kinases: targets for cancer therapy. *Nat. Rev. Cancer* 4, 361–370. doi: 10.1038/nrc1360

Günther, M., Juchum, M., Kelter, G., Fiebig, H., and Laufer, S. (2016). Lung cancer: EGFR inhibitors with low nanomolar activity against a therapy-resistant L858R/T790M/C797S mutant. *Angew. Chem. Int. Ed.* 55, 10890–10894. doi: 10.1002/anie.201603736

Günther, M., Lategahn, J., Juchum, M., Döring, E., Keul, M., Tumbrink, H. L., et al. (2017). Trisubstituted pyridinylimidazoles as potent inhibitors of the clinically resistant L858R/T790M/C797S EGFR mutant: targeting of both hydrophobic regions and the phosphate binding site. *J. Med. Chem.* 60, 5613–5637. doi: 10.1021/acs.jmedchem.7b00316

Han, C., Wan, L., Ji, H., Ding, K., Huang, Z., Lai, Y., et al. (2014). Synthesis and evaluation of 2-anilinopyrimidines bearing 3-aminopropamides as potential epidermal growth factor receptor inhibitors. *Eur. J. Med. Chem.* 77, 75–83. doi: 10.1016/j.ejmech.2014.02.032

Harrington, K. J., El-Hariry, I. A., Holford, C. S., Lusinchi, A., Nutting, C. M., Rosine, D., et al. (2009). Phase I study of lapatinib in combination with chemoradiation in patients with locally advanced squamous cell carcinoma of the head and neck. *J. Clin. Oncol.* 27, 1100–1107. doi: 10.1200/JCO.2008.17.5349

Huang, S. M., and Harari, P. M. (1999). Epidermal growth factor receptor inhibition in cancer therapy: biology, rationale and preliminary clinical results. *Invest. New Drugs* 17, 259–269. doi: 10.1023/A:1006384521198

Jia, Y., Yun, C. H., Park, E., Ercan, D., Manuia, M., Juarez, J., et al. (2016). Overcoming EGFR(T790M) and EGFR(C797S) resistance with mutant-selective allosteric inhibitors. *Nature* 534, 129–132. doi: 10.1038/nature17960

Juchum, M., Günther, M., Döring, E., Sievers-Engler, A., Lämmerhofer, M., and Laufer, S. (2017). Trisubstituted imidazoles with a rigidized hinge binding motif act as single digit nM inhibitors of clinically relevant EGFR L858R/T790M and L858R/T790M/C797S mutants: an example of target hopping. *J. Med. Chem.* 60, 4636–4656. doi: 10.1021/acs.jmedchem.7b00178

Kris, M. G., Natale, R. B., Herbst, R. S., Lynch, T. J., Prager, D., Belani, C. P., et al. (2003). Efficacy of gefitinib, an inhibitor of the epidermal growth factor receptor tyrosine kinase, in symptomatic patients with non-small cell lung cancer. *JAMA* 290, 2149–2158. doi: 10.1001/jama.290.16.2149

Moore, M. J., Goldstein, D., Hamm, J., Figer, A., Hecht, J. R., Gallinger, S., et al. (2007). Erlotinib plus gemcitabine compared with gemcitabine alone in patients with advanced pancreatic cancer: a phase III trial of the national cancer institute of Canada clinical trials group. *J. Clin. Oncol.* 25, 1960–1966. doi: 10.1200/JCO.2006.07.9525

Niederst, M. J., Hu, H., Mulvey, H. E., Lockerman, E. L., Garcia, A. R., Piotrowska, Z., et al. (2015). The allelic context of the C797S mutation acquired upon treatment with third generation EGFR inhibitors impacts sensitivity to subsequent treatment strategies. *Clin. Cancer Res.* 21, 3924–3933. doi: 10.1158/1078-0432.CCR-15-0560

Normanno, N., Bianco, C., De Luca, A., Maiello, M. R., and Salomon, D. S. (2003). Target-based agents against ErbB receptors and their ligands: a novel approach to cancer treatment. *Endocr. Relat. Cancer* 10, 1–21. doi: 10.1677/erc.0.0100001

Numao, N., Hemmi, H., Naujokaitis, S. A., Rabinovitz, M., and Beisler, J. A. (1981). Showdomycin analogues: synthesis and antitumor evaluation. *J. Med. Chem.* 24, 515–520. doi: 10.1021/jm00137a008

Ozvegy-Laczka, C., Cserepes, J., Elkind, N. B., and Sarkadi, B. (2005). Tyrosine kinase inhibitor resistance in cancer: role of ABC multidrug transporters. *Drug Resist. Updates* 8, 15–26. doi: 10.1016/j.drup.2005.02.002

Pao, W., and Chmielecki, J. (2010). Rational, biologically based treatment of EGFR-mutant non-small-cell lung cancer. *Nat. Rev. Cancer* 10, 760–774. doi: 10.1038/nrc2947

Park, H., Jung, H. Y., Mah, S., and Hong, S. (2017). Discovery of EGF receptor inhibitors that are selective for the d746-750/T790M/C797S mutant through structure-based *de novo* design. *Angew. Chem.* 56, 7634–7638. doi: 10.1002/anie.201703389

Piotrowska, Z., Niederst, M. J., Karlovich, C. A., Wakelee, H. A., Neal, J. W., Mino-Kenudson, M., et al. (2015). Heterogeneity underlies the emergence of EGFRT790 wild-type clones following treatment of T790M-positive cancers with a third-generation EGFR inhibitor. *Cancer Discov.* 5, 713–722. doi: 10.1158/2159-8290.CD-15-0399

Shie, J. J., Fang, J. M., Wang, S. Y., Tsai, K. C., Cheng, Y. S. E., Yang, A. S., et al. (2007). Synthesis of tamiflu and its phosphonate congeners possessing potent anti-influenza activity. *J. Am. Chem. Soc.* 129, 11892–11893. doi: 10.1021/ja073992i

Steuer, C. E., Khuri, F. R., and Ramalingam, S. S. (2015). The next generation of epidermal growth factor receptor tyrosine kinase inhibitors in the treatment of lung cancer. *Cancer* 121, E1–E6. doi: 10.1002/cncr.29139

Thress, K. S., Paweletz, C. P., Felip, E., Cho, B. C., Stetson, D., Dougherty, B., et al. (2015). Acquired EGFR C797S mutation mediates resistance to AZD9291 in non–small cell lung cancer harboring EGFR T790M. *Nat. Med.* 21, 560–562. doi: 10.1038/nm.3854

Traxler, P., and Furet, P. (1999). Strategies toward the design of novel and selective protein tyrosine kinase inhibitors. *Pharmacol. Ther.* 82, 195–206. doi: 10.1016/s0163-7258(98)00044-8

Walter, A. O., Sjin, R. T., Haringsma, H. J., Ohashi, K., Sun, J., Lee, K., et al. (2013). Discovery of a mutant-selective covalent inhibitor of EGFR that overcomes T790M-mediated resistance in NSCLC. *Cancer Discov.* 3, 1404–1415. doi: 10.1158/2159-8290.CD-13-0314

Zhou, W., Ercan, D., Chen, L., Yun, C. H., Li, D., Capelletti, M., et al. (2009). Novel mutant-selective EGFR kinase inhibitors against EGFR T790M. *Nature* 462, 1070–1074. doi: 10.1038/nature08622

10

Computer-Aided Drug Design in Epigenetics

***Wenchao Lu*[1,2†]*, Rukang Zhang*[1,2†]*, Hao Jiang*[1,2]*, Huimin Zhang*[1,3] *and Cheng Luo*[1,2*]**

[1] Drug Discovery and Design Center, CAS Key Laboratory of Receptor Research, State Key Laboratory of Drug Research, Shanghai Institute of Materia Medica, Chinese Academy of Sciences, Shanghai, China, [2] Department of Pharmacy, University of Chinese Academy of Sciences, Beijing, China, [3] School of Life Science and Technology, ShanghaiTech University, Shanghai, China

***Correspondence:**
Cheng Luo
cluo@simm.ac.cn

[†] These authors have contributed equally to this work.

Epigenetic dysfunction has been widely implicated in several diseases especially cancers thus highlights the therapeutic potential for chemical interventions in this field. With rapid development of computational methodologies and high-performance computational resources, computer-aided drug design has emerged as a promising strategy to speed up epigenetic drug discovery. Herein, we make a brief overview of major computational methods reported in the literature including druggability prediction, virtual screening, homology modeling, scaffold hopping, pharmacophore modeling, molecular dynamics simulations, quantum chemistry calculation, and 3D quantitative structure activity relationship that have been successfully applied in the design and discovery of epi-drugs and epi-probes. Finally, we discuss about major limitations of current virtual drug design strategies in epigenetics drug discovery and future directions in this field.

Keywords: drug discovery, epigenetics, small-molecule inhibitor, computer-aided drug design, virtual screening

INTRODUCTION

Covalent modifications on nucleosomes, the basic building blocks on chromatins, including methylation, acetylation, phosphorylation, and ubiquination specifically regulate downstream gene expression patterns in a context-dependent manner that form the fundamental molecular basis of epigenetics (Strahl and Allis, 2000; Berger, 2007). Dynamic regulation of epigenetic modification collections leads to different functional outcomes that plays a pivotal role in biological processes including genome reprogramming, gene transcription, DNA damage response and homeostatic regulation (Li, 2002; Vidanes et al., 2005; Kouzarides, 2007; Gut and Verdin, 2013). Epigenetic dysfunction is tightly related with the pathogenesis and progression of several diseases including malignant diseases especially cancers and chronic diseases such as immune-mediated diseases, neurodegenerative disorders and diabetes which underscoring the importance of these covalent modifications (Best and Carey, 2010; Dawson and Kouzarides, 2012; Tough et al., 2016; Hwang et al., 2017).

Proteins responsible to modulate epigenetic marks on nucleosomes could be roughly divided into three categories based on their relative function including writers (enzymes that deposit covalent modifications), erasers (enzymes that remove covalent modifications), and readers (proteins that recognize specific modifications and recruit chaperons). Encouraging success has been achieved in the development of epi-probes for dissecting epigenome in recent decades (Shortt et al., 2017). However, there is still formidable challenge for epigenetic drug discovery in both academia and industry due to complexity in epigenetics regulatory network and the limits in assays and drug development technologies. So far only seven epigenetic agents targeting two epigenetic enzymes (DNA methytransferases, histone deacetylases) have been approved for human use. The indications of approved epigenetic drugs are limited to malignant diseases such as myelodysplastic syndromes (MDS), acute myeloid leukemia (AML), chronic myelomonocytic leukemia (CML), peripheral T-cell lymphoma (PTCL), and cutaneous T-cell lymphoma (CTCL) while the applications of epigenetic drugs in chronic diseases treatment were less explored (Mann et al., 2007; Derissen et al., 2013; Laubach et al., 2015; Lee et al., 2015). Hence, there is urgent need to develop novel epigenetic drugs with multidisciplinary efforts and extensive collaborations that may accelerate the pace of drug discovery process.

With advanced development of computational methodologies, computer-aided drug design (CADD) has emerged as a burgeoning research filed (Zheng et al., 2013). Currently, many pharmaceuticals companies and research institutions all over the world have established their own CADD departments and continued efforts have been made toward the development and optimization of drug design methodologies and software (Kim et al., 2017). *In silico* druggability assessment helps researchers to identify more chemical-tractable targets and prioritize screening endeavor (Trosset and Vodovar, 2013). Based on rapid advancement of crystallography and successful applications of homology modeling, structure-based virtual screen (SBVS) has proven a useful method to quickly identify bioactive hits in early-stage discovery activities (Lounnas et al., 2013). Ligand-based drug design (LBDD) strategies like three dimensional quantitative structure activity relationship (3D-QSAR), 2D similarity-based searching, scaffold hopping and pharmacophore studies are also efficient approaches for hit enrichment and activity prediction based on available information of known inhibitors (Meena et al., 2011; Andrew et al., 2016; Yadav et al., 2017b). Moreover, quantum mechanical calculation and molecule dynamic (MD) simulation provide the in-depth understanding in protein catalytic mechanism that is quite useful mechanism-based drug design (Scheraga et al., 2007). *In silico* pharmacokinetic properties assessment allows the prediction of absorption, distribution, metabolism, elimination, and toxicity (ADMET) of drug candidates that is an important cheminformatics tool in drug design (Gaur et al., 2015; Yadav et al., 2016). Collectively, combined with the gained availability of diverse compound databases, these cost effective structure-based or ligand-based strategies significantly increase the efficiency in drug discovery and provide new horizons and promising avenues to conquer life-threatening diseases (**Figure 1**, **Table 1**).

Although these leading computational strategies have been successfully applied in traditional drug discovery pipeline, there are relatively few reports focusing on its contribution in epigenetic landscape (Li et al., 2015). In this review, we mainly focus on recent progress on the applications of these strategies and highlight representative studies and major contributions of computational approaches in this field. Other successful drug discovery studies using wet lab approaches are beyond the field of this review and not covered here that may also be interesting aspects in epigenetic-related studies.

WRITER

Epigenetic writers are the enzymes responsible for transferring methyl groups or acetyl groups to DNA, histone or other non-histone substrates from cofactors *S*-adenosyl-L-methionine (SAM) or acetyl coenzyme A (Ac-CoA). Based on their distinct functions, writers are usually divided into three categories, namely DNA methyltransferases (DNMTs), protein lysine/arginine methyltransferases (PKMTs/PRMTs) and histone acetyltransferases (HATs). These enzymes alter chromatin organization and contribute to downstream gene expression regulation through site-specific modification that are involved in the multiple function pathways (Gelato and Fischle, 2008). To elucidate their roles in physiological or pathological states, there has been increasing interest in the discovery of writer inhibitors through *in silico* approaches and many successful stories have been reported in the literature (**Figure 2**). In this section, we will present an overview of the current applications of computational methods used in hit identification targeting epigenetic writers.

DNA Methyltransferases

DNA methyltransferases catalyze DNA methylation by depositing a methyl group on the 5-position of the cytosine (Robertson, 2001). In mammalian cells, there are five members identified so far: DNMT1, DNMT2, DNMT3A, DNMT3B, and DNMT3L. Among them, DNMT1 is characterized as the maintenance methyltransferase that shows preference for hemimethylated DNA substrates while DNMT3A and DNMT3B belong to *de novo* methyltransferases subfamily that function in complex form and catalyze the methylation of unmethylated DNA (Okano et al., 1999; Goll and Bestor, 2005). In DNMTs, the founding member DNMT1 is the best studied. DNMT1 introduces a new methyl group into newly synthesized DNA strand in the context of CpG dinucleotide that maintains methylation patterns of template strand during DNA replication (Bestor, 2000; Auclair and Weber, 2012). Aberrant promoter DNA hypermethylation leads to silencing of tumor suppressor genes, which has been frequently observed in various carcinomas (Feinberg et al., 2006; Zhang and Xu, 2017). Therefore, DNMTs have become one of the most promising targets for cancer therapy and many computational approaches have evolved to fuel the development of epi-probes and epi-drugs targeting DNMTs (Medina-Franco et al., 2015).

Homology Modeling-Driven Studies

Homology modeling is a quite effective strategy especially when interested protein crystal structures are not available and it functions as the most valuable research tool to fill the sequence-structure gap for structure-based drug design (Dwivedi et al., 2015). The accuracy of homology models mainly depends on the sequence identity or similarity between the template protein and the protein to be modeled (Chothia and Lesk, 1986). As commonly accepted, homology models based on more than 50% of sequence identity with proteins whose structures have been experimentally acquired are usually very accurate and can be used for drug discovery purposes (Hillisch et al., 2004).

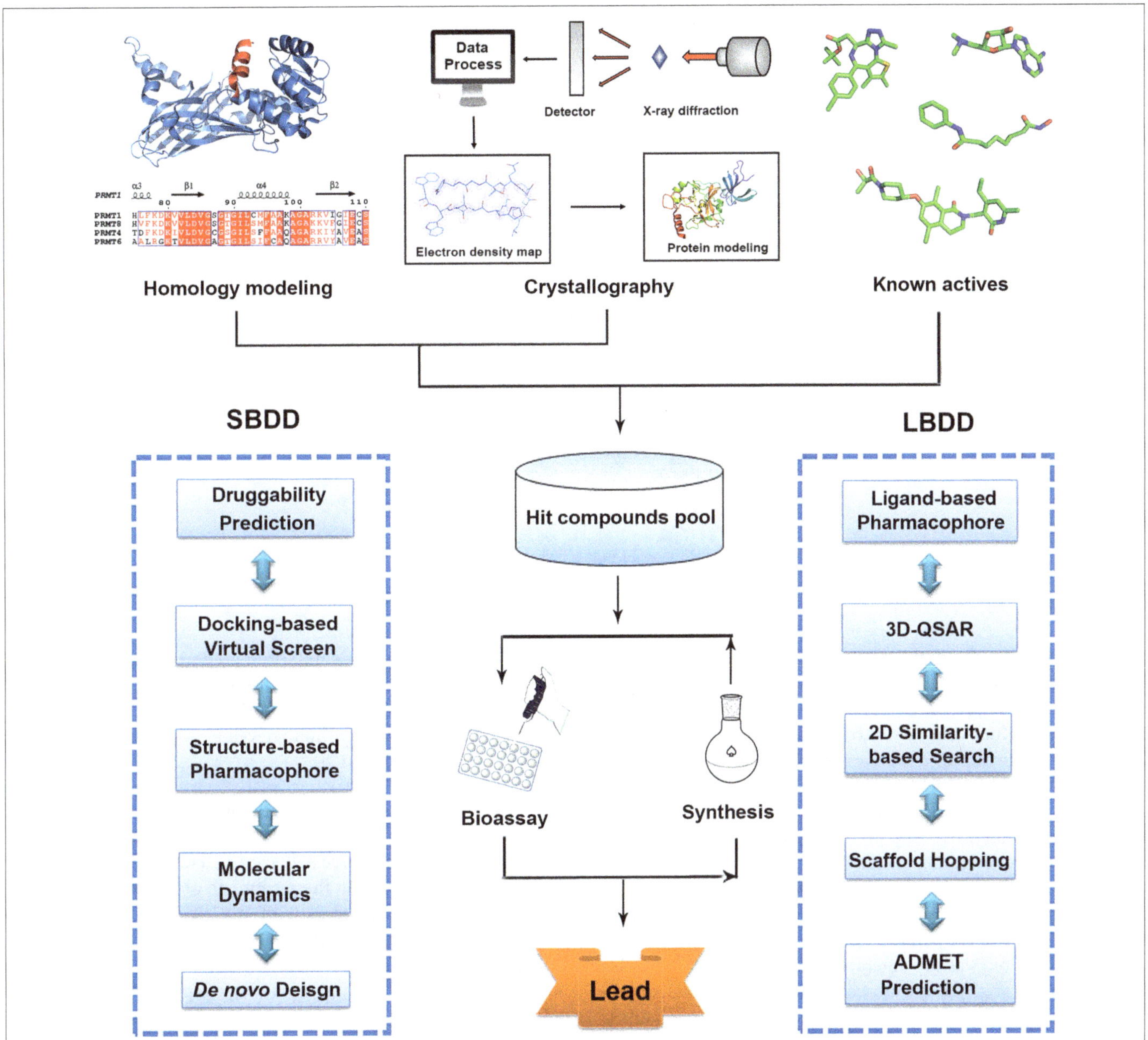

FIGURE 1 | Traditional workflow of structure-based drug design (SBDD) and ligand-based drug design (LBDD).

Since there was no DNMT1 crystal structure ever released until 2008, drug development against this therapeutic target progressed slowly (Syeda et al., 2011). To circumvent this, Siedlecki et al. built a homology model of human DNMT1 catalytic domain based on available structural information of M.HhaI, M.HaeIII, and DNMT2 in the MODELLER module of INSIGHT2000 (Siedlecki et al., 2003). In a follow-up study, based on this established homology model, Siedlecki and co-workers performed docking-based virtual screening of a diversity set containing 1,990 compounds from the National Cancer Institute (NCI) that represented more than 140,000 compounds using DOCK version 5.1.0. The screen resulted in the discovery of RG108 (compound 1 in **Figure 2**) that came out on top in biochemical assays (Brueckner et al., 2005; Siedlecki et al., 2006).

Similarly, Kuck et al. carried out virtual screening (VS) of a larger data set including more than 65,000 lead-like compounds based on the aforementioned DNMT1 homology model. Top-ranked compounds were re-scored by GLIDE, GOLD, and AUTODOCK followed by experimental tests. Among them, NSC14778 (compound 2 in **Figure 2**) presented inhibitory activities against DNMT1 and DNMT3B with the IC_{50} value of 92 and 17 μM, respectively while nanaomycin A (compound 3 in **Figure 2**) selectively inhibited DNMT3B with the IC_{50} value of 500 nM. To explain the selective inhibitory activities

TABLE 1 | The online public and commercial databases and compound collections used for virtual screening in epigenetics.

Database	Size	Website	Applications
ZINC	Over 35 million	http://zinc.docking.org	GCN5; KDM4A/C; HDAC1; BRD4/T; SIRT2-3
SPECS	~320,000	http://www.specs.net	DOT1L; DNMT1; SET7; DNMT3A; PRMT1; G9a; FTO; PRMT5; EZH2; HDAC8; LSD1; BRD4; Menin-MLL1
NCI	~260,000	https://cactus.nci.nih.gov/	DNMT1; Class I/IIa HDACs; KDM4A/B; BRD2
Maybridge	~56,000	http://www.maybridge.com	LSD1; HDAC2; HDAC8
ChemBridge	~1.1 million	http://www.chembridge.com	Type I PRMTs; PRMT5; p300/CBP; BRD4; Spindlin1; SIRT3
CoCoCo	~7 million	http://cococo.isof.cnr.it	SMYD3
Enamine	~2.4 million	http://www.enamine.net	LSD1; PRMT5
ChEMBL	~1.7 million	http://www.ebi.ac.uk/chembldb/index.php	GCN5; BRD4
ChemDiv	~1.5 million	http://www.chemdiv.com	PRMT5; BRD4; Spindlin1
Dictionary of Natural Products	~40,000	http://dnp.chemnetbase.com	BRD4
ASINEX	~87,000	http://www.asinex.com/libraries_synergy.html/	HDAC1
InterBioScreen	~550,000	https://www.ibscreen.com	HDAC1
eMolecules	Over 8 million	http://www.emolecules.com	BRD4; WDR5-MLL1
Life chemicals	~1.35 million	http://www.lifechemicals.com	BRD4
DrugBank	~10,000	http://www.drugbank.ca	SIRT3
WDI	~80,000	http://www.daylight.com/products/wdi.html	HDAC1; HDAC6

Data accessed in December 28, 2017.

of nanaomycin A, the authors established homology model of DNMT3B catalytic domain based on DNMT3A crystallographic structure, which provided structural basis for mechanism interpretation (Kuck et al., 2010a,b).

In order to further disclose the mechanism of action (MOA) of nanaomycin A, Caulfield and co-workers performed >100 ns molecular dynamic simulation using the CHARMM27 force field in NAMD version 2.62. The previously established DNMT3B homology model bound to nanaomycin A was used with either presence or absence of cofactor SAM in the simulation. The results suggested that nanaomycin A and SAM could bind to DNMT3B in a cooperative manner. Besides, nanaomycin A could form long-lasting interactions with key residues that involved in the methylation process which further validated the hypothesis supported by previous docking simulation (Caulfield and Medina-Franco, 2011).

High Throughput Virtual Screening

In 2014, through docking-based virtual screening based on the complex structure of mouse DNMT1 bound to *S*-adenosyl-L-homocysteine (SAH) (PDB ID: 4DA4), Chen et al. reported a novel non-nucleoside DNMT1 inhibitor DC_05 that showed significant selectivity toward other protein methyltransferases (Chen S. et al., 2014). Further medicinal chemistry optimization led to the discovery of more potent compound DC_517 (compound 4 in **Figure 2**) with the IC_{50} value of 1.7 μM. The putative binding models were generated based on molecular docking studies, which gave detailed interpretation of the structure-activity relationship (SAR).

In 2017, in order to identify novel DNMT3A inhibitors, Shao et al. conducted a multi-step docking-based virtual screening in combination with pharmacophore mapping. Through initial screening and follow-up similarity-based analog searching, the authors discovered novel DNMT3A inhibitor compound 40_3 (compound 5 in **Figure 2**) with the IC_{50} value of 41 μM, which may serve as the starting point to develop more potent DNMT3A inhibitors (Shao et al., 2017).

Quantum Mechanical Calculation

In 2012, based on the *ab initio* methods, Alcaro and co-workers developed the force field parameters implemented in the MacroModel package for the treatment of charge distribution and overall charge assignment of nucleic acids that undergo methylation. It gives essential insights related to the correct charge treatment and force field parameterization, which is an important issue in molecular modeling of epigenetic phenomena and shed light for the nucleic acids-related epigenetic functional study and in the development of DNA intercalating, subtype-selective DNMTs inhibitors (Alcaro et al., 2002).

Histone Methyltransferases

Histone methylation is one of the most important post-translational modifications on histones and results in either activation or repression depending on specific sites. The methylation marks could recruit different methyl-binding proteins and mediate downstream signaling pathways, which could be basically regulated by dynamic interplay between histone methyltransferases (HMTs) and demethyltransferases (HDMTs) (Martin and Zhang, 2005). Histone methyltransferases can be mainly divided into two categories based on their relative substrates: protein lysine methyltransferases and protein arginine N-methyltransferases (Li et al., 2012). Among them, PKMTs consist of SET domain-containing PKMTs (SUV, SET1, SET2, EZ, and RIZ) and non-SET domain-containing PKMT (DOT1L)

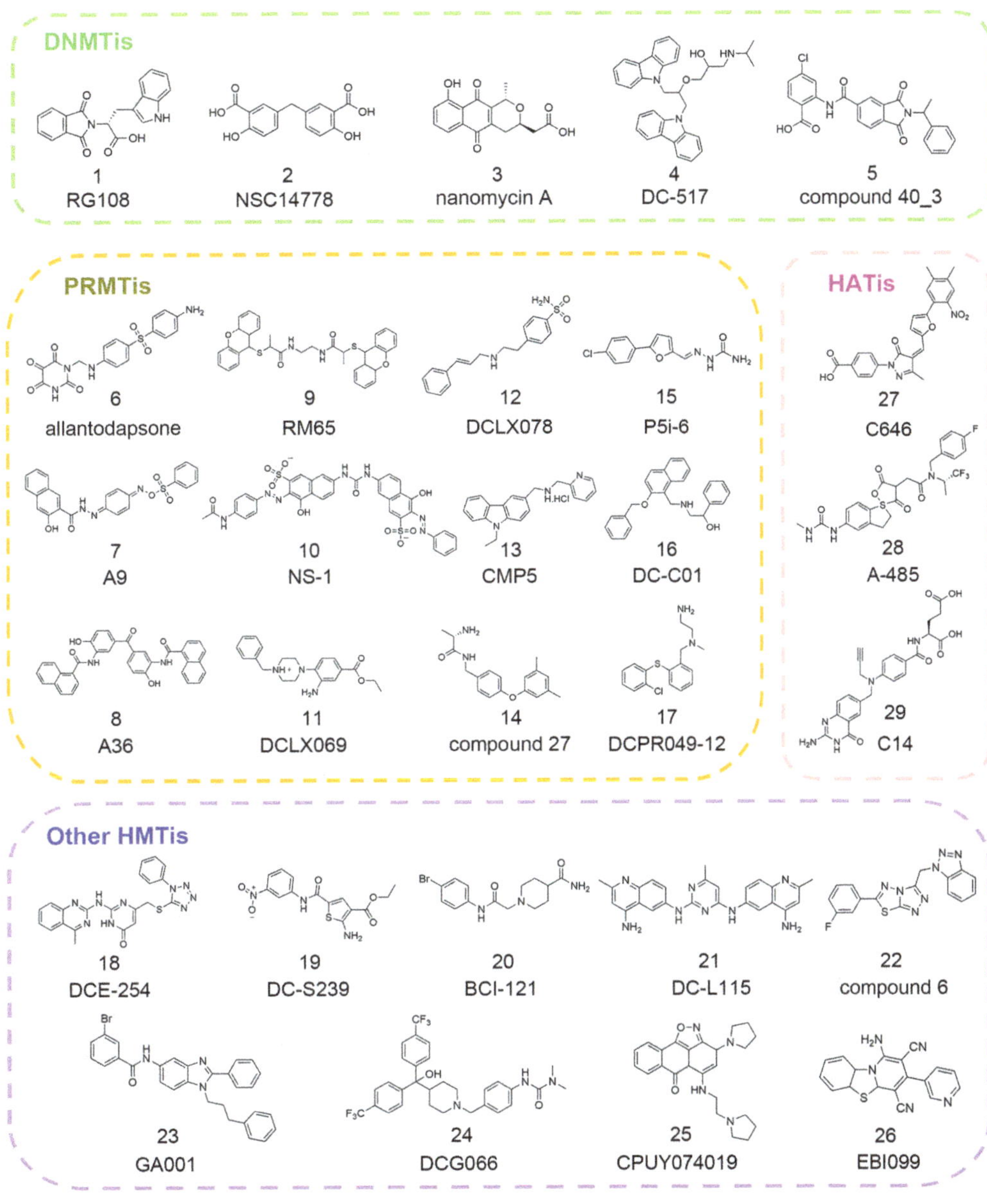

FIGURE 2 | Chemical structures of epigenetic writer inhibitors mentioned in this review.

(Kouzarides, 2002). As for PRMT family, it could be further classified into three subcategories: type I PRMTs responsible for arginine monomethylation and asymmetric dimethylation (PRMT1, 2, 4, 6, 8), type II PRMTs (PRMT5, 9) for arginine monomethylation and symmetrical dimethylation and type III PRMT (PRMT7) only with arginine monomethylation activity (Wolf, 2009). Emerging evidence demonstrated that deregulated alternations of methylation patterns were implicated in the pathogenesis of various cancers and other malignant diseases (Spannhoff et al., 2009; Jones et al., 2016). Consequently, continued efforts have been devoted to drug design for HMTs, which open up vast ranges of prospects for diseases treatment (**Table 2**).

Pharmacophore-Based Drug Discovery

With the increasing knowledge of known active molecules available in databases, pharmacophore modeling methods are receiving more attention in the era of rational drug design that could quickly extract the key steric and electronic features for ligand-receptor interactions (Guner et al., 2004; Yadav et al., 2010, 2012). In 2007, Spannhoff et al. presented first target-based virtual screening with NCI diversity set to discover novel PRMT1 inhibitors. The GRID-based pharmacophore model, the methodology originally introduced by Ortuso et al. in 2006, was applied as post-docking filter to analyze all preliminary docking solutions (Ortuso et al., 2006). The study resulted in the identification of allantodapsone (compound 6

TABLE 2 | The HMTs inhibitors derived based on virtual screening or high throughput screening.

Targets	Virtual screen			High throughput screen		
	I[a]	II[b]	III[c]	I	II	III
PRMT1	★			★		
PRMT3	★			★		
PRMT4	★			★		
PRMT5	★			★		
PRMT6	★			★		
DOT1L		★		★		
SUV420H1	–	–	–	★		
SUV420H2	–	–	–	★		
SMYD2	–	–	–	★		
SMYD3			★	★		
GLP	–	–	–	★		
G9a		★		★		
NSD2			★	–	–	–
SETD2	–	–	–	★		
SETD7		★		★		
SETD8		★		★		
EZH1	–	–	–	★		
EZH2			★	★		

[a]*The IC_{50} values smaller than 1 μM.*
[b]*The IC_{50} values at the range of 1–10 μM.*
[c]*The IC_{50} values at the range of 10–100 μM.*
The stars here denote that the IC_{50} value of the most potent compound against this target is in the corresponding range.

in **Figure 2**) with the IC_{50} value of 1.7 μM (Spannhoff et al., 2007a).

In the follow-up study, Heinke et al. expanded their work to a larger compound collection, the ChemBridge database containing 328,000 molecules (Heinke et al., 2009). Based on previously reported binding modes of allantodapsone, the pharmacophore models were generated in LigandScout with one HBD, one hydrogen bond acceptor (HBA), two hydrophobic/aromatic features, one included volume and 23 excluded volumes leading to the identification of nine compounds with PRMT1 inhibitory activity below 35 μM.

Ligand-based pharmacophore modeling is also a powerful tool in drug discovery campaigns. In 2012, Wang et al. constructed four rational pharmacophore models with HBA, HBD, and ring/aromatic (RA) as key chemical features based on 17 reported active molecules in Discovery Studio version 2.1. Then established models were used as the query to search theoretical-soluble small molecule library. Through cluster analysis in combination with biological assays, A9 and A36 (compounds 7–8 in **Figure 2**) were identified as PRMT1 inhibitors with the IC_{50} values of 41.7 and 12.0 μM, respectively (Wang et al., 2012). Kinetic analysis demonstrated that A9 was a peptide-competitive PRMT1 inhibitor whereas A36 was the non-competitive PRMT1 inhibitor that could be used as the parent compounds for further chemistry optimization.

The pharmacophore modeling has also been widely applied in hit identification targeting other HMTs. In 2016, aiming to identify novel EZH2 inhibitors, Wu et al. conducted ligand-based pharmacophore modeling based on validated EZH2 inhibitors (Wu et al., 2016). The reliability of constructed models was evaluated by enrichment capacity analysis using molecules in test sets. Based on the established models, they identified novel EZH2 inhibitors DCE_254 (compound 18 in **Figure 2**) with the IC_{50} value of 11 μM.

In 2015, through integrated structure-based pharmacophore-modeling and molecular docking, Meng et al. discovered a SET7 inhibitor, namely DC_S100 with the IC_{50} value of 30.0 μM (Meng et al., 2015). Docking-based SAR analysis followed by structure optimization led to the identification of DC-S239 (compound 19 in **Figure 2**), with the IC_{50} value of 4.6 μM. In addition, DC-S239 could dose-dependently inhibit the proliferation of MCF7, HL60, and MV4-11 with the IC_{50} values at micromolar range supporting its potential use in cellular context.

Molecular Dynamics Simulation

Molecular dynamics simulation is a useful theoretical technique to investigate the conformations and dynamic behaviors of biomolecules in long-time scale that provides atomic-level insight into the regulatory mechanism (Lindorff-Larsen et al., 2011; Okumura et al., 2018). To characterize the elusive roles of the N-terminal region and dimerization arms for PRMT1 activity, Zhou et al. performed MD simulations using GROMACS 4.3 package based on hPRMT1 homology model in monomer and dimer states (Zhou et al., 2015b). The simulations captured the dynamic correlations between the N-terminal region and dimerization arms. Moreover, the normalized covariance analysis and principal component analysis (PCA) were applied to analyze the energy landscape of different conformations at reduced dimensions. Through network topology analysis, a long-distance communication pathway was theoretically proposed which was further validated by biochemical mutational experiments. The simulations disclosed the underlying molecule mechanism of allosteric communication between the two regions and provided the rationale for mechanism-based PRMT subtype-selective inhibitors.

Molecule dynamic simulations could be not only wildly applied in protein dynamic regulation studies but also in MOA studies for small molecule inhibitors. In order to uncover the molecular basis of diamidine inhibitors for selective PRMT1 inhibition, Yan et al. conducted extensive MD simulations and molecular mechanics/Poisson–Boltzmann solvent-accessible surface area (MM/PBSA) calculation to analyze the interaction patterns in the binding cavity for the docking complex which provided the avenue to design more potent and specific inhibitors (Yan et al., 2014; Zhang et al., 2017a,b). A similar MD study was reported by Yang and co-workers to propose binding poses of identified PRMT1 inhibitors and circumvent the limitations introduced by inaccuracy of molecule docking methods (Yang et al., 2017).

High Throughput Virtual Screening

The big explosion of available structural information of HMTs has greatly facilitated the application of docking-based virtual screening (DBVS). In 2007, via virtual screening and 2D similarity-based analog searching, Spannhoff et al. identified RM65 (compound 9 in **Figure 2**) as the PRMT1 inhibitor with the IC_{50} value of 55.4 μM (Spannhoff et al., 2007b). In 2010, a similar study was reported by Feng and co-workers in structure-based virtual screening with 400,000 compounds. In this study, NS-1 (compound 10 in **Figure 2**) was identified as the PRMT1 inhibitor with an IC_{50} value of 12.7 μM which directly targeted the peptide substrates instead of enzymes (Feng et al., 2010). In 2014, Xie and co-workers used the combinatorial dockings methods including GLIDE and DOCK for *in silico* screen. The authors identified DCLX069 and DCLX078 (compounds 11–12 in **Figure 2**) with the IC_{50} values of 17.9 and 26.2 μM, respectively in biochemical assays (Xie et al., 2014).

A number of attempts have also been made to identify other PRMTis besides PRMT1 inhibitors. In 2015, Alinari et al. used comparative modeling and structure-based virtual screening with ChemBridge CNS-Set library of 10,000 small molecule compounds leading to the identification of first-in-class PRMT5 inhibitor CMP5 (compound 13 in **Figure 2**). In cellular context, CMP5 could selectively inhibit the proliferation and transformation of EBV-driven B-lymphocyte (Alinari et al., 2015). In 2016, Ferreira et al. started their work based on the two basic amine tails that mimicked the side chain of substrate arginine and established PRMT-focused virtual library. Through initial biochemical screening and structure-based optimization, the authors identified compound 27 (compound 14 in **Figure 2**) as the selective CARM1 inhibitor with an IC_{50} value of 0.05 μM and ligand efficiency of 0.43 (Ferreira de Freitas et al., 2016). In 2017, Ji et al. carried out molecular docking studies with semi-flexible docking methods in GOLD and identified selective PRMT5 inhibitor P5i-6 (compound 15 in **Figure 2**) with an IC_{50} of 0.57 μM (Ji et al., 2017). Similarly, Ye et al. identified PRMT5 inhibitor named DC_C01 (compound 16 in **Figure 2**) with the IC_{50} value of 2.8 μM via docking-based virtual screening and structure modification (Ye et al., 2017). Concurrent with the two studies described above, through hierarchical docking strategies and chemistry optimization, Chen et al. identified DCPR049_12 (compound 17 in **Figure 2**) with promising inhibitory activity for type I PRMT with the IC_{50} value at nanomolar range (Wang et al., 2017).

Besides PRMTs, docking-based virtual screening strategy was also applied in the epi-probe design for other HMTs. In 2015, in an attempt to search for SMYD3 inhibitors, Peserico et al. performed high-throughput virtual screening of the CoCoCo database containing nearly 260,000 molecules in GLIDE version 5.7 (Peserico et al., 2015). The study led to the identification of BCI-121 (compound 20 in **Figure 2**) as the best candidate for SMYD3 inhibition that could reduce global H3K4me2/3 and H4K5me levels in colorectal cancer. Similarly, Chen et al. identified the DOT1L inhibitor DC_L115 (compound 21 in **Figure 2**) with an IC_{50} value of 1.5 μM via structure-based virtual screening of approximately 200,000 molecules in SPECS database (Chen S. et al., 2016).

Very recently, Wang and co-workers developed a target-specific scoring function based on epsilon support vector regression (ε-SVR) named the SAM-score for SAM-dependent methyltransferases. Based on the built regression model, the authors identified compound 6 (compound 22 in **Figure 2**) as the DOT1L inhibitor with an IC_{50} of 8.3 μM (Wang et al., 2017). There are also some successful studies reported elsewhere for the discovery of other HMT inhibitors (compounds 23–26 in **Figure 2**) for G9a and SETD8 based on *in silico* approaches (Chen W. L. et al., 2016; Kondengaden et al., 2016; Milite et al., 2016).

Histone Acetyltransferases

Histone acetyltransferases (HATs) transfer acetyl groups onto N-terminal tails of core histone and consequently give rise to DNA relaxation, which is closely related to gene activation (Brown et al., 2000). HATs can be divided into four categories on the basis of their sequence similarities, including the GNAT family (GCN5 and PCAF), the MYST family (MOZ/MORF, YBF2/SAS3, SAS2, and TIP60), p300/CBP and RTT109 (Dancy and Cole, 2015). Recently, emerging evidence implicated that deregulation of HATs was closely correlated with tumorigenesis, neurological disorders and inflammatory diseases (Yang, 2004; Rajendrasozhan et al., 2009; Sheikh, 2014). Several HAT inhibitors have been reported, such as bi-substrate inhibitors, natural products, and small molecules. However, there is still a large gap between activities *in vitro* and their potential applications as therapeutic agents *in vivo* due to the lack of potency and selectivity for the current inhibitors which is a long-standing challenge in the field.

In 2010, Bowers et al. conducted structure-based, *in silico* screening approach with a screening set of *ca.* 500,000 commercially available compounds to identify the p300 inhibitor (Bowers et al., 2010). The compounds were scored and ranked based on ICM (Internal Coordinate Mechanics) score in the ICM-VLS software version 3.5. Then top 194 compounds were cherry-picked by visual inspection and purchased from ChemBridge for biochemical analysis. Among them, C646 (compound 27 in **Figure 2**) was identified with *K*i value of 400 nM. Further *in vitro* assay demonstrated that C646 was cofactor-competitive and selective p300 inhibitor. The detailed interaction patterns were confirmed by site-directed mutagenesis in accordance with the predicted computational model.

Very recently, Lasko and co-authors performed similar docking-based *in silico* screening with nearly 800,000 compounds and 1,300 available compounds were test in radioactive p300 acetylation assays (Lasko et al., 2017). Among them, hydantoin and a conjugated thiazolidinedione were identified with the IC_{50} values of 5.1 and 11.5 μM, respectively. More efforts were devoted to the optimization on hydantoin scaffold yielding A-485 (compound 28 in **Figure 2**) with an IC_{50} value of 60 nM. A-485 was a first-in-class highly potent, selective p300/CBP catalytic inhibitor and displayed significant selectivity against other HATs members. Besides, it inhibited proliferation across a broad range of cancer cell lines with specificity for hematological and prostate cell lineages and retarded tumor growth in xenograft models, which underscored the therapeutic potential targeting p300/CBP. Another small molecule discovered by virtual screening from ChEMBL bioassay database was C14 (compound 29 in **Figure 2**) with an IC_{50} value of 225 nM on PfGCN5 in parasite growth assay (Kumar et al., 2017). C14 displayed promising antimalarial activity and showed no effect on mammalian fibroblast cells supporting its safe use for further applications.

ERASER

Erasers are key modifying enzymes in charge of the removal of epigenetic marks that participate in dynamic regulation on gene expression patterns (Mosammaparast and Shi, 2010). Based on their different substrates and their relative functions, erasers could be divided into different families such as histone deacetylases (HDACs), RNA demethyltransferases, histone demethylases (HDMs), histone deubiquitinases, and so on (Arrowsmith et al., 2012). Among them, HDACs are the most studied targets for pharmacological interventions. So far, five epi-drugs targeting HDACs have been approved for clinical use and other HDAC inhibitors like entinostat and CUDC-907 have entered into clinical trials for advanced cancer treatment (Falkenberg and Johnstone, 2014; Li and Seto, 2016). In the following section, we will focus on representative computational work in drug discovery and related mechanism studies that expert in this field (**Figure 3**).

Histone Deacetylases

In mammalian cells, HDACs consist of 18 isoforms and are broadly classified into four categories based on their distinct structural features and subcellular localization: Class I (HDAC1, 2, 3, and 8), Class II (Class IIa HDAC4, 5, 7, 9, and Class IIb HDAC6, 10), Class III (NAD-dependent Sirtuins; SIRT1-7) and Class IV (HDAC11) (Gregoretti et al., 2004; Li and Seto, 2016). HDACs catalyze the deacetylation of histone as well as non-histone substrates and are implicated in fundamental physiological processes including gene transcription, cell cycle regulation, DNA damage response, and metabolism homeostasis (Bode and Dong, 2004; Minucci and Pelicci, 2006). There is a growing body of evidence that deregulation of HDACs activity is strongly correlated with the pathogenesis of several diseases including hematological malignancies and solid tumors that implicates the significance of target intervention (Minucci et al., 2001; Zhu et al., 2004; Buurman et al., 2012). Significant progress has been made in the development of HDAC inhibitors (HDACis) over the recent decades based on *in silico* approaches (Yanuar et al., 2016). The following chapters will focus on some representative studies using computational methods in this field, some of which are described below.

Quantum Mechanical Calculation

Hydroxamic acid moiety presented in most common HDACis is usually recognized as problematic fragment with poor pharmacokinetic profile. To rationally design non-hydroxamic acid HDACis with more favorable physico-chemical properties, Wang et al. performed density functional theory (DFT) calculations to investigate binding modes and related binding free energy of potential zinc binding groups (ZBGs) (Wang et al., 2007). In model active site, only the side chains of zinc-coordinated residues were kept for calculation including two formats and one imidazole that represented as the functional groups of zinc-coordinated histidine and two aspartic acid residues. The calculation results proposed alternatives with novel structural features that favored zinc binding including 3-hydroxy pyrones or β-amino ketones, which may be further utilized for medicinal chemistry optimization on current HDACis.

Apart from the applications in novel hit discovery, quantum mechanical calculation could also enable precise and solid interpretation into mechanism studies that facilitates the drug design of novel and specific HDACis. Finin et al. proposed that H143-D183 catalytic dyad was indispensable for HDAC8 enzymatic activity by abstracting proton from the bridged water molecule while Zhang et al. underscored the role of H142-D176 dyad in proton-shuttle process (Finnin et al., 1999; Wu et al., 2010). In addition, the controversial function of potassium ion near the active pocket present in HDAC crystal structures is also under debate (Gantt et al., 2010; Werbeck et al., 2014). Based on QM/MM simulations including the complete catalytic residues in the quantum region, Chen et al. explained disagreement for those observations and uncovered the unique catalytic mechanism of HDAC8. The results disclosed the inhibitory role of the potassium ion at the active site and uncovered the significance of the pK_a values of zinc-coordinated moiety in HDACis that would be of great value in developing potent and subtype-selective mechanism-based HDACis (Chen K. et al., 2014).

Quantitative Structure-Activity Relationship Analysis

QSAR analysis is a well-established ligand-based computational methodology to describe the quantitative relationship between compound biological activity and its physicochemical properties or structural features, which is the milestone progress in the era of rational drug design (Gupta, 2007; Yadav et al., 2013, 2017a). Since therapeutic value of HDACis has been addressed over recent years and many potent HDACis have been identified so far, comprehensive QSAR studies were conducted using different kinds of data sets to facilitate drug design and discovery against this drug-actionable target. In 2004, Wang et al. developed QSAR models based on hydroxamic acid-based HDACis and found statistically significant relationship between charge distribution, hydrophobicity, geometrical shape of compounds and its relative anti-proliferative activities for PC-3 cell lines (Wang et al., 2004). Since then, the number of QSAR modeling studies increased at a dramatic rate (Xie et al., 2004; Guo et al., 2005; Juvale et al., 2006; Chen et al., 2008; Kozikowski et al., 2008; Ragno et al., 2008).

The first QSAR studies used for virtual screening was reported by Tang and co-workers (Tang et al., 2009). Based on validated QSAR models, the authors screened the in-house library with *ca.* 9.5 million compounds and identified four novel scaffolds that favored HDACs inhibition (compounds 30–33 in **Figure 3**). In 2012, Xiang and colleagues developed pharmacophore and 3D-QSAR models on a series of (benz)imidazole inhibitors (Xiang et al., 2012). The results led to the discovery of 27 inhibitors with putative HDAC2 inhibitory activity. Later on, several groups employed QSAR modeling workflow for HDACis activity and selectivity prediction (Silvestri et al., 2012; Zhao et al., 2013b). In 2014, Kandakatla et al. conducted ligand based 3D-QSAR pharmacophore modeling and identified eight hit compounds from Maybridge and NCI databases as potential HDAC2 inhibitors (Kandakatla and Ramakrishnan, 2014). In

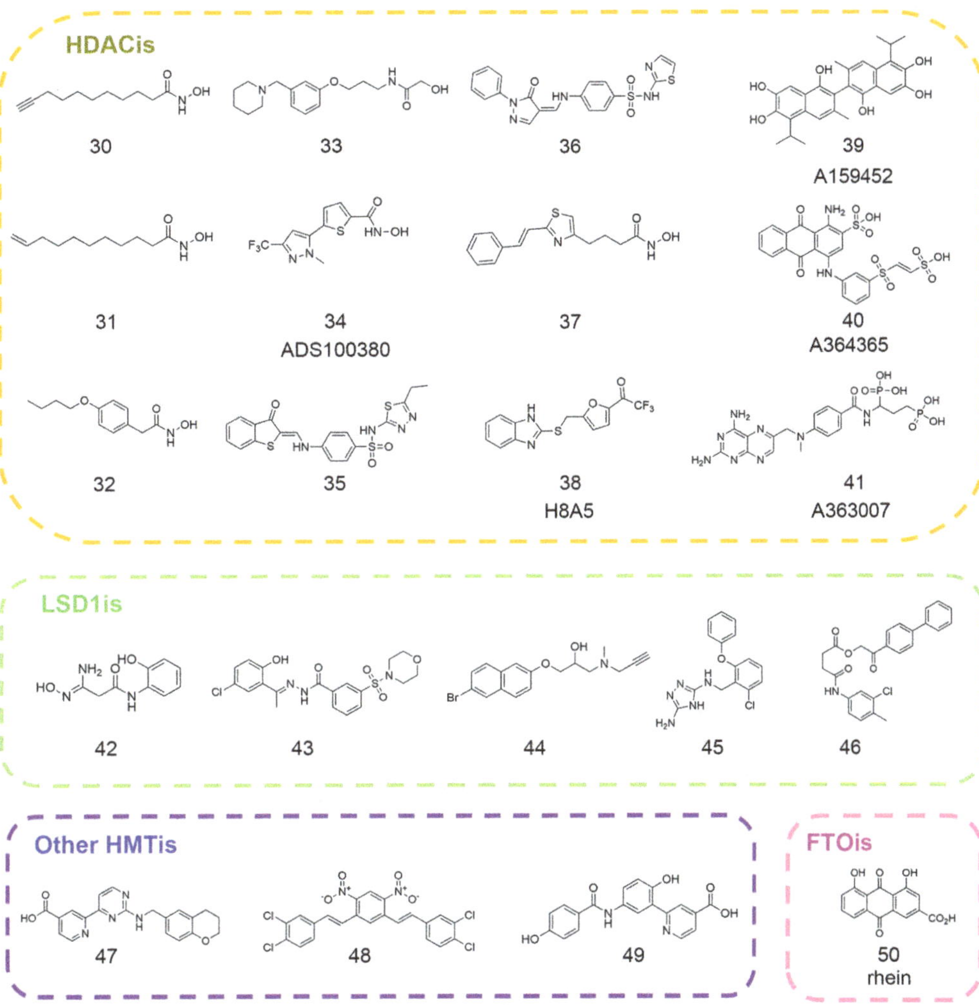

FIGURE 3 | Chemical structures of epigenetic eraser inhibitors mentioned in this review.

the same year, based on 79 previously published substrate-based SIRT1 inhibitors, Kokkonen and coworkers performed CoMFA studies that was successfully applied in the bioactivity prediction of 13 newly synthesized compounds (Kokkonen et al., 2014). Similarly, Cao et al. developed QSAR models using support vector classification and regression with scrupulous examination based on published HDAC8 inhibitors that was applied in next-round drug screening (Cao et al., 2016).

High Throughput Virtual Screening

In 2007, Price and colleagues initiated virtual screening with HDAC-focused library containing 644 hydroxamic acids (Price et al., 2007). The study resulted in the identification of ADS100380 (compound 34 in **Figure 3**) with an IC_{50} value of 0.75 μM followed by iterative optimization. Similarly, another successful application of structure-based virtual screen for the discovery of HDACis was carried out by Park et al. based on HDAC1 homology model (Park et al., 2010). The newly identified inhibitors (compounds 35–36 in **Figure 3**) presented novel chemotypes that had not yet been reported before with IC_{50} values at micromolar range. In 2016, Yoo et al. rationally designed selective HDAC6 inhibitors with the IC_{50} value of 0.199 μM (compound 37 in **Figure 3**) inspired by preliminary virtual screening efforts with LeadQuest chemical database containing 80,600 entries (Yoo et al., 2016). Very recently, Hu designed a versatile VS pipeline with better screening power for the rapid discovery of selective HDAC3 inhibitors (Hu et al., 2017). Many efforts have also been devoted to the discovery of Sirtuins inhibitors, the NAD-dependent class III histone deacetylases that was reported elsewhere (Salo et al., 2013; Kokkonen et al., 2015; Padmanabhan et al., 2016).

As commonly accepted, each computational approach may not perform optimally when applied alone due to complexity of epigenetic network and this highlighted the importance of various combined *in silico* approaches in epigenetic drug discovery. Hou et al. developed ZBG-based pharmacophore model with enhanced sensitivity for virtual screening leading to the identification of selective HDAC8 inhibitor H8-A5 (compound 38 in **Figure 3**) with the IC_{50} value of 1.8 μM. Then molecular docking followed by 50 ns MD simulation was performed to give detailed insight of the MOA of identified hits (Hou et al., 2015). In 2017, Ganai and co-workers employed top-down combinatorial strategy of molecule docking and molecular mechanics generalized born surface area (MM-GBSA), MD simulation and trajectory clustering, energetically-optimized pharmacophore. The authors identified distinct hot spots in highly homologous HDAC1 and HDAC2 that shed light on the development of specific HDAC2 inhibitors against neurological diseases (Ganai et al., 2017). Hsu and co-workers employed VS approach against classified NCI database leading to the identification of class IIa-selective HDACis (compounds 39–41 in **Figure 3**). Homology modeling was performed to generate HDAC5 and HDAC9 3D structures that provide atomic-resolution insight into the selectivity of these inhibitors (Hsu et al., 2017).

RNA Demethyltransferases

RNA methylation is one of most important chemical marks in epigenetic landscape among which N^6-methyladenosine (m6A) is the most abundant and conserved modification in eukaryotes (Desrosiers et al., 1974). Reversible N^6-methyladenosine could be dynamically regulated by related writers and erasers involved in gene expression, RNA splicing, transport, and stability (Fu et al., 2014). Fat mass and obesity-associated (FTO) enzyme is one of the RNA demethylases and depends on Fe (II) and α-KG cofactors for its oxidative demethylation activity (Jia et al., 2011). Genetic variations of *FTO* are functionally associated with human obesity and metabolic disorders (Frayling et al., 2007). Recent studies demonstrate that FTO is highly expressed in MLL-rearranged AML and plays pivotal role in leukemogenesis (Li et al., 2017). Collectively, these studies hold promise for drug design and development targeting FTO for therapeutic translation.

In order to gain detailed insight into molecular mechanism for its catalytic specificity, the complex crystal structure of FTO and 3-meT substrate was resolved, which laid foundations for structure-based drug design (Yadav et al., 2010). Chen et al. employed virtual screening strategy in an effort to identify inhibitors targeting FTO active site. After initial screening against the drug-like SPECS database in Dock version 4.0, the primary results were evaluated in Sybyl and revisited by AutoDock version 4.0. Then top 300 compounds were selected for cluster analysis to ensure scaffold diversity. Finally, 114 compounds were picked out for biochemical validation leading to the identification of natural product rhein (compound 50 in **Figure 3**) as the competitive FTO inhibitor. Further decomposed binding energy prediction highlighted the electrostatic interactions between R316 and rhein, which was validated by follow-up biophysical studies (Chen et al., 2012; Aik et al., 2013). Later on, more efforts have been devoted to the drug design and discovery of selective FTO inhibitors (Huang et al., 2015; Toh et al., 2015). These identified structurally different inhibitor collections may serve as the parent templates applied in ligand-based drug design approaches. The small molecule sets could be used to establish focused and biased libraries that may be useful for rational drug design against other RNA demethylases.

Histone Demethyltransferases

Histone demethylation remained ambiguous until the hallmark discovery of first lysine specific demethylase LSD1 in 2004 (Shi et al., 2004). These demethyltransferases catalyze lysine/arginine demethylation and function as transcription corepressor that is tightly associated with dynamic regulation of methylation patterns shaping the epigenome (Dimitrova et al., 2015). Since then, more histone demethylases have been identified and their biological relevance has been disclosed (Kooistra and Helin, 2012). Currently, histone demethylases could be mainly categorized into two subfamilies based on homology and substrate specificity: LSD demethylases (LSD1-2) and Jumonji C (JmjC) domain-containing demethylases (JHDMs) (Markolovic et al., 2016). Dysfunction of histone demethylases has been observed in malignant diseases especially cancers such as colorectal cancer, bladder cancer and lung cancer (Hayami et al., 2011; Højfeldt et al., 2013). Harris et al. delineated the potential oncogenic role of LSD1 (KDM1A) in leukemia using the mouse model of MLL-AF9 leukemia (Harris et al., 2012). In another study, the authors showed that KDM2B was highly expressed in leukemia samples and played central role in the etiology and progression of acute myeloid leukemia (He et al., 2011). Thus, histone demethylases were considered as putative epi-targets for discovering anticancer agents. In the following section, we will discuss the successful applications of computational approaches in the field.

High Throughput Virtual Screening

In order to pursue novel LSD1 inhibitors, Hazeldine et al. undertook the virtual screen strategy against Maybridge compound library. Sitemap was employed to assess the druggability of potential active chamber. Through high throughput virtual screen in GLIDE, the authors identified a total of 10 hits with GlideScore lower than −7.5 kcal/mol. The most effective compound (compound 42 in **Figure 3**) featuring amidoximes moiety displayed moderate *in vitro* activity with the IC_{50} value of 16.8 μM (Hazeldine et al., 2012). Later on, Sorna and co-workers reported structure-based docking studies with the ligand library containing 13 million compounds. High Throughput Virtual Screen (HTVS) protocol integrated in Schrödinger suite was applied and the database was subsequently refined by rule of five filters to weed out nonbinders and compounds with undesirable physicochemical parameters. Top 15% compounds were selected and re-ranked by combinatorial scoring with GLIDE, ICM, and GOLD to discard false positives. Based on chemical diversity analysis and visual inspection of initial docking results, 121 compounds were selected for biochemical validation and further medicinal chemistry optimization led to the identification of novel LSD1 inhibitor 12 (compound 43 in **Figure 3**) with the IC_{50} value of 0.013 μM (Sorna et al., 2013). Continued efforts have been made toward the discovery of potent, selective epi-probes against LSD1 and other histone demethylases (compounds 44–45,47 in **Figure 3**) based on computational approaches (Schmitt et al., 2013; Kutz et al., 2014; Roatsch et al., 2016). Chu et al. utilized GEMDOCK to screen the NCI database (~236,962 compounds) *in silico* and identified a selective KDM4A/KDM4B inhibitor (compound 48 in **Figure 3**) with the IC_{50} value at micromolar level (Chu et al., 2014). In 2016, Korczynska et al. performed molecular docking screens using ZINC fragment library (~600,000 commercially available fragments) in DOCK version 3.6 leading to the identification of 5-aminosalicylates as the KDM4C inhibitor with good ligand efficiency. Further docking analysis and fragment linking optimization yielded more potent inhibitor with K_i value of 43 nM (compound 49 in **Figure 3**) against KDM4C that highlighted the viable applications in fragment-based drug discovery (FBDD) (Korczynska et al., 2016).

3D-QSAR Pharmacophore Modeling

In 2015, Zhou et al. presented pharmacophore-based ligand mapping strategy against LSD1 using refined SPECS database (~171,143 small molecules) in Discovery Studio version 2.5. 3D conformations of 37 compounds with known activities (22 compounds for training set and 15 compounds for test set) were generated and used to generate pharmacophore in HypoGen module. The reliability of the pharmacophore model was verified by Fischer randomization test and decoy set prediction. Through combinatorial pharmacophore mapping and optimized docking in database screening, the authors identified XZ-09 (compound 46 in **Figure 3**) as a selective LSD1 inhibitor with the IC_{50} value of 2.4 μM that may serve as a lead compound for further optimization (Zhou et al., 2015a).

READER

The posttranslational modifications on histone tails with different modification states are recognized by specific epigenetic readers, which recruit effector modules to stimulate different functions. Until now there are several well-characterized epigenetic readers including acetyl-lysine readers, methyl-lysine readers, methyl-arginine readers, and phospho-serine readers. Among them, lysine acetylation and methylation related readers were studied extensively as drug targets in epi-drug design and discovery. The acetyl-lysine readers consist of bromodomains and the tandem PHD domains (Lange et al., 2008; Filippakopoulos et al., 2012). And the readers associated with lysine methylation include PHD zinc finger domains, WD40, Tudor, double/tandem Tudor, MBT, Ankyrin Repeats, zf-CW, PWWP, and chromodomains (Kim et al., 2006; Collins et al., 2008; Musselman and Kutateladze, 2009; He et al., 2010; Rona et al., 2016; Schapira et al., 2017). Emerging evidence demonstrated the dysfunction of epigenetic readers is implicated in various diseases such as cancer, intellectual disability, aging, autoimmune disease, inflammation and acquired immune deficiency syndrome (Baker et al., 2008; Greer and Shi, 2012; Jung et al., 2015). So far, several successful compounds selectively targeting epigenetic reader domains have been reported and some of them enter into clinical studies (Greschik et al., 2017). Herein, we focus on the computer-aided drug discovery in epigenetic readers and review the successful examples to illuminate the advantages and potential applications of computational drug design and discovery in this field (**Figure 4**).

Druggability Prediction

Based on the complex crystal structure information of epigenetic readers with their relative substrates or small molecule inhibitors, the druggability of these targets could be easily predicted by computational methods. Many pragmatic programs have been developed and applied to explore potential drug-actionable pocket and assess the druggability of these binding sites (Halgren, 2009; Fauman et al., 2011). In 2011, Santiago et al. conducted the systematic druggability prediction for methyl-lysine binding proteins (Santiago et al., 2011). Based on the terms like steric volume, enclosure and hydrophobicity of the pocket, the Dscores of potential pockets were calculated using SiteMap. The results revealed that the druggability of different of methyl-lysine readers was highly variable dependent on backbone motion and intramolecular interactions, among which chromodomains, WDR domains and PWWP domains were more targetable than others like Tudor and PHD domains for small molecule inhibitors.

In 2012, to explore the druggability for bromodomains, the acetyl-lysine binders, Vidler et al. retrieved the available crystal structures of 33 human bromodomains from the Protein Data Bank (PDB) and evaluated druggability in SiteMap (Vidler et al., 2012). Among them, bromodomain, and extra-terminal (BET) family was predicted as the highly druggable target, which was already proved by small molecule inhibitors studies, but it could not represent the whole bromodomain families. The authors classified 49 bromodomains into eight categories based on common binding site features and found that only one of them showed the comparable druggability with the BET family including CECR2, FALZ (A/B), GCN5L2, PCAF, TAF1 (A/B)(2), and TAF1L(2). Other groups were predicted with low scores suggesting to be challenging for epi-drug discovery. Collectively, these work uncovered novel druggable readers that were less explored before, which provided new opportunities for drug discovery.

Combinatorial *in Silico* Virtual Screen Approaches

With the rapid development of BET inhibitors, more complex crystal structures were obtained, which made structure-based virtual screen and chemical modifications more easily. Based on the well-known critical interactions between BET family and related inhibitors, many computational studies were performed to develop novel chemotypes for BET family.

In 2013, a high throughput virtual screening was performed with more than 7 million small molecules from the Dictionary of Natural Products, the ChEMBL database, and the ZINC database by Lucas and colleagues in order to discover novel inhibitors of BRD4(1) (Lucas et al., 2013). Based on standard precision and extra precision algorithm for molecular docking in GLIDE version 5.6, top-ranked 500 hits were clustered into 33 diverse categories. According to the prediction of several properties including physicochemical, pharmacokinetic, toxicological and binding promiscuity using various computational approaches,

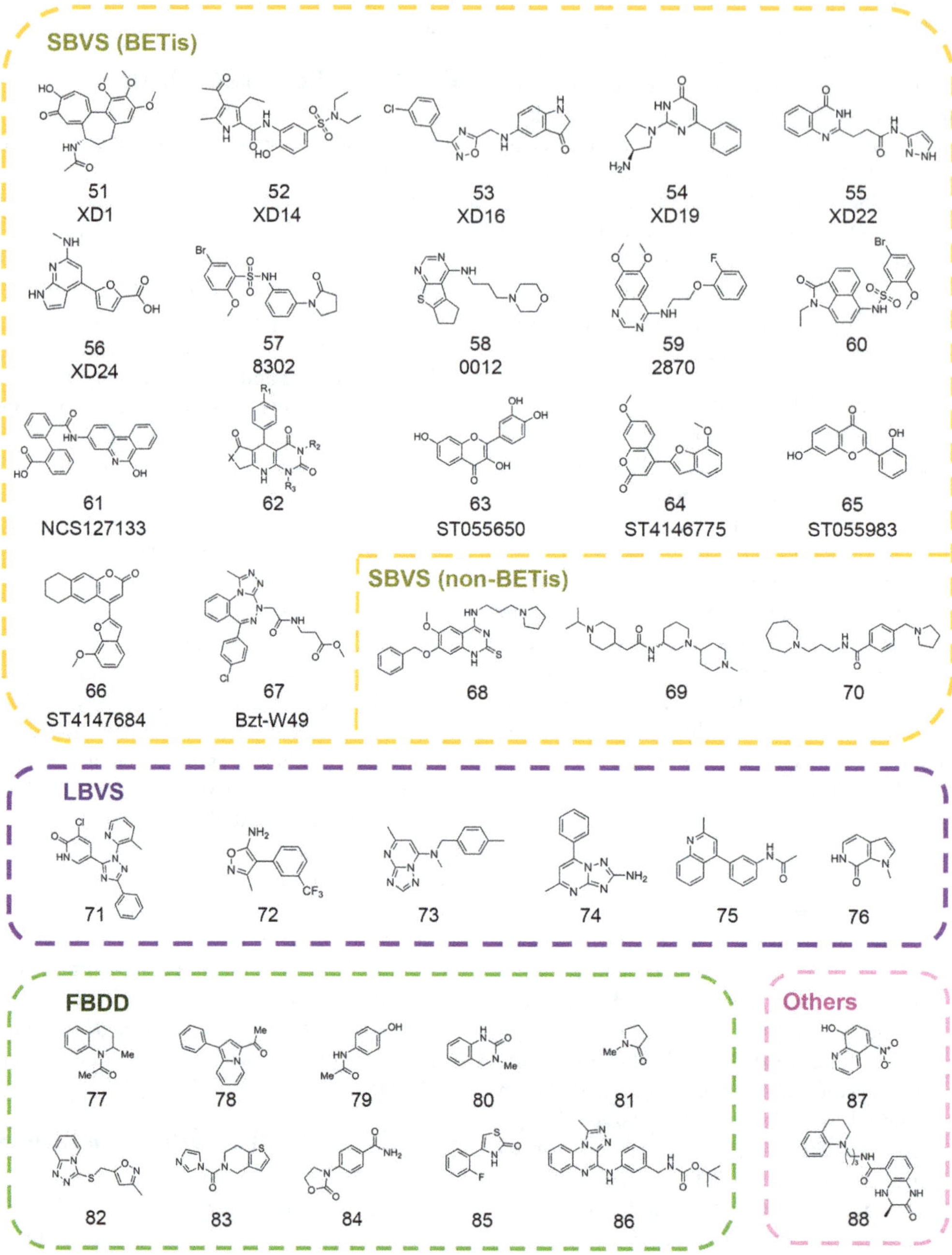

FIGURE 4 | Chemical structures of epigenetic reader inhibitors mentioned in this review.

22 candidate compounds were selected for further experimental validation. Finally, 7 compounds comprising 6 different novel scaffolds (compounds 51–56 in **Figure 4**) were identified with significant binding affinity. The subsequent resolved complex structures of BRD4(1) with XD14, XD1, and XD25 revealed the accurate binding modes consistent with the docking simulation.

In 2015, Allen et al. developed *in silico* screening approaches against kinases and bromodomains, which integrated machine learning and structure-based drug design strategies. At last several BRD4 inhibitors (compounds 57–58 in **Figure 4**) and one dual EGFR-BRD4 inhibitor (compound 59 in **Figure 4**) were identified (Allen et al., 2015). Similarly, Xue and co-authors performed another structure-based virtual screening against BET bromodomains (Xue et al., 2016). Approximately 10,000 compounds were firstly screened against BRD4(1) in GLIDE version 6.1. Through binding free energy assessment and cluster analysis, 15 representative compounds were chosen for biological evaluation. The results showed two compounds with benzo[*cd*]indol-2(1*H*)-one scaffold were identified as novel inhibitors targeting the BRD4(1). Before the optimization of this scaffold, binding modes of these two compounds were predicted by molecular docking in order to characterize the critical interactions. A 20 ns MD simulation was subsequently performed, which indicated the conformations were stable and reasonable for hit optimization. Further SAR analysis and resolved complex crystal structures provided guidance for hit optimization leading to the discovery of compound 85 (compound 60 in **Figure 4**) with high-potency biological activity.

Concomitantly, Tripathi et al. carried out a virtual screening against BRD2(2) using 1,700 compounds in NCI Diversity Set III library (Tripathi et al., 2016). The candidates were selected according to the free energy values, critical binding conformations, and ligand efficiency. Among them, crystal structure of compound NSC127133 (compound 61 in **Figure 4**) in complex with BRD2(2) was resolved, which displayed distinct structural features. In 2017, Ayoub et al. performed high throughput virtual screen with 6,000,000 compounds in ZINC database using the crystal structure of BRDT(1) (Ayoub et al., 2017). A dihydropyridopyrimidine scaffold (compound 62 in **Figure 4**) was identified with highly selectivity for BET family and submicromolar affinity for BRD4(1) and BRDT(1), which could be easily synthesized in one step.

With many new scaffolds uncovered from high throughput virtual screening, Raj et al. made an attempt to screen with flavonoids and derivatives instead of a common library with large collections of compounds (Raj et al., 2017). The followed ADMET properties analysis demonstrated the good drug-likeness properties of the identified compounds (compounds 63–66 in **Figure 4**) suggesting potential applications in the therapies for BET-related diseases. In another study, Deepak et al. designed three benzotriazepipne analogs using *in silico* tools with the aim to improve the selectivity between BET family members (Deepak et al., 2017). Combined with ensemble docking, MD simulation and binding energy calculation, compound Bzt-W49 (compound 67 in **Figure 4**) was synthesized and showed about 10-folds selectivity toward BRD4 compared to BRD2.

Besides the virtual screening efforts against BET family, drug discovery toward other readers has also progressed a lot in recent years. In 2016, a structure-based pharmacophore modeling combined with molecular docking were carried out to identify small molecule inhibitors of methyllysine reader protein Spindlin1 (Robaa et al., 2016). Several hits (compounds 68–70 in **Figure 4**) were subject to 2D-chemical similarity search and medicinal optimizations which improved the potency over 10-folds.

In addition to the *in silico* structure-based virtual screening against commercial libraries directly, the ligand-based computational methods would also help to improve the efficiency of virtual screening. In 2013, Vidler et al. carried out substructure searches for advanced enrichment of chemotypes in two branches (Vidler et al., 2013). For one thing, substructures that mimicked the acetyl-lysine moiety were searched in database. For another, similarity searching was performed to identify distinct chemotypes from known inhibitors using pharmacophore models, shape-based 2D fingerprint searches. The extensive set of substructures obtained was submitted to molecular docking in eMolecules database and manual selection for further experimental validation. Finally six novel hits (compounds 71–76 in **Figure 4**) including four unprecedented acetyl-lysine mimetics were identified. Structure-guided chemical modifications were performed based on complex crystal structures to improve the potency. In 2016, Hugle et al. screened PurchasableBoX library to select analog of previously identified bromodomain inhibitor XD14 (compound 52 in **Figure 4**) (Hügle et al., 2016). Several candidates were used to explore the SAR of XD14 and additional structural features of BRD4 through DFT calculation, atom-based QSAR and ligand-based pharmacophore, which offered the guidance for the development of novel BRD4(1) inhibitors.

Fragment-Based Drug Discovery

Fragment-based drug discovery has been widely practiced in drug discovery and some FBDD-derived drugs have entered into the clinical study (Erlanson et al., 2016). Many CADD integrated tools have been designed for scaffold replacement and fragment growing such as Molecular Operating Environment (MOE) developed by Chemical Computing Group, which could accelerate the pace of FBDD-guided drug discovery. In 2012, Chung et al. firstly built a fragment library that contained substructures with acetyl-lysine mimetic functional groups to identify novel BET inhibitors (Chung et al., 2012). The library was filtered to eliminate unsuitable substructures based on "rule of three" and predicted pK_a values. The remaining fragments were clustered and then representative members were selected in each cluster according to docking results. Coupled with follow-up experiments, Chung and colleagues identified several compounds (compounds 77–81 in **Figure 4**) with two novel fragment scaffolds, which significantly extended the chemotypes of current inhibitors.

In 2013, Zhao et al. built a fragment library to discover novel BRD4 inhibitors (Zhao et al., 2013a). The fragment compounds in ZINC database were filtered by particular rules including molecular weight $\leq$ 250 Da, rotatable bonds $\leq$ 5, log $P \leq 3.5$, and $1 \leq$ smallest set of small ring ≤ 4. According to the Tanimoto similarity calculated in Pipeline Pilot, 487 representative fragments were purchased to build the fragment library. Through molecular docking with established in-house library and crystallization experiments, 9 fragments were identified in the binding pocket of BRD4(1) in the solved crystal structures and four of them (compounds 82–85 in **Figure 4**) were presented in **Figure 4**. Further pharmacokinetic study showed the great potential for further drug development. In 2017, Ali et al. performed docking-based virtual screening with fragment-like database containing nearly 800,000 compounds from ZINC database in an effort to pursue BRD4 inhibitors (Ali et al., 2017). Finally, the authors unveiled the discovery of a novel scaffold (compound 86 in **Figure 4**) contained [1,2,4]triazolo[4,3-α]quinoxaline as BET inhibitors. Several rounds of chemical modification led to the synthesis of analogwith high potency and improved pharmacokinetic properties.

Target-Specific Scoring Function

Considering the better druggability for BET family, many efforts were devoted to the discovery of novel BET inhibitors.

However, the performance of either virtual screening or high throughput screening varies and shows high rate of false positives, which restricts the applications in this field. In order to improve enrichment factor in screening, a BRD4-specific score named BRD4LGR was developed through machine-learning-assisted approach by Xing et al. (Xing et al., 2017). First-round virtual screening was performed in GLIDE version 5.6 and 453 compounds were selected for *in vitro* evaluation resulting in a high false positive rate of 95%. Based on the first-round screening results and other reported studies, structure and activity data of 814 compounds was collected to construct specific scoring function. The authors identified critical molecular interaction features from reported complex structures and established logistic regression model to correlate the interaction features to potencies. Compared with GLIDE and PMF, BRD4LGR discriminated BRD4 inhibitors and non-inhibitors more effectively with high specificity and sensitivity. A second-round virtual screening using BRD4LGR identified 15 new active compounds with a lower FP rate at 85%. Beyond this, BRD4LGR was capable of interpreting key structure-activity relationships of BRD4 inhibitors, which would be quite valuable for chemistry optimization.

In a follow-up study, Jiang et al. employed virtual screening strategy with an in-house compound library containing 887 FDA-approved drugs using BRD4LGR scoring model (Jiang et al., 2017). The docking-based virtual screening coupled with similarity-based analog searching led to the discovery of nitroxoline (compound 87 in **Figure 4**) as a potent and novel BET inhibitor that was previously used to treat urinary tract infections. The successful application of BRD4LGR suggested potential use of nitroxoline in the treatment of BET family-related diseases.

Quantum Mechanical Calculations

Quantum mechanical calculations are commonly used to understand the nonbonding interactions, such as cation-π and hydrogen bond interactions. In order to explain the different affinity of 1,5-naphthyridine derivatives, Mirguet et al. carried out in vacuo QM calculations to calculate the bound conformations of several derivatives in their complex with BRD2 (Mirguet et al., 2014). The results showed that the differences in internal geometric energy might account for differences in relative bioactivity.

Besides, quantum mechanical calculations could be applied in combination with other computational studies in epi-probes discovery. In 2014, Rooney et al. identified two CREBBP bromodomain inhibitors with weak activity by *in silico* screen and biochemical assays (Rooney et al., 2014). Further structure-based chemical modifications led to the compound *(R)*-1 (compound 88 in **Figure 4**) with the IC_{50} value of 758 nM. The complex structure of (*R*)-1 and CREBBP bromodomain revealed an induced-fit pocket that didn't exist in apo-form. *(R)*-1 formed a cation-π interaction with R1173 to maintain the stability of the conformation. In an effort to rationalize the importance of the cation-π interaction, the authors undertook MD simulation in which the cation-π interaction was observed for 40% of the trajectory time. Then the strength of cation-π interaction was estimated by DFT calculations with the strength value of 3.2–4.7 kcal mol^{-1} in accordance with the experimentally measured average strengths involving lysine or arginine. Meanwhile, DFT calculations were also applied to confirm the significance of internal hydrogen bound in ligand conformation which were also applicable in other studies.

PROTEIN-PROTEIN INTERACTION

Epigenetic enzymes from the same protein subfamily often share similar catalytic core pockets and cofactors within family members, thus making it quite difficult to discover and design a selective inhibitor. A growing body of evidence suggests that a variety of protein–protein interactions (PPIs) are indispensable for integrity and oncogenic function of epigenetic enzymes. Therefore, these PPIs appear to be alternative drug targets to modulate chromatin state in epigenetic drug discovery. Due to the unique structural features of PPIs, which have large and flat contact surface and the lack of well-defined pockets, it remains challenging to explore small molecule inhibitors targeting epigenetic interactome (Wells and McClendon, 2007). However, with high-resolution protein complex structures resolved, advanced computational tools developed and renewed understanding of PPIs mechanisms, great progress has been made in the development of small molecule inhibitors (Scott et al., 2016). Here, we focus on the application of CADD methods, including structure-based virtual screening, scaffold hopping, structure-based pharmacophore modeling, and ligand-based pharmacophore profiling in the discovery and design of small molecule inhibitors targeting important epigenetic PPIs including EZH2-EED, WDR5-MLL1, and Menin–MLL1 (**Figure 5**).

EZH2-EED

Polycomb repressive complex 2 (PRC2) specifically trimethylates lysine 27 at histone H3, which is one of the cardinal marks for transcriptional repression (Simon and Kingston, 2009). Enhancer of zeste homolog 2 (EZH2) is the catalytic subunit of PRC2, which requires two additional subunits embryonic ectoderm development (EED) and suppressor of zeste 12 (SUZ12) for full functional activity (Czermin, 2002; Cao and Zhang, 2004). Aberrant PRC2 activity has been reported in the initiation and progression of wide range of cancers (Chang and Hung, 2012). Thus drug design and discovery targeting the PRC2 complex formation represents the unique strategy in chemical intervention.

Drug repositioning is an increasingly attractive strategy widely applied in biopharmaceutical companies to identify alterative therapeutic indications from approved drugs (Ashburn and Thor, 2004). In 2014, in order to pursue EZH2-EED inhibitors, Kong et al. utilized structure-based virtual screening approach to enrich the hits from in-house compound library containing *ca.* 1,000 existing drugs (Kong et al., 2014). The standard precision and extra precision mode in GLIDE version 5.5 were subsequently employed to perform docking-based virtual screening leading

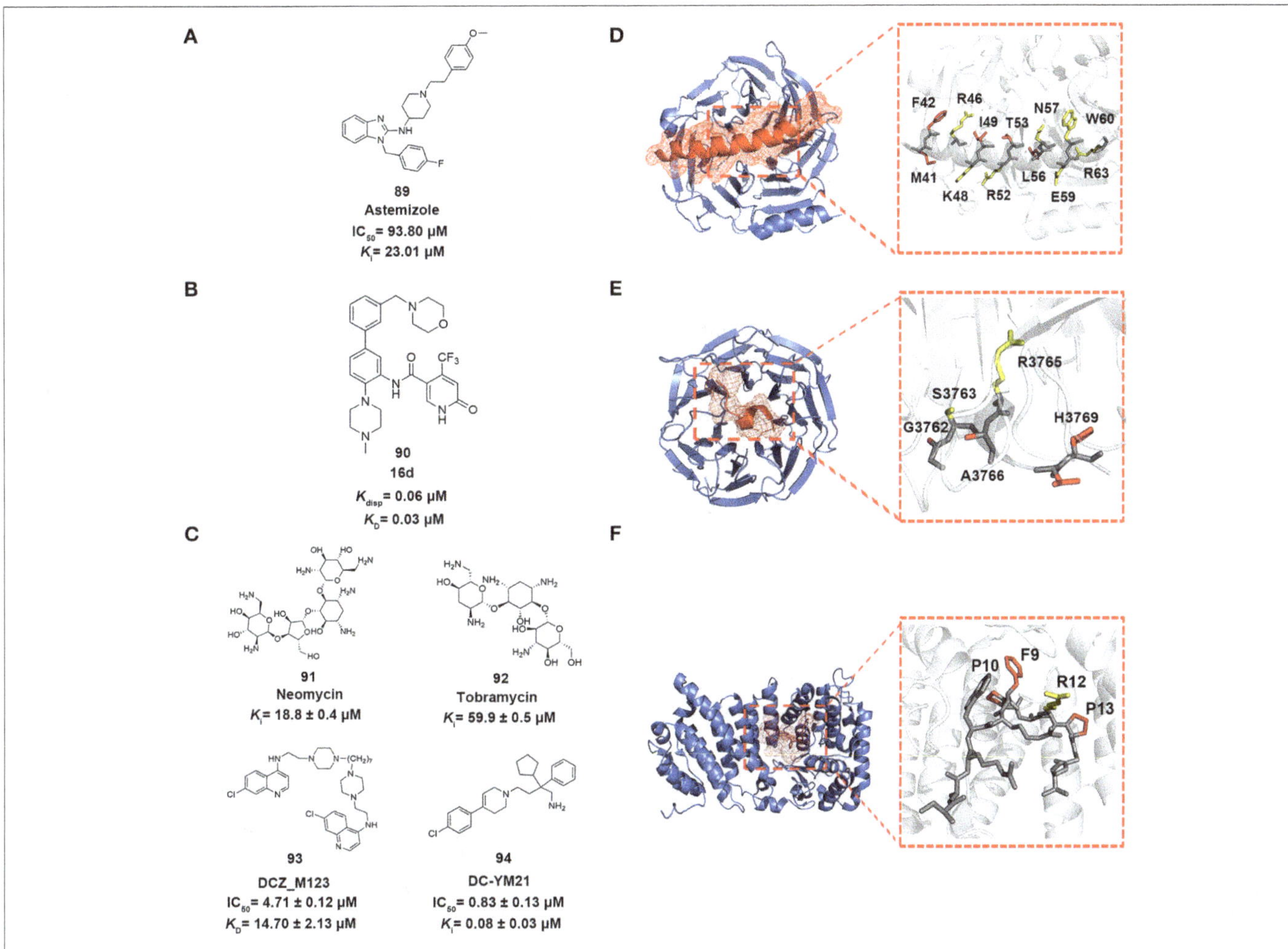

FIGURE 5 | Epigenetic PPI inhibitors. **(A–C)** Chemical structures of the inhibitors mentioned in this review. **(D–F)** The detailed interactions patterns of EZH2-EED (PDB code: 2QXV), WDR5-MLL1 (PDB code: 3EG6), and Menin-MLL1 (PDB code: 4GQ6). EED, WDR5, and Menin are represented in surface contours. The side chains of key residues involved in hydrophobic interactions are depicted in red while the ones involved in polar interactions are depicted in yellow.

to the identification of astemizole (compound 89 in **Figure 5**), a FDA-approved antihistamine drug as moderate EZH2-EED inhibitor with K_i value of 23.0 μM. Further biophysical assays and cellular studies demonstrated the competitive MOA of astemizole and its inhibition for intracellular PRC2 activity.

WDR5-MLL1

Mixed lineage leukemia 1 (MLL1) is the histone methyltransferase responsible for the H3K4 methylation. MLL1 interacts with many chaperons including WD repeat-containing protein 5 (WDR5), a common unit that is essential for the integrity of the catalytic core complex (Dou et al., 2006). Therapeutically targeting WDR5-MLL1 interaction by peptidomimetic inhibitors has been demonstrated as a promising strategy for MLL fusion-mediated acute leukemogenesis (Karatas et al., 2013).

In 2016, Getlik and co-workers designed focused library *in silico* guided by crystal structure information and initial SAR exploration on previously identified benzamides scaffold (Getlik et al., 2016). An exhaustive virtual enumeration was performed in Pipeline Pilot to search all accessible building blocks containing benzamides moieties. The set of compounds with poor physicochemical properties were removed by OICR HTS filters. About 1,200 acyl halides and 9,000 acids/esters were enumerated and used for further medium-throughput virtual screening. Subsequently, molecular docking was performed in GLIDE with one H-bond constraint to the side chain of S91 in WDR5. Through overall consideration of the docking score, binding pose, structural complexity and synthetic difficulty, 50 representative compounds were selected by visual inspection and prioritized as candidates for synthesis and verification. Finally, 4-(trifluoromethyl)pyridin-2(1*H*)-one moiety was discovered as better alternative in replacement of the benzamide moiety. Among the derivatives, the optimized antagonist 16 days (compound 90 in **Figure 5**) was the most potent inhibitor against WDR5-MLL1 with the K_{disp} value of 60 nM, which offered novel therapeutic options in the treatment of leukemia harboring MLL fusion proteins.

Menin-MLL1

The oncoprotein MLL1 can directly associate with cofactor Menin through N-terminal 43 amino acids including two Menin-binding motifs (MBMs), MBM1 (K_d = 53 ± 4.2 nM) and MBM2 (K_d = 1.4 ± 0.42 μM) (Grembecka et al., 2010). Menin-MLL1 interaction is required for oncogenic function of MLL fusion proteins and contributes to related leukemia pathogenesis (Yokoyama and Cleary, 2008; Huang et al., 2012). Thus, the Menin-MLL1 PPI interface has been spotlighted as a potential target for epi-drugs development against MLL-mediated leukemia.

In 2014, Li et al. employed structure-based pharmacophore modeling targeting the Menin–MLL1 interface based on the interaction patterns of Menin and MBM1 complex structure (PDB ID: 4GQ6) (Shi et al., 2012; Li et al., 2014). 10 best pharmacophore models were generated in Discovery Studio 3.0, considering the features of HBD, HBA, and hydrophobic group. Based on overall consideration of the fitness score in generated models, excluded volumes and hot spots analysis, one pharmacophore model with two hydrophobic groups and a hydrogen bond acceptor was selected as a query for follow-up virtual screening. Then an in-house library comprising 900 exiting drugs was built and queried by the constructed pharmacophore model. 29 compounds were finally selected for biochemical verification. Among them, two aminoglycoside antibiotics, neomycin and tobramycin (compounds 91–92 in **Figure 5**), were identified as Menin–MLL1 inhibitors in fluorescence polarization competition assay with binding affinities of 18.8 and 59.9 μM, respectively. Thermal shift assay and isothermal titration calorimetry validated the direct interactions between the two antibiotics and Menin. Molecular docking analysis indicated these antibiotics competitively occupied the binding site of MLL1 in the central cavity of Menin.

In 2016, Xu and co-workers conducted the structure-based molecular docking and ligand-based pharmacophore modeling to obtain Menin-MLL1 inhibitors (Xu et al., 2016). To establish the ligand data set, 74 previously reported inhibitors classified into three categories were collected and 5,000 decoy compounds were generated based on 10 compounds with best potency by DecoyFinder (Cereto-Massagué et al., 2012). For one thing, molecular docking with various constrained conditions was subsequently performed in GLIDE. According to the Glide score and enrichment factor (EF) values, non-constraint SP docking approach performed best and was more appropriate for SBVS that could well distinguish known inhibitors from decoys for Menin-MLL1 inhibitors. For another, ligand-based pharmacophore models with 4–6 pharmacophore features (HBA, HBD, hydrophobic group, aromatic ring and positively or negatively charged group) were generated from those collected inhibitors with pIC_{50} > 5.0. 3D-QSAR models were then developed based on the built pharmacophore models through partial least-squares (PLS) regression analysis. Through the joint LBVS and SBVS computational strategies, five compounds with novel scaffolds were identified as Menin-MLL1 inhibitors validated by fluorescence polarization assay. Among them, DCZ_M123 (compound 93 in **Figure 5**) showed the most potent inhibitory activity *in vitro* with the IC_{50} value of 4.7 μM and could effectively inhibit the growth of MLL leukemia cells by impairing the Menin-MLL1 interaction in cell-based assays.

Scaffold hopping was proposed as a promising strategy to look for novel molecular entities with similar three dimensional conformations and properties (Schneider et al., 1999). As a shape-based three dimensional structure superposition method, it has been extensively used to generate potential alternatives of known compounds based on the bioisosteric replacement of core motif within molecules (Sun et al., 2012; Lamberth, 2017). In 2016, Yue et al. applied a shape-based scaffold hopping approach to reposition approved drugs targeting the Menin-MLL1 interaction (Yue et al., 2016). In the study, reported bioactive conformations of representative Menin-MLL1 inhibitors MI-2-2 and MIV-6R (PDB code 4GQ4 and 4GO8, respectively) were used as query (Shi et al., 2012; He et al., 2014). An in-house library comprising ~1,600 existing drugs was aligned onto the query to perform 3D similarity searching using SHAFTS (Liu et al., 2011; Lu et al., 2011). A set of 12 top ranked compounds with SHAFTS similarity scores >1.2 (maximum 2.0) were selected for primary validation, which indicated that loperamide, previously used as anti-diarrhea agents, showed weak inhibition with the IC_{50} value of 69 μM. Further molecular docking analysis and medicinal chemistry optimization led to the identification of more potent loperamide-derived analog. Among them, DC_YM21 (compound 94 in **Figure 5**) presented nanomolar inhibitory activity of the same order of magnitude as the reported inhibitor MI-2-2.

FUTURE PERSPECTIVES

Computational methods are indispensable and creditable tools in both academia and industry that undoubtedly streamline the epi-drug and epi-probe discovery process. The focal point of this review is the state of art of CADD methods in epi-drug design and discovery framework over the past decades. Tremendous progress has been achieved in epigenetic drug discovery based on *in silico* approaches as we have mentioned above which unequivocally draws a positive picture in the field. However, it is widely accepted that these aforementioned hit-finding methodologies are far from perfect and not omnipotent in all situations. There are still formidable challenges that need to be overcome which limit the effective applications of current computational methods. Firstly, current molecular docking scoring functions rank the compounds collections with inherent poor prediction accuracy in novel target drug discovery whose function has just been unraveled not long ago (Sable and Jois, 2015). Secondly, traditional docking algorithms fail to take complicated factors into full consideration like protein flexibility, solvation, entropy, and dynamic inclusion of water molecules (Clark, 2008; Lavecchia and Di Giovanni, 2013). Thus, it's difficult to precisely predict the absolute binding energy for ligand-protein interactions based on current methodologies.

There are some reviews that investigate protein flexibility in detail (Barril and Fradera, 2006). However, the current computational methodology considering this issue is time-consuming that needs to be further improved. Thirdly, despite the fact that epigenetic enzymes have been actively pursued as potential drug targets, there is still conspicuous lack of potent chemical probes for a large number of knotty targets like HATs and epigenetic protein-protein interactions, which needs to be further explored. For these less well-studied epi-targets, there are few inhibitors with limited diversity of scaffolds ever reported that hinders the ligand-based drug design and development. For instance, PRMT5-MEP50 complex formation could enhance the stability and activity of PRMT5 and the PPI is essential for cancer cell invasion in lung cancer and breast cancer (Chen et al., 2017). Heterooctameric PRMT5-MEP50 complex structure has been resolved which enables structure-based drug design. Nonetheless, no chemical probes have ever been reported for such novel targets. Fourthly, the bioactivities of identified inhibitors vary considerably due to different assay platforms in differ different labs. Some of the reported inhibitors belong to pan-assay interference compounds and present non-specific interactions that have not been carefully examined (Dahlin et al., 2017). Overinterpretation of these results leads to misleading readouts and would go to the cul-de-sac in drug discovery process. Taken together, there are still many problems left unsolved which encourage the researcher to devote more drug discovery efforts in order to fill the vacancy in this field. To tackle with these issues, integrated SBVS and LBVS approaches should be applied to counterbalance their own limitations in a parallel manner in virtual screen campaigns. As for novel targets with fewer inhibitors ever reported, computational methods should be applied in synergy with experimental approaches. Multidisciplinary efforts shall be devoted to generate more diverse machine learning datasets for the establishment of target-customized scoring functions, which in turn help to exploit chemical space available in database as thoroughly as possible. Meanwhile, the researchers should carefully examine the biological data before interpreting the biological results. This appeals to the researchers to develop a reliable experimental platform to standardize current biochemical assays. It could be expected that with rapid development of computational power and methodologies, more epi-drugs and epi-probes will be developed in the near future, which could not only help to uncover the elusive role of each node in epigenetic regulatory network but also guide optimum therapeutic options in the treatment of epigenetic-related diseases.

AUTHOR CONTRIBUTIONS

WL, RZ, HJ, HZ, and CL wrote the manuscript. WL, RZ, and CL organized and revised the manuscript. All authors were involved in the preparation of the manuscript and approved the final version.

ACKNOWLEDGMENTS

We appreciate referees for comments on this review and apologize to those whose important work concerning this topic has not been cited herein due to the main focus of this review article. We gratefully acknowledge financial support from the National Natural Science Foundation of China (81625022, 21472208, and 81430084 to CL).

REFERENCES

Aik, W., Demetriades, M., Hamdan, M. K., Bagg, E. A., Yeoh, K. K., Lejeune, C., et al. (2013). Structural basis for inhibition of the fat mass and obesity associated protein (FTO). *J. Med. Chem.* 56, 3680–3688. doi: 10.1021/jm400193d

Alcaro, S., Ortuso, F., and Coleman, R. S. (2002). DNA cross-linking by azinomycin B: monte carlo simulations in the evaluation of sequence selectivity. *J. Med. Chem.* 45, 861–870. doi: 10.1021/jm011040w

Ali, I., Lee, J., Go, A., Choi, G., and Lee, K. (2017). Discovery of novel [1,2,4]triazolo[4,3-a]quinoxaline aminophenyl derivatives as BET inhibitors for cancer treatment. *Bioorg. Med. Chem. Lett.* 27, 4606–4613. doi: 10.1016/j.bmcl.2017.09.025

Alinari, L., Mahasenan, K. V., Yan, F., Karkhanis, V., Chung, J. H., Smith, E. M., et al. (2015). Selective inhibition of protein arginine methyltransferase 5 blocks initiation and maintenance of B-cell transformation. *Blood* 125, 2530–2543. doi: 10.1182/blood-2014-12-619783

Allen, B. K., Mehta, S., Ember, S. W., Schonbrunn, E., Ayad, N., and Schürer, S. C. (2015). Large-scale computational screening identifies first in class multitarget inhibitor of EGFR kinase and BRD4. *Sci. Rep.* 5:16924. doi: 10.1038/srep16924

Andrew, G., Mercader, P. R. D., and Sivakumar, P. M. (2016). *Chemometrics Applications and Research: QSAR in Medicinal Chemistry.* New York, NY: Apple Academic Press.

Arrowsmith, C. H., Bountra, C., Fish, P. V., Lee, K., and Schapira, M. (2012). Epigenetic protein families: a new frontier for drug discovery. *Nat. Rev. Drug Discov.* 11, 384–400. doi: 10.1038/nrd3674

Ashburn, T. T., and Thor, K. B. (2004). Drug repositioning: identifying and developing new uses for existing drugs. *Nat. Rev. Drug Discov.* 3, 673–683. doi: 10.1038/nrd1468

Auclair, G., and Weber, M. (2012). Mechanisms of DNA methylation and demethylation in mammals. *Biochimie* 94, 2202–2211. doi: 10.1016/j.biochi.2012.05.016

Ayoub, A. M., Hawk, L. M. L., Herzig, R. J., Jiang, J., Wisniewski, A. J., Gee, C. T., et al. (2017). BET bromodomain inhibitors with one-step synthesis discovered from virtual screen. *J. Med. Chem.* 60, 4805–4817. doi: 10.1021/acs.jmedchem.6b01336

Baker, L. A., Allis, C. D., and Wang, G. G. (2008). PHD fingers in human diseases: disorders arising from misinterpreting epigenetic marks. *Mutat. Res.* 647, 3–12. doi: 10.1016/j.mrfmmm.2008.07.004

Barril, X., and Fradera, X. (2006). Incorporating protein flexibility into docking and structure-based drug design. *Expert Opin. Drug Discov.* 1, 335–349. doi: 10.1517/17460441.1.4.335

Berger, S. L. (2007). The complex language of chromatin regulation during transcription. *Nature* 447, 407–412. doi: 10.1038/nature05915

Best, J. D., and Carey, N. (2010). Epigenetic therapies for non-oncology indications. *Drug Discov. Today* 15, 1008–1014. doi: 10.1016/j.drudis.2010.10.006

Bestor, T. H. (2000). The DNA methyltransferases of mammals. *Hum. Mol. Genet.* 9, 2395–2402. doi: 10.1093/hmg/9.16.2395

Bode, A. M., and Dong, Z. (2004). Post-translational modification of p53 in tumorigenesis. *Nat. Rev. Cancer* 4, 793–805. doi: 10.1038/nrc1455

Bowers, E. M., Yan, G., Mukherjee, C., Orry, A., Wang, L., Holbert, M. A., et al. (2010). Virtual ligand screening of the p300/CBP histone acetyltransferase:

identification of a selective small molecule inhibitor. *Chem. Biol.* 17, 471–482. doi: 10.1016/j.chembiol.2010.03.006

Brown, C. E., Lechner, T., Howe, L., and Workman, J. L. (2000). The many HATs of transcription coactivators. *Trends Biochem. Sci.* 25, 15–19. doi: 10.1016/S0968-0004(99)01516-9

Brueckner, B., Garcia Boy, R., Siedlecki, P., Musch, T., Kliem, H. C., Zielenkiewicz, P., et al. (2005). Epigenetic reactivation of tumor suppressor genes by a novel small-molecule inhibitor of human DNA methyltransferases. *Cancer Res.* 65, 6305–6311. doi: 10.1158/0008-5472.CAN-04-2957

Buurman, R., Gürlevik, E., Schäffer, V., Eilers, M., Sandbothe, M., Kreipe, H., et al. (2012). Histone deacetylases activate hepatocyte growth factor signaling by repressing microRNA-449 in hepatocellular carcinoma cells. *Gastroenterology* 143, 811-820 e815. doi: 10.1053/j.gastro.2012.05.033

Cao, G. P., Thangapandian, S., Son, M., Kumar, R., Choi, Y. J., Kim, Y., et al. (2016). QSAR modeling to design selective histone deacetylase 8 (HDAC8) inhibitors. *Arch. Pharm. Res.* 39, 1356–1369. doi: 10.1007/s12272-015-0705-5

Cao, R., and Zhang, Y. (2004). SUZ12 is required for both the histone methyltransferase activity and the silencing function of the EED-EZH2 complex. *Mol. Cell* 15, 57–67. doi: 10.1016/j.molcel.2004.06.020

Caulfield, T., and Medina-Franco, J. L. (2011). Molecular dynamics simulations of human DNA methyltransferase 3B with selective inhibitor nanaomycin A. *J. Struct. Biol.* 176, 185–191. doi: 10.1016/j.jsb.2011.07.015

Cereto-Massagué, A., Guasch, L., Valls, C., Mulero, M., Pujadas, G., and Garcia-Vallvé, S. (2012). DecoyFinder: an easy-to-use python GUI application for building target-specific decoy sets. *Bioinformatics* 28, 1661–1662. doi: 10.1093/bioinformatics/bts249

Chang, C. J., and Hung, M. C. (2012). The role of EZH2 in tumour progression. *Br. J. Cancer* 106, 243–247. doi: 10.1038/bjc.2011.551

Chen, B., Ye, F., Yu, L., Jia, G., Huang, X., Zhang, X., et al. (2012). Development of cell-active N6-methyladenosine RNA demethylase FTO inhibitor. *J. Am. Chem. Soc.* 134, 17963–17971. doi: 10.1021/ja3064149

Chen, H., Lorton, B., Gupta, V., and Shechter, D. (2017). A TGFbeta-PRMT5-MEP50 axis regulates cancer cell invasion through histone H3 and H4 arginine methylation coupled transcriptional activation and repression. *Oncogene* 36, 373–386. doi: 10.1038/onc.2016.205

Chen, K., Zhang, X., Wu, Y. D., and Wiest, O. (2014). Inhibition and mechanism of HDAC8 revisited. *J. Am. Chem. Soc.* 136, 11636–11643. doi: 10.1021/ja501548p

Chen, S., Li, L., Chen, Y., Hu, J., Liu, J., Liu, Y. C., et al. (2016). Identification of novel disruptor of telomeric silencing 1-like (DOT1L) inhibitors through structure-based virtual screening and biological assays. *J. Chem. Inf. Model.* 56, 527–534. doi: 10.1021/acs.jcim.5b00738

Chen, S., Wang, Y., Zhou, W., Li, S., Peng, J., Shi, Z., et al. (2014). Identifying novel selective non-nucleoside DNA methyltransferase 1 inhibitors through docking-based virtual screening. *J. Med. Chem.* 57, 9028–9041. doi: 10.1021/jm501134e

Chen, W. L., Wang, Z. H., Feng, T. T., Li, D. D., Wang, C. H., Xu, X. L., et al. (2016). Discovery, design and synthesis of 6H-anthra[1,9-cd]isoxazol-6-one scaffold as G9a inhibitor through a combination of shape-based virtual screening and structure-based molecular modification. *Bioorg. Med. Chem.* 24, 6102–6108. doi: 10.1016/j.bmc.2016.09.071

Chen, Y. D., Jiang, Y. J., Zhou, J. W., Yu, Q. S., and You, Q. D. (2008). Identification of ligand features essential for HDACs inhibitors by pharmacophore modeling. *J. Mol. Graph. Model.* 26, 1160–1168. doi: 10.1016/j.jmgm.2007.10.007

Chothia, C., and Lesk, A. M. (1986). The relation between the divergence of sequence and structure in proteins. *EMBO J.* 5, 823–826.

Chu, C. H., Wang, L. Y., Hsu, K. C., Chen, C. C., Cheng, H. H., Wang, S. M., et al. (2014). KDM4B as a target for prostate cancer: structural analysis and selective inhibition by a novel inhibitor. *J. Med. Chem.* 57, 5975–5985. doi: 10.1021/jm500249n

Chung, C. W., Dean, A. W., Woolven, J. M., and Bamborough, P. (2012). Fragment-based discovery of bromodomain inhibitors part 1: inhibitor binding modes and implications for lead discovery. *J. Med. Chem.* 55, 576–586. doi: 10.1021/jm201320w

Clark, D. E. (2008). What has virtual screening ever done for drug discovery? *Expert Opin. Drug Discov.* 3, 841–851. doi: 10.1517/17460441.3.8.841

Collins, R. E., Northrop, J. P., Horton, J. R., Lee, D. Y., Zhang, X., Stallcup, M. R., et al. (2008). The ankyrin repeats of G9a and GLP histone methyltransferases are mono- and dimethyllysine binding modules. *Nat. Struct. Mol. Biol.* 15, 245–250. doi: 10.1038/nsmb.1384

Czermin, B. (2002). Drosophila enhancer of Zeste/ESC complexes have a histone H3 methyltransferase activity that marks chromosomal polycomb sites. *Cell.* 11, 185–96. doi: 10.1016/S0092-8674(02)00975-3

Dahlin, J. L., Nelson, K. M., Strasser, J. M., Barsyte-Lovejoy, D., Szewczyk, M. M., Organ, S., et al. (2017). Assay interference and off-target liabilities of reported histone acetyltransferase inhibitors. *Nat. Commun.* 8, 1527. doi: 10.1038/s41467-017-01657-3

Dancy, B. M., and Cole, P. A. (2015). Protein lysine acetylation by p300/CBP. *Chem. Rev.* 115, 2419–2452. doi: 10.1021/cr500452k

Dawson, M. A., and Kouzarides, T. (2012). Cancer epigenetics: from mechanism to therapy. *Cell* 150, 12–27. doi: 10.1016/j.cell.2012.06.013

Deepak, V., Wang, B., Koot, D., Kasonga, A., Stander, X. X., Coetzee, M., et al. (2017). *In silico* design and bioevaluation of selective benzotriazepine BRD4 inhibitors with potent antiosteoclastogenic activity. *Chem. Biol. Drug Des.* 90, 97–111. doi: 10.1111/cbdd.12930

Derissen, E. J., Beijnen, J. H., and Schellens, J. H. (2013). Concise drug review: azacitidine and decitabine. *Oncologist* 18, 619–624. doi: 10.1634/theoncologist.2012-0465

Desrosiers, R., Friderici, K., and Rottman, F. (1974). Identification of methylated nucleosides in messenger RNA from Novikoff hepatoma cells. *Proc. Natl. Acad. Sci. U.S.A.* 71, 3971–3975. doi: 10.1073/pnas.71.10.3971

Dimitrova, E., Turberfield, A. H., and Klose, R. J. (2015). Histone demethylases in chromatin biology and beyond. *EMBO Rep.* 16, 1620–1639. doi: 10.15252/embr.201541113

Dou, Y., Milne, T. A., Ruthenburg, A. J., Lee, S., Lee, J. W., Verdine, G. L., et al. (2006). Regulation of MLL1 H3K4 methyltransferase activity by its core components. *Nat. Struct. Mol. Biol.* 13, 713–719. doi: 10.1038/nsmb1128

Dwivedi, G. R., Maurya, A., Yadav, D. K., Khan, F., Darokar, M. P., and Srivastava, S. K. (2015). Drug resistance reversal potential of ursolic acid derivatives against nalidixic acid- and multidrug-resistant *Escherichia coli*. *Chem. Biol. Drug Des.* 86, 272–283. doi: 10.1111/cbdd.12491

Erlanson, D. A., Fesik, S. W., Hubbard, R. E., Jahnke, W., and Jhoti, H. (2016). Twenty years on: the impact of fragments on drug discovery. *Nat. Rev. Drug Discov.* 15, 605–619. doi: 10.1038/nrd.2016.109

Falkenberg, K. J., and Johnstone, R. W. (2014). Histone deacetylases and their inhibitors in cancer, neurological diseases and immune disorders. *Nat. Rev. Drug Discov.*13, 673–691. doi: 10.1038/nrd4360

Fauman, E. B., Rai, B. K., and Huang, E. S. (2011). Structure-based druggability assessment - identifying suitable targets for small molecule therapeutics. *Curr. Opin. Chem. Biol.* 15, 463–468. doi: 10.1016/j.cbpa.2011.05.020

Feinberg, A. P., Ohlsson, R., and Henikoff, S. (2006). The epigenetic progenitor origin of human cancer. *Nat. Rev. Genet.* 7, 21–33. doi: 10.1038/nrg1748

Feng, Y., Li, M., Wang, B., and Zheng, Y. G. (2010). Discovery and mechanistic study of a class of protein arginine methylation inhibitors. *J. Med. Chem.* 53, 6028–6039. doi: 10.1021/jm100416n

Ferreira de Freitas, R., Eram, M. S., Smil, D., Szewczyk, M. M., Kennedy, S., Brown, P. J., et al. (2016). Discovery of a potent and selective coactivator associated arginine methyltransferase 1 (CARM1) inhibitor by virtual screening. *J. Med. Chem.* 59, 6838–6847. doi: 10.1021/acs.jmedchem.6b00668

Filippakopoulos, P., Picaud, S., Mangos, M., Keates, T., Lambert, J. P., Barsyte-Lovejoy, D., et al. (2012). Histone recognition and large-scale structural analysis of the human bromodomain family. *Cell* 149, 214–231. doi: 10.1016/j.cell.2012.02.013

Finnin, M. S., Donigian, J. R., Cohen, A., Richon, V. M., Rifkind, R. A., Marks, P. A., et al. (1999). Structures of a histone deacetylase homologue bound to the TSA and SAHA inhibitors. *Nature* 401, 188–193. doi: 10.1038/43710

Frayling, T. M., Timpson, N. J., Weedon, M. N., Zeggini, E., Freathy, R. M., Lindgren, C. M., et al. (2007). A common variant in the FTO gene is associated with body mass index and predisposes to childhood and adult obesity. *Science* 316, 889–894. doi: 10.1126/science.1141634

Fu, Y., Dominissini, D., Rechavi, G., and He, C. (2014). Gene expression regulation mediated through reversible mA RNA methylation. *Nat. Rev. Genet.* 15, 293–306. doi: 10.1038/nrg3724

Ganai, S. A., Abdullah, E., Rashid, R., and Altaf, M. (2017). Combinatorial *in silico* strategy towards identifying potential hotspots during inhibition of structurally identical HDAC1 and HDAC2 enzymes for effective chemotherapy against neurological disorders. *Front. Mol. Neurosci.* 10:357. doi: 10.3389/fnmol.2017.00357

Gantt, S. L., Joseph, C. G., and Fierke, C. A. (2010). Activation and inhibition of histone deacetylase 8 by monovalent cations. *J. Biol. Chem.* 285, 6036–6043. doi: 10.1074/jbc.M109.033399

Gaur, R., Yadav, D. K., Kumar, S., Darokar, M. P., Khan, F., and Bhakuni, R. S. (2015). Molecular modeling based semi-synthesis and *in vitro* evaluation of anticancer activity in indolyl chalcones. *Curr. Top. Med. Chem.* 15, 1003–1012. doi: 10.2174/1568026615666150317222059

Gelato, K. A., and Fischle, W. (2008). Role of histone modifications in defining chromatin structure and function. *Biol. Chem.* 389, 353–363. doi: 10.1515/BC.2008.048

Getlik, M., Smil, D., Zepeda-Velázquez, C., Bolshan, Y., Poda, G., Wu, H., et al. (2016). Structure-based optimization of a small molecule antagonist of the interaction between WD repeat-containing protein 5 (WDR5) and mixed-lineage leukemia 1 (MLL1). *J. Med. Chem.* 59, 2478–2496. doi: 10.1021/acs.jmedchem.5b01630

Goll, M. G., and Bestor, T. H. (2005). Eukaryotic cytosine methyltransferases. *Annu. Rev. Biochem.* 74, 481–514. doi: 10.1146/annurev.biochem.74.010904.153721

Greer, E. L., and Shi, Y. (2012). Histone methylation: a dynamic mark in health, disease and inheritance. *Nat. Rev. Genet.* 13, 343–357. doi: 10.1038/nrg3173

Gregoretti, I. V., Lee, Y. M., and Goodson, H. V. (2004). Molecular evolution of the histone deacetylase family: functional implications of phylogenetic analysis. *J. Mol. Biol.* 338, 17–31. doi: 10.1016/j.jmb.2004.02.006

Grembecka, J., Belcher, A. M., Hartley, T., and Cierpicki, T. (2010). Molecular basis of the mixed lineage leukemia-menin interaction: implications for targeting mixed lineage leukemias. *J. Biol. Chem.* 285, 40690–40698. doi: 10.1074/jbc.M110.172783

Greschik, H., Schüle, R., and Günther, T. (2017). Selective targeting of epigenetic reader domains. *Expert Opin. Drug Discov.* 12, 449–463. doi: 10.1080/17460441.2017.1303474

Guner, O., Clement, O., and Kurogi, Y. (2004). Pharmacophore modeling and three dimensional database searching for drug design using catalyst: Recent advances. *Curr. Med. Chem.* 11, 2991–3005. doi: 10.2174/0929867043364036

Guo, Y., Xiao, J., Guo, Z., Chu, F., Cheng, Y., and Wu, S. (2005). Exploration of a binding mode of indole amide analogues as potent histone deacetylase inhibitors and 3D-QSAR analyses. *Bioorg. Med. Chem.* 13, 5424–5434. doi: 10.1016/j.bmc.2005.05.016

Gupta, S. P. (2007). Quantitative structure-activity relationship studies on zinc-containing metalloproteinase inhibitors. *Chem. Rev.* 107, 3042–3087. doi: 10.1021/cr030448t

Gut, P., and Verdin, E. (2013). The nexus of chromatin regulation and intermediary metabolism. *Nature* 502, 489–498. doi: 10.1038/nature12752

Halgren, T. A. (2009). Identifying and characterizing binding sites and assessing druggability. *J. Chem. Inf. Model.* 49, 377–389. doi: 10.1021/ci800324m

Harris, W. J., Huang, X., Lynch, J. T., Spencer, G. J., Hitchin, J. R., Li, Y., et al. (2012). The histone demethylase KDM1A sustains the oncogenic potential of MLL-AF9 leukemia stem cells. *Cancer Cell* 21, 473–487. doi: 10.1016/j.ccr.2012.03.014

Hayami, S., Kelly, J. D., Cho, H. S., Yoshimatsu, M., Unoki, M., Tsunoda, T., et al. (2011). Overexpression of LSD1 contributes to human carcinogenesis through chromatin regulation in various cancers. *Int. J. Cancer* 128, 574–586. doi: 10.1002/ijc.25349

Hazeldine, S., Pachaiyappan, B., Steinbergs, N., Nowotarski, S., Hanson, A. S., Casero, R. A. Jr., et al. (2012). Low molecular weight amidoximes that act as potent inhibitors of lysine-specific demethylase 1. *J. Med. Chem.* 55, 7378–7391. doi: 10.1021/jm3002845

He, F., Umehara, T., Saito, K., Harada, T., Watanabe, S., Yabuki, T., et al. (2010). Structural insight into the zinc finger CW domain as a histone modification reader. *Structure* 18, 1127–1139. doi: 10.1016/j.str.2010.06.012

He, J., Anh, T. N., and Zhang, Y. (2011). KDM2b/JHDM1b, an H3K36me2-specific demethylase, is required for initiation and maintenance of acute myeloid leukemia. *Blood* 117, 3869–3880. doi: 10.1182/blood-2010-10-312736

He, S., Senter, T. J., Pollock, J., Han, C., Upadhyay, S. K., Purohit, T., et al. (2014). High-affinity small-molecule inhibitors of the menin-mixed lineage leukemia (MLL) interaction closely mimic a natural protein-protein interaction. *J. Med. Chem.* 57, 1543–1556. doi: 10.1021/jm401868d

Heinke, R., Spannhoff, A., Meier, R., Trojer, P., Bauer, I., Jung, M., et al. (2009). Virtual screening and biological characterization of novel histone arginine methyltransferase PRMT1 inhibitors. *ChemMedChem* 4, 69–77. doi: 10.1002/cmdc.200800301

Hillisch, A., Pineda, L. F., and Hilgenfeld, R. (2004). Utility of homology models in the drug discovery process. *Drug Discov. Today* 9, 659–669. doi: 10.1016/S1359-6446(04)03196-4

Højfeldt, J. W., Agger, K., and Helin, K. (2013). Histone lysine demethylases as targets for anticancer therapy. *Nat. Rev. Drug Discov.* 12, 917–930. doi: 10.1038/nrd4154

Hou, X., Du, J., Liu, R., Zhou, Y., Li, M., Xu, W., et al. (2015). Enhancing the sensitivity of pharmacophore-based virtual screening by incorporating customized ZBG features: a case study using histone deacetylase 8. *J. Chem. Inf. Model.* 55, 861–871. doi: 10.1021/ci500762z

Hsu, K. C., Liu, C. Y., Lin, T. E., Hsieh, J. H., Sung, T. Y., Tseng, H. J., et al. (2017). Novel class IIa-selective histone deacetylase inhibitors discovered using an *in silico* virtual screening approach. *Sci. Rep.* 7:3228. doi: 10.1038/s41598-017-03417-1

Hu, H., Xia, J., Wang, D., Wang, X. S., and Wu, S. (2017). A thoroughly validated virtual screening strategy for discovery of novel HDAC3 inhibitors. *Int. J. Mol. Sci.* 18:137. doi: 10.3390/ijms18010137

Huang, J., Gurung, B., Wan, B., Matkar, S., Veniaminova, N. A., Wan, K., et al. (2012). The same pocket in menin binds both MLL and JUND but has opposite effects on transcription. *Nature* 482, 542–546. doi: 10.1038/nature10806

Huang, Y., Yan, J., Li, Q., Li, J., Gong, S., Zhou, H., et al. (2015). Meclofenamic acid selectively inhibits FTO demethylation of m6A over ALKBH5. *Nucleic Acids Res.* 43, 373–384. doi: 10.1093/nar/gku1276

Hügle, M., Lucas, X., Weitzel, G., Ostrovskyi, D., Breit, B., Gerhardt, S., et al. (2016). 4-Acyl pyrrole derivatives yield novel vectors for designing inhibitors of the Acetyl-lysine recognition site of BRD4. *J. Med. Chem.* 59, 1518–1530. doi: 10.1021/acs.jmedchem.5b01267

Hwang, J. Y., Aromolaran, K. A., and Zukin, R. S. (2017). The emerging field of epigenetics in neurodegeneration and neuroprotection. *Nat. Rev. Neurosci.* 18, 347–361. doi: 10.1038/nrn.2017.46

Ji, S., Ma, S., Wang, W. J., Huang, S. Z., Wang, T. Q., Xiang, R., et al. (2017). Discovery of selective protein arginine methyltransferase 5 inhibitors and biological evaluations. *Chem. Biol. Drug Des.* 89, 585–598. doi: 10.1111/cbdd.12881

Jia, G., Fu, Y., Zhao, X., Dai, Q., Zheng, G., Yang, Y., et al. (2011). N6-methyladenosine in nuclear RNA is a major substrate of the obesity-associated FTO. *Nat. Chem. Biol.* 7, 885–887. doi: 10.1038/nchembio.687

Jiang, H., Xing, J., Wang, C., Zhang, H., Yue, L., Wan, X., et al. (2017). Discovery of novel BET inhibitors by drug repurposing of nitroxoline and its analogues. *Org. Biomol. Chem.* 15, 9352–9361. doi: 10.1039/C7OB02369C

Jones, P. A., Issa, J. P., and Baylin, S. (2016). Targeting the cancer epigenome for therapy. *Nat. Rev. Genet.* 17, 630–641. doi: 10.1038/nrg.2016.93

Jung, M., Gelato, K. A., Fernández-Montalván, A., Siegel, S., and Haendler, B. (2015). Targeting BET bromodomains for cancer treatment. *Epigenomics* 7, 487–501. doi: 10.2217/epi.14.91

Juvale, D. C., Kulkarni, V. V., Deokar, H. S., Wagh, N. K., Padhye, S. B., and Kulkarni, V. M. (2006). 3D-QSAR of histone deacetylase inhibitors: hydroxamate analogues. *Org. Biomol. Chem.* 4, 2858–2868. doi: 10.1039/b606365a

Kandakatla, N., and Ramakrishnan, G. (2014). Ligand based pharmacophore modeling and virtual screening studies to design novel HDAC2 inhibitors. *Adv. Bioinformatics* 2014:812148. doi: 10.1155/2014/812148

Karatas, H. T. E. C., Cao, F., Chen, Y., Bernard, D., Liu, L., Wang, S., et al. (2013). High-affinity, small-molecule peptidomimetic inhibitors of MLL1/WDR5 protein-protein interaction. *J. Am. Chem. Soc.* 135, 669–682. doi: 10.1021/ja306028q

Kim, H., Jang, C., Yadav, D. K., and Kim, M. H. (2017). The comparison of automated clustering algorithms for resampling representative conformer ensembles with RMSD matrix. *J. Cheminformatics* 9:21. doi: 10.1186/s13321-017-0208-0

Kim, J., Daniel, J., Espejo, A., Lake, A., Krishna, M., Xia, L., et al. (2006). Tudor, MBT and chromo domains gauge the degree of lysine methylation. *EMBO Rep.* 7, 397–403. doi: 10.1038/sj.embor.7400625

Kokkonen, P., Kokkola, T., Suuronen, T., Poso, A., Jarho, E., and Lahtela-Kakkonen, M. (2015). Virtual screening approach of sirtuin inhibitors results in two new scaffolds. *Eur. J. Pharm. Sci.* 76, 27–32. doi: 10.1016/j.ejps.2015.04.025

Kokkonen, P., Mellini, P., Nyrhilä, O., Rahnasto-Rilla, M., Suuronen, T., Kiviranta, P., et al. (2014). Quantitative insights for the design of substrate-based SIRT1 inhibitors. *Eur. J. Pharm. Sci.* 59, 12–19. doi: 10.1016/j.ejps.2014.04.003

Kondengaden, S. M., Luo, L. F., Huang, K., Zhu, M., Zang, L., Bataba, E., et al. (2016). Discovery of novel small molecule inhibitors of lysine methyltransferase G9a and their mechanism in leukemia cell lines. *Eur. J. Med. Chem.* 122, 382–393. doi: 10.1016/j.ejmech.2016.06.028

Kong, X., Chen, L., Jiao, L., Jiang, X., Lian, F., Lu, J., et al. (2014). Astemizole arrests the proliferation of cancer cells by disrupting the EZH2-EED interaction of polycomb repressive complex 2. *J. Med. Chem.* 57, 9512–9521. doi: 10.1021/jm501230c

Kooistra, S. M., and Helin, K. (2012). Molecular mechanisms and potential functions of histone demethylases. *Nat. Rev. Mol. Cell Biol.* 13, 297–311. doi: 10.1038/nrm3327

Korczynska, M., Le, D. D., Younger, N., Gregori-Puigjané, E., Tumber, A., Krojer, T., et al. (2016). Docking and linking of fragments to discover jumonji histone demethylase inhibitors. *J. Med. Chem.* 59, 1580–1598. doi: 10.1021/acs.jmedchem.5b01527

Kouzarides, T. (2002). Histone methylation in transcriptional control. *Curr. Opin. Genet. Dev.* 12, 198–209. doi: 10.1016/S0959-437X(02)00287-3

Kouzarides, T. (2007). Chromatin modifications and their function. *Cell* 128, 693–705. doi: 10.1016/j.cell.2007.02.005

Kozikowski, A. P., Chen, Y., Gaysin, A. M., Savoy, D. N., Billadeau, D. D., and Kim, K. H. (2008). Chemistry, biology, and QSAR studies of substituted biaryl hydroxamates and mercaptoacetamides as HDAC inhibitors-nanomolar-potency inhibitors of pancreatic cancer cell growth. *ChemMedChem* 3, 487–501. doi: 10.1002/cmdc.200700314

Kuck, D., Caulfield, T., Lyko, F., and Medina-Franco, J. L. (2010a). Nanaomycin A selectively inhibits DNMT3B and reactivates silenced tumor suppressor genes in human cancer cells. *Mol. Cancer Ther.* 9, 3015–3023. doi: 10.1158/1535-7163.MCT-10-0609

Kuck, D., Singh, N., Lyko, F., and Medina-Franco, J. L. (2010b). Novel and selective DNA methyltransferase inhibitors: docking-based virtual screening and experimental evaluation. *Bioorg. Med. Chem.* 18, 822–829. doi: 10.1016/j.bmc.2009.11.050

Kumar, A., Bhowmick, K., Vikramdeo, K. S., Mondal, N., Subbarao, N., and Dhar, S. K. (2017). Designing novel inhibitors against histone acetyltransferase (HAT: GCN5) of *Plasmodium falciparum*. *Eur. J. Med. Chem.* 138, 26–37. doi: 10.1016/j.ejmech.2017.06.009

Kutz, C. J., Holshouser, S. L., Marrow, E. A., and Woster, P. M. (2014). 3,5-Diamino-1,2,4-triazoles as a novel scaffold for potent, reversible LSD1 (KDM1A) inhibitors. *Medchemcomm* 5, 1863–1870. doi: 10.1039/C4MD00283K

Lamberth, C. (2017). Agrochemical lead optimization by scaffold hopping. *Pest Manag. Sci.* 4, 282–292. doi: 10.1002/ps.4755

Lange, M., Kaynak, B., Forster, U. B., Tönjes, M., Fischer, J. J., Grimm, C., et al. (2008). Regulation of muscle development by DPF3, a novel histone acetylation and methylation reader of the BAF chromatin remodeling complex. *Genes Dev.* 22, 2370–2384. doi: 10.1101/gad.471408

Lasko, L. M., Jakob, C. G., Edalji, R. P., Qiu, W., Montgomery, D., Digiammarino, E. L., et al. (2017). Discovery of a selective catalytic p300/CBP inhibitor that targets lineage-specific tumours. *Nature* 550, 128–132. doi: 10.1038/nature24028

Laubach, J. P., Moreau, P., San-Miguel, J. F., and Richardson, P. G. (2015). Panobinostat for the treatment of multiple myeloma. *Clin. Cancer. Res.* 21, 4767–4773. doi: 10.1158/1078-0432.CCR-15-0530

Lavecchia, A., and Di Giovanni, C. (2013). Virtual screening strategies in drug discovery: a critical review. *Curr. Med. Chem.* 20, 2839–2860. doi: 10.2174/09298673113209990001

Lee, H. Z., Kwitkowski, V. E., Del Valle, P. L., Ricci, M. S., Saber, H., Habtemariam, B. A., et al. (2015). FDA approval: belinostat for the treatment of patients with relapsed or refractory peripheral T-cell lymphoma. *Clin. Cancer Res.* 21, 2666–2670. doi: 10.1158/1078-0432.CCR-14-3119

Li, E. (2002). Chromatin modification and epigenetic reprogramming in mammalian development. *Nat. Rev. Genet.* 3, 662–673. doi: 10.1038/nrg887

Li, G. B., Yang, L. L., Yuan, Y., Zou, J., Cao, Y., Yang, S. Y., et al. (2015). Virtual screening in small molecule discovery for epigenetic targets. *Methods* 71, 158–166. doi: 10.1016/j.ymeth.2014.11.010

Li, K. K., Luo, C., Wang, D., Jiang, H., and Zheng, Y. G. (2012). Chemical and biochemical approaches in the study of histone methylation and demethylation. *Med. Res. Rev.* 32, 815–867. doi: 10.1002/mrr.20228

Li, L., Zhou, R., Geng, H., Yue, L., Ye, F., Xie, Y., et al. (2014). Discovery of two aminoglycoside antibiotics as inhibitors targeting the menin-mixed lineage leukaemia interface. *Bioorg. Med. Chem. Lett.* 24, 2090–2093. doi: 10.1016/j.bmcl.2014.03.055

Li, Y., and Seto, E. (2016). HDACs and HDAC inhibitors in cancer development and therapy. *Cold Spring Harb. Perspect. Med.* 6:a026831. doi: 10.1101/cshperspect.a026831

Li, Z., Weng, H., Su, R., Weng, X., Zuo, Z., Li, C., et al. (2017). FTO Plays an oncogenic role in acute myeloid leukemia as a N-Methyladenosine RNA demethylase. *Cancer Cell* 31, 127–141. doi: 10.1016/j.ccell.2016.11.017

Lindorff-Larsen, K., Piana, S., Dror, R. O., and Shaw, D. E. (2011). How fast-folding proteins fold. *Science* 334, 517–520. doi: 10.1126/science.1208351

Liu, X., Jiang, H., and Li, H. (2011). SHAFTS: a hybrid approach for 3D molecular similarity calculation. 1. method and assessment of virtual screening. *J. Chem. Inf. Model.* 51, 2372–2385. doi: 10.1021/ci200060s

Lounnas, V., Ritschel, T., Kelder, J., McGuire, R., Bywater, R. P., and Foloppe, N. (2013). Current progress in structure-based rational drug design marks a new mindset in drug discovery. *Comput. Struct. Biotechnol. J.* 5:e201302011. doi: 10.5936/csbj.201302011

Lu, W., Cao, X., Xue, M., Liu, K., Zhao, Z., Shen, H. X., et al. (2011). SHAFTS: A hybrid approach for 3D molecular similarity calculation. 2. prospective case study in the discovery of diverse p90 Ribosomal S6 Protein Kinase 2 inhibitors to suppress cell migration. *J. Med. Chem.* 51, 3564–3574. doi: 10.1021/jm200139j

Lucas, X., Wohlwend, D., Hügle, M., Schmidtkunz, K., Gerhardt, S., Schüle, R., et al. (2013). 4-Acyl pyrroles: mimicking acetylated lysines in histone code reading. *Angew. Chem. Int. Ed Engl.* 52, 14055–14059. doi: 10.1002/anie.201307652

Mann, B. S., Johnson, J. R., He, K., Sridhara, R., Abraham, S., Booth, B. P., et al. (2007). Vorinostat for treatment of cutaneous manifestations of advanced primary cutaneous T-cell lymphoma. *Clin. Cancer Res.* 13, 2318–2322. doi: 10.1158/1078-0432.CCR-06-2672

Markolovic, S., Leissing, T. M., Chowdhury, R., Wilkins, S. E., Lu, X., and Schofield, C. J. (2016). Structure-function relationships of human JmjC oxygenases-demethylases versus hydroxylases. *Curr. Opin. Struct. Biol.* 41, 62–72. doi: 10.1016/j.sbi.2016.05.013

Martin, C., and Zhang, Y. (2005). The diverse functions of histone lysine methylation. *Nat. Rev. Mol. Cell Biol.* 6, 838–849. doi: 10.1038/nrm1761

Medina-Franco, J. L., Méndez-Lucio, O., Dueñas-González, A., and Yoo, J. (2015). Discovery and development of DNA methyltransferase inhibitors using *in silico* approaches. *Drug Discov. Today* 20, 569–577. doi: 10.1016/j.drudis.2014.12.007

Meena, A., Yadav, D. K., Srivastava, A., Khan, F., Chanda, D., and Chattopadhyay, S. K. (2011). *In silico* exploration of anti-inflammatory activity of natural coumarinolignoids. *Chem. Biol. Drug Des.* 78, 567–579. doi: 10.1111/j.1747-0285.2011.01173.x

Meng, F., Cheng, S., Ding, H., Liu, S., Liu, Y., Zhu, K., et al. (2015). Discovery and optimization of novel, selective histone methyltransferase SET7 inhibitors by pharmacophore- and docking-based virtual screening. *J. Med. Chem.* 58, 8166–8181. doi: 10.1021/acs.jmedchem.5b01154

Milite, C., Feoli, A., Viviano, M., Rescigno, D., Mai, A., Castellano, S., et al. (2016). Progress in the development of lysine methyltransferase SETD8 inhibitors. *ChemMedChem* 11, 1680–1685. doi: 10.1002/cmdc.201600272

Minucci, S., and Pelicci, P. G. (2006). Histone deacetylase inhibitors and the promise of epigenetic (and more) treatments for cancer. *Nat. Rev. Cancer* 6, 38–51. doi: 10.1038/nrc1779

Minucci, S., Nervi, C., Lo Coco, F., and Pelicci, P. G. (2001). Histone deacetylases: a common molecular target for differentiation treatment of acute myeloid leukemias? *Oncogene* 20, 3110–3115. doi: 10.1038/sj.onc.1204336

Mirguet, O., Lamotte, Y., Chung, C. W., Bamborough, P., Delannée, D., Bouillot, A., et al. (2014). Naphthyridines as novel BET family bromodomain inhibitors. *ChemMedChem* 9, 580–589. doi: 10.1002/cmdc.201300259

Mosammaparast, N., and Shi, Y. (2010). Reversal of histone methylation: biochemical and molecular mechanisms of histone demethylases. *Annu. Rev. Biochem.* 79, 155–179. doi: 10.1146/annurev.biochem.78.070907.103946

Musselman, C. A., and Kutateladze, T. G. (2009). PHD fingers: epigenetic effectors and potential drug targets. *Mol. Interv.* 9, 314–323. doi: 10.1124/mi.9.6.7

Okano, M., Bell, D. W., Haber, D. A., and Li, E. (1999). DNA methyltransferases Dnmt3a and Dnmt3b are essential for de novo methylation and mammalian development. *Cell* 99, 247–257. doi: 10.1016/S0092-8674(00)81656-6

Okumura, H., Higashi, M., Yoshida, Y., Sato, H., and Akiyama, R. (2018). Theoretical approaches for dynamical ordering of biomolecular systems. *Biochim. Biophys. Acta* 1862, 212–228. doi: 10.1016/j.bbagen.2017.10.001

Ortuso, F., Langer, T., and Alcaro, S. (2006). GBPM: GRID-based pharmacophore model: concept and application studies to protein-protein recognition. *Bioinformatics* 22, 1449–1455. doi: 10.1093/bioinformatics/btl115

Padmanabhan, B., Ramu, M., Mathur, S., Unni, S., and Thiyagarajan, S. (2016). Identification of new inhibitors for human SIRT1: an *in-silico* approach. *Med. Chem.* 12, 347–361. doi: 10.2174/1573406412666160107111612

Park, H., Kim, S., Kim, Y. E., and Lim, S. J. (2010). A structure-based virtual screening approach toward the discovery of histone deacetylase inhibitors: identification of promising zinc-chelating groups. *ChemMedChem* 5, 591–597. doi: 10.1002/cmdc.200900500

Peserico, A., Germani, A., Sanese, P., Barbosa, A. J., Di Virgilio, V., Fittipaldi, R., et al. (2015). A SMYD3 small-molecule inhibitor impairing cancer cell growth. *J. Cell. Physiol.* 230, 2447–2460. doi: 10.1002/jcp.24975

Price, S., Bordogna, W., Bull, R. J., Clark, D. E., Crackett, P. H., Dyke, H. J., et al. (2007). Identification and optimisation of a series of substituted 5-(1H-pyrazol-3-yl)-thiophene-2-hydroxamic acids as potent histone deacetylase (HDAC) inhibitors. *Bioorg. Med. Chem. Lett.* 17, 370–375. doi: 10.1016/j.bmcl.2006.10.048

Ragno, R., Simeoni, S., Rotili, D., Caroli, A., Botta, G., Brosch, G., et al. (2008). Class II-selective histone deacetylase inhibitors. Part 2: alignment-independent GRIND 3-D QSAR, homology and docking studies. *Eur. J. Med. Chem.* 43, 621–632. doi: 10.1016/j.ejmech.2007.05.004

Raj, U., Kumar, H., and Varadwaj, P. K. (2017). Molecular docking and dynamics simulation study of flavonoids as BET bromodomain inhibitors. *J. Biomol. Struct. Dyn.* 35, 2351–2362. doi: 10.1080/07391102.2016.1217276

Rajendrasozhan, S., Yao, H., and Rahman, I. (2009). Current perspectives on role of chromatin modifications and deacetylases in lung inflammation in COPD. *COPD* 6, 291–297. doi: 10.1080/15412550903049132

Roatsch, M., Robaa, D., Pippel, M., Nettleship, J. E., Reddivari, Y., Bird, L. E., et al. (2016). Substituted 2-(2-aminopyrimidin-4-yl)pyridine-4-carboxylates as potent inhibitors of JumonjiC domain-containing histone demethylases. *Future Med. Chem.* 8, 1553–1571. doi: 10.4155/fmc.15.188

Robaa, D., Wagner, T., Luise, C., Carlino, L., McMillan, J., Flaig, R., et al. (2016). Identification and structure-activity relationship studies of small-molecule inhibitors of the methyllysine reader protein spindlin1. *ChemMedChem* 11, 2327–2338. doi: 10.1002/cmdc.201600362

Robertson, K. D. (2001). DNA methylation, methyltransferases, and cancer. *Oncogene* 20, 3139–3155. doi: 10.1038/sj.onc.1204341

Rona, G. B., Eleutherio, E. C. A., and Pinheiro, A. S. (2016). PWWP domains and their modes of sensing DNA and histone methylated lysines. *Biophys. Rev.* 8, 63–74. doi: 10.1007/s12551-015-0190-6

Rooney, T. P., Filippakopoulos, P., Fedorov, O., Picaud, S., Cortopassi, W. A., Hay, D. A., et al. (2014). A series of potent CREBBP bromodomain ligands reveals an induced-fit pocket stabilized by a cation-pi interaction. *Angew. Chem. Int. Ed Engl.* 53, 6126–6130. doi: 10.1002/anie.201402750

Sable, R., and Jois, S. (2015). Surfing the protein-protein interaction surface using docking methods: application to the design of PPI inhibitors. *Molecules* 20, 11569–11603. doi: 10.3390/molecules200611569

Salo, H. S., Laitinen, T., Poso, A., Jarho, E., and Lahtela-Kakkonen, M. (2013). Identification of novel SIRT3 inhibitor scaffolds by virtual screening. *Bioorg. Med. Chem. Lett.* 23, 2990–2995. doi: 10.1016/j.bmcl.2013.03.033

Santiago, C., Nguyen, K., and Schapira, M. (2011). Druggability of methyl-lysine binding sites. *J. Comput. Aided Mol. Des.* 25, 1171–1178. doi: 10.1007/s10822-011-9505-2

Schapira, M., Tyers, M., Torrent, M., and Arrowsmith, C. H. (2017). WD40 repeat domain proteins: a novel target class? *Nat. Rev. Drug Discov.* 16, 773–786. doi: 10.1038/nrd.2017.179

Scheraga, H. A., Khalili, M., and Liwo, A. (2007). Protein-folding dynamics: overview of molecular simulation techniques. *Annu. Rev. Phys. Chem.* 58, 57–83. doi: 10.1146/annurev.physchem.58.032806.104614

Schmitt, M. L., Hauser, A. T., Carlino, L., Pippel, M., Schulz-Fincke, J., Metzger, E., et al. (2013). Nonpeptidic propargylamines as inhibitors of lysine specific demethylase 1 (LSD1) with cellular activity. *J. Med. Chem.* 56, 7334–7342. doi: 10.1021/jm400792m

Schneider, G., Neidhart, W., Giller, T., and Schmid, G. (1999). Scaffold-Hopping by topological pharmacophore search: a contribution to virtual screening. *Angew. Chem. Int. Ed.* 38, 2894–2896. doi: 10.1002/(SICI)1521-3773(19991004)38:19<2894::AID-ANIE2894>3.0.CO;2-F

Scott, D. E., Bayly, A. R., Abell, C., and Skidmore, J. (2016). Small molecules, big targets: drug discovery faces the protein-protein interaction challenge. *Nat. Rev. Drug Discov.* 15, 533–550. doi: 10.1038/nrd.2016.29

Shao, Z., Xu, P., Xu, W., Li, L., Liu, S., Zhang, R., et al. (2017). Discovery of novel DNA methyltransferase 3A inhibitors via structure-based virtual screening and biological assays. *Bioorg. Med. Chem. Lett.* 27, 342–346. doi: 10.1016/j.bmcl.2016.11.023

Sheikh, B. N. (2014). Crafting the brain - role of histone acetyltransferases in neural development and disease. *Cell Tissue Res.* 356, 553–573. doi: 10.1007/s00441-014-1835-7

Shi, A., Murai, M. J., He, S., Lund, G., Hartley, T., Purohit, T., et al. (2012). Structural insights into inhibition of the bivalent menin-MLL interaction by small molecules in leukemia. *Blood* 120, 4461–4469. doi: 10.1182/blood-2012-05-429274

Shi, Y., Lan, F., Matson, C., Mulligan, P., Whetstine, J. R., Cole, P. A., et al. (2004). Histone demethylation mediated by the nuclear amine oxidase homolog LSD1. *Cell* 119, 941–953. doi: 10.1016/j.cell.2004.12.012

Shortt, J., Ott, C. J., Johnstone, R. W., and Bradner, J. E. (2017). A chemical probe toolbox for dissecting the cancer epigenome. *Nat. Rev. Cancer* 17, 160–183. doi: 10.1038/nrc.2016.148

Siedlecki, P., Garcia Boy, R., Comagic, S., Schirrmacher, R., Wiessler, M., Zielenkiewicz, P., et al. (2003). Establishment and functional validation of a structural homology model for human DNA methyltransferase 1. *Biochem. Biophys. Res. Commun.* 306, 558–563. doi: 10.1016/S0006-291X(03)01000-3

Siedlecki, P., Garcia Boy, R., Musch, T., Brueckner, B., Suhai, S., Lyko, F., et al. (2006). Discovery of two novel, small-molecule inhibitors of DNA methylation. *J. Med. Chem.* 49, 678–683. doi: 10.1021/jm050844z

Silvestri, L., Ballante, F., Mai, A., Marshall, G. R., and Ragno, R. (2012). Histone deacetylase inhibitors: structure-based modeling and isoform-selectivity prediction. *J. Chem. Inf. Model.* 52, 2215–2235. doi: 10.1021/ci300160y

Simon, J. A., and Kingston, R. E. (2009). Mechanisms of polycomb gene silencing: knowns and unknowns. *Nat. Rev. Mol. Cell Biol.* 10, 697–708. doi: 10.1038/nrm2763

Sorna, V., Theisen, E. R., Stephens, B., Warner, S. L., Bearss, D. J., Vankayalapati, H., et al. (2013). High-throughput virtual screening identifies novel N'-(1-phenylethylidene)-benzohydrazides as potent, specific, and reversible LSD1 inhibitors. *J. Med. Chem.* 56, 9496–9508. doi: 10.1021/jm400870h

Spannhoff, A., Heinke, R., Bauer, I., Trojer, P., Metzger, E., Gust, R., et al. (2007a). Target-based approach to inhibitors of histone arginine methyltransferases. *J. Med. Chem.* 50, 2319–2325. doi: 10.1021/jm061250e

Spannhoff, A., Machmur, R., Heinke, R., Trojer, P., Bauer, I., Brosch, G., et al. (2007b). A novel arginine methyltransferase inhibitor with cellular activity. *Bioorg. Med. Chem. Lett.* 17, 4150–4153. doi: 10.1016/j.bmcl.2007.05.088

Spannhoff, A., Sippl, W., and Jung, M. (2009). Cancer treatment of the future: inhibitors of histone methyltransferases. *Int. J. Biochem. Cell Biol.* 41, 4–11. doi: 10.1016/j.biocel.2008.07.024

Strahl, B. D., and Allis, C. D. (2000). The language of covalent histone modifications. *Nature* 403, 41–45. doi: 10.1038/47412

Sun, H., Tawa, G., and Wallqvist, A. (2012). Classification of scaffold-hopping approaches. *Drug Discov. Today* 17, 310–324. doi: 10.1016/j.drudis.2011.10.024

Syeda, F., Fagan, R. L., Wean, M., Avvakumov, G. V., Walker, J. R., Xue, S., et al. (2011). The replication focus targeting sequence (RFTS) domain is a DNA-competitive inhibitor of Dnmt1. *J. Biol. Chem.* 286, 15344–15351. doi: 10.1074/jbc.M110.209882

Tang, H., Wang, X. S., Huang, X. P., Roth, B. L., Butler, K. V., Kozikowski, A. P., et al. (2009). Novel inhibitors of human histone deacetylase (HDAC)

identified by QSAR modeling of known inhibitors, virtual screening, and experimental validation. *J. Chem. Inf. Model.* 49, 461–476. doi: 10.1021/ci800366f

Toh, J. D. W., Sun, L., Lau, L. Z. M., Tan, J., Low, J. J. A., Tang, C. W. Q., et al. (2015). A strategy based on nucleotide specificity leads to a subfamily-selective and cell-active inhibitor of N-methyladenosine demethylase FTO. *Chem. Sci.* 6, 112–122. doi: 10.1039/C4SC02554G

Tough, D. F., Tak, P. P., Tarakhovsky, A., and Prinjha, R. K. (2016). Epigenetic drug discovery: breaking through the immune barrier. *Nat. Rev. Drug Discov.* 15, 835–853. doi: 10.1038/nrd.2016.185

Tripathi, S., Mathur, S., Deshmukh, P., Manjula, R., and Padmanabhan, B. (2016). A novel phenanthridionone based scaffold as a potential inhibitor of the BRD2 bromodomain: crystal structure of the complex. *PLoS ONE* 11:e0156344. doi: 10.1371/journal.pone.0156344

Trosset, J. Y., and Vodovar, N. (2013). Structure-based target druggability assessment. *Methods Mol. Biol.* 986, 141–164. doi: 10.1007/978-1-62703-311-4_10

Vidanes, G. M., Bonilla, C. Y., and Toczyski, D. P. (2005). Complicated tails: histone modifications and the DNA damage response. *Cell* 121, 973–976. doi: 10.1016/j.cell.2005.06.013

Vidler, L. R., Brown, N., Knapp, S., and Hoelder, S. (2012). Druggability analysis and structural classification of bromodomain acetyl-lysine binding sites. *J. Med. Chem.* 55, 7346–7359. doi: 10.1021/jm300346w

Vidler, L. R., Filippakopoulos, P., Fedorov, O., Picaud, S., Martin, S., Tomsett, M., et al. (2013). Discovery of novel small-molecule inhibitors of BRD4 using structure-based virtual screening. *J. Med. Chem.* 56, 8073–8088. doi: 10.1021/jm,4011302

Wang, C., Jiang, H., Jin, J., Xie, Y., Chen, Z., Zhang, H., et al. (2017). Development of potent type i protein arginine methyltransferase (PRMT) inhibitors of leukemia cell proliferation. *J. Med. Chem.* 60, 8888–8905. doi: 10.1021/acs.jmedchem.7b01134

Wang, D., Helquist, P., and Wiest, O. (2007). Zinc binding in HDAC inhibitors: A DFT study. *J. Org. Chem.* 72, 5446–5449. doi: 10.1021/jo070739s

Wang, D. F., Wiest, O., Helquist, P., Lan-Hargest, H. Y., and Wiech, N. L. (2004). QSAR Studies of PC-3 cell line inhibition activity of TSA and SAHA-like hydroxamic acids. *Bioorg. Med. Chem. Lett.* 14, 707–711. doi: 10.1016/j.bmcl.2003.11.062

Wang, J., Chen, L., Sinha, S. H., Liang, Z., Chai, H., Muniyan, S., et al. (2012). Pharmacophore-based virtual screening and biological evaluation of small molecule inhibitors for protein arginine methylation. *J. Med. Chem.* 55, 7978–7987. doi: 10.1021/jm300521m

Wells, J. A., and McClendon, C. L. (2007). Reaching for high-hanging fruit in drug discovery at protein-protein interfaces. *Nature* 450, 1001–1009. doi: 10.1038/nature06526

Werbeck, N. D., Kirkpatrick, J., Reinstein, J., and Hansen, D. F. (2014). Using N-ammonium to characterise and map potassium binding sites in proteins by NMR spectroscopy. *Chembiochem* 15, 543–548. doi: 10.1002/cbic.201300700

Wolf, S. S. (2009). The protein arginine methyltransferase family: an update about function, new perspectives and the physiological role in humans. *Cell. Mol. Life Sci.* 66, 2109–2121. doi: 10.1007/s00018-009-0010-x

Wu, R., Wang, S., Zhou, N., Cao, Z., and Zhang, Y. (2010). A proton-shuttle reaction mechanism for histone deacetylase 8 and the catalytic role of metal ions. *J. Am. Chem. Soc.* 132, 9471–9479. doi: 10.1021/ja103932d

Wu, Y., Hu, J., Ding, H., Chen, L., Zhang, Y., Liu, R., et al. (2016). Identification of novel EZH2 inhibitors through pharmacophore-based virtual screening and biological assays. *Bioorg. Med. Chem. Lett.* 26, 3813–3817. doi: 10.1016/j.bmcl.2016.05.018

Xiang, Y., Hou, Z., and Zhang, Z. (2012). Pharmacophore and QSAR studies to design novel histone deacetylase 2 inhibitors. *Chem. Biol. Drug Des.* 79, 760–770. doi: 10.1111/j.1747-0285.2012.01341.x

Xie, A., Liao, C., Li, Z., Ning, Z., Hu, W., Lu, X., et al. (2004). Quantitative structure-activity relationship study of histone deacetylase inhibitors. *Curr. Med. Chem. Anticancer. Agents* 4, 273–299. doi: 10.2174/1568011043352948

Xie, Y., Zhou, R., Lian, F., Liu, Y., Chen, L., Shi, Z., et al. (2014). Virtual screening and biological evaluation of novel small molecular inhibitors against protein arginine methyltransferase 1 (PRMT1). *Org. Biomol. Chem.* 12, 9665–9673. doi: 10.1039/C4OB01591F

Xing, J., Lu, W., Liu, R., Wang, Y., Xie, Y., Zhang, H., et al. (2017). Machine-learning-assisted approach for discovering novel inhibitors targeting bromodomain-containing protein 4. *J. Chem. Inf. Model.* 57, 1677–1690. doi: 10.1021/acs.jcim.7b00098

Xu, Y., Yue, L., Wang, Y., Xing, J., Chen, Z., Shi, Z., et al. (2016). Discovery of novel inhibitors targeting the menin-mixed lineage leukemia interface using pharmacophore- and docking-based virtual screening. *J. Chem. Inf. Model.* 56, 1847–1855. doi: 10.1021/acs.jcim.6b00185

Xue, X., Zhang, Y., Liu, Z., Song, M., Xing, Y., Xiang, Q., et al. (2016). Discovery of Benzo[cd]indol-2(1H)-ones as potent and specific BET bromodomain inhibitors: structure-based virtual screening, optimization, and biological evaluation. *J. Med. Chem.* 59, 1565–1579. doi: 10.1021/acs.jmedchem.5b01511

Yadav, D. K., Kalani, K., Khan, F., and Srivastava, S. K. (2013). QSAR and docking based semi-synthesis and *in vitro* evaluation of 18 beta-glycyrrhetinic acid derivatives against human lung cancer cell line A-549. *Med. Chem.* 9, 1073–1084. doi: 10.2174/1573406411309080009

Yadav, D. K., Khan, F., and Negi, A. S. (2012). Pharmacophore modeling, molecular docking, QSAR, and *in silico* ADMET studies of gallic acid derivatives for immunomodulatory activity. *J. Mol. Model.* 18, 2513–2525. doi: 10.1007/s00894-011-1265-3

Yadav, D. K., Kumar, S., Saloni., Singh, H., Kim, M. H., Sharma, P., et al. (2017a). Molecular docking, QSAR and ADMET studies of withanolide analogs against breast cancer. *Drug Des. Dev. Ther.* 11, 1859–1870. doi: 10.2147/DDDT.S130601

Yadav, D. K., Meena, A., Srivastava, A., Chanda, D., Khan, F., and Chattopadhyay, S. K. (2010). Development of QSAR model for immunomodulatory activity of natural coumarinolignoids. *Drug Des. Dev. Ther.* 4, 173–186. doi: 10.2147/DDDT.S10875

Yadav, D. K., Rai, R., Kumar, N., Singh, S., Misra, S., Sharma, P., et al. (2016). New arylated benzo[h]quinolines induce anti-cancer activity by oxidative stress-mediated DNA damage. *Sci. Rep.* 6:38128. doi: 10.1038/srep38128

Yadav, D. K., Saloni., Sharma, P., Misra, S., Singh, H., Mancera, R. L., et al. (2017b). Studies of the benzopyran class of selective COX-2 inhibitors using 3D-QSAR and molecular docking. *Arch. Pharm. Res.* doi: 10.1007/s12272-017-0945-7. [Epub ahead of print].

Yan, L., Yan, C., Qian, K., Su, H., Kofsky-Wofford, S. A., Lee, W. C., et al. (2014). Diamidine compounds for selective inhibition of protein arginine methyltransferase 1. *J. Med. Chem.* 57, 2611–2622. doi: 10.1021/jm401884z

Yang, H., Ouyang, Y., Ma, H., Cong, H., Zhuang, C., Lok, W. T., et al. (2017). Design and synthesis of novel PRMT1 inhibitors and investigation of their binding preferences using molecular modelling. *Bioorg. Med. Chem. Lett.* 27, 4635–4642. doi: 10.1016/j.bmcl.2017.09.016

Yang, X. J. (2004). The diverse superfamily of lysine acetyltransferases and their roles in leukemia and other diseases. *Nucleic Acids Res.* 32, 959–976. doi: 10.1093/nar/gkh252

Yanuar, A., Azminah, E. Y., Andika, E. Y., Erlina, L., and Syahdi, R. R. (2016). *In silico* approach to finding new active compounds from histone deacetylase (HDAC) family. *Curr. Pharm. Des.* 22, 3488–3497. doi: 10.2174/1381612822666160414142514

Ye, Y., Zhang, B., Mao, R., Zhang, C., Wang, Y., Xing, J., et al. (2017). Discovery and optimization of selective inhibitors of protein arginine methyltransferase 5 by docking-based virtual screening. *Org. Biomol. Chem.* 15, 3648–3661. doi: 10.1039/C7OB00070G

Yokoyama, A., and Cleary, M. L. (2008). Menin critically links MLL proteins with LEDGF on cancer-associated target genes. *Cancer Cell* 14, 36–46. doi: 10.1016/j.ccr.2008.05.003

Yoo, J., Kim, S. J., Son, D., Seo, H., Baek, S. Y., Maeng, C. Y., et al. (2016). Computer-aided identification of new histone deacetylase 6 selective inhibitor with anti-sepsis activity. *Eur. J. Med. Chem.* 116, 126–135. doi: 10.1016/j.ejmech.2016.03.046

Yue, L., Du, J., Ye, F., Chen, Z., Li, L., Lian, F., et al. (2016). Identification of novel small-molecule inhibitors targeting menin-MLL interaction, repurposing the antidiarrheal loperamide. *Org. Biomol. Chem.* 14, 8503–8519. doi: 10.1039/C6OB01248E

Zhang, J., Qian, K., Yan, C., He, M., Jassim, B. A., Ivanov, I., et al. (2017a). Discovery of decamidine as a new and potent PRMT1 inhibitor. *Medchemcomm* 8, 440–444. doi: 10.1039/C6MD00573J

Zhang, W. Y., Lu, W. C., Jiang, H., Lv, Z. B., Xie, Y. Q., Lian, F. L., et al. (2017b). Discovery of alkyl bis(oxy)dibenzimidamide derivatives as novel protein arginine methyltransferase 1 (PRMT1) inhibitors. *Chem. Biol. Drug Des.* 90, 1260–1270. doi: 10.1111/cbdd.13047

Zhang, W., and Xu, J. (2017). DNA methyltransferases and their roles in tumorigenesis. *Biomark. Res.* 5:1. doi: 10.1186/s40364-017-0081-z

Zhao, L., Cao, D., Chen, T., Wang, Y., Miao, Z., Xu, Y., et al. (2013a). Fragment-based drug discovery of 2-thiazolidinones as inhibitors of the histone reader BRD4 bromodomain. *J. Med. Chem.* 56, 3833–3851. doi: 10.1021/jm301793a

Zhao, L., Xiang, Y., Song, J., and Zhang, Z. (2013b). A novel two-step QSAR modeling work flow to predict selectivity and activity of HDAC inhibitors. *Bioorg. Med. Chem. Lett.* 23, 929–933. doi: 10.1016/j.bmcl.2012.12.067

Zheng, M., Liu, X., Xu, Y., Li, H., Luo, C., and Jiang, H. (2013). Computational methods for drug design and discovery: focus on China. *Trends Pharmacol. Sci.* 34, 549–559. doi: 10.1016/j.tips.2013.08.004

Zhou, C., Kang, D., Xu, Y., Zhang, L., and Zha, X. (2015a). Identification of novel selective lysine-specific demethylase 1 (LSD1) inhibitors using a pharmacophore-based virtual screening combined with docking. *Chem. Biol. Drug Des.* 85, 659–671. doi: 10.1111/cbdd.12461

Zhou, R., Xie, Y., Hu, H., Hu, G., Patel, V. S., Zhang, J., et al. (2015b). Molecular mechanism underlying PRMT1 dimerization for SAM binding and methylase activity. *J. Chem. Inf. Model.* 55, 2623–2632. doi: 10.1021/acs.jcim.5b00454

Zhu, P., Martin, E., Mengwasser, J., Schlag, P., Janssen, K. P., and Göttlicher, M. (2004). Induction of HDAC2 expression upon loss of APC in colorectal tumorigenesis. *Cancer Cell* 5, 455–463. doi: 10.1016/S1535-6108(04)00114-X

11

Reverse Screening Methods to Search for the Protein Targets of Chemopreventive Compounds

Hongbin Huang[1,2†]*, Guigui Zhang*[1,3†]*, Yuquan Zhou*[1,2]*, Chenru Lin*[1,3]*, Suling Chen*[1,2]*, Yutong Lin*[1,3]*, Shangkang Mai*[1,2] *and Zunnan Huang*[1,3*]

[1] *Key Laboratory for Medical Molecular Diagnostics of Guangdong Province, Dongguan Scientific Research Center, Guangdong Medical University, Dongguan, China,* [2] *The Second School of Clinical Medicine, Guangdong Medical University, Dongguan, China,* [3] *School of Pharmacy, Guangdong Medical University, Dongguan, China*

Correspondence:
Zunnan Huang
zn_huang@yahoo.com

† *These authors have contributed equally to this work.*

This article is a systematic review of reverse screening methods used to search for the protein targets of chemopreventive compounds or drugs. Typical chemopreventive compounds include components of traditional Chinese medicine, natural compounds and Food and Drug Administration (FDA)-approved drugs. Such compounds are somewhat selective but are predisposed to bind multiple protein targets distributed throughout diverse signaling pathways in human cells. In contrast to conventional virtual screening, which identifies the ligands of a targeted protein from a compound database, reverse screening is used to identify the potential targets or unintended targets of a given compound from a large number of receptors by examining their known ligands or crystal structures. This method, also known as *in silico* or computational target fishing, is highly valuable for discovering the target receptors of query molecules from terrestrial or marine natural products, exploring the molecular mechanisms of chemopreventive compounds, finding alternative indications of existing drugs by drug repositioning, and detecting adverse drug reactions and drug toxicity. Reverse screening can be divided into three major groups: shape screening, pharmacophore screening and reverse docking. Several large software packages, such as Schrödinger and Discovery Studio; typical software/network services such as ChemMapper, PharmMapper, idTarget, and INVDOCK; and practical databases of known target ligands and receptor crystal structures, such as ChEMBL, BindingDB, and the Protein Data Bank (PDB), are available for use in these computational methods. Different programs, online services and databases have different applications and constraints. Here, we conducted a systematic analysis and multilevel classification of the computational programs, online services and compound libraries available for shape screening, pharmacophore screening and reverse docking to enable non-specialist users to quickly learn and grasp the types of calculations used in protein target fishing. In addition, we review the main features of these methods, programs and databases and provide a variety of examples illustrating the application of one or a combination of reverse screening methods for accurate target prediction.

Keywords: drug design, reverse screening, shape similarity, pharmacophore modeling, reverse docking, methodology, online service, screening databases

INTRODUCTION

New drugs can be designed via traditional receptor structure-based virtual screening, which enables the discovery of bioactive compounds that bind the target protein, but they can also originate from reverse virtual screening, which finds the unknown protein targets of active compounds or additional targets of existing drugs (drug repositioning; Hurle et al., 2013). Among the 84 drug products introduced to the market in 2013, new indications of existing drugs accounted for 20%, implying that drug repositioning plays a key role in drug discovery (Graul et al., 2014; Li J. et al., 2016). The majority of drugs or bioactive compounds exert their functions by interacting with protein targets. With an increasing number of drugs showing the ability to target multiple proteins, target identification plays an important role in the fields of drug discovery and biomedical research (Wang J. et al., 2016). Many reverse screening methods can be used to search for the protein targets of molecules (Ziegler et al., 2013), although the earliest approaches involved expensive and time-consuming biological assays (Drews, 1997). However, with the continuous development of Big Data and computational techniques, computer-aided reverse screening methods are playing an increasingly important role in the prediction of the off-target effects and side effects of drugs as well as in drug repositioning (Rognan, 2010; Liu et al., 2014; Schomburg and Rarey, 2014).

These computational methods can be divided into three classes according to their underlying principles: shape screening, pharmacophore screening, and reverse docking. In the absence of receptor crystal structures, shape or pharmacophore screening facilitates the discovery of the potential targets of a query molecule by comparing its overall shape or key pharmacophore features with those of the compounds from a ligand database annotated with target information (Schuffenhauer et al., 2003; Hawkins et al., 2007; Chen et al., 2009). The annotated targets of the matched ligands can then be considered potential targets of the query molecule. Reverse docking, in contrast to the traditional molecular docking used to find the ligands of a target protein, refers to the successive docking of a query molecule into the active pocket of each protein from a protein 3D structure database based on spatial and energy principles to identify protein targets with strong binding affinity as potential targets of the query molecule (Li et al., 2013). Reverse screening methods are important computational techniques for identifying new

---

Abbreviations: 4-HT, 4-Hydroxy-tamoxifen; 5-Aza-dC, 5′-Aza-2′-deoxycytidine; 5-HT1AR, 5-Hydroxytryptamine 1A receptor; 5-HT2A, 5-Hydroxytryptamine receptor 2A; 67DiOHC8S, 6,7-Dihydroxycoumarin-8-sulfate; 6BIO, 6-Bromo-indirubin-3′oxime; ABL, BCR-ABL tyrosine kinase; ACE, Angiotensin converting enzyme; ACHE, Acetylcholinesterase; ACM2, Muscarinic acetylcholine receptor 2; ADA, Adenosine deaminase; ADH, Alcohol dehydrogenase; AdrA3, Adenosine receptors A3; ADRB1, Human beta-1 adrenergic receptor; AGS-IV, Astragaloside IV; AKR1B1, Aldo-keto reductase family 1, member B1; ANXA5, Annexin A5; Apaf-1, Apoptotic protease activating factor-1; APH(2′)-Iva, Aminoglycoside-2′-phosphotransferase type Iva; AR, Aldose reductase; AR′, Androgen receptor; ASA, Aspirin; BACE1, ASC, Astragalus Salvia compound; Beta-secretase 1; BBR, Berberine; Braf, B-raf kinase; Bub1, Human spindle checkpoint kinase Bub1; CA, Carnosic acid; CA1, Carbonic anhydrase 1; CA2, Carbonic anhydrase 2; CaM, Calmodulin; CASP-3, Cysteinyl aspartate specific proteinase 3; CB1, Cannabinoid receptor 1; CB2, Cannabinoid receptor 2; CBS, Cystathionine beta-synthase; c-di-GMP, Cyclic diguanylate monophosphate; CDK2, Cyclin dependent kinase-2; CHS, Chitin synthase; CK2, Casein kinase 2; CN, Calcineurin; CO, Curculigo orchioides; Complex I, NADH:ubiquinone oxidoreductase; COMT, Catechol-O-methyltransferase; COX-1, Prostaglandin G/H synthase 1; COX1, Cyclooxygenase-1; COX2, Cyclooxygenase-2; CT, Cryptotanshinone; CYP450, Cytochrome p450; D2R, Dopamine D2 receptor; DAPDC, Diaminopimelate decarboxylase; DAPH, Dialkylphosphorylhydrazone; DHFR, Dihydrofolate reductase; DHODH, Dihydroorotate dehydrogenase; DIP, Dipyridamole; DPD, Dihydropyrimidine dehydrogenase; DPP-IV, Dipeptidyl peptidase IV; DRD2, Dopamine receptor D2; EB1, Microtubule-associated protein RP/EB family member 1; EGFR, Epidermal growth factor receptor; EphA7, Ephrin receptor EphA7; ErbB-1, ErbB-1 tyrosine kinase; ErbB-2, ErbB-2 tyrosine kinase; ERK1, Extracellular regulated protein kinases 1; ERR-γ, Estrogen-related receptor-γ; ERα, Human estrogen receptor alpha; ESR1, Estrogen receptor alpha; ESR2, Estrogen receptor beta; FAK, Focal adhesion kinase; FGFR-4, Fibroblast growth factor receptor 4; GAD, Ganoderic acid D; GAPDH, Glyceraldehyde-3-phosphate Dehydrogenase; GBA3, Cytosolic beta-glucosidase; GCN5, General control non-derepressible 5; GCR, Glucocorticoid receptor; GFW, Guizhi Fuling Wan; GK, Glucokinase; GMP reductase, Guanosine 5′-monophosphate oxidoreductase; GPX1, Glutathione peroxidase 1; GR, Glucocorticoid receptor; GR′, Glutathione reductase; GS, β(1,3)-Glucan synthase; GSH-S, Glutathione synthetase; GSK3β, Glycogen synthase kinase-3 beta; GST, Glutathione S-transferase; GSTA1, Glutathione S-transferase A1; GSTP1, Glutathione s-transferase PI-1; GTPase, Guanosine triphosphatase; GTs, Ganoderma triterpenes; HDAC2, Histone deacetylase 2; HDPR, 6-hydroxyl-1,6-dihydropurine ribonucleoside; HEXB, beta-Hexosaminidase; HGFR, Hepatocyte Growth Factor Receptor; HGPRT, Hypoxanthine-guanine phosphoribosyltransferase; HIV-1 PR, HIV-1 protease; HMGCR, 3-Hydroxy-3-methylglutaryl-coenzyme A reductase; HpPDF, H. pylori PDF; HPRT, Hypoxanthine phosphoribosyltransferase; HRAS, Harvey rat sarcoma; HRH4, Histamine receptor H4; HSD11B1, 11 beta-Hydroxysteroid dehydrogenase type 1; HSPA8, Heat shock protein family A member 8; HSYA, Hydroxysafflor yellow A; IDO, Indoleamine 2,3-dioxygenase; IDV, Indinavir; I-FABP, Intestinal fatty acid binding protein; IGF1-R, Insulin-like growth factor 1 receptor; IL-2, Interleukin-2; IMPDHII, Inosine 5′-monophosphate dehydrogenase II; JNK, c-Jun N-terminal kinase; LCN-2, Lipocalin-2; LDH, L-lactate dehydrogenase; LTA4H, Leukotriene A4 hydrolase; lysC, Lysozyme C; MAO-B, Monoamine oxidase B; MAP2K1, Mitogen-activated protein kinase kinase 1; MAPK-14, Mitogen-activated protein kinase 14; MCDF, 6-Methyl-1,3,8-trichlorodibenzofuran; MDM2, Mouse double minute 2 homolog; MEK1, Mitogen-activated protein kinase 1; MIF, Migration inhibitory factor; MMP3, Metalloproteinase 3; MMP8, Metalloproteinase 8; MPO, Myeloperoxidase; MTX, Methotrexate; NBP, DL-3-n-Butylphthalide; NF-kB, Nuclear factor kB; NK2 receptor, Neurokinin NK2 receptors; NMT, N-myristoyltransferase; NQO1, NAD(P)H quinone oxidoreductases; Nrf2, Nuclear factor erythroid 2-related factor 2; OBA, Obacunone; OPRK, Kappa opioid receptor; OSC, Oxidosqualene cyclase; p38 MAPK, p38 Mitogen-activated protein kinase; PARP1, Poly [ADP-ribose] polymerase 1; PAs, Pyrrolizidine alkaloids; PBP4, Penicillin binding protein 4; PDE4, Phosphodiesterase 4; PDF, Peptide deformylase; PDGFR, Platelet-Derived Growth Factor Receptor; PDK1, Phosphoinositide-dependent kinase-1; PEPCK, Phosphoenolpyruvate carboxykinase; PGS, Phenolic acid glycoside sulfate; PI-3K, Phosphoinositide 3-kinase; PKA, cAMP-dependent protein kinase; PLA2, Phospholipase A2; PLMF1, Periodic leaf movement factor 1; POLB, DNA polymerase beta; PPARγ, Peroxisome proliferator-activated receptor γ; PPARδ, Peroxisome proliferator-activated receptor delta; PRDX3, Thioredoxin-dependent peroxide reductase mitochondrial precursor; PRIMA-1, P53 reactivation and induction of massive apoptosis; PTP1B, Protein tyrosine phosphatase 1B; PTPNT1, Protein tyrosine phosphatase non-receptor type 1; RA, Rosmarinic acid; RARα, Retinoic acid receptor alpha; REN, Renin; SAA, Salvianolic acid A; SB, Salvianolic acid B; SFJD, Shufengjiedu Capsule; SHBG, Sex hormone-binding globulin; SND, Sini decoction; STAT3, Signal transducer and activator of transcription 3; SULT1E1, Estrogen sulfotransferase; TCDD, 2,3,7,8-tetrachlorodibenzo-p-dioxin; TDP1, Tyrosyl-DNA phosphodiesterase 1; THRa, Human thyroid hormone receptor alpha; TOP1, DNA topoisomerase 1; UA, Ursolic acid; TrxR, Thioredoxin reductase; VEGFR-2, Vascular endothelial growth factor receptor; VGKC, Voltage gated potassium channel; WB, Wentilactone B; XO, Xanthine oxidase.

macromolecular targets of existing drugs or active molecules and for analyzing their functional mechanisms or side effects (Patel et al., 2015). Based on the principles of the methods and the availability of existing large-scale small-molecule [e.g., ChEMBL, the European Molecular Biology Laboratory (Gaulton et al., 2017)] or macromolecule (e.g., the PDB; Rose et al., 2015) databases, researchers worldwide have developed a variety of software and online services for predicting the protein targets of small molecules. Representative examples include SEA (Keiser et al., 2007), PharmMapper (Liu et al., 2010) and INVDOCK (Chen and Zhi, 2001), which are among the earliest tools for shape screening, pharmacophore screening and reverse docking, respectively. In recent years, these three methods have been widely used in the prediction of protein targets to clarify the molecular mechanisms of active small molecules against various diseases (Kharkar et al., 2014; Cereto-Massagué et al., 2015). Many of these molecules are derived from Chinese herbal medicine, and while their pharmacological or biological activities are known, their cellular and molecular mechanisms remain unclear. For example, Lim et al. (2014) used shape screening to determine that curcumin (compound **1**, **Figure 1**), extracted from Zingiberaceae, suppresses the proliferation of human colon cancer cells by targeting cyclin dependent kinase 2 (CDK2). Marine compounds are another class of bioactive small molecules. For example, wentilactone B (WB, compound **2**) is a tetranorditerpenoid derivative extracted from the marine algae-derived endophytic fungus *Aspergillus wentii* EN-48. Zhang et al. (2013) used reverse docking to discover that this small molecule induces G2/M phase arrest and apoptosis of human hepatocellular carcinoma cells by co-targeting the Ras/Raf/MAPK proteins in their signaling pathways.

Here, we begin by introducing the basic principles of these three types of reverse screening methods, i.e., shape screening, pharmacophore screening and reverse docking, for the prediction of the protein targets of small molecules. Then, representative and classical software and online services for each method as well as the relevant databases are hierarchically categorized and systematically presented. Finally, we reviewed nearly all articles on the applications of these methods since 2000 and selected some typical examples to illustrate the use of these methods. By statistically analyzing these articles, we reveal the trends in the application of these three methods for computer-aided protein target prediction. In addition, we discuss their shortcomings and possible solutions as well as previous reviews of these reverse screening approaches for predicting the protein targets of small molecules.

METHODS

Reverse screening to search for unknown targets, unintended targets, or secondary targets of small-molecule drugs can be achieved by shape similarity screening, pharmacophore model screening, or reverse protein-ligand docking (**Figure 2**). These three different calculation approaches are complementary and can be used in conjunction with each other. By comparison, shape, and pharmacophore screening are simpler and faster, while reverse docking is more complex and slower. We will introduce these three methods in detail in the following sections.

Shape Screening

The basic principle of shape screening, from a two-dimensional (2D) perspective, is that structurally similar molecules may have similar bioactivity by targeting the same proteins. From a three-dimensional (3D) perspective, the basic principle is that molecules with similar volumes may have the potential to bind effectively to spaces of the same or similar size (considering the ligand-induced fit effect; Koshland, 1958) in the active pockets of proteins (Shang et al., 2017). To use shape screening to predict the targets of small molecules, a small-molecule ligand database annotated with protein targets is necessary. Then, the overall shape similarity of a query molecule to each ligand in the database can be measured individually. Finally, the protein targets for matched molecules with high similarity scores can be considered potential targets of the query molecule (Schuffenhauer et al., 2003). Shape screening involves two levels of mapping: the first mapping between the query molecule and the ligands in the database and the second mapping between the matched ligands in the database and their annotated protein targets (**Figure 2**).

Shape similarity comparison is based on the 2D or 3D topological structures of small molecules. Notably, 2D methods were originally created to obtain more of the same part between paired molecules, whereas 3D methods can be used to enhance scaffold diversity (Nettles et al., 2006). A universal descriptor for molecular similarity comparison in 2D methods is FingerPrint2D (FP2), which employs a simple bit vector to represent a variety of chemical characteristics and is encoded in a variety of software and databases (Bender et al., 2004). The most frequently used type of FP2 is extended-connectivity fingerprints (ECFPs), which are circular fingerprints. ECFPs symbolize circular atomic neighborhoods based on the Morgan algorithm and are designed especially for structural activity modeling (Rogers and Hahn, 2010). They have variable length: for example, ECFP4 refers to a diameter of 4 and ECFP6 to a diameter of 6 (Glem et al., 2006), both of which are encoded in TargetHunter (Wang L. et al., 2013). Molecular ACCess System (MACCS; Durant et al., 2002) is another commonly used FP2. It is a structure key-based fingerprint and is encoded in the 2D approach of the ChemMapper server (Gong et al., 2013). In addition to FP2, other descriptors are based on 2D topologies or paths, including the daylight fingerprint (http://www.daylight.com) encoded in ChemProt 3.0 (Kringelum et al., 2016) and the MDL structural key, another 2D descriptor (Durant et al., 2002). Structural matching based on 3D topology mainly compares the 3D geometries of the molecules, sometimes with the addition of pharmacophores (Lo et al., 2016), ElectroShapes (Armstrong et al., 2010), Spectrophores (Smusz et al., 2015), or other additional information. For example, WEGA (Yan et al., 2013) and gWEGA (Yan et al., 2014) compare only the volumes of two molecules, but SHAFTS (Lu et al., 2011), encoded in ChemMapper, incorporates pharmacophore matching when calculating the volume similarity.

The similarity of the descriptors in both 2D and 3D methods can be measured by the Tanimoto coefficient. The Tanimoto coefficient represents the ratio of the union to the intersection of the shapes of two molecules (Salim et al., 2003). For example, TargetHunter uses the Tanimoto coefficient to calculate the similarity among molecular fingerprints (Wang L. et al., 2013). The City-Block distance (CBD, also called the Manhattan or Hamming distance), which represents the difference between the sum of two molecular shapes and twice the overlap of two molecular shapes, can also be used to calculate the molecular similarity (Awale and Reymond, 2014). For example, SwissTargetPrediction uses this formula to calculate ElectroShape vectors in 3D comparisons (Gfeller et al., 2014).

Shape screening can be divided into two subclasses: indirect target prediction and direct target prediction. Indirect target prediction indicates that the potential targets of the query molecule are manually selected from the annotated protein targets of the matched database ligands. ROCS (Rush et al., 2005) and TargetHunter (Wang L. et al., 2013) are representative examples. These programs merely calculate the similarity scores between the query molecule and the matched ligands in the database but cannot reveal the complex relationships among the annotated protein targets of multiple matched ligands. In general, the annotated targets of any database ligand are not unique, and a protein target may also be annotated with multiple compounds (Rognan, 2010). Therefore, these programs can have high rates of false positives in target prediction and low accuracy in target searching.

Direct target prediction not only calculates the similarity score between the query molecules and the ligands in the database but also estimates the probability that the annotated targets of the matched ligands are targets of the query molecule. This extra process can reduce the false positive rate of target prediction and improve the accuracy of the target search. The probability that the annotated targets of the matched ligands are targets of the query molecule can be evaluated by multiple computational models or algorithms (the dotted line in **Figure 2**). For example, ChemMapper (Gong et al., 2013), which is based on a compound-protein network constructed from the top similar structures and their annotated targets, employs a random walk algorithm (Köhler et al., 2008) to calculate the probabilities of interaction between the query structure and the annotated targets of the hit compounds. In addition, SwissTargetPrediction (Gfeller et al., 2014) and CSNAP3D (Lo et al., 2016) use a cross-validation method and a network algorithm, respectively, to assess the probabilities that the annotated targets of the matched ligands are targets of the query molecule.

Because shape screening is based on the comparison of overall molecular shape, it may not be suitable for predicting the potential targets of molecules that are excessively large or

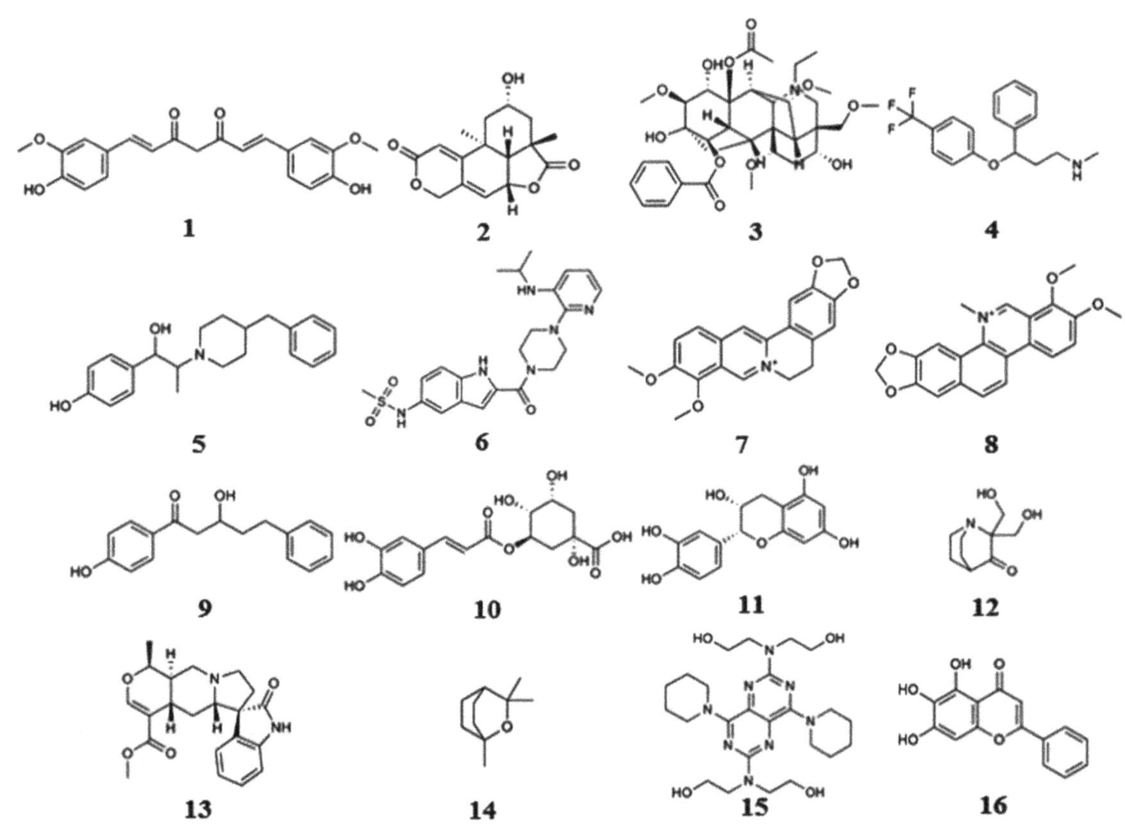

FIGURE 1 | Compounds described in the manuscript.

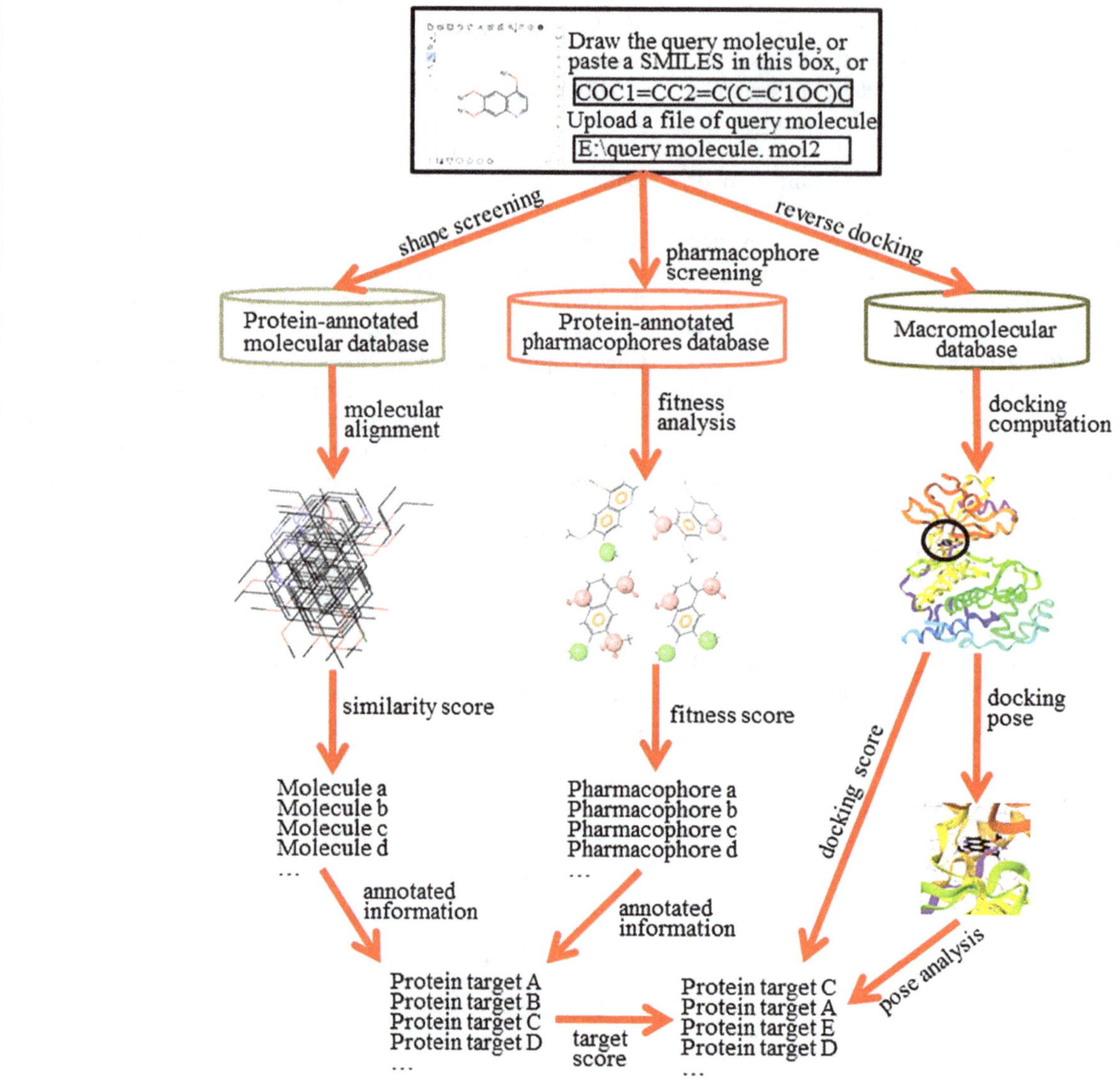

FIGURE 2 | The principle and workflow of shape screening, pharmacophore screening, and reverse docking.

small. Judging the potential targets of an oversized molecule is difficult because its best matched ligands usually show a low similarity score, and selecting the potential targets of an undersized molecule is difficult because its matched ligands are numerous with high similarity scores. Shape screening is suitable for predicting potential targets whose available inhibitors have sizes similar to that of the query molecule but is less fit for finding novel targets whose current inhibitors differ greatly in size from the query molecule but whose active pocket space is easily adjusted to bind diverse ligands due to a strong induced-fit effect.

Pharmacophore Screening

The basic principle of pharmacophore screening is that the binding of certain drugs with their protein targets is primarily determined by key functional pharmacophores (Rognan, 2010). Thus, the matching of these important pharmacophores can be used to search for new targets of small-molecule drugs (Fang and Wang, 2002). A pharmacophore is the spatial arrangement of functional characteristics that allows molecules to interact with target proteins in a particular binding mode, such as a hydrophobic center (H), hydrogen bond acceptor vector (HBA), hydrogen bond donor vector (HBD), positively charged center (P), or negatively charged center (N) (Kurogi and Güner, 2001). A pharmacophore model is the combination of pharmacophores in a pattern of ligand-protein interaction that give the final pharmacological effect (Leach et al., 2010). Similar to a ligand database for shape screening, a pharmacophore database also requires annotation with target protein information. In pharmacophore screening, the pharmacophore features of the query molecule are successively matched with the features of the pharmacophore models in the database. A higher matching degree indicates that the annotated protein target of the matched pharmacophore model has greater potential to be a target of the query molecule (Steindl et al., 2006). Pharmacophore screening also undergoes two levels of mapping: the first mapping is between the pharmacophore models of the query molecule and of the ligands in the database, and the second mapping is between the matched pharmacophore models of the ligands in the database and their annotated protein targets (**Figure 2**).

The pharmacophore database is built by pharmacophore modeling. The three construction methods are the use of ligands only, receptor structures only, or co-crystallized complex structures, which can be defined as ligand-based, structure-based and complex-based pharmacophore modeling, respectively. Ligand-based pharmacophore modeling was initially designed and is often used for traditional ligand-based virtual screening; an example is the quantitative structure–activity relationship (QSAR; Pulla et al., 2016). The most substantial common features shared by a group of active molecules can be easily extracted by using this method to form a good pharmacophore model to guide the further optimization of active compounds (Leach et al., 2010; Gaurav and Gautam, 2014). However, this approach is seldom used in reverse pharmacophore modeling due to the arbitrariness of pharmacophore models based on a single protein-annotated ligand.

The other two main methods, the use of only receptor structures and the use of protein-ligand complex structures, are forms of structure-based pharmacophore modeling (Gaurav and Gautam, 2014). In receptor-based methods, the pharmacophore features are first extracted from potential binding sites detected by specific protocols, and the pharmacophore models are then derived from the clustering of interaction point information and further refined or validated by using the input of the known ligands and their available or even calculated binding data (Chen and Lai, 2006). For instance, Pocket v.2 (Chen and Lai, 2006) and Catalyst SBP in Discovery Studio (DS) (BIOVIA, 2017) can both produce this type of pharmacophore database. In complex-based methods, pharmacophore models are simply generated via knowledge-based topological rules by using all features, such as hydrogen bonding information, charge, and hydrophobic contacts, based on the interactions between the co-crystallized ligands and receptor atoms (Sutter et al., 2011; Meslamani et al., 2012). Complex-based pharmacophore modeling is commonly used to construct pharmacophore databases, such as PharmaDB in Discovery Studio (Meslamani et al., 2012) and PharmTargetDB in PharmMapper (Liu et al., 2010), due to the stronger association between the built pharmacophore models and the experimentally verified ligand-protein interactions, which can improve the accuracy of target prediction.

The matching process between a pharmacophore model of the query molecule and the pharmacophore models in the pharmacophore database considers the alignment of two core components: pharmacophore feature types and the positions of the feature types (Wolber and Langer, 2005). The alignment of feature types is the matching between the pharmacophore features shared by the query molecule and the database ligands, such as matching between a hydrophobic feature in the molecular structure and those in database ligand pharmacophore models. The alignment of the feature positions is the pairwise matching of the distances between the fitted feature types in the pharmacophore models (Kabsch, 1976). For example, PharmMapper groups pharmacophores into triplets (e.g., H-H-H, H-HBA-HBD) and uses the vertexes of a triangle to represent the pharmacophore feature types and the side length of the triangle to measure the relative positions of these feature types (Liu et al., 2010).

In pharmacophore screening, the pairwise fitness score between pharmacophore models can be used directly as a basis for target evaluation. The fitness score includes the scores obtained from both the alignments between feature types and the alignments between the positions of each pair of pharmacophore models from the query molecule and database ligands. Higher fitness scores indicate higher probabilities (Wang X. et al., 2016). In addition, other matching information, such as the number of matched features and overall shape similarity, can also be used as additional references for target evaluation (Khedkar et al., 2007). If the pharmacophore scoring process does not consider the overall shape of the query molecules, it will be more likely to find pseudo protein targets with high fitness scores for a smaller query molecule because its limited pharmacophore features can be easily matched in the database (Wang X. et al., 2016). Thus, the target score must be recalculated to improve the prediction accuracy (the dotted line in **Figure 2**). For example, PharmMapper utilizes a normalized fitness score to re-rank the potential targets by standardizing a normal distribution of the fitness score to achieve a higher accuracy (Wang X. et al., 2017).

Since the construction of the pharmacophore database by structure-based pharmacophore modeling is not easy, the development of corresponding tools based on this principle has been somewhat limited. However, compared with shape screening, pharmacophore screening can improve the accuracy of prediction because it focuses on matching the key pharmacophore functional groups. In addition, it can ignore the total size of the molecule. As a result, pharmacophore screening can be used to search for potential targets of a query molecule with a large or small volume and can also be employed to find novel protein targets capable of binding a large diversity of ligands. Although PharmTargetDB, the PharmMapper in-house repository, does incorporate protein structural information, a pharmacophore database can be built to use ligands only. That is, constructing a pharmacophore database based on ligands with currently unavailable target structures is also useful for pharmacophore screening.

Reverse Docking

The basic principle of reverse docking is that the binding strength of a small-molecule ligand and a potential protein target is determined by their interaction energy (docking energy). To use reverse docking to predict the targets of a query molecule, a structure grid database of a large number of protein targets is normally required. Then, the query molecule is individually docked with each protein structure in the database. Each docking score is calculated. Finally, the protein targets are sorted according to their docking energy. Generally, a higher rank indicates a greater probability that the protein is a target of the query molecule. In contrast to shape screening and pharmacophore screening, reverse docking involves one level of mapping, which reflects the direct relationship between the query molecule and the target proteins (**Figure 2**). However, it is a complex process that includes recognition of a binding site, construction of the docking grid, a molecular docking algorithm, docking score calculation and target evaluation, among other steps (Lee et al., 2016).

In most cases, the active site of a protein is already known and can be determined from its co-crystallized small-molecule ligand. However, for some *apo*-form structures without co-crystallized ligands, the docking program must first recognize the active binding site of these proteins. If the *apo*-form structure is from a protein for which other co-crystallized structures are available, its active site can also be identified from those protein structures with co-crystallized ligands. Otherwise, *de novo* detection of the active site of the *apo*-form structure is required. The literature describes multiple ways to achieve this task. For example, Wang et al. (2012) uses the "divide-and-conquer" method in idTarget to search the surface structure of the entire protein and possible allosteric structures to find potential binding sites. Kuntz et al. (1982) describes a method that was later used in INVDOCK (Chen and Zhi, 2001) to define a binding site by a group of overlapping probe spheres of certain radii, which fill up a cavity and whose inward-facing surfaces cover the van der Waals surfaces of the protein atoms at the interface. Active site recognition is very useful in attempts to dock a query molecule into cavities other than the binding pockets of known ligands, which can increase the diversity of the binding between the query molecule and protein targets and improve the accuracy of reverse docking.

The database of protein targets used in reverse docking can be a library of protein crystal structure grids with recognized binding sites determined by co-crystallized ligands or available cavities. We can build these databases by continuously downloading a series of protein crystal structures from the Protein Data Bank (PDB); the time-consuming human-computer interaction processes (such as the deletion of water molecules, the addition of hydrogen atoms, and energy optimization) can be accomplished by using a molecular docking program, and the protein structure grids are finally generated. Traditional molecular docking programs, such as DOCK (Allen et al., 2015), AutoDock (Di Muzio et al., 2017), Schrödinger (Schrödinger, 2018) and Discovery Studio (BIOVIA, 2017), can be used to construct a custom target database for reverse docking to search for potential targets of a small molecule. Alternatively, the protein target database can also be a simply processed, automatically constructed protein structure database, and the grids can be generated after the programmed identification of active sites in the process of reverse docking; an example is the idTarget in-house database (Wang et al., 2012). Notably, the lack of a universal protein structure grid database and the need to build a new one for each docking program are the main reasons that reverse docking cannot be used as often as traditional structure-based virtual screening.

At present, reverse screening uses two main types of molecular docking techniques, originally developed in DOCK and AutoDock. DOCK (Ewing et al., 2001) adopts a "geometry matching method" to perform molecular docking by complementing the geometric shape of the docking ligands with that of the protein active site, usually including hydrogen binding sites and locally accessible sites (Shoichet et al., 2010). The matching process is performed by an "anchor and grow algorithm," in which the anchor is a rigid portion of the ligand that is used to initialize a pruned conformation search, and grow refers to the generation of multiple conformations of the remaining segments to simulate the flexible docking of the ligand (Ewing et al., 2001). AutoDock uses a "docking simulation method" that employs the "genetic algorithm" to sample the conformations of a docking molecule inside a grid of the receptor binding pocket (Willett, 1995). In this algorithm, the molecule starts randomly at the receptor surface and undergoes orientation, translation and rotation to cause conformational changes until the ideal binding pose with the best binding energy is found (Morris et al., 2015). Among three reverse docking programs, INVDOCK (Chen and Zhi, 2001) and TarFisDock (Li et al., 2006) use the DOCK geometry matching method for molecular docking, while idTarget uses the AutoDock genetic algorithm for reverse docking (Wang et al., 2012).

Currently, almost all molecular docking programs can perform flexible-ligand docking due to the small size of the ligands; however, these programs still have difficulty in performing molecular docking with a fully flexible protein. Therefore, depending on the flexibility of the receptor proteins, reverse docking can also be classified into two types: rigid protein docking and semi-flexible protein docking. Although reverse docking with a rigid receptor is fast, it ignores ligand/receptor-induced fit effects. An example of a rigid protein docking program for reverse screening is TarFisDock (Li et al., 2006). Reverse docking with semi-flexible receptors can be achieved by various methods such as side-chain rotations (Liu H. et al., 2015), stretching of active pocket residues (Halgren et al., 2004), and ensemble docking (Lorber and Shoichet, 1998). For example, INVDOCK allows the amino acid residues of the receptor binding sites to rotate with the entry of the ligand, thereby simulating the ligand induced-fit conformational changes of receptors (Chen and Zhi, 2001). idTarget uses the docking of a query molecule into an ensemble of different receptor crystal structures after clustering (Wang et al., 2012) and thus simulates semi-flexible receptor docking by possible binding of the molecule with the distinct locations of the active pocket residues of the receptor in its different structures.

The docking score between a query molecule and receptors is an evaluation criterion for ranking its potential targets in reverse screening. Docking energy is a major method of scoring docking poses and normally refers to the interaction energy between the ligand and protein but may also include the energy of the ligand or the energies of both the ligand and the protein (or a part of the protein such as the binding pocket). For example, INVDOCK evaluates the docking structure by calculating the interaction energy between the ligand and receptor (Chen and Zhi, 2001), whereas idTarget scores the docking pose by calculating the energy of the ligand, the protein binding pocket and the interaction between them (Wang et al., 2012). According to the principle that the most stable structure has the lowest energy, a more negative docking energy results in stronger binding between the ligand and protein. The docking energy is calculated based on energy functions, which are mainly divided into three types: molecular mechanics energy functions, empirical energy functions, and semi-empirical energy functions. The molecular mechanics energy functions are more comprehensive and are rigorously defined by the sum of terms with clear physical meaning, including bond stretching, angle bending, torsion angles, van der Waals forces, electrostatic interactions, desolvation, or hydrophobic interactions, conformational entropy, and potentially others (Huang and Zou, 2010; Wang et al., 2011). In reality, the molecular mechanics energy functions used in the docking programs may include only some of these terms. For example, TarFisDock uses energy functions including only van der Waals and electrostatic interaction terms (Li et al., 2006). Empirical energy functions comprise weighted energy terms whose coefficients are obtained by reproducing the binding affinities of a benchmark data set of protein-ligand complexes (Gilson et al., 1997; Gilson and Zhou, 2007). For example, INVDOCK uses an empirical energy function based on simple contact terms, including hydrogen bond and non-bond terms, to calculate the ligand-protein interactive energy as the binding affinity (Chen and Zhi, 2001). Semi-empirical energy functions combine some molecular mechanics energy terms with empirical weights and/or empirical functional forms and have been widely used in computational docking methods (Raha and Merz, 2005). For example, idTarget follows the AutoDock 4 robust scoring functions (Huey et al., 2007) and employs a semi-empirical free energy function that includes hydrogen bonding, electrostatics, desolvation, and torsional entropy, whose weighting coefficients are derived from regression analysis of the experimental binding affinity information (Wang et al., 2011). In addition, reverse docking allows visual assessment of the docking poses by analyzing the number of hydrogen bonds, the presence or absence of critical hydrogen bonds and pi-pi conjugation, etc., as in traditional virtual screening, to further assist target evaluation for a more accurate prediction.

Reverse docking considers key elements of both shape screening and pharmacophore modeling. It determines whether or not the size of a query molecule can fit inside the binding pocket of a protein target by docking and scores the interaction of the key pharmacophore groups in the molecule and the targets to perform target evaluation. Thus, reverse docking could be the most comprehensive of the three methods in principle. However, similar to traditional molecular docking, it also has the following shortcomings: incompleteness of the search space, inaccuracy of the scoring function, and extensive calculation (Lee et al., 2016). Relative to traditional docking, reverse docking has the additional problem that the sizes of the active pockets of proteins defined by co-crystallized ligands are inconsistent. Even if the docking pockets can be defined as being a universally equal size, the residue density of different protein binding pockets may vary, resulting in differences in the calculation ranges for the binding interaction energies. Therefore, reverse docking suffers from a rationality problem, as it is unable to normalize binding energies for the correct sorting of potential targets. Nevertheless, reverse docking can serve as an effective method to complement shape and pharmacophore screening when the protein structures are available.

Software and Online Services

Many software programs, some of which are available as online services, can be used for reverse screening to predict protein targets of small molecules, but the numbers of online tools available for the three methods are quite different. Shape screening tools are the most numerous and include more than a dozen, such as ChemProt (Kringelum et al., 2016), ROCS (Rush et al., 2005), ChemMapper (Gong et al., 2013), and the SEA search server (Keiser et al., 2007). They are listed in the outer ring of **Figure 3**. By contrast, the only tool available for pharmacophore screening is PharmMapper (Liu et al., 2010), as shown in the inner ring of **Figure 3**. The main tools available for target searching by reverse docking are TarFisDock (Li et al., 2006), idTarget (Wang et al., 2012) and INVDOCK (Chen and Zhi, 2001), which are illustrated in the middle ring of **Figure 3**. A few large software packages, such as Schrödinger and Discovery Studio, also contain related modules that perform reverse screening, but they can be used only for the indirect prediction of potential targets of small molecules. These tools require users to build their own databases or perform other relevant processing steps. We have summarized the basic information on these tools, organized according to their characteristics, in **Table 1**. In addition, for each type of software and online service,

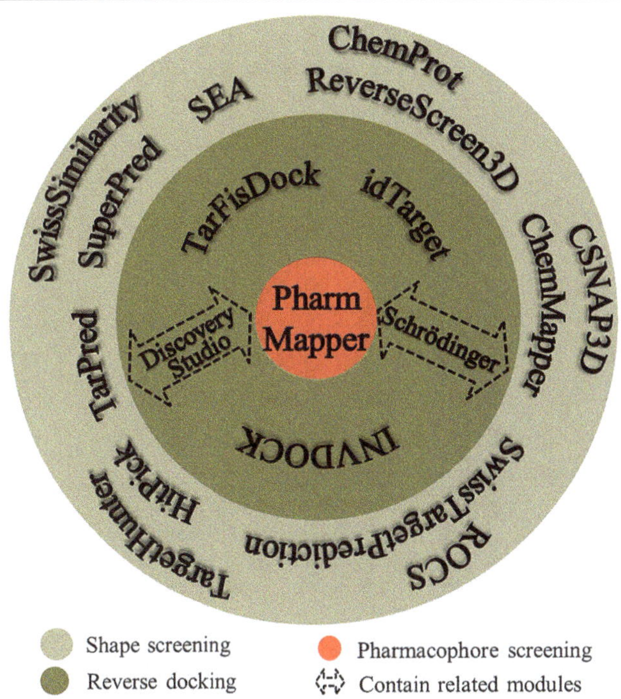

FIGURE 3 | Software and online services for shape screening, pharmacophore screening, and reverse docking.

TABLE 1 | Characteristics of reverse screening tools.

Name	Required format	Search method	Coverage	Reference website	First version	Last version	State
SuperPred	SMILES, Pubchem-Name	2D similarity	341,000 compounds, 1800 targets, 665,000 compound-target interactions	http://prediction.charite.de/	2014	2014	Accessible
HitPick	SMILES	1NN similarity searching and Laplacian-modified naïve Bayesian target models	145,549 chemical-protein interactions collected from STITCH 3.1	http://mips.helmholtz-muenchen.de/hitpick/cgi-bin/index.cgi?content=targetPrediction.html	2013	2013	Accessible
ChemMapper	SMILES, MOL2, SDF, SMI	SHAFTS, USR, FP2, MACCS, and random walk algorithm	Nearly 300,000 chemical structures and >3 million compounds	http://lilab.ecust.edu.cn/chemmapper/	2013	2016	Accessible
SEA server	SMILES	FP2 and BLAST-like model	Hundreds of target-ligand sets	http://sea.bkslab.org/	2007	2007	Accessible
ReverseScreen3D	SMILES	Hybrid 2D&3D	Automatically updated from RCSB PDB	http://www.modeling.leeds.ac.uk/ReverseScreen3D	2011	2011	Inaccessible
TarPred	SMILES	KNN-based data fusion with molecular similarity	533 individual targets with 179,807 active ligands	http://202.127.19.75:5555/	2015	2015	Inaccessible
SwissTargetPrediction	SMILES	Five species, FP2, 3D similarity	280,000 compounds and >2000 targets	http://www.swisstargetprediction.ch/index.php	2014	2014	Accessible
SwissSimilarity	SMILES	FP2, five 3D methods	>30 chemical databases covering drugs, bioactive compounds, etc.	http://www.swisssimilarity.ch/	2016	2016	Accessible
ChemProt	SMILES, name	MACCS, FP2, daylight-like fingerprints	>1.7 million unique chemicals and >20,000 proteins	http://potentia.cbs.dtu.dk/ChemProt/	2011	2016	Accessible
TargetHunter	SMILES	ECFP6, ECFP4, FP2	CHEMBL Version 22	http://www.cbligand.org/TargetHunter/	2013	2016	accessible
CSNAP3D	SMILES, SDF	3D similarity, network algorithms	Based on CHEMBL database	http://services.mbi.ucla.edu/CSNAP/index.html	2016	2016	accessible
ROCS	SDF, MOL2, PDB	3D similarity	User prepared	https://www.eyesopen.com/rocs	2006	2017	Accessible
PharmMapper	MOL2, SDF	Pharmacophores	23,236 proteins covering >53,000 pharmacophore models	http://lilab.ecust.edu.cn/pharmmapper/	2010	2017	Accessible
TarFisDock	MOL2	DOCK4.0	Based on the PDTD, which contains 1207 entries covering 841 known and potential drug targets	http://www.dddc.ac.cn/tarfisdock/	2006	2008	Inaccessible
idTarget	PDB, MOL2, pdbqt, cif	MeDock, divide-and-conquer	All protein structures in the PDB	http://idtarget.rcas.sinica.edu.tw	2012	2012	Accessible
INVDOCK	NA	DOCK	An in-house database (9000 protein and nucleic acid entries)	http://bidd.nus.edu.sg/group/softwares/invdock.htm	2001	NA	Accessible
Discovery Studio	SDF, MOL2, PDB	Pharmacophores	140,000 receptor-ligand pharmacophore models.	http://accelrys.com/products/collaborative-science/biovia-discovery-studio/pharmacophore-and-ligand-based-design.html	2012	2017	Accessible

we have provided more detailed descriptions of a few classic representatives.

Shape Screening

At present, many online services are available to search for targets of small-molecule drugs by shape screening. According to whether these services and software programs can directly sort the potential protein targets by probability or not, we classified them into direct target prediction tools, such as SuperPred (Dunkel et al., 2008), HitPick (Liu et al., 2013), ChemMapper, SEA search server, ReverseScreen3D (Kinnings and Jackson, 2011), TarPred (Liu et al., 2015a), and SwissTargetPrediction, and indirect target prediction tools, such as SwissSimilarity (Zoete et al., 2016), ChemProt, TargetHunter (Wang L. et al., 2013), CSNAP3D (Lo et al., 2016), and ROCS. These categories, respectively, are located on the inside and outside of the outer ring in **Figure 3**. A brief introduction to these services, including their input and output formats, shape similarity calculation methods, database information and website links, is provided in **Table 1**. Because indirect target prediction services require the manual selection of protein targets, we do not provide a more detailed overview of these tools here. We chose the SEA search server among the direct target prediction services as a representative for further description because it is the oldest and most widely used shape-screening service (Keiser et al., 2007).

As a web-based target prediction tool, SEA was developed in 2007, and it performs quantitative classification and target association based on the chemical similarity of protein-related ligands (Keiser et al., 2007). SEA supports only the SMILES format for the input of query molecules for target prediction. After receiving the relevant information about the query compound, SEA performs a pairwise comparison of a 2D similarity metric in a collection of ~65,000 ligands annotated with drug targets, in which most annotations contain hundreds of ligands (Keiser et al., 2007). SEA then clusters the ligands based on their chemical similarity into hundreds of sets, relating their corresponding annotated targets to each other quantitatively, and further uses a model resembling that of BLAST (Mount, 2007) to link these sets together in a minimal spanning tree (Keiser et al., 2007). Next, a statistical model is used to rank the significance (*E*-value) of the resulting similarity scores of each set in the minimum spanning tree. Finally, SEA produces a list of Max Tanimoto coefficients (MaxTc) and *E*-values. A larger similarity score (maxTC) with smaller significance score (*E*-value) indicate a higher rank, and there is a greater probability that the protein is a potential target.

Pharmacophore Screening

PharmMapper, the only web server to screen the potential protein targets of a query molecule based on pharmacophore modeling (**Figure 3**), was developed in 2010 (Liu et al., 2010; Wang X. et al., 2017). PharmMapper uses a triangle hashing mapping method to match the pharmacophore models between the compound and the internal database ligands to predict potential protein targets of a query molecule (Liu et al., 2010). A brief introduction to this online tool is also given in **Table 1**, including the input and output formats, database information and website link. Its in-house database, PharmTargetDB, will be described in detail in the Databases section. PharmMapper supports the Tripos Mol2, MDL and SDF formats for the input of a 2D or 3D query molecule structure to begin a job. Next, PharmMapper flexibly aligns the molecule with each protein pharmacophore model in its database and calculates the fit score between the query molecule and the pharmacophore models (Liu et al., 2010). Subsequently, PharmMapper ranks candidate targets according to the fit score (Liu et al., 2010) or according to normalized fit scores standardized by using a two-dimensional Z-transformation algorithm on the ligand and pharmacophore target dimensions (Wang X. et al., 2016), and records the aligned pharmacophore pose for the query molecule and targets. With the default setting, the top 300 target hits of the prioritizing list are outputted, and users can select candidate proteins based on both these fit scores and the aligned pose for further bioassay experiments (Liu et al., 2010; Wang X. et al., 2017).

Reverse Docking

TarFisDock, idTarget, and INVDOCK (**Figure 3**) are three reverse docking programs that are currently widely used in predicting the targets and mechanisms of various active biomolecules. A brief introduction to these tools is given in **Table 1**, including the input and output formats, database information and website links. Here, we will also provide a slightly more detailed description of these three tools.

TarFisDock, a web-based tool for predicting the potential binding targets of a given ligand, was first released in 2006 (Li et al., 2006) and last updated in 2008 (Gao et al., 2008). TarFisDock uses reverse docking to search for all possible protein binding partners of small molecules from a potential drug target database called PDTD (Li et al., 2006), which will be described further in the Databases section. This program supports only the mol2 format for the input of the query molecule. TarFisDock (Li et al., 2006) uses the docking program DOCK 4.0 to perform molecular docking between the given molecule and each protein in the PDTD, and it calculates their binding energy based on van der Waals and electrostatic interaction terms by using the Amber force field (Weiner et al., 1984). TarFisDock can output a list of the top 2, 5, or 10% target hits according to binding energy. The main limitation of TarFisDock is the insufficient number of target proteins in the PDTD. The PDTD initially released in 2006 contained only 698 protein structures (Li et al., 2006) and was expanded to contain >830 protein targets in 2008 (Gao et al., 2008). TarFisDock considers the flexibility of the small molecules but has yet to consider the flexibility of the protein targets.

In 2012, the web server idTarget (Wang et al., 2012) was developed to predict the potential binding targets of small molecules via a divide-and-conquer reverse docking approach. To improve the efficiency of target prediction, idTarget uses a contraction-and-expansion strategy to differentiate the protein structures at different levels for molecular docking into the families of homologous structures by clustering almost all of the protein structures deposited in the PDB (Wang et al., 2012). idTarget supports multiple coordinate formats, including pdbqt and mol2, for the input of the given molecule. Then, the program uses MEDock (Chang et al., 2005) to initially generate a large number of conformations of the query molecule and directly orient them inside the grid box of the binding site for molecular docking (Wang et al., 2012). Subsequently, idTarget assesses the binding pose by using semi-empirical score functions derived from quantum chemical charge models and robust regression analysis (Wang et al., 2012). Finally, the program outputs two sets of results, both of which are ranked in ascending order of the predicted binding free energy (ΔG^{Pred}). One set of results is listed according to the names of the proteins, while the other is listed according to the names of the homologous families (Wang et al., 2012). In addition, idTarget provides two modes for searching binding poses, scanning mode and fast mode (Wang et al., 2012). In "scanning mode," molecular docking is performed individually for each protein structure in the database. In "fast mode," the ligand is docked simultaneously to the binding sites of the superposed homologous protein structures, and the binding poses are further minimized by adaptive local sampling (Shindyalov and Bourne, 1998). The fast mode performs quick searches via docking between the ligand and the common binding sites after the protein structures of each homologous family are pre-aligned, but the scanning mode does not limit the docking conformation searches to these predetermined binding sites (Wang et al., 2012). Both modes uses the strategy of ensemble docking (Lorber and Shoichet, 1998) to consider the flexibility of the receptor indirectly (Wang et al., 2012).

INVDOCK (Chen and Zhi, 2001), an online service for ligand-protein reverse docking that runs on both Windows and Unix platforms, was developed in 2001. INVDOCK has an in-house protein target database of 9000 protein and nucleic acid entries (Chen and Zhi, 2001). It supports standard 3D ligand structure files, such as the SDF and MOL formats. INVDOCK sets cavities on the protein surface that are covered by a large portion of spherical probes as active binding pockets. The automatic docking is performed by multi-configuration shape matching between the molecule and cavities. Then, torsion optimization and energy minimization are performed on the molecule and on the protein residues in the binding region (Chen and Zhi, 2001). Finally, the simplified DOCK scoring method is used to score the binding energy, and the protein targets are ranked in ascending order by the ligand-protein interaction energy function (ΔE_{LP}; Chen and Zhi, 2001). INVDOCK also considers the flexibility of the protein via a limited torsion space sampling of rotatable bonds in the side chains of the target residues at the binding site (Chen and Zhi, 2001).

Integrated Software Suites

Some drug design software suites, such as Schrödinger (2018) and Discovery Studio (BIOVIA, 2017), can also be used in shape screening, pharmacophore screening, and reverse docking to predict the protein targets of small molecules.

The Schrödinger modules for reverse screening are "Shape Screening," "Pharmacophore Modeling," and "Docking". However, Schrödinger does not provide any ligand or protein database that can be used for reverse screening, and thus, users must provide the databases themselves. "Shape Screening" and "Pharmacophore Modeling" require a protein-annotated ligand database that can be generated by a simple process from the ligand library Ligand Expo, which can be downloaded from the PDB database (Feng et al., 2004; Rose et al., 2015). Each small-molecule ligand in this library is annotated with its co-crystallized protein target information. The protein structure grid database for reverse docking can be constructed by users via grid generation by the "Docking" module after the "Protein Presentation Wizard" is used to pre-process the protein crystal structure coordinates from the PDB, such as to remove water molecules and add hydrogens. Then, reverse docking can be performed by using "Glide Cross Docking" to dock a given molecule with multiple proteins simultaneously. Although the number of proteins for simultaneous docking in "Glide Cross Docking" is limited (normally $\sim$ 50), users can write their own scripts to run reverse docking for one ligand and many proteins. We have performed several reverse screening tasks by using these modules in the Schrödinger software package (Kim et al., 2014; Lim et al., 2014; Wang Z. et al., 2016).

The "Pharmacophore" and "Receptor-Ligand Interaction" modules of Discovery Studio can be used for reverse screening. Users can select shape screening or pharmacophore screening by using the "Ligand Profiler" tool in the "Pharmacophore" module. This tool allows users to upload a database or use the Ligand Profiler Pharmacophore Database, PharmaDB, provided in the software. This database is generated from an annotated database of druggable binding sites called scPDB (Desaphy et al., 2015) based on the PDB and contains the molecular structure and corresponding pharmacophores for calculation of the shape and pharmacophore similarity. The protein crystal structure database for reverse docking must be prepared by the user. These crystal structures can be defined by the "Define and Edit Binding Site" in the "Tools" menu of the "Receptor-Ligand Interaction" module. "Libdock Batch Mode" in the "Protocols" menu of the "Receptor-Ligand Interaction" module can be used for batch docking and has the same effect as reverse docking. Because of the different algorithms and databases needed, the advantages and disadvantages of these two software suites for reverse screening have yet to be evaluated.

Databases

Databases, whether protein-annotated ligand structure/pharmacophore databases or protein structure grid databases, are key elements of reverse screening. Although reverse screening has been under development for nearly two decades, no general or benchmarked database is available for use in different methods or programs. Here, we have classified the existing relevant databases at different levels (**Figure 4**). The first class of databases is associated with software built by software developers and used for program running. We call these databases "software databases" or "direct databases" (shown at the bottom layer of **Figure 4**). Each database in this class is named for its corresponding software or referred to as the software in-house database. The second class of databases provides resources describing annotated ligands or target structures, but the users must process and collect these resources to construct direct databases for reverse screening. We call these

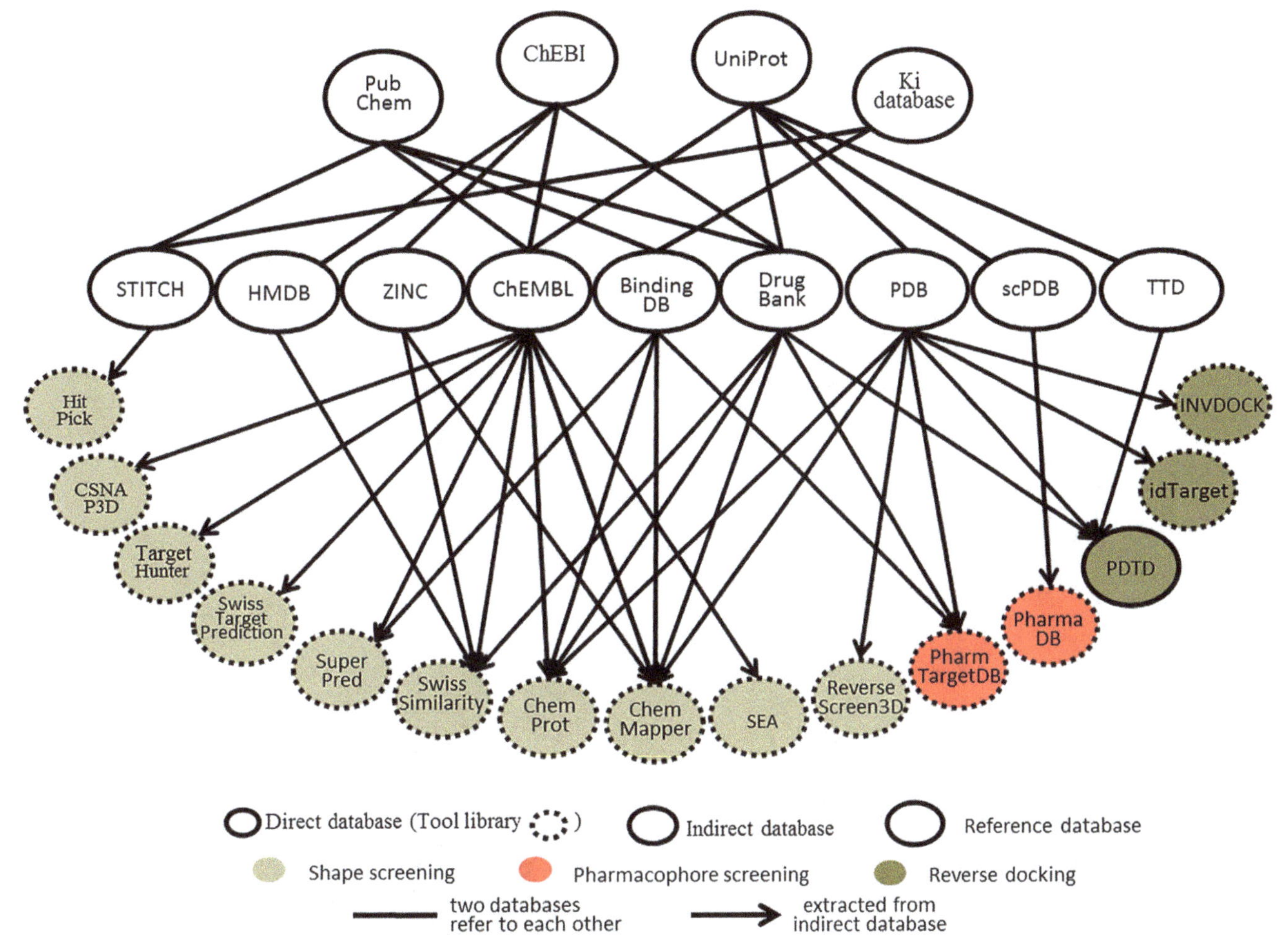

FIGURE 4 | The relationships among direct databases, indirect databases, and reference databases used in reverse screening.

databases "indirect databases" (shown in the middle layer of **Figure 4**), and examples include the PDB (Rose et al., 2015) and ZINC (Sterling and Irwin, 2015). The third class of databases can provide a large amount of information about ligands or proteins that can be used for reverse screening, but collecting and organizing the information from these databases to construct direct databases is difficult. However, we can use them to search for various information resources, such as additional targets, the bioactivities of matched molecules, or the signaling pathways of potential target proteins for further analysis of the reverse screening results. We call these databases "reference databases" (shown in the upper layer of **Figure 4**); examples include PubChem (Kim et al., 2016) and UniProt (Pundir et al., 2015). Relevant information on several direct databases used for reverse screening can be found in **Table 1**. In addition, information on indirect and reference databases, including the database coverage and website links, is listed in **Table 2**. In the following paragraphs, we provide a slightly more detailed introduction to these three classes of databases and their relationships with each other.

Direct Databases

Direct Databases Used in Shape Screening

Each online service for shape screening has its own in-house database, except ROCS (Rush et al., 2005), which requires users to prepare their own protein-annotated ligand databases (Mori et al., 2015). The database information for 12 shape-screening software programs is shown in the "coverage" column of **Table 1**. Among the 11 direct databases, TargetHunter, CSNAP3D and ReverseScreen3D do not give specific capacity data; for the former two, the information is not published, and the latter is noted only as updated with updates to the RCSB PDB, according to the literature (Kinnings and Jackson, 2011).

Figure 4 shows 10 direct databases with clear sources, including HitPick, CSNAP3D, TargetHunter, SwissTargetPrediction, SuperPred, SwissSimilarity, ChemProt, ChemMapper, SEA, and ReverseScreen3D. These databases are basically constructed by extracting data from indirect databases (**Figure 4**). For example, ChemMapper is built from several public databases, including ChEMBL (Gaulton et al., 2017), DrugBank (Law et al., 2014), BindingDB (Gilson et al.,

TABLE 2 | Characteristics of indirect and reference databases.

Database name	Aims	Coverage	Website	Last update
INDIRECT DATABASE				
STITCH	A database of known and predicted interactions between chemicals and proteins	9.6 million proteins, 0.5 million chemicals	http://stitch.embl.de/	2017
HMDB	A comprehensive, high-quality, freely accessible online database of small-molecule metabolites found in the human body	74,507 metabolite entries, 5,701 protein sequences linked to metabolite entries	http://www.hmdb.ca/	2017
ZINC	Database of commercially available compounds for virtual screening	>100 million purchasable compounds	http://zinc15.docking.org/	2015
ChEMBL	An open large-scale bioactivity database	2,101,843 compound records, 1,735,442 distinct compounds	https://www.ebi.ac.uk/chembl/	2017
BindingDB	Database of measured binding affinities	2037 FDA-approved small-molecule drugs, 241 FDA-approved biotech (protein/peptide) drugs, 96 nutraceuticals, >6000 experimental drugs	https://www.bindingdb.org/bind/index.jsp	2011
DrugBank	Database combining detailed drug data with comprehensive drug target information	8,261 drug entries, 4,338 non-redundant protein sequences	https://www.drugbank.ca/	2017
PDB	Crystal structures of macromolecules and ligands	133,093 macromolecular structures, 53,025 citations, 23,711 ligands	http://www.rcsb.org/pdb/home/home.do	2017
scPDB	Druggable binding sites from the PDB	9283 entries, 3678 proteins, 5608 ligands	http://bioinfo-pharma.u-strasbg.fr/scPDB/	2013
TTD	Information on therapeutic protein and nucleic acid targets, relevant diseases, pathway information and the corresponding drugs	2,589 targets, 31,614 drugs, 20,278 small molecules, 653 antisense drugs	http://bidd.nus.edu.sg/group/cjttd/	2011
REFERENCE DATABASE				
PubChem	Information on chemical substances and their biological activities	>235 million substance descriptions, 90 million unique chemical structures, 230 million bioactivity outcomes from over one million biological assay experiments	https://pubchem.ncbi.nlm.nih.gov/	2017
CHEBI	A database and ontology of molecular entities focused on "small" chemical compounds	>52,450 compounds	http://www.ebi.ac.uk/chebi/	2017
UniProt	Resource for protein sequences and functional information	Swiss-Prot (555,100), TrEMBL (88,032,926)	http://www.uniprot.org/	2017
PDSP Ki database	A unique resource in the public domain that provides information on the abilities of drugs to interact with an expanding number of molecular targets	60,231 annotated ligands	https://kidbdev.med.unc.edu/databases/kidb.php	2017

2016), KEGG (http://www.kegg.jp/kegg/) and the PDB. It collects bioactive targets and pharmacological information on small molecules, each of which has various pre-generated conformations for 3D similarity screening (Gong et al., 2013). ChemProt 3.0 (Kringelum et al., 2016) includes all chemical-protein interaction data from the available open source databases, including ChEMBL (version 19), BindingDB, the Psychoactive Drug Screening Program (PDSP) Ki database (Roth et al., 2000), and DrugBank, as well as clinical information from the Anatomical Therapeutic Chemical (ATC) Classification System (Wang Y. C. et al., 2013) and side effect data from Sider (Kuhn et al., 2016). The SwissSimilarity database gathers protein-annotated ligands mainly from four indirect databases, namely, HMDB (Wishart et al., 2009), ZINC, ChEMBL, and DrugBank, as well as from some reference databases, such as Chemical Entries of Biological Interest (ChEBI; Hastings et al., 2016). The SuperPred (Nickel et al., 2014) database consists of a large data set of ligand-target interactions from two indirect databases, ChEMBL and BindingDB. The CSNAP3D (Lo et al., 2016), Target Hunter (Wang L. et al., 2013), SwissTargetPrediction (Gfeller et al., 2014), and SEA (Keiser et al., 2007) databases are all constructed by taking ligands with protein target information from ChEMBL. The HitPick (Liu et al., 2013) database collects information from the STITCH database (Szklarczyk et al., 2015), and the information in ReverseScreen3D (Kinnings and Jackson, 2011) is extracted from the PDB database. In addition, the TarPred (Liu et al., 2015a) database, which is not shown in **Figure 4**, is a compound-target-disease database built by gathering information from the Comparative Toxicogenomics Database (CTD; Davis et al., 2017) and UniProt.

Direct Databases Used in Pharmacophore Screening

Two direct databases used for pharmacophore screening are shown in **Figure 4**. PharmTargetDB is the in-house database of the PharmMapper server (Liu et al., 2010), and PharmaDB (Meslamani et al., 2012) is the direct database deposited and used in Discovery Studio. Since these two databases are updated when the software updates, the different versions of PharmTargetDB and PharmaDB have different data capacities. The numbers of pharmacophore models in the newest versions are also shown in **Table 1**.

The pharmacophore models in PharmTargetDB are derived from the DrugBank, BindingDB, PDB, and PDTD databases. These models are built by extracting pharmacophore features within cavities by using the receptor-based pharmacophore modeling program Pocket 2.0 (Chen and Lai, 2006) after the binding sites of given protein structures are detected and ranked based on their druggability scores by using the software CAVITY (Yuan et al., 2013) for binding site detection (Wang X. et al., 2017). The original version of PharmTargetDB contained more than 7,000 pharmacophore models built from co-crystallized complex structures of protein targets (Liu et al., 2010). A new version of PharmMapper was published in 2017 (Wang X. et al., 2017), and the new PharmTargetDB is six times larger than the previous one, with a total of 23,236 proteins covering 51,431 pharmacophore models. PharmaDB is the pharmacodynamics database for Discovery Studio drug design software, and its pharmacophore models are constructed by using the Receptor-Ligand Pharmacophore Generation Protocol with default settings based on the binding information of ligand and protein complexes in the scPDB database. The original version of PharmaDB contained 68,056 pharmacophore models annotated with receptor information (Meslamani et al., 2012). The latest version of PharmaDB includes 140,000 pharmacophore models (BIOVIA, 2017), and users can utilize it in Discovery Studio to perform rapid reverse pharmacophore screening to search for protein targets of small molecules.

Direct Databases Used in Reverse Docking

The direct databases used in reverse docking are collections of target structure grids, which are usually generated from protein crystal structures by using docking programs or their auxiliary software tools. Before grid generation, the target crystal structures downloaded from the PDB must be preprocessed to remove ions and waters, add hydrogens and define the binding pocket. The original 3D protein structures can also be downloaded from some PDB derivative databases, such as the PDBbind-CN Database (Liu Z. et al., 2015), where all valid ligand-protein structures in the PDB are identified and collected.

PDTD, INVDOCK, and idTarget are the three direct databases used for reverse docking shown in **Figure 4**. Among them, PDTD is the only open database, and it can be downloaded as a compressed file, which is then decompressed as a collection of two types of structure files. The first type is the preprocessed protein structure file in the PDB and mol2 formats, and the second type is the active site structure file in PDB format. These two types of structure files for any PDB entry can be downloaded independently and viewed using the molecular visualization tool plug-in (Gao et al., 2008). Currently, this database contains more than 1,100 protein entries with 3D structures in the PDB and covers 841 diverse drug targets associated with diseases, biological functions, and signaling pathways (Gao et al., 2008). The binding (active) sites of these protein structures were defined by a data set of amino acid residues within 6.5 Å of the bound ligand (Gao et al., 2008). The INVDOCK and idTarget databases are not published but are the in-house databases of the corresponding programs. In addition, in contrast to the binding sites defined by the co-crystallized ligands in the PDTD, the binding sites in the INVDOCK and idTarget databases are generated from the available cavities by a search performed with spherical probes. The protein structures in these two databases also originate from the PDB. The INVDOCK in-house database, constructed in 2001, collects 9000 proteins and nucleic acid structures from the PDB database (Chen and Zhi, 2001). Each receptor structure grid in this database is constructed by first calculating the inward-facing surface covering the interface of van der Waals surfaces of the receptor crystal structure with a probe sphere 1.4 Å in radius. The binding site is then defined as the surrounding space within 15 Å of the center of the cavity formed by the combination of neighboring spheres covered by protein atoms in more than 50% of directions. Finally, grid generation is performed (Chen and Zhi, 2001). The idTarget database collects all protein structures in the PDB and is regularly updated when the PDB updates (Wang et al., 2012). The binding sites of each protein in the database are dynamically determined, and the grids are constructed by the "divide-and-conquer" method according to the size of the query molecule (Wang et al., 2012). Theoretically, idTarget could be the most extensive and complete database among the three for reverse docking.

Indirect Databases

Indirect databases are rich in ligand and target information and can be simply processed to build direct databases for reverse screening. Nine indirect databases are shown in the middle layer of **Figure 4**, and a brief introduction to these databases, including the coverage, update time and website link, is given in **Table 2**. Among these nine indirect databases, ZINC, ChEMBL, BindingDB, and DrugBank mainly include structural information on ligands and their target annotations, whereas the PDB, scPDB, and Therapeutic Target Database (TTD) mainly provide 3D structures of proteins with ligand binding information. The 15 direct and in-house software-associated databases used for reverse screening are essentially extracted or constructed from these indirect databases. These indirect databases are also extensively linked to reference databases. For example, DrugBank and ChEMBL have mutual data exchange with PubChem, ChEBI, and UniProt. BindingDB (Gilson et al., 2016) collects data from the PubChem and PDSP Ki databases. The scPDB and PDB share protein information with UniProt, including sequences and crystal structures. In addition, HMDB (Wishart et al., 2007) and ZINC share compound information with ChEBI, and the TTD database collects its information on therapeutic protein targets from UniProt.

Users can employ indirect databases to build their own databases when they use large commercial software suites for molecular drug design, such as Schrödinger and Discovery Studio, to perform reverse screening. For example, users can collect small molecules with explicit target annotation from the DrugBank, ChEMBL, and ZINC databases to construct a ligand database for shape screening. They can also use ligand-protein binding information from the BindingDB, scPDB, and PDB databases to build a pharmacophore model database for pharmacophore screening or a protein structure grid database for reverse docking. Notably, Ligand Expo (Feng et al., 2004) from the PDB can be easily used to build in-house program databases for shape or pharmacophore screening after non-ligand small molecules, including metal ions and solvent molecules, are removed. In addition, a collection of protein crystal structures downloaded from the PDB can be used to generate a protein structure grid database for reverse screening. In fact, we built our own databases for use in Schrödinger based on this Ligand Expo database and the protein structures in the PDB, and we then performed shape screening and reverse docking to search for the protein targets of several natural compounds (Kim et al., 2014; Lim et al., 2014; Wang Z. et al., 2016).

Reference Databases

Reference databases normally contain a very large amount of information on small-molecule compounds and proteins. However, extracting the rich information resources from these databases to establish direct databases for reverse screening can be difficult for users. Nevertheless, we can utilize these databases to search for additional information on the matched molecules and their potential protein targets from reverse screening results.

The four main reference databases, PubChem, ChEBI, PDSP Ki, and UniProt, which are closely associated with the nine indirect databases, are shown in the upper layer of **Figure 4**. A brief introduction to these four databases is also provided in **Table 2**. PubChem consists of three interrelated sub-databases: substances, compounds, and bioassays. The first two sub-databases provide information on the chemical structure and other properties of small molecules, and the sub-database of bioassays gives information on their pharmacological properties and biological targets (Kim et al., 2016). ChEBI is a freely available dictionary of molecular entities focused on "small" chemical compounds. ChEBI and ChEMBL are both sites of the European Molecular Biology Laboratories, and their data occasionally overlap. Compared with ChEMBL, ChEBI is more focused on "molecular entity" information, such as the chemical and biological roles and applications of a small molecule, rather than on biological target information (Hastings et al., 2013, 2016). The PDSP Ki database is a unique open resource that provides information on the ability of drugs to interact with increasing numbers of molecular targets. The key data in this database are the Ki activity data on ligands internally derived or from published articles, but it also includes information on protein-annotated ligand structures, protein-ligand affinities, and article sources (Roth et al., 2000). UniProt (Pundir et al., 2015) is a freely accessible resource of protein sequence and function information extracted from gene sequencing and published literature that undergoes quality assurance by curator-evaluated computational analysis (Poux et al., 2017).

The PubChem, ChEBI, UniProt, and Ki databases are the four major reference databases used by researchers. However, more reference databases containing information on proteins or ligands are available, and readers who are interested in learning about them can read two further database review papers authored by Zhang Y. et al. (2011) and Moura Barbosa and Del Rio (2012).

Applications

We reviewed nearly all articles on the applications of shape, pharmacophore screening and reverse docking in searching for the potential targets of small molecules published since 2000 and conducted a systematic analysis. In addition, we have provided slightly more detailed descriptions of some representative examples of the application of existing services to drug discovery. In reviewing these previous studies, we found two approaches to method application: the use of a single method and the use of combined methods. In general, shape screening, pharmacophore screening and reverse docking have all been successfully applied individually. However, these methods have their own limitations in terms of features and application scopes, as mentioned above. The majority of newer examples involve the combined application of multiple methods. Finally, it is noted that all the compounds as examples for illustration in this section are shown in **Figure 1**.

Shape Screening

Shape-screening services have a wide range of applications. **Table 3** shows 18 examples of the use of SEA, TargetHunter, ROCS, SwissTargetPrediction, etc. to perform shape screening for molecular target prediction. Here, even if an article involves several query molecules, we still present them as one example.

Reverse screening based on shape similarity has multiple types of applications. First, it is used to search for the targets of molecules from Chinese herbal medicine. For instance, using TargetHunter, Zhang et al. predicted human beta-1 adrenergic receptor (ADRB1) as the protein target of aconitine (compound **3**), an experimentally active component of Sini Decoction in the treatment of cardiovascular disease, and this prediction has been experimentally verified (Zhang H. et al., 2016). Shape screening is also helpful for drug repositioning and for clarifying the mechanisms of action of existing drugs. For example, Keiser et al. conducted shape screening using SEA to reposition 3,665 FDA-approved and investigational drugs, and they successfully predicted unintended targets of several drugs, such as the antagonism of the β1 receptor by the transporter inhibitor prozac (compound **4**), the inhibition of the 5-HT transporter by the ion channel drug vadilex (compound **5**), and the antagonism of the histamine H4 receptor by the enzyme inhibitor rescriptor (compound **6**; Keiser et al., 2009).

Pharmacophore Screening

Reverse screening based on pharmacophore modeling is also widely used to search for the targets of components of various Chinese traditional medicines. **Table 4** shows 27 examples of the use of PharmMapper and Discovery Studio to perform pharmacophore screening for the prediction of molecular targets.

For example, Liu et al. used PharmMapper to predict p38, glucocorticoid receptor (GR) and dihydroorotate dehydrogenase (DHODH) as potential targets of berberine (BBR, compound 7) and further elucidated the possible molecular mechanisms by which these protein targets participate in the anti-melanoma activity of BBR (Liu et al., 2017). Lei et al. employed the Pharmacophore module of Discovery Studio 3.5 in reverse screening and found that the isoquinoline alkaloids (such as compound **8**) extracted from Macleaya cordata (Bo Luo Hui) might target macrophage migration inhibitory factor (MIF), potentially leading to the broad-spectrum antitumor effects of the plant (Lei et al., 2015).

Reverse Docking

Reverse screening based on molecular docking is widely used to search for the targets of small molecules to elucidate their mechanisms of action. **Tables 5**, **6** show 25 and 20 examples with and without experimental validation, respectively, of the application of reverse docking to the prediction of molecular targets by using TarFisDock, idTarget, INVDOCK, and conventional virtual screening software such as DOCK, MDock, and AutoDock.

For example, several research groups used INVDOCK to predict that p53 (Lu et al., 2010), calmodulin (CaM; Ma et al., 2013), annexin A5 (ANXA5) and heat shock protein family A member 8 (HSPA8; Lu et al., 2012) might be protein targets of the broad-spectrum anticancer drug BBR (compound 7).

TABLE 3 | Applications of shape screening in predicting protein targets of small molecules.

Query molecule	Target information	Reverse screening tool	References
EXPERIMENTALLY VERIFIED			
Prozac[1], Vadilex[2], Rescriptor[3]	β1 receptor[1], 5-HT transporter[2], HRH4[3]	SEA	Keiser et al., 2009
Wuweizi (compound 11/12)	GBA3[11,12], SHBG[11,12]	SEA	Wang et al., 2015
Lignan	5-HT1AR	SEA	Zheng et al., 2015
Plumbagin	TrxR, GR'	SEA	Hwang et al., 2015
Obacunone	MIF	SEA	Gao et al., 2018
5-aza-dC	HDM2	SuperPred	Putri et al., 2017
Sini decoction (aconitine[1], liquiritin[2], 6-gingerol[3])	ADRB1[1], ACE[2], HMGCR[1,3]	TargetHunter	Zhang H. et al., 2016
Salvinorin A*	OPRK, CB1, CB2, DRD2	TargetHunter	Xu et al., 2016b
NOT EXPERIMENTALLY VERIFIED			
NBP	NQO1, IDO, NADH-ubiquinone oxidoreductase	SEA	Wang Y. et al., 2017
Quinoline derivative (83b1)	PPARδ	SEA	Pun et al., 2017
Tributyltin (Ch-409)	RamC	SwissTargetPrediction	Waseem et al., 2017
Xeronine	Adr A3, TDP1, muscleblind-like proteins 1	SwissTargetPrediction	Sanni et al., 2017
KNOWN TARGETS COMPUTATIONALLY VERIFIED			
Methadone[1], emetine[2], loperamide[3]	Muscarinic M3[1], α2 adrenergic[2], NK2 receptors[3]	SEA	Keiser et al., 2007
CID 46907796	Nrf2	TargetHunter	Wang L. et al., 2013
Chlorotrianisene	COX-1, ESR1	SwissTargetPrediction	Gfeller et al., 2014
Entecavir	POLB	TarPred	Liu et al., 2015a
Taxol mimetics	Tubulin	CSNAP3D	Lo et al., 2016
Caffeine	D2R	ChemProt	Kringelum et al., 2016

**Target prediction confirmed by the literature. Superscript values denotes that the protein targets in the second column correspond to the query molecules in the first column respectively.*

TABLE 4 | Applications of pharmacophore screening in predicting protein targets of small molecules.

Query molecule	Target information	Reverse screening tools	References
EXPERIMENTALLY VERIFIED			
CT	MAP2K1	PharmMapper	Yuan et al., 2014
Arctigenin	PDK1	PharmMapper	Fang et al., 2015
HSYA	XO	PharmMapper	Xu et al., 2016a
ZYZ-488	Apaf-1	PharmMapper	Wang Y. et al., 2016
NCI 748494/1	c-Met kinase	PharmMapper	El-Wakil et al., 2017
UA	CASP-3, JNK2, ERK1	PharmMapper	Ma et al., 2017
BBR	GR, p38, DHODH	PharmMapper	Liu et al., 2017
5,7-dihydroxy-4′-methoxy-8-prenylflavanone	AChE	PharmMapper	Das et al., 2017
Phytoestrogens (genistein[1], daidzein[2], secoisolariciresinol[3])	AKR1B1[1], H-Ras[2], GSTP1[3]	PharmMapper	Dutta et al., 2017
NOT EXPERIMENTALLY VERIFIED			
MCDF	GR	PharmMapper	Chitrala and Yeguvapalli, 2014
Capsaicin	CA2	PharmMapper	Ye et al., 2015
SID 242078875	DPP-IV, PTP1B, PEPCK, GSK-3B, GK	PharmMapper	Krishnasamy and Muthusamy, 2016
Flavanoid analogs	CDK2	PharmMapper	Simon et al., 2017
Chalcones and chalcone-like compounds	Cysteine proteases	PharmMapper	Gomes et al., 2017
16E-arylideno-nitrogen mustard hybrids(3/4)	GRs	PharmMapper	Acharya et al., 2018
Components of CO	ESR1, ESR2, HSD11B1, cortisone reductase	PharmMapper	Wang N. et al., 2017
N-substituted tetrahydro-β-carboline imidazolium salt derivatives	MEK-1	PharmMapper	Liang et al., 2017
ASC	AKR1B1, ALB, AR, BACE1, CDK2, F2	PharmMapper	Zeng et al., 2017a
GFW compounds	F2, MMP3, CA2, AKR1B, CDK2	PharmMapper	Zeng et al., 2017b
Thiadiazole compounds	c-Met	PharmMapper	Meshram et al., 2017
Components in SFJD	Multi-targets in ERK pathway	PharmMapper	Li et al., 2017
Isoquinoline alkaloids	MIF, ZipA-FtsZ, GAPDH, etc.	Discovery Studio 3.5	Lei et al., 2015
Six GTs	GCN5, CDK2	Discovery Studio 4.0	Shao et al., 2016
Pinctada fucata oligopeptide	5HT2A, BACE-1	Discovery Studio	Chen et al., 2017
KOWN TARGETS COMPUTATIONALLY VERIFIED			
Tamoxifen	ERRγ	PharmMapper	Liu et al., 2010
S-adenosyl-L-homocysteine	Modification methylase TaqI	PharmMapper	Wang X. et al., 2016
Kanamycin	APH(2′)-Iva	PharmMapper	Wang X. et al., 2017

**Target prediction confirmed by the literature. Superscript values denotes that the protein targets in the second column correspond to the query molecules in the first column respectively.*

Zhang et al. employed TarFisDock in the reverse docking of 19 compounds extracted from the traditional Chinese medicines Bacopa monnieri (L.) Wettst and Daphne odora Thunb. Var. Marginata, and they concluded that five of the compounds (such as compound **9**) might target dipeptidyl peptidase IV (DPP-IV), thus accounting for the effectiveness of these medicines in the treatment of diabetes and their anti-inflammatory effects (Zhang S. et al., 2011). Scafuri et al. (2016) applied idTarget to predict that the proteins guanosine triphosphatase (GTPase), guanosine 5′-monophosphate oxidoreductase (GMP reductase) and hypoxanthine-guanine phosphoribosyltransferase (HGPRT) might be key targets of apple polyphenols (such as compound **10** and **11**), resulting in their cancer-preventive effects. Grinter et al. used MDock to fish for the protein targets of the compound PRIMA-1 (compound **12**) in the PDTD database and discovered that PRIMA-1 could inhibit the cholesterol synthetic pathway by directly binding with oxidosqualene cyclase (OSC), considerably reducing the viability of BT-474 and T47-D breast cancer cells (Grinter et al., 2011).

Hybrid Applications

The combinations of methods include shape screening with reverse docking, shape screening with pharmacophore screening, pharmacophore screening with reverse docking, and the combination of all three methods. **Table 7** shows 22 examples of the use of these four combinations to predict molecular targets.

Eight target prediction examples were performed by combining shape similarity and molecular docking. Kozielewicz et al. employed ReverseScreen3D and TarFisDock to predict the targets of oxindole pentacyclic alkaloids (such as compound **13**) and found that the biological ability of these compounds to induce cancer cell apoptosis may potentially involve the inhibition of several important targets, including dihydrofolate reductase (DHFR) and mouse double minute 2 homolog

TABLE 5 | Applications of reverse docking in predicting protein targets of small molecules with experimental verification.

Query molecule	Target information	Reverse screening tools	References
Triptonide[1], triptolide[2], triptriolide[3]	ERα[1,2,3]	AutoDock 4.2	Liu et al., 2015b
c-di-GMP	Human LCN2 protein	DOCK 6	Li et al., 2015
Derivatives of indirubin (6BIO)	PDK1	GlamDock	Zahler et al., 2007
DAPH	Hexokinase	GOLD	Da Matta et al., 2015
Apple polyphenols	GMP reductase, GTPase H-ras, HGPRT	idTarget	Scafuri et al., 2016
Anti-HIV drugs (Pis, NRTIs)*	POLB, TOP1, etc.	INVDOCK	Ji et al., 2006
Analgesics*	ErbB-2, PLA2, GSH-S	INVDOCK	Pan et al., 2014
GAD	EphA7, EB1, PRDX3	INVDOCK	Yue et al., 2008
BBR	p53	INVDOCK	Lu et al., 2010
SB	EGFR	INVDOCK	Feng et al., 2011
BBR	HSPA8, ANXA5	INVDOCK	Lu et al., 2012
AGS-IV	CN, ACE, JNK	INVDOCK	Zhao et al., 2012
SB*	ACE, REN	INVDOCK	Ye et al., 2012
WB	CDK2, PAK4, BRaf1	INVDOCK	Zhang et al., 2013
BBR	CaM	INVDOCK	Ma et al., 2013
Ophiobolin O	GSK3β	INVDOCK	Lv et al., 2015
PRIMA-1	OSC	Mdock	Grinter et al., 2011
Meranzin	COX1, COX2, PPARγ	SELNERGY	Do et al., 2007
Tofisopam	PDE4	SELNERGY	Bernard et al., 2008
Anti-*Helicobacter pylori* drugs (compound 1/2)	HpPDF[1,2]	TarFisDock	Cai et al., 2006
[6]-gingerol	LTA4H	TarFisDock	Jeong et al., 2009
5 of 19 natural products	DPP-IV	TarFisDock	Zhang S. et al., 2011
Bezafibrate	CDK2	TarFisDock	Liu et al., 2015c
Bicyclol	IMPDHII	TarFisDock	Zhang Y. W. et al., 2016
Esculentoside A	CK2	TarFisDock	Li Y. et al., 2016

**Target prediction confirmed by the literature. Superscript values denotes that the protein targets in the second column correspond to the query molecules in the first column respectively.*

(MDM2; Kozielewicz et al., 2014). The combination of shape screening and pharmacophore screening has been applied in three instances to predict molecular targets. Biplab Bhattacharjee and Jhinuk Chatterjee used PharmMapper and ReverseScreen3D to perform reverse screening and demonstrated that eucalyptol (compound **14**), the effective component of cardamom, might target CASP-3 and cAMP-dependent protein kinase (PKA), resulting in its anti-apoptosis, anti-inflammation, anti-proliferation, anti-invasion and anti-angiogenesis activities in cancer prevention (Bhattacharjee and Chatterjee, 2013). The combination of pharmacophore modeling and reverse docking has been used most frequently to predict the targets of small molecules, as shown by the 10 applications given in **Table 7**. For example, Ge et al. used PharmMapper and idTarget in reverse screening and predicted that dihydropyrimidine dehydrogenase (DPD) and human spindle checkpoint kinase Bub1 were the potential unintended or secondary targets of the antithrombotic agent dipyridamole (DIP, compound **15**), resulting in its anti-cancer activity (Ge et al., 2016). Finally, one application combined all three methods for reverse screening. Gao et al. used the Pharmacophore Modeling and Docking modules in Schrödinger as well as RerverseScreen3D jointly to predict molecular targets and found that baicalein (compound **16**), an anti-Parkinson disease drug, played a protective role in the nervous system by targeting catechol-O-methyltransferase (COMT) and monoamine oxidase B (MAO-B); these targets were confirmed experimentally (Gao et al., 2013).

DISCUSSION

Comparison of the Applications of the Three Types of Reverse Screening Software and Online Services in the Prediction of Small-Molecule Targets

To provide a better understanding of the application of reverse screening for small-molecule target prediction, we collected as many reverse screening tools and databases as possible, most of which have been updated since 2016 (**Tables 1**, **2**). In addition, we counted the number of applications of these three methods since 2000, the number of applications of their representative software programs, and the application trends over the years. All information is shown in **Tables 3–7** and **Figures 5A,B**.

Different types of reverse screening tools have characteristic features. Many software programs and online services are based on shape similarity, and they have a rich supply of ligand databases. These shape screening tools have rapidly updated in-house databases, can screen large chemical databases rapidly, and therefore can be used for large-scale preliminary reverse screening. Although shape-screening methods have the smallest number of applications, a slow upward trend is evident in recent years (**Figure 5A**). Notably, few studies have applied TarPred, SwissSimilarity, and ChemMapper. The main software and online services based on pharmacophore modeling are PharmMapper and Discovery Studio, each with its own

TABLE 6 | Applications of reverse docking in predicting protein targets of small molecules without experimental verification.

Query molecule	Target information	Reverse screening tool	Reference
NOT EXPERIMENTALLY VERIFIED			
Tea polyphenols	LTA4 hydrolase	Autodock, TarFisDock	Zheng et al., 2011
4 compounds	PBP4	Autodock Vina	Sarangi et al., 2015
Lenalidomide	VEGFR-2, erbB-3, FGFR-4, ABL, p38MAPK, MMP-3	Autodock	Hu et al., 2017
Torcetrapib	PDGFR, HGFR, IL-2, ErbB1	Discovery Studio	Fan et al., 2012
Melamine and cyanuric acid	GPX1, HEXB, LDH, lys C	INVDOCK	Ma et al., 2011
PAs	GSTA1, GPX1	INVDOCK	Yan et al., 2016
Icariin	PI3K, AChE	INVDOCK	Cui et al., 2016
Dioscin	TOP1	MDock	Yin et al., 2015
Ginsenosides	MEK1, EGFR, thrombin, Aurora A	Schrödinger	Park and Cho, 2017
TCDD	MMP8, MMP3, OSC, MPO	TarFisDock	Oliveroverbel et al., 2010
Ganoderic acid	HIV-1 proteasein	TarFisDock	Akbar and Yam, 2011
Fullerene derivatives	HPRT, BACE1	TarFisDock	Gupta et al., 2011
Alpha lipoic acid	LTA4 hydrolase, VGKC	TarFisDock	Maldonado-Rojas, 2011
Aryl-aminopyridine derivatives	CDK2, aurora kinase, KIT receptor	TarFisDock	Erić et al., 2012
KNOWN TARGETS COMPUTATIONALLY VERIFIED			
4-HT, vitamin E	ER, GST	INVDOCK	Chen and Zhi, 2001
ASA[1], gentamicin[2], ibuprofen[3], IDV[4], neomycin[5], penicillin G[6], 4-HT[7], vitamin C[8]	Antithrombin[1], CA1[2,5], SULT1E1[3], IFABP[4], GST[6], ADH[7], alphaamylase[8]	INVDOCK	Chen and Ung, 2001
Biotin[1], 4-HT[2], HDPR[3], methotrexate[4]	Streptavidin[1], ERa[2], ADA[3], DHFR[4]	GOLD	Paul et al., 2004
ε-viniferin	PDE4	SELNERGY	Do et al., 2005
Vitamin E[1], 4-HT[2]	AChE[1], DHFR[2]	TarFisDock	Li et al., 2006
DRV[1], 6BIO[2], N-(4-aminobiphenyl-3-yl)-benzamide[3]	HDAC2[1], HIV-1 PR[2], CDK2[3]	idTarget	Wang et al., 2012

**Target prediction confirmed by the literature. Superscript values denotes that the protein targets in the second column correspond to the query molecules in the first column respectively.*

pharmacophore database. PharmMapper is a free online service, whereas Discovery Studio is commercial software, leading to more widespread use of PharmMapper. Among the three reverse screening methods, pharmacophore modeling has the fewest applications before 2016 (**Figures 5A,B**), but its application exhibited a significantly escalating trend in 2017 (**Figures 5A,B**). The reverse docking method has been applied the most; however, the applications of reverse docking have shown a downward trend in recent years. The possible reasons are that some online services, such as TarFisDock, have undergone limited expansion of the existing protein crystal structure grid database, while others, such as idTarget, have a long computational time and high computational cost. **Figure 5A** also illustrates the trend of the practical applications of hybrid methods, with a slow rise in the use of combinations of multiple reverse screening methods for target prediction in recent years.

In addition, we downloaded from PubChem or sketched in Schrödinger the structures of 57 small-molecule ligands whose targets were predicted by reverse screening and further verified experimentally, as reported in these application articles. We used the Cluster Analysis Module in Schrödinger via the two-tiered drop-down menu of Maestro's Scripts/Cheminformatics/Clustering of Ligands and a pop-up window titled Clustering based on Volume Overlap to conduct a cluster analysis of these small molecules. **Figure 6** shows representative compounds in the 28 clusters we obtained. Their targets were predicted separately by shape screening, pharmacophore screening and reverse docking. By comparing the structures of these molecules, we may be able to summarize some rules regarding the application ranges of each type of method according to the structures of the query molecules. For example, shape screening may be suitable for a query molecule whose structure shows stereoscopic sense even in a two-dimensional structural view and that is neither very large nor very small (Compounds **3** and **17–23**). Pharmacophore screening is appropriate for query molecules whose structures contain diverse pharmacophore functional groups with a good balance between them (compounds **24–30**). Reverse docking is suitable for the most diverse range of query molecules (compounds **31–39**). We hope that this type of cluster analysis can provide some guidance for the effective use of reverse screening to predict small-molecule targets in the future.

Deficiencies in Current Reverse Screening Methods and Potential Solutions

Each reverse screening tool has its own characteristics and appropriate application scope in terms of principle, algorithm and program. However, we need to know the application scopes of these tools in order to select the most appropriate software for making accurate predictions. Thus, a horizontal comparison can provide a better understanding of the advantages and

TABLE 7 | Applications of hybrid screening in predicting protein targets of small molecules.

Query molecule	Target information	Method	Reverse screening tool	References
EXPERIMENTALLY VERIFIED				
Rosemary components (carnosol,CA,UA,RA)*	CDK2, MAPK-14, AR', PPARγ	RD&PS	PharmMapper, idTarget	Deshmukh et al., 2013
DIP*	DPD, Bub1	RD&PS	PharmMapper, idTarget	Ge et al., 2016
Magnaporthe oryzae inhibitor C1	CYP450, NMT, GS, CHS	RD&PS	PharmMapper, TarFisDock	Chen et al., 2016
SAA*	AR	RD&PS	DRAR-CPI, PharmMapper	Chen and Cui, 2017
Curcumin	CDK2	RD&SS	Schrödinger	Lim et al., 2014
Naproxen	PI 3-K	RD&SS	Schrödinger	Kim et al., 2014
GV2–20	CA2	RD&SS	ROCS, AutoDock	Mori et al., 2015
Kinetin	Chitinase	RD&SS	idTarget, ReverseScreen3D	Kumar et al., 2015
Glabridin	Braf, MEK1/2	RD&SS	Schrödinger	Wang Z. et al., 2016
Macrocyclic amidinoureas	Chitinase	RD&SS	ROCS, OEDocking	Maccari et al., 2017
α-FMH	GST	PS&SS	PharmMapper, ReverseScreen3D	Considine et al., 2017
Baicalein	COMT, MAO-B	RD&PS&SS	Schrödinger, ReverseScreen3D	Gao et al., 2013
NOT EXPERIMENTALLY VERIFIED				
Saffron bioactive ingredients (picrocrocin)	HSP 90-α	RD&PS	PharmMapper, idTarget	Bhattacharjee et al., 2012
Danshensu	GTPase Hras	RD&PS	PharmMapper, idTarget	Chen and Ren, 2014
Tanshinone IIA	RARα	RD&PS	PharmMapper, AutoDock Vina	Chen, 2014
2-thiazolylimino-5-benzylidin-thiazolidin-4-one	COX2, AChE, AR, THRα	RD&PS	PharmMapper, TarFisDock	Iyer et al., 2015
Glycopentalone	CDK-2, VEGFR-2	RD&PS	AutoDock4.2, PharmMapper	Gurung et al., 2016
PGS[1], PLMF1[2], 67DiOHC8S[3]	GSTA1[1], PTPNT1[2,3], CBS[3]	RD&PS	PharmMapper, DRAR-CPI	Pereira et al., 2017
Oxindole pentacyclic alkaloids	DHFR, MDM2	RD&SS	TarFisDock, ReverseScreen3D	Kozielewicz et al., 2014
Quercetin	PARP1	RD&SS	SHAFTS, idTarget	Carvalho et al., 2017
Cardamom bioactive components (eucalyptol)	CASP-3, PKA	PS&SS	PharmMapper, ReverseScreen3D	Bhattacharjee and Chatterjee, 2013
Amai alkaloid and pyridine derivatives in maca	AR', CA2, ERα, MAPK14, etc.	PS&SS	Discovery Studio4.5	Yi et al., 2016

**Target prediction confirmed by the literature. Superscript values denotes that the protein targets in the second column correspond to the query molecules in the first column respectively.*

disadvantages of these reverse screening tools and their in-house databases. Some clear deficiencies are present in the programs and in-house databases of current reverse screening tools, making a comparison of the efficiency or the accuracy of target prediction by these tools difficult. None of the online services has a general interface module that can be used to upload and recognize user databases. Because these tools cannot use external databases, evaluating the methods or services based on benchmark databases is infeasible. However, researchers may be able to test the pros and cons of these tools in a way that does not require a benchmark database: we may not need to know the superiority of these tools over each other but may instead need to learn their practical uses and application scopes so that they can be better applied in real-life practice. This comparison requires studies to select some benchmarking query compounds whose known targets represent a large category and whose secondary targets or non-targets have also been studied thoroughly. We can use evaluation indexes such as the enrichment factor and receiver operating characteristic (ROC) curve (Truchon and Bayly, 2007) to assess the practical effects of reverse screening tools on the prediction of targets within this large category for other small molecules, thus achieving a horizontal comparison of existing software and online services. This theory is not yet perfected, and successful examples of this approach remain lacking, but it may provide prospects for developing assessments of reverse screening methods and tools.

Moreover, reverse screening servers also lack general-type databases, and their in-house databases are not publicized. We cannot learn the inclusion and exclusion criteria for building these direct databases. Almost all direct databases are bound to the corresponding software, and we are unable to conduct potential data mining. The resources of different online services are also undisclosed, and the services cannot refer to each other's databases. Hence, we encourage the developers of all software and online services to disclose their own databases and their construction processes to facilitate user comprehension and utilization. Only in this way can these software databases be better applied in practice, and this approach could also promote the production of more excellent protein-annotated ligand or target structure grid databases for reverse screening.

Previous Reviews and Prospective Studies on Reverse Screening in Molecular Target Prediction

To date, five reviews of reverse screening are available in the literature, which we will discuss briefly below. Readers can also peruse these reviews to deepen their understanding of molecule target prediction algorithms. We will not address other reviews that involve the use of experimental methods or a combination of computational and experimental methods to predict molecular targets (Schenone et al., 2013).

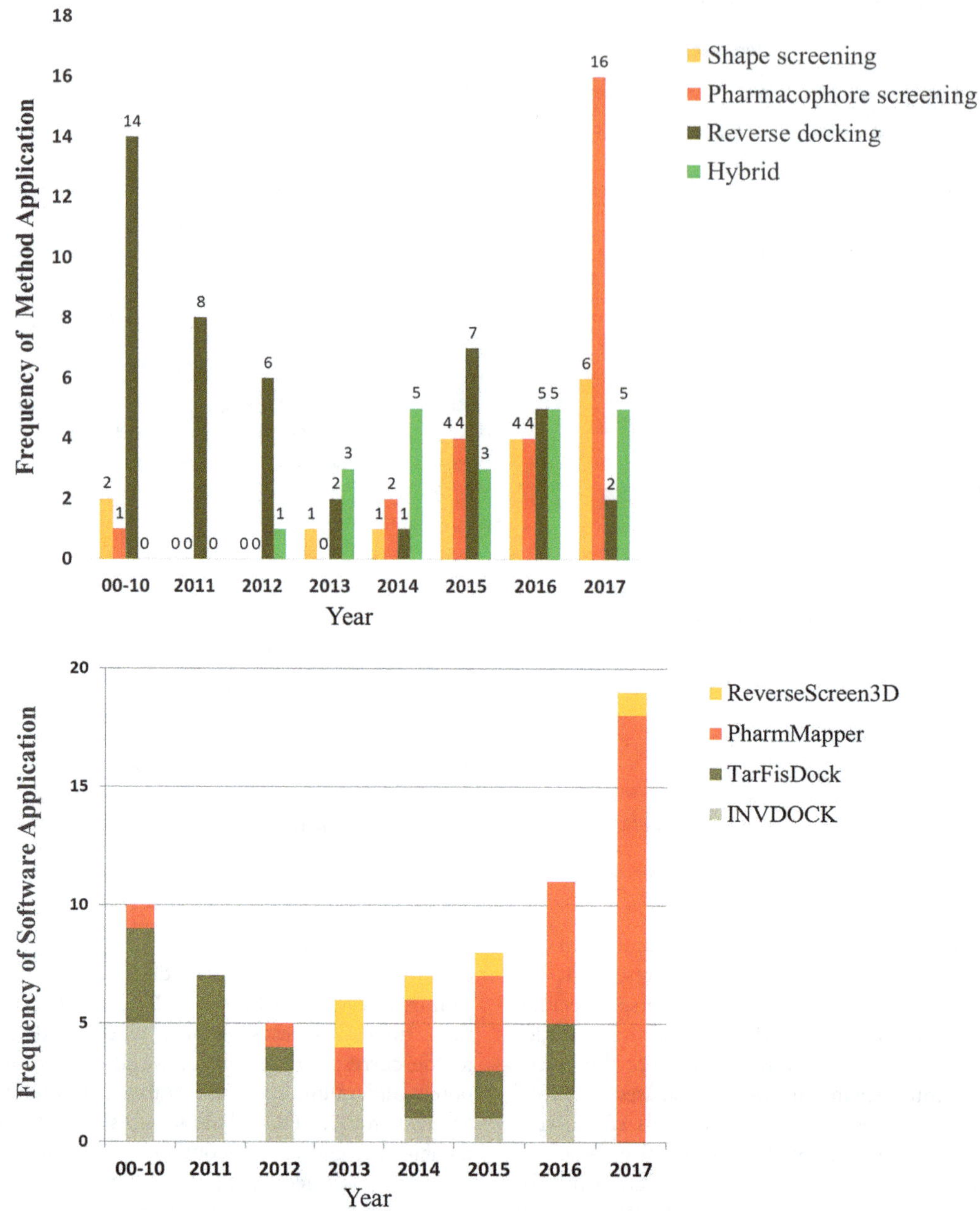

FIGURE 5 | The number and trend of applications using the three reverse screening methods and representative software since the year 2000.

Three of the five reviews are similar to our work and provide broad overviews of in silico target fishing. They describe the principles, databases and software involved in computer-aided small-molecule target prediction in terms of different aspects, perspectives and levels (Rognan, 2010; Zheng et al., 2013; Cereto-Massagué et al., 2015). Cereto-Massagué et al. (2015) categorize the methods of target fishing into four classes according to computational principles: molecular similarity methods, protein structure-based methods, data mining/machine learning methods, and methods based on the analysis of bioactivity spectra. Our review covers the principles and applications of the first two classes, molecular similarity and protein structure, but does not address the latter two categories of machine learning and bioactivity spectra. Therefore, readers can review the article by Cereto-Massagué et al. carefully if they are interested in the calculation methods used in those latter two categories. Rognan et al. (Rognan, 2010) describe only protein structure-based approaches and further classify them into protein-ligand docking, structure-based pharmacophore searches, binding site similarity measurements, and protein-ligand fingerprints. Based on the principle of receptor structure-based screening, the authors describe these four sub-methods in detail and discuss their pros and cons for target fishing and ligand profiling. That review features descriptions of protein pocket similarity

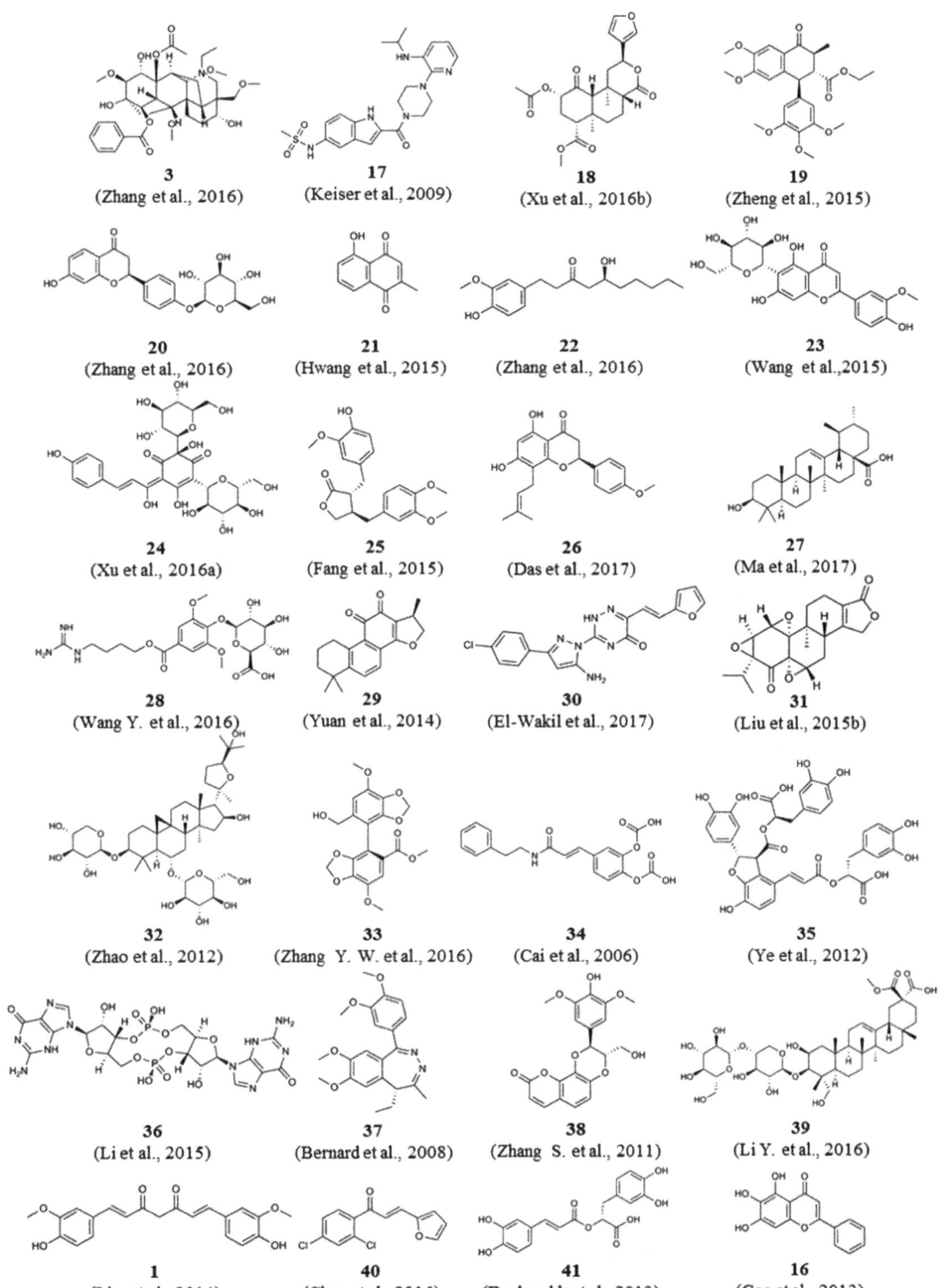

FIGURE 6 | Twenty-eight representative compounds obtained by the clustering of 57 bioactive compounds for target prediction by different reverse screening methods.

matching and the molecular fingerprinting of protein-ligand interaction information, which is worth reading and comparing to our paper. In addition, Zheng et al. (2013) provide a comprehensive overview of computer-aided drug design methods, including conventional (forward) virtual screening and reverse screening, in terms of five aspects: drug target prediction, drug repositioning, protein-ligand interaction, virtual screening and lead optimization, and ADME/T (absorption, distribution, metabolism, excretion, and toxicity) property prediction. The three reverse screening methods we reviewed are closely related to drug target prediction, drug repositioning and protein-ligand interaction. The above review can help readers systematically study and understand the field of computer-aided virtual screening in drug design.

The other two reviews address only reverse docking and its applications. Specifically, Kharkar et al. (2014) give a detailed description of reverse docking programs and their target databases and further discuss the applications of reverse docking in target identification and the prediction of target functions and off-target effects. Lee et al. (2016) summarize target databases, software programs and services and discuss the application of reverse docking in small-molecule target recognition and drug discovery. They also professionally discuss four issues related to reverse docking that remain to be solved: the standardization of database construction, the inclusion of receptor flexibility, the time-consuming nature of flexible receptor docking, and the inaccuracy of binding free energy calculations and ligand binding pose prediction. Readers may refer to these two reviews for a more comprehensive understanding of reverse docking methods.

CONCLUSION

In this review article, based on previous studies, we selected the three most commonly used types of reverse screening methods, i.e., methods based on shape similarity, pharmacophore modeling and molecular docking, and provided a detailed and comprehensive introduction, including a description of the principles underlying each method and a systematic classification of software, online services, and databases. In addition, we collected nearly all the articles related to the application of computer-aided target reverse screening prediction published since 2000 and analyzed the possible relationships or correlations between compound structures and screening methods by using cluster analysis. The purpose of this review is to help readers quickly understand these three methods and the characteristics of the software and online services based on these methods, to familiarize readers with the status and applications of the different levels of ligand and protein databases used in reverse screening and to provide a better understanding of how existing tools can be applied to molecule target prediction. We strongly believe that more accurate predictions resulting from the familiarity of users with the existing online services and databases will increase the importance of reverse screening in drug repositioning and future research on the pharmacodynamics and pharmacological mechanisms of bioactive compounds.

AUTHOR CONTRIBUTIONS

HH, GZ, YZ, CL, SC, YL, and SM: Information retrieval and analysis and reverse tools identification and classification; HH, GZ, LC, YL, and ZH: Database classification; HH, GZ, YZ, and ZH: Reference classification; HH, GZ, YZ, LC, SC, YL, SM, and ZH: Manuscript writing; HH, GZ, and ZH: Manuscript revision; HH, GZ, SC, YL, and ZH: Figure processing and table processing; HH, GZ, CL, and ZH: Cluster analysis; ZH: Manuscript guidance, communication work, and financial support.

ACKNOWLEDGMENTS

This work was supported by the National Natural Science Foundation of China (31770774), the Natural Science Foundation of Guangdong Province, China (2015A030313518), the Provincial Major Project of Basic or Applied Research in Natural Science, Guangdong Provincial Education Department (2016KZDXM038), and the 2013 Sail Plan The Introduction of the Shortage of Top-Notch Talent Project (YueRenCaiBan [2014] 1). We also thank American Journal Experts (AJE) for their help in revising English language.

REFERENCES

Acharya, P. C., Bansal, R., and Kharkar, P. S. (2018). Hybrids of steroid and nitrogen mustard as antiproliferative agents: synthesis, *in vitro* evaluation and *in silico* inverse screening. *Drug Res.* 68, 100–103. doi: 10.1055/s-0043-118538

Akbar, R., and Yam, W. K. (2011). Interaction of ganoderic acid on HIV related target: molecular docking studies. *Bioinformation* 7:413. doi: 10.6026/97320630007413

Allen, W. J., Balius, T. E., Mukherjee, S., Brozell, S. R., Moustakas, D. T., Lang, P. T., et al. (2015). DOCK 6: impact of new features and current docking performance. *J. Comput. Chem.* 36, 1132–1156. doi: 10.1002/jcc.23905

Armstrong, M. S., Morris, G. M., Finn, P. W., Sharma, R., Moretti, L., Cooper, R. I., et al. (2010). ElectroShape: fast molecular similarity calculations incorporating shape, chirality and electrostatics. *J. Comput. Aided Mol. Des.* 24, 789–801. doi: 10.1007/s10822-010-9374-0

Awale, M., and Reymond, J. L. (2014). A multi-fingerprint browser for the ZINC database. *Nucleic Acids Res.* 42, W234–W239. doi: 10.1093/nar/gku379

Bender, A., Mussa, H. Y., Glen, R. C., and Reiling, S. (2004). Molecular similarity searching using atom environments, information-based feature selection, and a naive Bayesian classifier. *J. Chem. Inf. Comput. Sci.* 44, 170–178. doi: 10.1021/ci034207y

Bernard, P., Dufresne-Favetta, C., Favetta, P., Do, Q. T., Himbert, F., Zubrzycki, S., et al. (2008). Application of drug repositioning strategy to TOFISOPAM. *Curr. Med. Chem.* 15, 3196–3203. doi: 10.2174/092986708786848488

Bhattacharjee, B., and Chatterjee, J. (2013). Identification of proapoptopic, anti-inflammatory, anti- proliferative, anti-invasive and anti-angiogenic targets of essential oils in cardamom by dual reverse virtual screening and binding pose analysis. *Asian Pac. J. Cancer Prev.* 14, 3735–3742. doi: 10.7314/APJCP.2013.14.6.3735

Bhattacharjee, B., Vijayasarathy, S., Karunakar, P., and Chatterjee, J. (2012). Comparative reverse screening approach to identify potential anti-neoplastic targets of saffron functional components and binding mode. *Asian Pac. J. Cancer Prev.* 13, 5605–5611. doi: 10.7314/APJCP.2012.13.11.5605

BIOVIA (2017). *Discovery Studio Modeling Environment, Release 2017.* San Diego, CA: Dassault Systèmes

Cai, J., Han, C., Hu, T., Zhang, J., Wu, D., Wang, F., et al. (2006). Peptide deformylase is a potential target for anti-*Helicobacter pylori* drugs: reverse docking, enzymatic assay, and X-ray crystallography validation. *Protein Sci.* 15, 2071–2081. doi: 10.1110/ps.062238406

Carvalho, D., Paulino, M., Polticelli, F., Arredondo, F., Williams, R. J., and Abincarriquiry, J. A. (2017). Structural evidence of quercetin multi-target bioactivity: a reverse virtual screening strategy. *Eur. J. Pharm. Sci.* 106, 393–403. doi: 10.1016/j.ejps.2017.06.028

Cereto-Massagué, A., Ojeda, M. J., Valls, C., Mulero, M., Pujadas, G., and Garcia-Vallve, S. (2015). Tools for *in silico* target fishing. *Methods* 71, 98–103. doi: 10.1016/j.ymeth.2014.09.006

Chang, D. T., Oyang, Y. J., and Lin, J. H. (2005). MEDock: a web server for efficient prediction of ligand binding sites based on a novel optimization algorithm. *Nucleic Acids Res.* 33, W233–W238. doi: 10.1093/nar/gki586

Chen, H., Wang, X., Hong, J., Rui, L., and Hou, T. (2016). Discovery of the molecular mechanisms of the novel chalcone-based Magnaporthe oryzae inhibitor C1 using transcriptomic profiling and co-expression network analysis. *Springerplus* 5:1851. doi: 10.1186/s40064-016-3385-9

Chen, J., and Lai, L. (2006). Pocket v.2: further developments on receptor-based pharmacophore modeling. *J. Chem. Inf. Model.* 46, 2684–2691. doi: 10.1021/ci600246s

Chen, S. J. (2014). A potential target of Tanshinone IIA for acute promyelocytic leukemia revealed by inverse docking and drug repurposing. *Asian Pac. J. Cancer Prev.* 15, 4301–4305. doi: 10.7314/APJCP.2014.15.10.4301

Chen, S. J., and Cui, M. C. (2017). Systematic understanding of the mechanism of salvianolic acid A via computational target fishing. *Molecules* 22:E644. doi: 10.3390/molecules22040644

Chen, S. J., and Ren, J. L. (2014). Identification of a potential anticancer target of danshensu by inverse docking. *Asian Pac. J. Cancer Prev.* 15, 111–116. doi: 10.7314/APJCP.2014.15.1.111

Chen, Y. K., Qiao, L. S., Huo, X. Q., Zhang, X., Han, N., and Zhang, Y. L. (2017). [Pharmacological mechanism analysis of oligopeptide from Pinctada fucata based on *in silico* proteolysis and protein interaction network]. *Zhongguo Zhong Yao Za Zhi* 42, 3417–3423. doi: 10.19540/j.cnki.cjcmm.20170731.002

Chen, Y. Z., and Ung, C. Y. (2001). Prediction of potential toxicity and side effect protein targets of a small molecule by a ligand-protein inverse docking approach. *J. Mol. Graph. Model.* 20, 199–218. doi: 10.1016/S1093-3263(01)00109-7

Chen, Y. Z., and Zhi, D. G. (2001). Ligand-protein inverse docking and its potential use in the computer search of protein targets of a small molecule. *Proteins* 43, 217–226. doi: 10.1002/1097-0134(20010501)43:2<217::AID-PROT1032>3.0.CO;2-G

Chen, Z., Li, H. L., Zhang, Q. J., Bao, X. G., Yu, K. Q., Luo, X. M., et al. (2009). Pharmacophore-based virtual screening versus docking-based virtual screening: a benchmark comparison against eight targets. *Acta Pharmacol. Sin.* 30, 1694–1708. doi: 10.1038/aps.2009.159

Chitrala, K. N., and Yeguvapalli, S. (2014). Computational prediction and analysis of breast cancer targets for 6-methyl-1, 3, 8-trichlorodibenzofuran. *PLoS ONE* 9:e109185. doi: 10.1371/journal.pone.0109185

Considine, K. L., Stefanidis, L., Grozinger, K. G., Audie, J., and Alper, B. J. (2017). Efficient synthesis of α-fluoromethylhistidine di-hydrochloride and demonstration of its efficacy as a glutathione S-transferase inhibitor. *Bioorg. Med. Chem. Lett.* 27, 1335–1340. doi: 10.1016/j.bmcl.2017.02.024

Cui, Z., Sheng, Z., Yan, X., Cao, Z., and Tang, K. (2016). *In silico* insight into potential anti-Alzheimer's disease mechanisms of Icariin. *Int. J. Mol. Sci.* 17:E113. doi: 10.3390/ijms17010113

Da Matta, C. B., de Queiroz, A. C., Santos, M. S., Alexandre-Moreira, M. S., Gonçalves, V. T., Del Cistia C. N., et al. (2015). Novel dialkylphosphorylhydrazones: synthesis, leishmanicidal evaluation and theoretical investigation of the proposed mechanism of action. *Eur. J. Med. Chem.* 101, 1–12. doi: 10.1016/j.ejmech.2015.06.014

Das, S., Laskar, M. A., Sarker, S. D., Choudhury, M. D., Choudhury, P. R., Mitra, A., et al. (2017). Prediction of anti-Alzheimer's activity of flavonoids targeting acetylcholinesterase *in silico*. *Phytochem. Anal.* 28, 324–331. doi: 10.1002/pca.2679

Davis, A. P., Grondin, C. J., Johnson, R. J., Sciaky, D., King, B. L., McMorran, R., et al. (2017). The comparative toxicogenomics database: update 2017. *Nucleic Acids Res.* 45, D972–D978. doi: 10.1093/nar/gkw838

Desaphy, J., Bret, G., Rognan, D., and Kellenberger, E. (2015). sc-PDB: a 3D-database of ligandable binding sites—10 years on. *Nucleic Acids Res* 43, D399–D404. doi: 10.1093/nar/gku928

Deshmukh, D. S., Madagi, S., and Savadatti, V. (2013). Identification of potential anti-tumorigenic targets for rosemary components using dual reverse screening approaches. *Int. J. Pharm. Bio. Sci.* 3, 399–408.

Di Muzio, E., Toti, D., and Polticelli, F. (2017). DockingApp: a user friendly interface for facilitated docking simulations with AutoDock Vina. *J. Comput. Aided Mol. Des.* 31, 213–218. doi: 10.1007/s10822-016-0006-1

Do, Q. T., Lamy, C., Renimel, I., Sauvan, N., André, P., Himbert, F., et al. (2007). Reverse pharmacognosy: identifying biological properties for plants by means of their molecule constituents: application to meranzin. *Planta Med.* 73, 1235–1240. doi: 10.1055/s-2007-990216

Do, Q. T., Renimel, I., Andre, P., Lugnier, C., Muller, C. D., and Bernard, P. (2005). Reverse pharmacognosy: application of selnergy, a new tool for lead discovery. The example of epsilon-viniferin. *Curr. Drug Discov. Technol.* 2, 161–167. doi: 10.2174/1570163054866873

Drews, J. (1997). Strategic choices facing the pharmaceutical industry: a case for innovation. *Drug Discov. Today* 2, 72–78. doi: 10.1016/S1359-6446(96)10051-9

Dunkel, M., Gunther, S., Ahmed, J., Wittig, B., and Preissner, R. (2008). SuperPred: drug classification and target prediction. *Nucleic Acids Res.* 36, W55–W59. doi: 10.1093/nar/gkn307

Durant, J. L., Leland, B. A., Henry, D. R., and Nourse, J. G. (2002). Reoptimization of MDL keys for use in drug discovery. *J. Chem. Inf. Comput. Sci.* 42, 1273–1280. doi: 10.1021/ci010132r

Dutta, S., Kharkar, P. S., Sahu, N. U., and Khanna, A. (2017). Molecular docking prediction and *in vitro* studies elucidate anti-cancer activity of phytoestrogens. *Life Sci.* 185, 73–84. doi: 10.1016/j.lfs.2017.07.015

El-Wakil, M. H., Ashour, H. M., Saudi, M. N., Hassan, A. M., and Labouta, I. M. (2017). Target identification, lead optimization and antitumor evaluation of some new 1,2,4-triazines as c-Met kinase inhibitors. *Bioorg. Chem.* 73, 154–169. doi: 10.1016/j.bioorg.2017.06.009

Erić, S., Ke, S., Barata, T., Solmajer, T., Antić Stankovic, J., Juranic, Z., et al. (2012). Target fishing and docking studies of the novel derivatives of aryl-aminopyridines with potential anticancer activity. *Bioorg. Med. Chem.* 20, 5220–5228. doi: 10.1016/j.bmc.2012.06.051

Ewing, T. J., Makino, S., Skillman, A. G., and Kuntz, I. D. (2001). DOCK 4.0: search strategies for automated molecular docking of flexible molecule databases. *J. Comput. Aided Mol. Des.* 15, 411–428. doi: 10.1023/A:1011115820450

Fan, S., Qiang, G., Pan, Z., Xin, L., Lu, T., Yan, P., et al. (2012). Clarifying off-target effects for torcetrapib using network pharmacology and reverse docking approach. *BMC Syst. Biol.* 6:152. doi: 10.1186/1752-0509-6-152

Fang, R., Cui, Q., Sun, J., Duan, X., Ma, X., Wang, W., et al. (2015). PDK1/Akt/PDE4D axis identified as a target for asthma remedy synergistic with beta2 AR agonists by a natural agent arctigenin. *Allergy* 70, 1622–1632. doi: 10.1111/all.12763

Fang, X., and Wang, S. (2002). A web-based 3D-database pharmacophore searching tool for drug discovery. *J. Chem. Inf. Comput. Sci.* 42, 192–198. doi: 10.1021/ci010083i

Feng, L. X., Jing, C. J., Tang, K. L., Tao, L., Cao, Z. W., Wu, W. Y., et al. (2011). Clarifying the signal network of salvianolic acid B using proteomic assay and bioinformatic analysis. *Proteomics* 11, 1473–1485. doi: 10.1002/pmic.201000482

Feng, Z., Chen, L., Maddula, H., Akcan, O., Oughtred, R., Berman, H. M., et al. (2004). Ligand depot: a data warehouse for ligands bound to macromolecules. *Bioinformatics* 20, 2153–2155. doi: 10.1093/bioinformatics/bth214

Gao, L., Fang, J. S., Bai, X. Y., Zhou, D., Wang, Y. T., Liu, A. L., et al. (2013). *In silico* target fishing for the potential targets and molecular mechanisms of baicalein as an antiparkinsonian agent: discovery of the protective effects on NMDA receptor-mediated neurotoxicity. *Chem. Biol. Drug Des.* 81, 675–687. doi: 10.1111/cbdd.12127

Gao, Y., Hou, R., Liu, F., Liu, H., Fei, Q., Han, Y., et al. (2018). Obacunone causes sustained expression of MKP-1 thus inactivating p38 MAPK to suppress pro-inflammatory mediators through intracellular MIF. *J. Cell. Biochem.* 119, 837–849. doi: 10.1002/jcb.26248

Gao, Z., Li, H., Zhang, H., Liu, X., Kang, L., Luo, X., et al. (2008). PDTD: a web-accessible protein database for drug target identification. *BMC Bioinformatics* 9:104. doi: 10.1186/1471-2105-9-104

Gaulton, A., Hersey, A., Nowotka, M., Bento, A. P., Chambers, J., Mendez, D., et al. (2017). The ChEMBL database in 2017. 45, D945–D954. doi: 10.1093/nar/gkw1074

Gaurav, A., and Gautam, V. (2014). Structure-based three-dimensional pharmacophores as an alternative to traditional methodologies.

J. Recep. Lig. Channel Res. 7, 27–38. doi: 10.2147/JRLCR.S46845

Ge, S. M., Zhan, D. L., Zhang, S. H., Song, L. Q., and Han, W. W. (2016). Reverse screening approach to identify potential anti-cancer targets of dipyridamole. *Am. J. Transl. Res.* 8, 5187–5198.

Gfeller, D., Grosdidier, A., Wirth, M., Daina, A., Michielin, O., and Zoete, V. (2014). SwissTargetPrediction: a web server for target prediction of bioactive small molecules. *Nucleic Acids Res.* 42, W32–W38. doi: 10.1093/nar/gku293

Gilson, M. K., Given, J. A., Bush, B. L., and McCammon, J. A. (1997). The statistical-thermodynamic basis for computation of binding affinities: a critical review. *Biophys. J.* 72, 1047–1069. doi: 10.1016/S0006-3495(97)78756-3

Gilson, M. K., Liu, T., Baitaluk, M., Nicola, G., Hwang, L., and Chong, J. (2016). BindingDB in 2015: a public database for medicinal chemistry, computational chemistry and systems pharmacology. *Nucleic Acids Res.* 44, D1045–D1053. doi: 10.1093/nar/gkv1072

Gilson, M. K., and Zhou, H. X. (2007). Calculation of protein-ligand binding affinities. *Annu. Rev. Biophys. Biomol. Struct.* 36, 21–42. doi: 10.1146/annurev.biophys.36.040306.132550

Glem, R. C., Bender, A., Arnby, C. H., Carlsson, L., Boyer, S., and Smith, J. (2006). Circular fingerprints: flexible molecular descriptors with applications from physical chemistry to ADME. *IDrugs* 9, 199–204.

Gomes, M. N., Alcântara, L. M., Neves, B. J., Melo-Filho, C. C., Freitas-Junior, L. H., Moraes, C. B., et al. (2017). Computer-aided discovery of two novel chalcone-like compounds active and selective against Leishmania infantum. *Bioorg. Med. Chem. Lett.* 27, 2459–2464. doi: 10.1016/j.bmcl.2017.04.010

Gong, J., Cai, C., Liu, X., Ku, X., Jiang, H., Gao, D., et al. (2013). ChemMapper: a versatile web server for exploring pharmacology and chemical structure association based on molecular 3D similarity method. *Bioinformatics* 29, 1827–1829. doi: 10.1093/bioinformatics/btt270

Graul, A. I., Cruces, E., and Stringer, M. (2014). The year's new drugs and biologics, 2013 Part I. *Drugs Today* 50, 51–100. doi: 10.1358/dot.2014.50.1.2116673

Grinter, S. Z., Liang, Y., Huang, S. Y., Hyder, S. M., and Zou, X. (2011). An inverse docking approach for identifying new potential anti-cancer targets. *J. Mol. Graph. Model.* 29, 795–799. doi: 10.1016/j.jmgm.2011.01.002

Gupta, S. K., Dhawan, A., and Shanker, R. (2011). *In silico* approaches: prediction of biological targets for fullerene derivatives. *J. Biomed. Nanotechnol.* 7, 91–92. doi: 10.1166/jbn.2011.1217

Gurung, A. B., Ali, M. A., Bhattacharjee, A., Al-Anazi, K. M., Farah, M. A., Al-Hemaid, F. M., et al. (2016). Target fishing of glycopentalone using integrated inverse docking and reverse pharmacophore mapping approach. *Genet. Mol. Res.* 15. doi: 10.4238/gmr.15038544

Halgren, T. A., Murphy, R. B., Friesner, R. A., Beard, H. S., Frye, L. L., Pollard, W. T., et al. (2004). Glide: a new approach for rapid, accurate docking and scoring. 2. Enrichment factors in database screening. *J. Med. Chem.* 47, 1750–1759. doi: 10.1021/jm030644s

Hastings, J., de Matos, P., Dekker, A., Ennis, M., Harsha, B., Kale, N., et al. (2013). The ChEBI reference database and ontology for biologically relevant chemistry: enhancements for 2013. *Nucleic Acids Res.* 41, D456–D463. doi: 10.1093/nar/gks1146

Hastings, J., Owen, G., Dekker, A., Ennis, M., Kale, N., Muthukrishnan, V., et al. (2016). ChEBI in 2016: improved services and an expanding collection of metabolites. *Nucleic Acids Res.* 44, D1214–D1219. doi: 10.1093/nar/gkv1031

Hawkins, P. C., Skillman, A. G., and Nicholls, A. (2007). Comparison of shape-matching and docking as virtual screening tools. *J. Med. Chem.* 50, 74–82. doi: 10.1021/jm0603365

Hu, S., Yuan, L., Hong, Y., and Li, Z. (2017). Design, synthesis and biological evaluation of Lenalidomide derivatives as tumor angiogenesis inhibitor. *Bioorg. Med. Chem. Lett.* 27, 4075–4081. doi: 10.1016/j.bmcl.2017.07.046

Huang, S. Y., and Zou, X. (2010). Inclusion of solvation and entropy in the knowledge-based scoring function for protein-ligand interactions. *J. Chem. Inf. Model.* 50, 262–273. doi: 10.1021/ci9002987

Huey, R., Morris, G. M., Olson, A. J., and Goodsell, D. S. (2007). A semiempirical free energy force field with charge-based desolvation. *J. Comput. Chem.* 28, 1145–1152. doi: 10.1002/jcc.20634

Hurle, M. R., Yang, L., Xie, Q., Rajpal, D. K., Sanseau, P., and Agarwal, P. (2013). Computational drug repositioning: from data to therapeutics. *Clin. Pharmacol. Ther.* 93, 335–341. doi: 10.1038/clpt.2013.1

Hwang, G. H., Ryu, J. M., Jeon, Y. J., Choi, J., Han, H. J., Lee, Y. M., et al. (2015). The role of thioredoxin reductase and glutathione reductase in plumbagin-induced, reactive oxygen species-mediated apoptosis in cancer cell lines. *Eur. J. Pharmacol.* 765, 384–393. doi: 10.1016/j.ejphar.2015.08.058

Iyer, P., Bolla, J., Kumar, V., Gill, M. S., and Sobhia, M. E. (2015). *In silico* identification of targets for a novel scaffold, 2-thiazolylimino-5-benzylidin-thiazolidin-4-one. *Mol. Divers.* 19, 1–16. doi: 10.1007/s11030-015-9578-2

Jeong, C. H., Bode, A. M., Pugliese, A., Cho, Y. Y., Kim, H. G., Shim, J. H., et al. (2009). [6]-Gingerol suppresses colon cancer growth by targeting leukotriene A4 hydrolase. *Cancer Res.* 69, 5584–5591. doi: 10.1158/0008-5472.CAN-09-0491

Ji, Z. L., Wang, Y., Yu, L., Han, L. Y., Zheng, C. J., and Chen, Y. Z. (2006). *In silico* search of putative adverse drug reaction related proteins as a potential tool for facilitating drug adverse effect prediction. *Toxicol. Lett.* 164, 104–112. doi: 10.1016/j.toxlet.2005.11.017

Kabsch, W. (1976). A solution for the best rotation to relate two sets of vectors. *Acta Crystallogr. A* 32, 922–923. doi: 10.1107/S0567739476001873

Keiser, M. J., Roth, B. L., Armbruster, B. N., Ernsberger, P., Irwin, J. J., and Shoichet, B. K. (2007). Relating protein pharmacology by ligand chemistry. *Nat. Biotechnol.* 25, 197–206. doi: 10.1038/nbt1284

Keiser, M. J., Setola, V., Irwin, J. J., Laggner, C., Abbas, A. I., Hufeisen, S. J., et al. (2009). Predicting new molecular targets for known drugs. *Nature* 462, 175–181. doi: 10.1038/nature08506

Kharkar, P. S., Warrier, S., and Gaud, R. S. (2014). Reverse docking: a powerful tool for drug repositioning and drug rescue. *Future Med. Chem.* 6, 333–342. doi: 10.4155/fmc.13.207

Khedkar, S. A., Malde, A. K., Coutinho, E. C., and Srivastava, S. (2007). Pharmacophore modeling in drug discovery and development: an overview. *Med. Chem.* 3, 187–197. doi: 10.2174/157340607780059521

Kim, M. S., Kim, J. E., Lim, D. Y., Huang, Z., Chen, H., Langfald, A., et al. (2014). Naproxen induces cell-cycle arrest and apoptosis in human urinary bladder cancer cell lines and chemically induced cancers by targeting PI3K. *Cancer Prev. Res.* 7, 236–245. doi: 10.1158/1940-6207.CAPR-13-0288

Kim, S., Thiessen, P. A., Bolton, E. E., Chen, J., Fu, G., Gindulyte, A., et al. (2016). PubChem substance and compound databases. *Nucleic Acids Res.* 44, D1202–D1213. doi: 10.1093/nar/gkv951

Kinnings, S. L., and Jackson, R. M. (2011). ReverseScreen3D: a structure-based ligand matching method to identify protein targets. *J. Chem. Inf. Model.* 51, 624–634. doi: 10.1021/ci1003174

Köhler, S., Bauer, S., Horn, D., and Robinson, P. N. (2008). Walking the interactome for prioritization of candidate disease genes. *Am. J. Hum. Genet.* 82, 949–958. doi: 10.1016/j.ajhg.2008.02.013

Koshland, D. E. (1958). Application of a theory of enzyme specificity to protein synthesis. *Proc. Natl. Acad. Sci. U.S.A.* 44, 98–104. doi: 10.1073/pnas.44.2.98

Kozielewicz, P., Paradowska, K., Erić, S., Wawer, I., and Zloh, M. (2014). Insights into mechanism of anticancer activity of pentacyclic oxindole alkaloids of Uncaria tomentosa by means of a computational reverse virtual screening and molecular docking approach. *Monatsh. Chem.* 145, 1201–1211. doi: 10.1007/s00706-014-1212-y

Kringelum, J., Kjaerulff, S. K., Brunak, S., Lund, O., Oprea, T. I., and Taboureau, O. (2016). ChemProt-3.0: a global chemical biology diseases mapping. *Database* 2016:bav123. doi: 10.1093/database/bav123

Krishnasamy, G., and Muthusamy, K. (2016). A computational study on role of 6-(hydroxymethyl)-3-[3,4,5-trihydroxy-6-[(3,4,5-trihydroxyoxan-2-yl)oxymethyl]oxan-2-yl]oxyoxane-2,4,5-triol in the regulation of blood glucose level. J. Biomol. Struct. Dyn. 34, 2599–2618. doi: 10.1080/07391102.2015.1124289

Kuhn, M., Letunic, I., Jensen, L. J., and Bork, P. (2016). The SIDER database of drugs and side effects. *Nucleic Acids Res.* 44, D1075–D1079. doi: 10.1093/nar/gkv1075

Kumar, S. P., Parmar, V. R., Jasrai, Y. T., and Pandya, H. A. (2015). Prediction of protein targets of kinetin using *in silico* and *in vitro* methods: a case study on spinach seed germination mechanism. *J. Chem. Biol.* 8, 95–105. doi: 10.1007/s12154-015-0135-3

Kuntz, I. D., Blaney, J. M., Oatley, S. J., Langridge, R., and Ferrin, T. E. (1982). A geometric approach to macromolecule-ligand interactions. *J. Mol. Biol.* 161, 269–288. doi: 10.1016/0022-2836(82)90153-X

Kurogi, Y., and Güner, O. F. (2001). Pharmacophore modeling and three-dimensional database searching for drug design using catalyst. *Curr. Med. Chem.* 8, 1035–1055. doi: 10.2174/0929867013372481

Law, V., Knox, C., Djoumbou, Y., Jewison, T., Guo, A. C., Liu, Y., et al. (2014). DrugBank 4.0: shedding new light on drug metabolism. *Nucleic Acids Res.* 42, D1091–D1097. doi: 10.1093/nar/gkt1068

Leach, A. R., Gillet, V. J., Lewis, R. A., and Taylor, R. (2010). Three-dimensional pharmacophore methods in drug discovery. *J. Med. Chem.* 53, 539–558. doi: 10.1021/jm900817u

Lee, A., Lee, K., and Kim, D. (2016). Using reverse docking for target identification and its applications for drug discovery. *Expert Opin. Drug Discov.* 11, 707–715. doi: 10.1080/17460441.2016.1190706

Lei, Q., Liu, H., Peng, Y., and Xiao, P. (2015). *In silico* target fishing and pharmacological profiling for the isoquinoline alkaloids of Macleaya cordata (Bo Luo Hui). *Chin. Med.* 10:37. doi: 10.1186/s13020-015-0067-4

Li, G. B., Yang, L. L., Xu, Y., Wang, W. J., Li, L. L., and Yang, S. Y. (2013). A combined molecular docking-based and pharmacophore-based target prediction strategy with a probabilistic fusion method for target ranking. *J. Mol. Graph. Model.* 44, 278–285. doi: 10.1016/j.jmgm.2013.07.005

Li, Y., Cao, Y., Xu, J., Qiu, L., Xu, W., Li, J., et al. (2016). Esculentoside A suppresses lipopolysaccharide-induced pro-inflammatory molecule production partially by casein kinase 2. *J. Ethnopharmacol.* 198, 15–23. doi: 10.1016/j.jep

Li, H., Gao, Z., Kang, L., Zhang, H., Yang, K., Yu, K., et al. (2006). TarFisDock: a web server for identifying drug targets with docking approach. *Nucleic Acids Res.* 34, W219–W224. doi: 10.1093/nar/gkl114

Li, J., Zheng, S., Chen, B., Butte, A. J., Swamidass, S. J., and Lu, Z. (2016). A survey of current trends in computational drug repositioning. *Brief. Bioinformatics* 17, 2–12. doi: 10.1093/bib/bbv020

Li, W., Cui, T., Hu, L., Wang, Z., Li, Z., and He, Z. G. (2015). Cyclic diguanylate monophosphate directly binds to human siderocalin and inhibits its antibacterial activity. *Nat. Commun.* 6:8330. doi: 10.1038/ncomms9330

Li, Y., Chang, N., Han, Y., Zhou, M., Gao, J., Hou, Y., et al. (2017). Anti-inflammatory effects of Shufengjiedu capsule for upper respiratory infection via the ERK pathway. *Biomed. Pharmacother.* 94, 758–766. doi: 10.1016/j.biopha.2017.07.118

Liang, J., Wang, M., Li, X., He, X., Cao, C., and Meng, F. (2017). Determination of structural requirements of N-substituted tetrahydro-beta-carboline imidazolium salt derivatives using *in silico* approaches for designing MEK-1 inhibitors. *Molecules* 22:E1020. doi: 10.3390/molecules22061020

Lim, T. G., Lee, S. Y., Huang, Z., Lim, D. Y., Chen, H., Jung, S. K., et al. (2014). Curcumin suppresses proliferation of colon cancer cells by targeting CDK2. *Cancer Prev. Res.* 7, 466–474. doi: 10.1158/1940-6207.CAPR-13-0387

Liu, B., Fu, X. Q., Li, T., Su, T., Guo, H., Zhu, P. L., et al. (2017). Computational and experimental prediction of molecules involved in the anti-melanoma action of berberine. *J. Ethnopharmacol.* 208, 225–235. doi: 10.1016/j.jep.2017.07.023

Liu, H., Lin, F., Yang, J. L., Wang, H. R., and Liu, X. L. (2015). Applying side-chain flexibility in motifs for protein docking. *Genomics Insights* 8, 1–10. doi: 10.4137/GEI.S29821

Liu, X., Gao, Y., Peng, J., Xu, Y., Wang, Y., Zhou, N., et al. (2015a). TarPred: a web application for predicting therapeutic and side effect targets of chemical compounds. *Bioinformatics.* 31, 2049–2051. doi: 10.1093/bioinformatics/btv099

Liu, X., Ouyang, S., Yu, B., Liu, Y., Huang, K., Gong, J., et al. (2010). PharmMapper server: a web server for potential drug target identification using pharmacophore mapping approach. *Nucleic Acids Res.* 38, W609–W614. doi: 10.1093/nar/gkq300

Liu, X., Vogt, I., Haque, T., and Campillos, M. (2013). HitPick: a web server for hit identification and target prediction of chemical screenings. *Bioinformatics.* 29, 1910–1912. doi: 10.1093/bioinformatics/btt303

Liu, X., Wang, K., Duan, N., Lan, Y., Ma, P., Zheng, H., et al. (2015b). Computational prediction and experimental validation of low-affinity target of triptolide and its analogues. *RSC Adv.* 5, 34572–34579. doi: 10.1039/C4RA17009A

Liu, X., Xu, Y., Li, S., Wang, Y., Peng, J., Luo, C., et al. (2014). *In silico* target fishing: addressing a "Big Data" problem by ligand-based similarity rankings with data fusion. *J. Cheminform.* 6:33. doi: 10.1186/1758-2946-6-33

Liu, X., Yang, X., Chen, X., Zhang, Y., Pan, X., Wang, G., et al. (2015c). Expression profiling identifies bezafibrate as potential therapeutic drug for lung adenocarcinoma. *J. Cancer* 6, 1214–1221. doi: 10.7150/jca.12191

Liu, Z., Li, J., Liu, J., Liu, Y., Nie, W., Han, L., et al. (2015). Cross-mapping of protein - ligand binding data between ChEMBL and PDBbind. *Mol. Inform.* 34, 568–576. doi: 10.1002/minf.201500010

Lo, Y. C., Senese, S., Damoiseaux, R., and Torres, J. Z. (2016). 3D chemical similarity networks for structure-based target prediction and scaffold hopping. *ACS Chem. Biol.* 11, 2244–2253. doi: 10.1021/acschembio.6b00253

Lorber, D. M., and Shoichet, B. K. (1998). Flexible ligand docking using conformational ensembles. *Protein Sci.* 7, 938–950. doi: 10.1002/pro.5560070411

Lu, B., Hu, M., Liu, K., and Peng, J. (2010). Cytotoxicity of berberine on human cervical carcinoma HeLa cells through mitochondria, death receptor and MAPK pathways, and *in-silico* drug-target prediction. *Toxicol. In Vitro* 24, 1482–1490. doi: 10.1016/j.tiv.2010.07.017

Lu, B., Zhao, J., Xu, L., Xu, Y., Wang, X., and Peng, J. (2012). Identification of molecular target proteins in berberine-treated cervix adenocarcinoma HeLa cells by proteomic and bioinformatic analyses. *Phytother. Res.* 26, 646–656. doi: 10.1002/ptr.3615

Lu, W., Liu, X., Cao, X., Xue, M., Liu, K., Zhao, Z., et al. (2011). SHAFTS: a hybrid approach for 3D molecular similarity calculation. 2. Prospective case study in the discovery of diverse p90 ribosomal S6 protein kinase 2 inhibitors to suppress cell migration. *J. Med. Chem.* 54, 3564–3574. doi: 10.1021/jm200139j

Lv, C., Qin, W., Zhu, T., Wei, S., Hong, K., Zhu, W., et al. (2015). Ophiobolin O isolated from Aspergillus ustus induces G1 arrest of MCF-7 cells through interaction with AKT/GSK3β/cyclin D1 signaling. *Mar. Drugs* 13:431. doi: 10.3390/md13010431

Ma, C., Kang, H., Liu, Q., Zhu, R., and Cao, Z. (2011). Insight into potential toxicity mechanisms of melamine: an *in silico* study. *Toxicology* 283, 96–100. doi: 10.1016/j.tox.2011.02.009

Ma, C., Tang, K., Liu, Q., Zhu, R., and Cao, Z. (2013). Calmodulin as a potential target by which berberine induces cell cycle arrest in human hepatoma Bel7402 cells. *Chem. Biol. Drug Des.* 81, 775–783. doi: 10.1111/cbdd.12124

Ma, X., Zhang, Y., Wang, Z., Shen, Y., Zhang, M., Nie, Q., et al. (2017). Ursolic acid, a natural nutraceutical agent, targets caspase3 and alleviates inflammation-associated downstream signal transduction. *Mol. Nutr. Food Res.* 61, 1–9. doi: 10.1002/mnfr.201700332

Maccari, G., Deodato, D., Fiorucci, D., Orofino, F., Truglio, G. I., Pasero, C., et al. (2017). Design and synthesis of a novel inhibitor of T. Viride chitinase through an *in silico* target fishing protocol. *Bioorg. Med. Chem. Lett.* 27, 3332–3336. doi: 10.1016/j.bmcl.2017.06.016

Maldonado-Rojas, W., Verbel, J. O., and Zuniga, C. O., (2011). Searching of protein targets for alpha lipoic acid. *J. Braz. Chem. Soc.* 22, 2250–2259. doi: 10.1590/S0103-50532011001200003

Meshram, R. J., Baladhye, V. B., Gacche, R. N., Karale, B. K., and Gaikar, R. B. (2017). Pharmacophore mapping approach for drug target identification: a chemical synthesis and *in silico* study on novel thiadiazole compounds. *J. Clin. Diagn. Res.* 11, Kf01–kf08. doi: 10.7860/JCDR/2017/22761.9925

Meslamani, J., Li, J., Sutter, J., Stevens, A., Bertrand, H. O., and Rognan, D. (2012). Protein-ligand-based pharmacophores: generation and utility assessment in computational ligand profiling. *J. Chem. Inf. Model.* 52, 943–955. doi: 10.1021/ci300083r

Mori, M., Cau, Y., Vignaroli, G., Laurenzana, I., Caivano, A., Vullo, D., et al. (2015). Hit recycling: discovery of a potent carbonic anhydrase inhibitor by *in silico* target fishing. *ACS Chem. Biol.* 10, 1964–1969. doi: 10.1021/acschembio.5b00337

Morris, G. M., Goodsell, D. S., Halliday, R. S., Huey, R., Hart, W. E., Belew, R. K., et al. (2015). Automated docking using a Lamarckian genetic algorithm and an empirical binding free energy function. *J Comput Chem* 19, 1639-1662. doi: 10.1002/(SICI)1096-987X(19981115)19:14<1639::AID-JCC10>3.0.CO;2-B

Mount, D. W. (2007). Using the Basic Local Alignment Search Tool (BLAST). *CSH Protoc* 2007:pdb.top17. doi: 10.1101/pdb.top17

Moura Barbosa, A. J., and Del Rio, A. (2012). Freely accessible databases of commercial compounds for high- throughput virtual screenings. *Curr. Top. Med. Chem.* 12, 866–877. doi: 10.2174/156802612800166710

Nettles, J. H., Jenkins, J. L., Bender, A., Deng, Z., Davies, J. W., and Glick, M. (2006). Bridging chemical and biological space: "target fishing" using 2D and 3D molecular descriptors. *J. Med. Chem.* 49, 6802–6810. doi: 10.1021/jm060902w

Nickel, J., Gohlke, B. O., Erehman, J., Banerjee, P., Rong, W. W., Goede, A., et al. (2014). SuperPred: update on drug classification and target prediction. *Nucleic Acids Res.* 42, W26–W31. doi: 10.1093/nar/gku477

Oliveroverbel, J., Cabarcasmontalvo, M., and Ortegazúñiga, C. (2010). Theoretical targets for TCDD: a bioinformatics approach. *Chemosphere* 80, 1160–1166. doi: 10.1016/j.chemosphere.2010.06.020

Pan, J. B., Ji, N., Pan, W., Hong, R., Wang, H., and Ji, Z. L. (2014). High-throughput identification of off-targets for the mechanistic study of severe adverse drug reactions induced by analgesics. *Toxicol. Appl. Pharmacol.* 274, 24–34. doi: 10.1016/j.taap.2013.10.017

Park, K., and Cho, A. E. (2017). Using reverse docking to identify potential targets for ginsenosides. *J. Ginseng Res.* 41, 534–539. doi: 10.1016/j.jgr.2016.10.005

Patel, H., Lucas, X., Bendik, I., Günther, S., and Merfort, I. (2015). Target fishing by cross-docking to explain polypharmacological effects. *ChemMedChem* 10, 1209–1217. doi: 10.1002/cmdc.201500123

Paul, N., Kellenberger, E., Bret, G., Müller, P., and Rognan, D. (2004). Recovering the true targets of specific ligands by virtual screening of the protein data bank. *Proteins* 54, 671–680. doi: 10.1002/prot.10625

Pereira, A. S. P., Bester, M. J., and Apostolides, Z. (2017). Exploring the anti-proliferative activity of Pelargonium sidoides DC with *in silico* target identification and network pharmacology. *Mol. Divers.* (Suppl 6), 1–12. doi: 10.1007/s11030-017-9769-0

Poux, S., Arighi, C. N., Magrane, M., Bateman, A., Wei, C. H., Lu, Z., et al. (2017). On expert curation and scalability: Uniprotkb/Swiss-Prot as a case study. *Bioinformatics* 33, 3454–3460. doi: 10.1093/bioinformatics/btx439

Pulla, V. K., Sriram, D. S., Viswanadha, S., Sriram, D., and Yogeeswari, P. (2016). Energy-based pharmacophore and three-dimensional quantitative structure–activity relationship (3D-QSAR) modeling combined with virtual screening to identify novel small-molecule inhibitors of silent mating-type information regulation 2 homologue 1 (SIRT1). *J. Chem. Inf. Model.* 56, 173–187. doi: 10.1021/acs.jcim.5b00220

Pun, I. H., Chan, D., Chan, S. H., Chung, P. Y., Zhou, Y. Y., Law, S., et al. (2017). Anti-cancer effects of a novel quinoline derivative 83b1 on human esophageal squamous cell carcinoma through down-regulation of COX-2 mRNA and PGE2. *Cancer Res. Treat.* 49, 219–229. doi: 10.4143/crt.2016.190

Pundir, S., Magrane, M., Martin, M. J., and O'Donovan, C. (2015). Searching and navigating uniprot databases. *Curr. Protoc. Bioinformatics 50*, 1.27, 21–10. doi: 10.1002/0471250953.bi0127s50

Putri, J. F., Widodo, N., Sakamoto, K., Kaul, S. C., and Wadhwa, R. (2017). Induction of senescence in cancer cells by 5'-Aza-2'-deoxycytidine: bioinformatics and experimental insights to its targets. *Comput. Biol. Chem.* 70, 49–55. doi: 10.1016/j.compbiolchem.2017.08.003

Raha, K., and Merz, K. M. Jr. (2005). Large-scale validation of a quantum mechanics based scoring function: predicting the binding affinity and the binding mode of a diverse set of protein-ligand complexes. *J. Med. Chem.* 48, 4558–4575. doi: 10.1021/jm048973n

Rogers, D., and Hahn, M. (2010). Extended-connectivity fingerprints. *J. Chem. Inf. Model.* 50, 742–754. doi: 10.1021/ci100050t

Rognan, D. (2010). Structure-based approaches to target fishing and ligand profiling. *Mol. Inform.* 29, 176–187. doi: 10.1002/minf.200900081

Rose, P. W., Prlic, A., Bi, C., Bluhm, W. F., Christie, C. H., Dutta, S., et al. (2015). The RCSB Protein Data Bank: views of structural biology for basic and applied research and education. 43, D345–D356. doi: 10.1093/nar/gku1214

Roth, B. L., Lopez, E., Patel, S., and Kroeze, W. K. (2000). The multiplicity of serotonin receptors: uselessly diverse molecules or an embarrassment of riches? *Neuroscientist* 6, 252–262. doi: 10.1177/107385840000600408

Rush, T. S. III, Grant, J. A., Mosyak, L., and Nicholls, A. (2005). A shape-based 3-D scaffold hopping method and its application to a bacterial protein-protein interaction. *J. Med. Chem.* 48, 1489–1495. doi: 10.1021/jm040163o

Salim, N., Holliday, J., and Willett, P. (2003). Combination of fingerprint-based similarity coefficients using data fusion. *J. Chem. Inf. Comput. Sci.* 43, 435–442. doi: 10.1021/ci025596j

Sanni, D. M., Fatoki, T. H., Kolawole, A. O., and Akinmoladun, A. C. (2017). Xeronine structure and function: computational comparative mastery of its mystery. *In Silico Pharmacol* 5:8. doi: 10.1007/s40203-017-0028-y

Sarangi, A. N., Lohani, M., and Aggarwal, R. (2015). Proteome mining for drug target identification in Listeria monocytogenes strain EGD-e and structure-based virtual screening of a candidate drug target penicillin binding protein 4. *J. Microbiol. Methods* 111, 9–18. doi: 10.1016/j.mimet.2015.01.011

Scafuri, B., Marabotti, A., Carbone, V., Minasi, P., Dotolo, S., and Facchiano, A. (2016). A theoretical study on predicted protein targets of apple polyphenols and possible mechanisms of chemoprevention in colorectal cancer. *Sci. Rep.* 6:32516. doi: 10.1038/srep32516

Schenone, M., Dancik, V., Wagner, B. K., and Clemons, P. A. (2013). Target identification and mechanism of action in chemical biology and drug discovery. *Nat. Chem. Biol.* 9, 232–240. doi: 10.1038/nchembio.1199

Schomburg, K. T., and Rarey, M. (2014). What is the potential of structure-based target prediction methods? *Future Med. Chem.* 6, 1987–1989. doi: 10.4155/fmc.14.135

Schrödinger (2018). *Small-Molecule Drug Discovery Suite 2018-1*. New York, NY: Schrödinger, LLC.

Schuffenhauer, A., Floersheim, P., Acklin, P., and Jacoby, E. (2003). Similarity metrics for ligands reflecting the similarity of the target proteins. *J. Chem. Inf. Comput. Sci.* 43, 391–405. doi: 10.1021/ci025569t

Shang, J., Dai, X., Li, Y., Pistolozzi, M., and Wang, L. (2017). HybridSim-VS: a web server for large-scale ligand-based virtual screening using hybrid similarity recognition techniques. *Bioinformatics* 33, 3480–3481. doi: 10.1093/bioinformatics/btx418

Shao, Y., Qiao, L., Wu, L., Sun, X., Zhu, D., Yang, G., et al. (2016). Structure identification and anti-cancer pharmacological prediction of triterpenes from ganoderma lucidum. *Molecules* 21: E678. doi: 10.3390/molecules21050678

Shindyalov, I. N., and Bourne, P. E. (1998). Protein structure alignment by incremental combinatorial extension (CE) of the optimal path. *Protein Eng.* 11, 739–747. doi: 10.1093/protein/11.9.739

Shoichet, B. K., Kuntz, I. D., and Bodian, D. L. (2010). Molecular docking using shape descriptors. *J. Comput. Chem.* 13, 380–397. doi: 10.1002/jcc.540130311

Simon, L., Imane, A., Srinivasan, K. K., Pathak, L., and Daoud, I. (2017). *In silico* drug-designing studies on flavanoids as anticolon cancer agents: pharmacophore mapping, molecular docking, and monte carlo method-based QSAR modeling. *Interdiscip. Sci.* 9, 445–458. doi: 10.1007/s12539-016-0169-4

Smusz, S., Mordalski, S., Witek, J., Rataj, K., Kafel, R., and Bojarski, A. J. (2015). Multi-step protocol for automatic evaluation of docking results based on machine learning methods–a case study of serotonin receptors 5-HT(6) and 5-HT(7). *J. Chem. Inf. Model.* 55, 823–832. doi: 10.1021/ci500564b

Steindl, T. M., Schuster, D., Laggner, C., and Langer, T. (2006). Parallel screening: a novel concept in pharmacophore modeling and virtual screening. *J. Chem. Inf. Model.* 46, 2146–2157. doi: 10.1021/ci6002043

Sterling, T., and Irwin, J. J. (2015). ZINC 15–ligand discovery for everyone. *J. Chem. Inf. Model.* 55, 2324–2337. doi: 10.1021/acs.jcim.5b00559

Sutter, J., Li, J., Maynard, A. J., Goupil, A., Luu, T., and Nadassy, K. (2011). New features that improve the pharmacophore tools from Accelrys. *Curr. Comput. Aided Drug Des.* 7, 173–180. doi: 10.2174/157340911796504305

Szklarczyk, D., Franceschini, A., Wyder, S., Forslund, K., Heller, D., Huerta-Cepas, J., et al. (2015). STRING v10: protein-protein interaction networks, integrated over the tree of life. *Nucleic Acids Res.* 43, D447–D452. doi: 10.1093/nar/gku1003

Truchon, J. F., and Bayly, C. I. (2007). Evaluating virtual screening methods: good and bad metrics for the "early recognition" problem. *J. Chem. Inf. Model.* 47, 488–508. doi: 10.1021/ci600426e

Wang, J. C., Chu, P. Y., Chen, C. M., and Lin, J. H. (2012). idTarget: a web server for identifying protein targets of small chemical molecules with robust scoring functions and a divide-and-conquer docking approach. *Nucleic Acids Res.* 40, W393–W399. doi: 10.1093/nar/gks496

Wang, S. Y., Fu, L. L., Zhang, S. Y., Tian, M., Zhang, L., Zheng, Y. X. et al. (2015). *In silico* analysis and experimental validation of active compounds from fructus Schisandrae chinensis in protection from hepatic injury. *Cell Prolifer.* 48, 86–94. doi: 10.1111/cpr.12157

Wang, J. C., Lin, J. H., Chen, C. M., Perryman, A. L., and Olson, A. J. (2011). Robust scoring functions for protein-ligand interactions with quantum chemical charge models. *J. Chem. Inf. Model.* 51, 2528–2537. doi: 10.1021/ci200220v

Wang, J., Gao, L., Lee, Y. M., Kalesh, K. A., Ong, Y. S., Lim, J., et al. (2016). Target identification of natural and traditional medicines with quantitative chemical proteomics approaches. *Pharmacol. Ther.* 162, 10–22. doi: 10.1016/j.pharmthera.2016.01.010

Wang, L., Ma, C., Wipf, P., Liu, H., Su, W., and Xie, X. Q. (2013). TargetHunter: an *in silico* target identification tool for predicting therapeutic potential of small organic molecules based on chemogenomic database. *AAPS J.* 15, 395–406. doi: 10.1208/s12248-012-9449-z

Wang, N., Zhao, G., Zhang, Y., Wang, X., Zhao, L., Xu, P., et al. (2017). A network pharmacology approach to determine the active components and potential targets of curculigo orchioides in the treatment of osteoporosis. *Med. Sci. Monit.* 23, 5113–5122. doi: 10.12659/MSM.904264

Wang, X., Pan, C., Gong, J., Liu, X., and Li, H. (2016). Enhancing the enrichment of pharmacophore-based target prediction for the polypharmacological profiles of drugs. *J. Chem. Inf. Model.* 56, 1175–1183. doi: 10.1021/acs.jcim.5b00690

Wang, X., Shen, Y., Wang, S., Li, S., Zhang, W., Liu, X., et al. (2017). PharmMapper 2017 update: a web server for potential drug target identification with a comprehensive target pharmacophore database. *Nucleic Acids Res.* 45, W356–W360. doi: 10.1093/nar/gkx374

Wang, Y., Cao, Y., Zhu, Q., Gu, X., and Zhu, Y. Z. (2016). The discovery of a novel inhibitor of apoptotic protease activating factor-1 (Apaf-1) for ischemic heart: synthesis, activity and target identification. *Sci. Rep.* 6:29820. doi: 10.1038/srep29820

Wang, Y. C., Chen, S. L., Deng, N. Y., and Wang, Y. (2013). Network predicting drug's anatomical therapeutic chemical code. *Bioinformatics* 29, 1317–1324. doi: 10.1093/bioinformatics/btt158

Wang, Y., Qi, W., Zhang, L., Ying, Z., Sha, O., Li, C., et al. (2017). The novel targets of DL-3-n-butylphthalide predicted by similarity ensemble approach in combination with molecular docking study. *Quant. Imaging Med. Surg.* 7, 532–536. doi: 10.21037/qims.2017.10.08

Wang, Z., Luo, S., Wan, Z., Chen, C., Zhang, X., Li, B., et al. (2016). Glabridin arrests cell cycle and inhibits proliferation of hepatocellular carcinoma by suppressing braf/MEK signaling pathway. *Tumour Biol.* 37, 5837–5846. doi: 10.1007/s13277-015-4177-5

Waseem, D., Butt, A. F., Haq, I. U., Bhatti, M. H., and Khan, G. M. (2017). Carboxylate derivatives of tributyltin (IV) complexes as anticancer and antileishmanial agents. *Daru* 25:8. doi: 10.1186/s40199-017-0174-0

Weiner, S. J., Kollman, P. A., Case, D. A., Singh, U. C., Ghio, C., Alagona, G., et al. (1984). A new force field for molecular mechanical simulation of nucleic acids and proteins. *J. Am. Chem. Soc.* 106, 765–784. doi: 10.1021/ja00315a051

Willett, P. (1995). Genetic algorithms in molecular recognition and design. *Trends Biotechnol.* 13, 516–521. doi: 10.1016/S0167-7799(00)89015-0

Wishart, D. S., Knox, C., Guo, A. C., Eisner, R., Young, N., Gautam, B., et al. (2009). HMDB: a knowledgebase for the human metabolome. *Nucleic Acids Res.* 37, D603–D610. doi: 10.1093/nar/gkn810

Wishart, D. S., Tzur, D., Knox, C., Eisner, R., Guo, A. C., Young, N., et al. (2007). HMDB: the Human Metabolome Database. *Nucleic Acids Res.* 35, D521–D526. doi: 10.1093/nar/gkl923

Wolber, G., and Langer, T. (2005). LigandScout: 3-D pharmacophores derived from protein-bound ligands and their use as virtual screening filters. *J. Chem. Inf. Model.* 45, 160–169. doi: 10.1021/ci049885e

Xu, X., Guo, Y., Zhao, J., Wang, N., Ding, J., and Liu, Q. (2016a). Hydroxysafflor yellow A inhibits LPS-induced NLRP3 inflammasome activation via binding to xanthine oxidase in mouse RAW264.7 macrophages. *Mediators Inflamm.* 2016:8172706. doi: 10.1155/2016/8172706

Xu, X., Ma, S., Feng, Z., Hu, G., Wang, L., and Xie, X. Q. (2016b). Chemogenomics knowledgebase and systems pharmacology for hallucinogen target identification-Salvinorin A as a case study. *J. Mol. Graph. Model.* 70, 284–295. doi: 10.1016/j.jmgm.2016.08.001

Yan, X., Kang, H., Feng, J., Yang, Y., Tang, K., Zhu, R., et al. (2016). Identification of toxic pyrrolizidine alkaloids and their common hepatotoxicity mechanism. *Int. J. Mol. Sci.* 17:318. doi: 10.3390/ijms17030318

Yan, X., Li, J., Gu, Q., and Xu, J. (2014). gWEGA: GPU-accelerated WEGA for molecular superposition and shape comparison. *J. Comput. Chem.* 35, 1122–1130. doi: 10.1002/jcc.23603

Yan, X., Li, J., Liu, Z., Zheng, M., Ge, H., and Xu, J. (2013). Enhancing molecular shape comparison by weighted Gaussian functions. *J. Chem. Inf. Model.* 53, 1967–1978. doi: 10.1021/ci300601q

Ye, L., He, Y., Ye, H., Liu, X., Yang, L., Cao, Z., et al. (2012). Pathway-pathway network-based study of the therapeutic mechanisms by which salvianolic acid B regulates cardiovascular diseases. *Chin. Sci. Bull.* 57, 1672–1679. doi: 10.1007/s11434-012-5142-y

Ye, X. Y., Ling, Q. Z., and Chen, S. J. (2015). Identification of a potential target of capsaicin by computational target fishing. *Evid. Based Complement. Alternat. Med.* 2015:983951. doi: 10.1155/2015/983951

Yi, F., Tan, X. L., Yan, X., and Liu, H. B. (2016). *In silico* profiling for secondary metabolites from Lepidium meyenii (maca) by the pharmacophore and ligand-shape-based joint approach. *Chin. Med.* 11:42. doi: 10.1186/s13020-016-0112-y

Yin, L., Zheng, L., Xu, L., Dong, D., Han, X., Qi, Y., et al. (2015). *In-silico* prediction of drug targets, biological activities, signal pathways and regulating networks of dioscin based on bioinformatics. *BMC Complement. Altern. Med.* 15, 1–17. doi: 10.1186/s12906-015-0579-6

Yuan, D. P., Long, J., Lu, Y., Lin, J., and Tong, L. (2014). The forecast of anticancer targets of cryptotanshinone based on reverse pharmacophore-based screening technology. *Chin. J. Nat. Med.* 12, 12443–448. doi: 10.1016/S1875-5364(14)60069-8

Yuan, Y., Pei, J., and Lai, L. (2013). Binding site detection and druggability prediction of protein targets for structure-based drug design. *Curr. Pharm. Des.* 19, 2326–2333. doi: 10.2174/1381612811319120019

Yue, Q. X., Cao, Z. W., Guan, S. H., Liu, X. H., Tao, L., Wu, W. Y., et al. (2008). Proteomics characterization of the cytotoxicity mechanism of ganoderic acid D and computer-automated estimation of the possible drug target network. *Mol. Cell. Proteomics* 7, 949–961. doi: 10.1074/mcp.M700259-MCP200

Zahler, S., Tietze, S., Totzke, F., Kubbutat, M., Meijer, L., Vollmar, A. M., et al. (2007). Inverse *in silico* screening for identification of kinase inhibitor targets. *Chem. Biol.* 14, 1207–1214. doi: 10.1016/j.chembiol.2007.10.010

Zeng, L., Yang, K., and Ge, J. (2017a). Uncovering the pharmacological mechanism of astragalus salvia compound on pregnancy-induced hypertension syndrome by a network pharmacology approach. *Sci. Rep.* 7:16849. doi: 10.1038/s41598-017-17139-x

Zeng, L., Yang, K., Liu, H., and Zhang, G. (2017b). A network pharmacology approach to investigate the pharmacological effects of Guizhi Fuling Wan on uterine fibroids. *Exp. Ther. Med.* 14, 4697–4710. doi: 10.3892/etm.2017.5170

Zhang, H., Ma, S., Feng, Z., Wang, D., Li, C., Cao, Y., et al. (2016). Cardiovascular disease chemogenomics knowledgebase-guided target identification and drug synergy mechanism study of an herbal formula. *Sci. Rep.* 6:33963. doi: 10.1038/srep33963

Zhang, S., Lu, W., Liu, X., Diao, Y., Bai, F., Wang, L., et al. (2011). Fast and effective identification of the bioactive compounds and their targets from medicinal plants via computational chemical biology approach. *Med. Chem. Commun.* 2, 471–477. doi: 10.1039/c0md00245c

Zhang, Y., Zhu, Y., and He, F. (2011). An overview of human protein databases and their application to functional proteomics in health and disease. *Sci. China Life Sci.* 54, 988–998. doi: 10.1007/s11427-011-4247-x

Zhang, Z., Miao, L., Lv, C., Sun, H., Wei, S., Wang, B., et al. (2013). Wentilactone B induces G2/M phase arrest and apoptosis via the Ras/Raf/MAPK signaling pathway in human hepatoma SMMC-7721 cells. *Cell Death Dis.* 4:e657. doi: 10.1038/cddis.2013.182

Zhang, Y. W., Guo, Y. S., Bao, X. Q., Sun, H., and Zhang, D. (2016). Bicyclol promotes toll-like 2 receptor recruiting inosine 5′-monophosphate dehydrogenase II to exert its anti-inflammatory effect. *J. Asian Nat. Prod. Res.* 18, 475–485. doi: 10.1080/10286020.2015.1131678

Zhao, J., Yang, P., Li, F., Tao, L., Ding, H., Rui, Y., et al. (2012). Therapeutic effects of astragaloside iv on myocardial injuries: multi-target identification and network analysis. *PLoS ONE* 7:e44938. doi: 10.1371/journal.pone.0044938

Zheng, M., Liu, X., Xu, Y., Li, H., Luo, C., and Jiang, H. (2013). Computational methods for drug design and discovery: focus on China. *Trends Pharmacol. Sci.* 34, 549–559. doi: 10.1016/j.tips.2013.08.004

Zheng, R., Chen, T. S., and Lu, T. (2011). A comparative reverse docking strategy to identify potential antineoplastic targets of tea functional components and binding mode. *Int. J. Mol. Sci.* 12, 5200–5212. doi: 10.3390/ijms12085200

Zheng, Y., Wu, J., Feng, X., Jia, Y., Huang, J., Hao, Z., et al. (2015). *In silico* analysis and experimental validation of lignan extracts from kadsura longipedunculata for potential 5-HT1AR agonists. *PLoS ONE* 10:e0130055. doi: 10.1371/journal.pone.0130055

Ziegler, S., Pries, V., Hedberg, C., and Waldmann, H. (2013). Target identification for small bioactive molecules: finding the needle in the haystack. *Angew Chem. Int. Edit* 52, 2744–2792. doi: 10.1002/anie.201208749

Zoete, V., Daina, A., Bovigny, C., and Michielin, O. (2016). SwissSimilarity: a web tool for low to ultra high throughput ligand-based virtual screening. *J. Chem. Inf. Model.* 56, 1399–1404. doi: 10.1021/acs.jcim.6b00174

12

Structure-Activity Relationship Analysis of 3-Phenylcoumarin-Based Monoamine Oxidase B Inhibitors

Sanna Rauhamäki[1], Pekka A. Postila[1], Sanna Niinivehmas[1], Sami Kortet[1,2], Emmi Schildt[1,2], Mira Pasanen[1], Elangovan Manivannan[1,3], Mira Ahinko[1], Pasi Koskimies[4], Niina Nyberg[5], Pasi Huuskonen[5], Elina Multamäki[1], Markku Pasanen[5], Risto O. Juvonen[5], Hannu Raunio[5], Juhani Huuskonen[2] and Olli T. Pentikäinen[1,6]**

[1] Computational Bioscience Laboratory, Department of Biological and Environmental Science & Nanoscience Center, University of Jyväskylä, Jyväskylä, Finland, [2] Department of Chemistry & Nanoscience Center, University of Jyväskylä, Jyväskylä, Finland, [3] School of Pharmacy, Devi Ahilya University, Madhya Pradesh, India, [4] Forendo Pharma Ltd., Turku, Finland, [5] School of Pharmacy, University of Eastern Finland, Kuopio, Finland, [6] MedChem.fi, Institute of Biomedicine, University of Turku, Turku, Finland

***Correspondence:**
Juhani Huuskonen
juhani.s-p.huuskonen@jyu.fi
Olli T. Pentikäinen
olli.pentikainen@utu.fi

Monoamine oxidase B (MAO-B) catalyzes deamination of monoamines such as neurotransmitters dopamine and norepinephrine. Accordingly, small-molecule MAO-B inhibitors potentially alleviate the symptoms of dopamine-linked neuropathologies such as depression or Parkinson's disease. Coumarin with a functionalized 3-phenyl ring system is a promising scaffold for building potent MAO-B inhibitors. Here, a vast set of 3-phenylcoumarin derivatives was designed using virtual combinatorial chemistry or rationally *de novo* and synthesized using microwave chemistry. The derivatives inhibited the MAO-B at 100 nM–1 μM. The IC_{50} value of the most potent derivative **1** was 56 nM. A docking-based structure-activity relationship analysis summarizes the atom-level determinants of the MAO-B inhibition by the derivatives. Finally, the cross-reactivity of the derivatives was tested against monoamine oxidase A and a specific subset of enzymes linked to estradiol metabolism, known to have coumarin-based inhibitors. Overall, the results indicate that the 3-phenylcoumarins, especially derivative **1**, present unique pharmacological features worth considering in future drug development.

Keywords: 3-phenylcoumarin, monoamine oxidase B (MAO-B), structure-activity relationship (SAR), virtual drug design, Parkinson's disease

INTRODUCTION

During neuronal signaling, neurotransmitters are released from the presynaptic cell into the synaptic cleft, from where they bind into their specific receptors embedded on the postsynaptic membrane. The membrane lipid bilayer, especially its anionic phospholipid constituents, has been suggested to play a role in the small-molecule entry processes with the receptors (Orłowski et al., 2012; Postila et al., 2016; Mokkila et al., 2017). Moreover, to assure that the neurotransmission remains transient, the neurotransmitters are removed quickly from the synaptic cleft via enzymatic degradation and cellular uptake.

When inside the neuron, monoamine neurotransmitters such as norepinephrine and dopamine are either recycled or destined for deactivation through oxidative deamination ($RCH_2NHR' + H_2O + O_2 = RCHO + R'NH_2 + H_2O_2$) by monoamine oxidases A (MAO-A; E.C. 1.4.3.4) and B (MAO-B; E.C. 1.4.3.4). These enzymes are integral monotopic proteins that anchor themselves as dimers onto the mitochondrial outer membrane surface by protruding their α-helical C-termini into the lipid bilayer (**Figure 1A**). Moreover, both subtypes A and B deaminate preferentially their respective substrates to aldehydes: MAO-A catalyzes serotonin, norepinephrine, and to some extent dopamine; and MAO-B catalyzes dopamine, phenethylamine, benzylamine and to a lesser extent norepinephrine (Shih et al., 1999; Edmondson et al., 2005; Gaweska and Fitzpatrick, 2011).

The MAO-B, which is the target of this study, is connected to neurodegenerative disorders such as Alzheimer's disease but also mental disorders such as schizophrenia, anorexia nervosa, depression and attention deficit disorder. In all of these conditions, the involvement of MAO-B in the metabolism of dopamine and other amines is in a key role (Youdim et al., 2006; Carradori and Silvestri, 2015). For instance, due to gliosis associated with Parkinson's disease, increased levels of MAO-B speed up degradation of dopamine in the motor neurons. MAO-B inhibitors decrease the degradation and boost dopamine concentration in the synapse. Thus, instead of introducing more dopamine, the neurotransmitter levels are elevated by inhibiting MAO-B. As a result, MAO-B inhibitors such as selegiline are used in treatment of Parkinson's disease, moreover, their neuroprotective effects can benefit Alzheimer's disease patients (Youdim et al., 2006). Due to these hepatotoxic effects of irreversibly binding MAO inhibitors, reversible inhibitors such as moclobemide were developed (Youdim et al., 2006; Finberg and Rabey, 2016). The MAO inhibitors can exhibit selectivity toward MAO-A (moclobemide) or MAO-B (pargyline, selegiline) or be non-selective (phenelzine, tranylcypromine). The selectivity, which can be lost in high dosages, is important for avoiding MAO-A inhibition related cheese effect (Youdim et al., 2006; Finberg and Rabey, 2016).

A vast amount of different types of MAO inhibitors are described in the literature and for example the ChEMBL database lists inhibition data for thousands of compounds. The specific problem in the development of MAO-specific ligands is that the promising compounds have potential to become active on other amine oxidases such as vascular adhesion protein 1 (Nurminen et al., 2010, 2011). Here, the aim was to probe the MAO-B activity and selectivity effects of different substitutions on the coumarin core by focusing, especially, on the 3-phenylcoumarin (or 3-arylcoumarin). Notably, there exist two X-ray crystal structures with structurally related coumarin analogs in which 3-chlorobenzyloxy groups are attached at the C7-position (**Figures 1B–D**). The studied set of 3-phenylcoumarin derivatives with different R1-R7 groups (**Figure 1E**) introduced in this study make an important addition to the earlier studies in which the potential of coumarin core, including 61 3-phenylcoumarin derivatives (Matos et al., 2009b, 2010, 2011a,b; Santana et al., 2010; Serra et al., 2012; Viña et al., 2012a,b), to block MAO-A and MAO-B has been explored (Borges et al., 2005; Catto et al., 2006; Matos et al., 2009a, 2010, 2011a; Serra et al., 2012; Ferino et al., 2013; Joao Matos et al., 2013; Patil et al., 2013). The compounds were designed using virtual combinatorial chemistry or rationally *de novo* and binding were probed via molecular docking prior to synthesis or *in vitro* testing.

Initially, 52 derivatives of the 3-phenylcoumarin core were synthesized and tested here for the first time for MAO-B inhibition using a specifically tailored spectrophotometric assay (Supplementary Table S1) (Holt et al., 1997). Next, 24 of the derivatives (**Figure 2**, **Table 1**), producing >70% inhibition at 10 μM, were selected for further analysis. These derivatives inhibited MAO-B at a ∼100 nM to ∼1 μM range, while the most potent derivative **1** produces ∼50–60 nM inhibition (**Table 1**, **Figure 2**). Finally, the potency of the derivatives for inhibiting estrogen receptor (ER), 17-β-hydroxysteroid dehydrogenase 1 (HSD1), aromatase (CYP19A1), and cytochrome P450 1A2 (CYP1A2), the topics of both our prior (Niinivehmas et al., 2016) and ongoing studies, was also considered. A docking-based structure-activity relationship (SAR) analysis (**Figure 2**) was performed with all of the synthetized 3-phenylcoumarins focusing mainly on the 24 most potent compounds.

In short, this study explores thoroughly the pharmacological potential of 3-phenylcoumarin (**Figure 1E**) for blocking the MAO-B activity (**Table 1**, Supplementary Table S1) and, furthermore, explains the basis of the inhibitory effect on the atom level.

MATERIALS AND METHODS

Virtual Combinatorial Chemistry

The 3-phenylcoumarin was chosen as the scaffold of interest for building new MAO-B-specific inhibitors (see section The Alignment of the 3-Phenylcoumarin Scaffold at the Active Site). The analogs were designed using virtual combinatorial chemistry or virtual synthesis. In the initial stages, methoxy group was included at the R1 or R2 position (**Figure 1E**) in the coumarin core due to its predicted favorability at the active site. The R4-R7 substituents of the 3-phenyl ring (**Figure 1E**) were designed by combining phenylacetic acid with either 6-methoxycoumarin or 7-methoxycoumarin. The preliminary combinatorial compound library was generated using MAESTRO version 9.3 CombiGlide (CombiGlide, version 2.8, Schrödinger, LLC, New York, NY, USA) and Combinatorial Screening module. The compounds were docked with GLIDE and scored using GlideScore. Some of these derivatives with promising potency and selectivity profile in this study (**8, 10, 25, 37**) were eventually synthesized, albeit using different chemistry (see section Chemical Procedure), and tested *in vitro*. Majority of the final derivatives were designed *de novo* after performing the initial docking simulations with the virtual synthesis products.

Abbreviations: MAO-A, monoamine oxidase A; MAO-B, monoamine oxidase B; HSD1 or 17-β-HSD1, 17-β-hydroxysteroid dehydrogenase 1; ER, estrogen receptor; CYP1A2, cytochrome P450 1A2; CYP19A1, aromatase; SAR, structure-activity relationship.

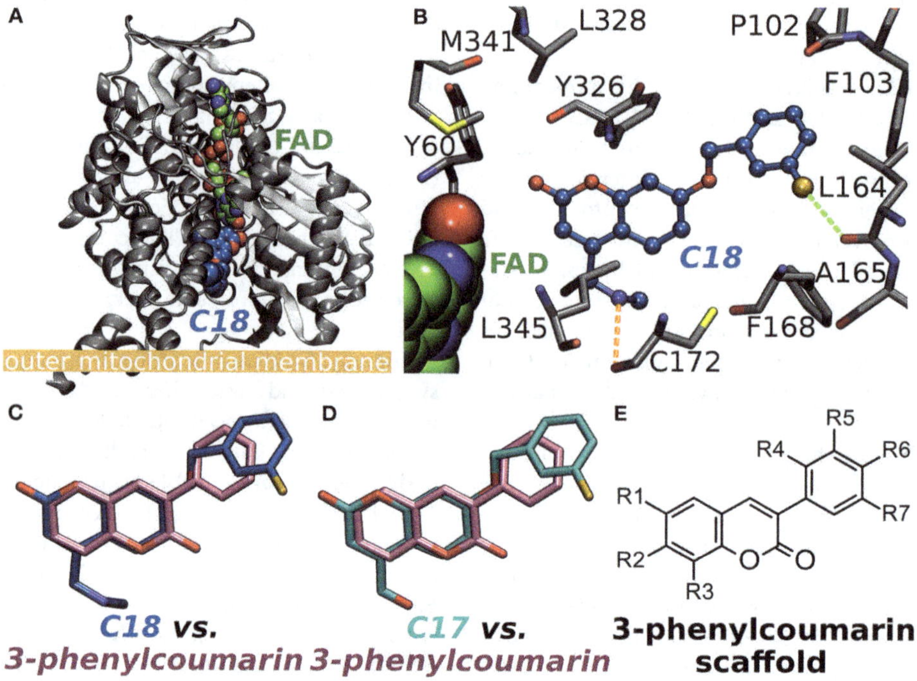

FIGURE 1 | Monoamine oxidase B structure and the small-molecule inhibitors. **(A)** The cytoplasmic MAO-B monomer (gray cartoon; PDB: 2V61; A-chain) (Binda et al., 2007) is anchored by its C-terminal helix onto the outer mitochondrial membrane [thick orange line; from the OPM database (Lomize et al., 2006)]. The bound inhibitor 7-(3-chlorobenzyloxy)-4-(methylamino)methyl-coumarin (*C18* in PDB: 2V61; blue backbone) and the cofactor flavin adenine dinucleotide (FAD; green backbone) are shown as CPK models. **(B)** A close up of the MAO-B active site with *C18* (blue backbone; ball-and-stick model) shows the small-molecule forming a halogen bond (green dotted line) and an H-bond (orange dotted line) with the main chain oxygen atoms of Leu164 and Cys172 (ball-and-stick models with gray backbone), respectively. The binding poses of the coumarin-based inhibitors **(C)** *C18* and **(D)** 7-(3-chlorobenzyloxy)-4-carboxaldehyde-coumarin (*C17* in PDB: 2V60) (Binda et al., 2007) are highly similar with the 3-phenylcoumarin scaffold pose produced by molecular docking. Notably, the coumarin ring is reversed for the established inhibitors in comparison to the docking-based pose of the scaffold. Moreover, the phenyl rings of *C17* and *C18* are attached via ether bonds to the coumarin's C7-position instead of C3-position used with the inhibitors introduced in this study. **(E)** The 2D structure of the 3-phenylcoumarin scaffold indicating the positions of the functional R1-R7 groups.

Chemical Procedure

All reactions were carried out using commercial materials (Sigma-Aldrich, Mannheim, Germany) and reagents without further purification unless otherwise noted. Reaction mixtures were heated by the CEM Discover microwave apparatus. All reactions were monitored by thin layer chromatography (TLC) on silica gel plates. ^{1}H NMR and ^{13}C NMR data was recorded on a Bruker Avance 400 MHz spectrometer or Bruker Avance III 300 MHz spectrometer. Chemical shifts are expressed in parts per million values (ppm) and are designated as s (singlet), br s (broad singlet), d (doublet), dd (double doublet), and t (triplet). Coupling constants (*J*) are expressed as values in hertz (Hz). The mass spectra were recorded using Micromass LCT ESI-TOF equipment. Elemental analyses were done with Elementar Vario EL III elemental analyzer. The coumarin derivatives were synthesized using Perkin-Oglialor condensation reaction. The method was developed from the earlier published procedures and transferred to microwave reactor and it was published earlier by authors (Niinivehmas et al., 2016).

A typical procedure: A mixture of salicylaldehyde derivative (2 mmol) and phenyl acetic acid derivative (2.1 mmol), acetic acid anhydride (0.6 ml), and triethylamine (0.36 ml) were placed in a microwave reactor tube and this mixture was heated at 100–170°C with microwave apparatus (100–200 W) for 10–20 min. After cooling, 2 ml of 10% $NaHCO_3$ solution was added and the precipitate was filtered, dried and recrystallized from $EtOH/H_2O$ or acetone/H_2O mixture. The acetyl group(s) were removed by treating the compound with 2 M MeOH/NaOH(aq) (1:1) solution for 30–60 min at r.t. The solution was acidified with 2 M HCl(aq,) and the precipitate was filtered and recrystallized if needed.

Based on the elemental analysis and/or ^{1}H-NMR the purity of compounds was >95%.

6-methoxy-3-(4-(trifluoromethyl)phenyl)-2H-chromen-2-one (1). Yield: 76%; ^{1}H-NMR (400 MHz, $CDCl_3$) δ: 3.86 (s, 3H, CH_3O-), 6.99 (s, 1H, H-5), 7.14 (d, 1H, J^3 = 7.7 Hz, H-7), 7.29 (d, J^3 = 8.9 Hz, H-8), 7.69 (d, 2H, J^3 = 7.9 Hz, H-2', H-6'), 7.58 (m, 3H, H-4, H-3', H-5'); ^{13}C-NMR (100.6 MHz, $CDCl_3$) δ: 55.99, 110.24, 117.73, 119.78, 120.02, 125.51 (q, J^{C-F} = 4 Hz), 127.37, 129.05, 130.85 (q, J^{C-F} = 32 Hz), 138.41, 140.88, 148.33, 156.44, 160.42. HRMS(ESI): calc. for $C_{17}H_{11}F_3O_3Na_1$ 343.0558, found 343.0574; elemental anal. for $C_{17}H_{11}F_3O_3$, calc. C% 63.76, H% 3.46, found C% 63.25, H% 3.51.

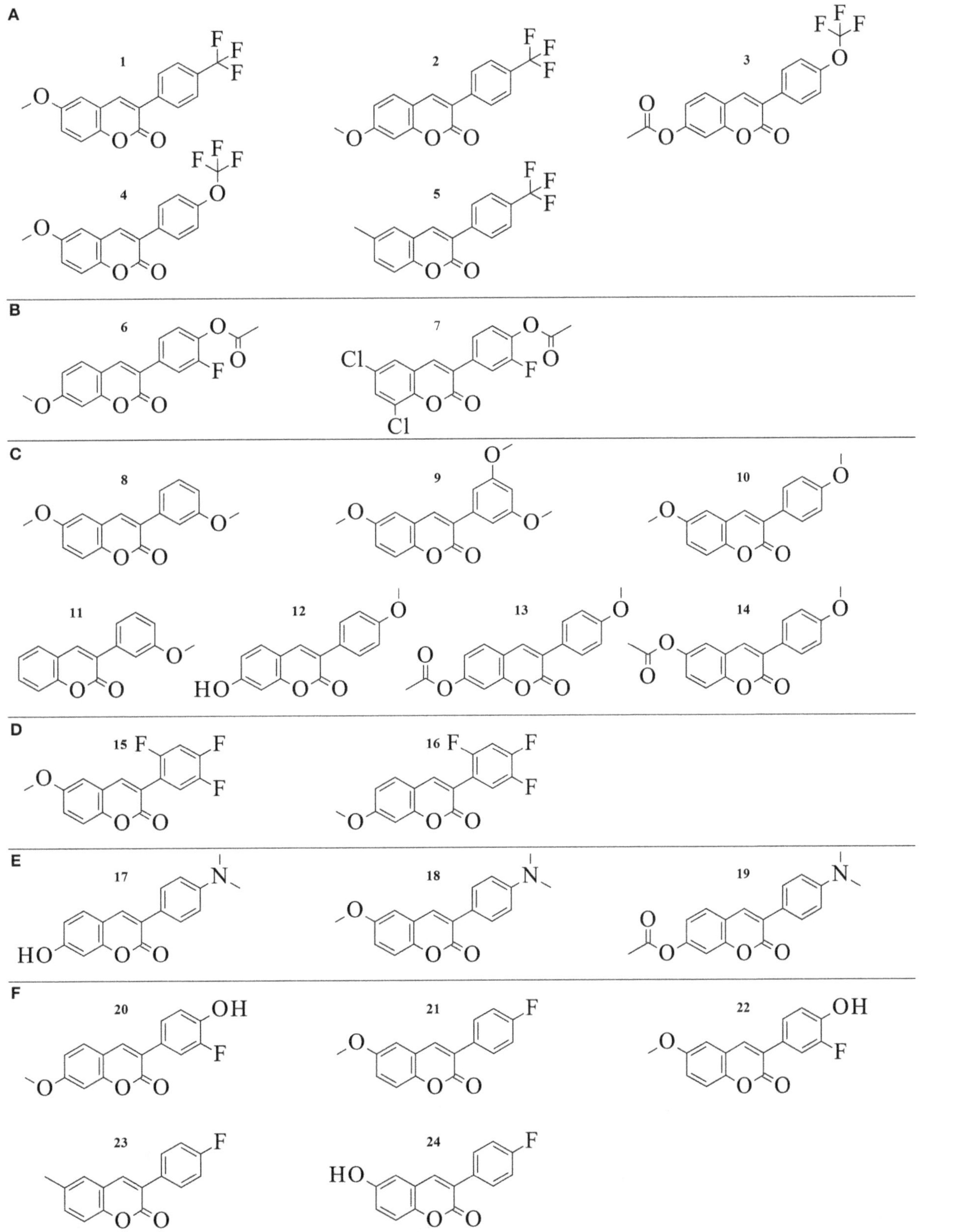

FIGURE 2 | 2D structures of the 24 3-phenylcoumarin derivatives producing at least 70% MAO-B inhibition. The compounds are grouped to **(A–F)** groups based on the chemical similarity of the R1-R7 substituents (**Figure 1E**). See **Table 1** for the detailed activity data.

TABLE 1 | The activity data on the 24 most potent 3-phenylcoumarin derivatives.

Group	ID	MAO-B inhibition IC_{50} nM	QPlogPo/w	MAO-B inhibition % (10 μM)	MAO-A inhibition % (100 μM)	ER inhibition % (10 μM)	HSD1 inhibition % (1 μM)	CYP1A2 inhibition IC_{50} μM
Control	c	61[(1)]	2.43[(1)]	102.00[(1)]	100.89[(2)]	106.60[(3)]	N/A	N/A
A	01	56	4.08	99.53	0.00	N/A	0	124.00
	02	138	4.11	99.58	0.00	N/A	1	N/A
	03	141	3.33	100.44	22.03	N/A	0	280.00
	04	317	4.22	101.96	0.00	N/A	0	7.00
	05	343	4.35	105.33	0.00	1.08	0	171.00
B	06	189	2.47	99.92	0.00	N/A	21	N/A
	07	888	3.36	91.01	0.00	N/A	0	46.00
C	08	231	3.11	111.93	0.00	0	0	2.30
	09	255	3.21	80.21	0.00	N/A	0	84.00
	10	400	3.15	97.57	10.14	N/A	0	15.00
	11	798	3.06	90.33	0.00	0.29	4	1.60
	12	955	2.49	85.89	24.57	91.34	3	170.00
	13	1946	2.41	85.89	2.48	N/A	0	570.00
	14	8476	2.34	75.75	N/A	N/A	1	87.51
D	15	292	3.73	87.16	0.00	0	12	3.00
	16	1433	3.71	77.63	N/A	8.80	33	4.50
E	17	384	2.80	90.14	4.74	N/A	5	35.00
	18	617	3.49	93.86	0.00	0	1	17.00
	19	866	2.79	85.41	0.00	N/A	15	370.00
F	20	391	2.71	100.82	0.00	86.10	46	30.00
	21	433	3.32	88.77	0.00	0	0	3.00
	22	831	2.73	94.86	0.00	55.38	54	1.50
	23	902	3.58	83.49	0.00	0	11	3.00
	24	1058	2.61	89.10	14.18	0	20	3.00

*N/A = not available. Controls: [(1)]pargyline, [(2)]clorgyline, [(3)]kit control. The compounds are grouped (A–F) based on the chemical similarity of the R1–R7 substituents (**Figure 1E**).*

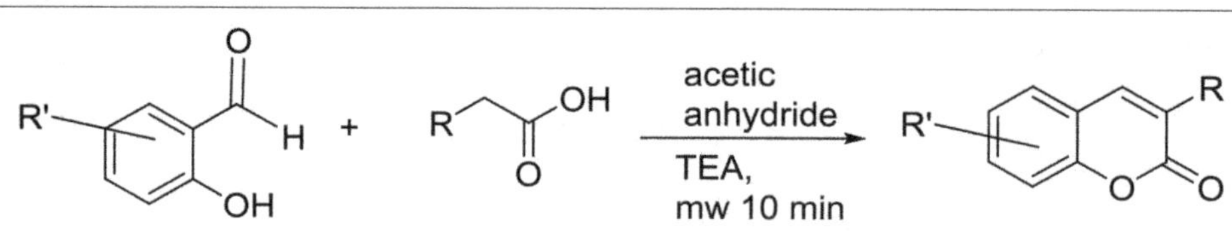

SCHEME 1 | The synthesis of 3-phenylcoumarin analogs.

6-methoxy-3-(4-(trifluoromethyl)phenyl)-2H-chromen-2-one (2). Yield: 80%; ^{1}H-NMR (300 MHz, d^6-DSMO) δ: 3.88 (s, 3H, CH_3O-), 6.99 (s, 1H, J^3 = 8.7 Hz, J^4 = 2.4 Hz, H-6), 7.03 (d, 1H, J^4 = 2.4 Hz, H-7), 7.71 (d, J^3 = 8.6 Hz, H-8), 7.79 (d, 2H, J^3 = 8.3 Hz, H-2', H-6'), 7.93 (d, 2H, H-3', H-5'), 8.32 (s, 1H, H-4); ^{13}C-NMR (75.5 MHz, d^6-DMSO) δ: 55.97, 100.25, 112.80, 121.57, 122.38, 120.02, 124.97 (q, J^{C-F} = 4 Hz), 128.29 (q, J^{C-F} = 32 Hz), 128.97, 129.99, 139.01, 142.10, 155.09, 159.62, 162.82. HRMS(ESI) calc for $C_{17}H_{11}F_3O_3Na_1$ [M + Na]$^+$: 343.05525, found 343.05610.

2-oxo-3-(4-(trifluoromethoxy)phenyl)-2H-chromen-7-yl acetate (3). (Dobelmann-Mara et al., 2017) Yield: 54%; %; ^{1}H-NMR (400 MHz, d^6-DMSO) δ: 2.27 (s, 3H, $CH_3C(O)O$-), 7.20 (dd, 1H, J^3 = Hz, J^4 = Hz, H-6), 7.33 (d, 1H, J^4 = Hz, H-8), 7.47 (d, 2H, J^3 = Hz, H-3', H-5'), 7.81 (d, 1H, J^3 = 8.4 Hz, H-5), 8.32 (s, 1H, H-4); ^{13}C-NMR (100 MHz, d^6-DMSO) δ: 20.86 109.74, 117.23, 118.88, 120.75, 124.84, 129.42, 129.60, 130.52, 133.85, 140.73, 148.35, 152.90, 153.55, 159.40, 168.78; HRMS(ESI) calc. for $C_{18}H_{11}F_3O_5Na_1$ [M + Na]$^+$ 387.0457, found 387.0481.

6-methoxy-3-(4-(trifluoromethoxy)phenyl)-2H-chromen-2-one (4). Yield: 52%; ^{1}H-NMR (400 MHz, $CDCl_3$) δ: 3.86 (s, 3H, CH_3O-), 6.98 (d, 1H, $J^4 = 3$ Hz, H-5), 7.12 (dd, $J^3 = 9.1$ Hz, $J^4 = 3$ Hz, H-7), 7.27-7.30 (m, 3H, H-8, H-3', H-5'), 7.74 (d, 2H, $J^3 = 8.9$ Hz, H-2', H-6'); 7.77 (s, 1H, H-4); ^{13}C-NMR (100 MHz, $CDCl_3$) δ: 55.99, 110.16, 117.70, 119.68, 119.92, 120.97, 127.41, 130.26, 133.51, 140.20, 148.21, 149.67, 156.41, 160.65. HRMS(ESI) calc for $C_{17}H_{11}F_3O_4Na_1$ $[M + Na]^+$: 359.05071, found 359.05260. elemental anal. for $C_{17}H_{11}F_3O_4 \cdot 0.5H_2O$, calc. C% 59.14, H% 3.50, found C% 58.99, H% 3.25.

6-methyl-3-(4-(trifluoromethyl)phenyl)-2H-chromen-2-one (5). Yield: 54%; ^{1}H-NMR (400 MHz, $CDCl_3$) δ: 7.27 (d, 1H, $J^4 = 2.2$ Hz, H-5), 7.35-7.38 (m, 2H, H-7, H-8), 7.70 (d, $J^3 = 8.2$ Hz, H-2', H-6'), 7.82 (m, 3H, H-4, H-3', H-5'); ^{13}C-NMR (100 MHz, $CDCl_3$) δ: 20.92, 116.46, 119.22, 122.80, 125.53 (q, $J^{C-F} = 4$ Hz), 126.98, 128.07, 129.05, 130.80 (q, $J^{C-F} = 33$ Hz), 133.29, 134.62, 138.50, 141.08, 152.04 160.53; HRMS(ESI) calc for $C_{17}H_{12}Cl_2O_4Na_1$ $[M + Na]^+$: 373.0005, found 372.9998.

2-fluoro-4-(7-methoxy-2-oxo-2H-chromen-3-yl)phenyl acetate (6). Yield 75%; ^{1}H-NMR (400 MHz, d^6-DMSO) δ: 2.35 (s, 3H, $CH_3C(O)O$-Ph), 3.88 (s, 3H, CH_3O-Ph), 6.99 (dd, 1H, $J^3 = 8.6$ Hz, $J^4 = 2.4$ Hz, H-6), 7.05 (d, 1H, $J^4 = 2.4$ Hz, H-8), 7.37 (dd, $J^3 = 9.3$ Hz, $J^{H-F} = 8.3$ Hz, H-5'), 7.62 (ddd, 1H, $J^3 = 8.5$ Hz, $J^4 = 2.1$ Hz, $J^{H-F} = 0.8$ Hz, H-6'), 7.68 (d, $J = 8.6$ Hz, 1H, H-5), 7.74 (dd, $J^{H-F} = 12.1$ Hz, $J^4 = 2.0$ Hz, H-3'), 8.31 (s, 1H, H-4); ^{13}C-NMR (100 MHz, d^6-DMSO) δ: 20.19, 55.97, 100.25, 112.79, 116.35 (d, $J^{C-F} = 20.3$ Hz), 121.02, 121.03, 123.83, 124.79 (d, $J^{C-F} = 3.2$ Hz), 129.86, 134.24 (d, $J^{C-F} = 7.7$ Hz), 137.20 (d, $J^{C-F} = 13.1$ Hz), 141.55, 153.00 ($J^{C-F} = 246.1$ Hz), 154.92, 159.65, 162.69, 168.19. HRMS(ESI) calc for $C_{18}H_{13}F_1O_5Na_1$ $[M + Na]^+$: 351.06447, found 351.06240; elemental anal. for $C_{18}H_{13}F_1O_5$ C% 65.85, H% 3.99, found C% 65.28 H% 4.02.

4-(6,8-dichloro-2-oxo-2H-chromen-3-yl)-2-fluorophenyl acetate (7). Yield 58%; ^{1}H-NMR (400 MHz, d^6-DMSO) δ: 2.36 (s, 3H, $CH_3C(O)O$-), 7.43 (dd, $J^3 = 9.3$ Hz, $J^{H-F} = 8.3$ Hz, H-5'), 7.67 (ddd, 1H, $J^3 = 8.4$ Hz, $J^4 = 2.1$ Hz, $J^{H-F} = 0.8$ Hz, H-6'), 7.74 (dd, $J^{H-F} = 11.8$ Hz, $J^4 = 2.0$ Hz, H-3'), 7.84 (d, 1H, $J^4 = 2.4$ Hz, H-7), 7.97 (d, 1H, $J^4 = 2.4$ Hz, H-5), 8.32 (s, 1H, H-4); ^{13}C-NMR (100 MHz, d^6-DMSO) δ: 20.72, 117.23 (d, $J^{C-F} = 21$ Hz), 121.13, 122.17, 124.65, 125.74 (d, $J^{C-F} = 3.3$ Hz), 127.29, 128.80, 131.47, 133.70 (d, $J^{C-F} = 7.7$ Hz), 138.50 (d, $J^{C-F} = 12.9$ Hz), 140.12, 147.94, 152.30, 154.75. 158.73; HRMS(ESI): calc. for $C_{17}H_9Cl_2F_1O_4Na_1$ $[M + Na]^+$: 388.9760, found 388. 9762.

6-methoxy-3-(3-methoxyphenyl)-2H-chromen-2-one (8). Yield 78%; ^{1}H-NMR (400 MHz, $CDCl_3$) δ: 3.85 (s, 3H, CH_3O-Ph), 3.86 (s, 3H, CH_3O-Ph), 6.93-6.97 (m, 2H, H-4', H-5), 7.10 (dd, 1H, $J^3 = 9.0$, Hz, $J^4 = 1.9$ Hz, H-7), 7.25-7.29 (m, 3H, H-8, H-2', H-6'), 7.35 (t, 1H, $J^3 = 8.2$ Hz, H-5'), 7.76 (s, 1H, H-4); ^{13}C-NMR (100 MHz, $CDCl_3$) δ: 55.69, 56.18, 110.28, 114.57, 114.88, 117.78, 119.55, 120.28, 121.26, 128.80, 129.79, 136.43, 140.13, 148.34, 156.47, 159.88, 160.91; HRMS(ESI): calc. for $C_{17}H_{14}O_4Na_1$ $[M + Na]^+$: 305.07898, found 305.07950; elemental anal. for $C_{14}H_{14}O_4$ calc. C% 72.33, H% 5.00, found C% 72.41, H% 4.88.

3-(3,5-dimethoxyphenyl)-6-methoxy-2H-chromen-2-one (9). (Vilar et al., 2006) Yield 59%; ^{1}H-NMR (400 MHz, d^6-DMSO) δ: 3.79 (s, 6H, CH_3O-Ph), 3.82 (s, 3H, CH_3O-Ph), 6.56 (t, 1H, $J^4 = 2.3$ Hz, H-4'), 6.89 (d, 2H, $J^4 = 2.3$ Hz, H-2', H-6'), 7.20 (dd, 1H, $J^3 = 9.0$ Hz, $J^4 = 3.0$ Hz, H-7), 7.31 (d, 1H, $J^4 = 3.0$ Hz, H-5), 7.36 (d, 1H, $J^3 = 9.0$ Hz, H-8), 8.23 (s, 1H, H-4); ^{13}C-NMR (100 MHz, d^6-DMSO) δ: 55.30, 55.66, 100.48, 106.71, 110.69, 116.90, 119.36, 119.78, 126.75, 136.44, 140.66, 147.33, 155.62, 159.53, 160.16; HRMS(ESI): calc. for $C_{18}H_{16}O_5Na_1$ $[M + Na]^+$: 335.08954, found 305.09010; elemental anal. for $C_{14}H_{14}O_4$ calc. C% 69.22, H% 5.16, found C% 68.80, H% 5.14.

6-methoxy-3-(4-methoxyphenyl)-2H-chromen-2-one (10). (Prendergast, 2001; Ferino et al., 2013) Yield 79%; ^{1}H-NMR (400 MHz, $CDCl_3$) δ: 3.847 (s, 3H, CH_3O-Ph), 3.852 (s, 3H, CH_3O-Ph), 6.95-6.98 (m, 3H, H-5, H-3', H-5'), 7.07 (dd, 1H, $J^3 = 9.0$ Hz, $J^4 = 2.9$ Hz, H-7), 7.27 (d, 1H, $J^4 = 8.8$ Hz, H-5), 7.66 (d, 2H, $J^3 = 8.9$ Hz, H-2', H-6'), 7.70 (s, 1H, H-4); ^{13}C-NMR (100 MHz, $CDCl_3$) δ:55.69, 56.16, 110.11, 114.23, 117.69, 119.05, 120.51, 127.47, 128.49, 130.18, 138.63, 148.11, 156.44, 160.49, 161.24; HRMS(ESI): calc. for $C_{17}H_{14}O_4Na_1$ $[M + Na]^+$: 305.07898, found 305.07910; elemental anal. for $C_{17}H_{14}O_4$ calc. C% 72.33, H% 5.00, found C% 72.34, H% 4.86.

3-(3-methoxyphenyl)-2H-chromen-2-one (11). (Kirkiacharian et al., 1999) Yield 81%; ^{1}H-NMR (400 MHz, $CDCl_3$) δ: 3.86 (s, 3H, CH_3O-Ph), 6.95 (ddd, 1H, $J^3 = 8.2$ Hz, $J^4 = 2.3$ Hz, $J^4 = 2.5$ Hz, H-4'), 7.26-7.37 (m, 5H, H-6, H-8, H-2', H-5', H-6'), 7.51-7.53 (m, 2H, H-5, H-7), 7.81 (s, 1H, H-4); ^{13}C-NMR (100 MHz, $CDCl_3$) δ: 55.69, 114.56, 114.86, 116.76, 119.94, 121.24, 124.81, 128.26, 128.49, 129.80, 131.76, 136.35, 140.28, 153.85, 159.88, 160.76; HRMS(ESI): calc. for $C_{16}H_{12}O_3Na_1$ $[M + Na]^+$: 275.06841, found 275.06540; elemental anal. for $C_{16}H_{12}O_3$ calc. C% 76.18, H% 4.79, found C% 75.94, H% 4.67.

7-hydroxy-3-(4-methoxyphenyl)-2H-chromen-2-one (12). (Prendergast, 2001) Yield 81%; ^{1}H-NMR (400 MHz, d^6-DMSO) δ: 3.79 (s, 3H, CH_3O-Ph), 6.74 (s, 1H, H-8), 6.81 (d, 1H, $J^3 = 8.5$ Hz, H-6), 6.99 (d, 2H, $J^3 = 8.3$ Hz, H-3', H-5'), 7.57 (d, 1H, $J^3 = 8.4$ Hz, H-5), 7.65 (d, 2H, $J^3 = 8.3$ Hz, H-2, H-6'), 8.08 (s, 1H, H-4), 10.54 (s, 1H, HO-Ph); ^{13}C-NMR (100 MHz, d^6-DMSO) δ: 55.18, 101.66, 112.10, 113.29, 113.61, 121.84, 127.30, 129.48, 129.70, 139.73, 154.63, 159.14, 160.20, 160.88; HRMS(ESI): calc. for $C_{16}H_{12}O_4Na_1$ $[M + Na]^+$: 291.06333, found 291.06160.

3-(4-methoxyphenyl)-2-oxo-2H-chromen-7-yl acetate (13). (Bhandri et al., 1949) Yield 67%; ^{1}H-NMR (400 MHz, d^6-DMSO) δ: 7.02 (d, 2H, $J^3 = 7.8$ Hz, H-3', H-5'), 7.17 (d, 1H, $J^3 = 8.3$ Hz, H-6), 7.29 (d, 1H, H-8), 7.69 (d, 2H, $J^3 = 7.8$ Hz, H-2', H-6'), 7.79 (d, 1H, $J^3 = 8.2$ Hz, H-5), 8.19 (s, 1H, H-4); ^{13}C-NMR (100 MHz, d^6-DMSO) δ: 20.85, 55.22, 109.57, 113.68, 117.49, 118.68, 125.69, 126.72, 129.19, 129.75, 138.62, 152.36, 153.15, 159.59, 168.81; HRMS (ESI): Calc for $C_{18}H_{14}O_5Na_1$ $[M + Na]^+$: 333.07389, found 333.07220. Elemental analysis for $C_{18}H_{14}O_5$ calc C% 69.67 H% 4.55, found C% 69.58 H% 4.52.

3-(4-methoxyphenyl)-2-oxo-2H-chromen-6-yl acetate (14). Yield 34%; 1H-NMR (300 MHz, d6-DMSO) δ: 2.31 (s, 3H, CH3C(O)O-), 3.81 (s, 3H, CH3O-), 7.03 (d, 2H, J3 = 8.7 Hz, H-3', H-5'), 7.37 (dd, 1H, J3 = 8.9 Hz, J4 = 2.5 Hz, H-7), 7.47 (d, 1H, J3 = 8.9 Hz, H-8), 7.54 (d, 1H, J4 = 2.5 Hz, H-5), 7.70 (d, 2H, J3 = 8.7 Hz, H-2', H-6'), 8.15 (s, 1H, H-5); 13C-NMR (75 MHz, d6-DMSO) δ: 20.73, 55.21, 113.68, 116.83, 120.07, 120.53, 125.00, 126.61, 127.03, 129.84, 138.30, 146.39, 150.18, 159.64, 159.71, 169.22. HRMS (ESI): Calc for C18H14O5 [M + H]+: 311.0914, found 311.0908.

6-methoxy-3-(2,4,5-trifluorophenyl)-2H-chromen-2-one (15). Yield 80%; ^{1}H-NMR (400 MHz, d^6-DMSO) δ: 3.81 (s, 3H, CH_3O-Ph), 7.26 (dd, 1H, $J^3 = 9.0$ Hz, $J^4 = 3.0$ Hz, H-7), 7.31 (d, 1H, $J^4 = 3.0$ Hz, H-5), 7.41 (d, 1H, $J^3 = 9.0$ Hz, H-8), 7.64-7.77 (m, 2H, H-2', H-6'), 8.18 (s, 1H, H-4); ^{13}C-NMR (100 MHz, d^6-DMSO) δ: 55.73, 106.31 (dd, $J^{C-F} = 21$ Hz, $J^{C-F} = 22$ Hz), 110.90, 117.25, 119.12, 119.39, 119.55, 120.07, 120.91, 143.74, 145.70 (d, $J^{C-F} = 242$ Hz), 147.64, 149.34 ($J^{C-F} = 252$ Hz), 155.13 ($J^{C-F} = 248$ Hz), 155.79, 158.78. HRMS (ESI): Calc for $C_{16}H_9F_3O_3Na_1$ [M + Na]$^+$: 329.04015, found 329.04090. Elemental analysis for $C_{16}H_9F_3O_3$: calc C% 62.75 H% 2.96, found C% 62.62 H% 3.15.

7-methoxy-3-(2,4,5-trifluorophenyl)-2H-chromen-2-one (16). Yield 85 %; ^{1}H-NMR (300 MHz, d^6-DMSO) δ: 3.88 (s, 3H, CH_3O-Ph), 7.00 (dd, 1H, $J^3 = 8.6$ Hz, $J^4 = 2.4$ Hz, H-6), 7.06 (d, 1H, $J^4 = 2.3$ Hz, H-8), 7.61-7.6 (m, 3H, H-5, H-2', H-6'), 8.17 (s, 1H, H-4); ^{13}C-NMR (75.5 MHz, d^6-DMSO) δ: 56.02, 100.49, 106.21 (dd, $J^{C-F} = 21$ Hz, $J^{C-F} = 21$ Hz), 112.24, 112.85, 116.85, 119.30, 119.57, 129.95, 144.06, 145.67 (d, $J^{C-F} = 242$ Hz), 148.93 (d, $J^{C-F} = 250$) Hz, 155.10 (d, $J^{C-F} = 245$ Hz), 155.22, 158.89, 162.98; HRMS (ESI): Calc for $C_{16}H_9F_3O_3Na_1$ [M + Na]$^+$: 329.04015, found 329.03980.

3-(4-(dimethylamino)phenyl)-7-hydroxy-2H-chromen-2-one (17). (Kirkiacharian et al., 2003) In the first step 7-acetoxy-3-(4-(dimethylamino)phenyl)-2*H*-chromen-2one was obtained. Yield: 70%; ^{1}H-NMR (400 MHz, d^6-DMSO) δ: 2.31 (s, 3H, $CH_3C(O)O$-Ph), 2.95 (s, 6H, $(CH_3)_2N$-Ph), 6.77 (d, $J^3 = 9.0$ Hz, 2H, H-2', H-6'), 7.14 (dd, $J^3 = 8.4$ Hz, $J^4 = 2.2$ Hz, 1H, H-5), 7.26 (d, $J^4 = 2.2$ Hz, 1H, H-8), 7.63 (d, $J^3 = 9.0$ Hz, 2H, H-3', H-5') 7.76 (d, $J^3 = 8.5$ Hz, 1H, H-5), 8.11 (s, 1H, H-4); ^{13}C-NMR (100.6 MHz, d^6-DMSO) δ: 20.85, 39.84, 109.44, 111.58, 117.76, 118.57, 121.57, 126.00, 128.82, 129.11, 136.46, 150.45, 151.90, 152.77, 159.74, 168.85. In the second step 7-hydroxy-3-(4-(dimethylamino)phenyl)-2*H*-chromen-2one was obtained. Yield: 85% yellow solid; ^{1}H-NMR (400 MHz, d^6-DMSO) δ: 2.94 (s, 6H, $(CH_3)_2N$-), 6.72 (d, $J^4 = 2.3$ Hz, 1H, H-8), 6.75 (d, $J^3 = 9.0$ Hz, 2H, H-2', H-6'), 6.79 (dd, $J^3 = 8.4$ Hz, $J^4 = 2.3$ Hz, 1H, H-5),), 7.55 (d, $J^3 = 8.5$ Hz, 1H, H-5), 7.58 (d, $J^3 = 9.0$ Hz, 2H, H-3', H-5'), 7.99 (s, 1H, H-4); ^{13}C-NMR (100.6 MHz, d^6-DMSO) δ: 39.92, 101.59, 112.33, 113.16, 122.30, 122.32, 129.34, 137.83, 150.07, 154.27, 160.30, 160.41; HRMS (ESI): Calc for $C_{17}H_{15}N_1O_3Na_1$ [M + Na]$^+$: 304.09496, found 304.09480; elemental anal. for $C_{17}H_{15}N_1O_3$, calc. C% 72.58, H% 5.37, N% 4.98, found C% 72.45, H% 5.40, N% 5.15.

3-(4-(dimethylamino)phenyl)-6-methoxy-2H-chromen-2-one (18). Yield 55%; ^{1}H-NMR (400 MHz, d^6-DMSO) δ: 2.96 (s, 6H, $(CH_3)_2N$-Ph), 3.81 (s, 3H, CH_3O-Ph), 6.77 (d, 2H, $J^3 =$ Hz, H-3', H-5'), 7.14 (dd, 1H, $J^3 = 3.0$ Hz, $J^4 = 9.0$ Hz, H-7), 7.28 (d, 1H, $J^4 = 3.0$ Hz, H-5), 7.33 (d, 1H, $J^3 = 9.0$ Hz, H-8), 7.63 (d, 2H, $J^3 = 9.0$ Hz, H-2', H-6'), 8.06 (s, 1H, H-4); ^{13}C-NMR (100.6 MHz, d^6-DMSO) δ: 39.93, 110.27, 111.59, 116.68, 118.16, 120.35, 121.73, 126.96, 129.15, 136.79, 146.79, 150.46, 155.59, 160.06; HRMS (ESI): Calc for $C_{18}H_{17}N_1O_3Na_1$ [M + Na]$^+$: 318.11061, found 318.11050; elemental anal. for $C_{18}H_{17}N_1O_3$, calc. C% 73.20, H% 5.80, N% 4.74, found C% 72.75, H% 5.83, N% 4.45.

3-(4-(dimethylamino)phenyl)-2-oxo-2H-chromen-7-yl acetate (19). Yield 70%; ^{1}H-NMR (400 MHz, d^6-DMSO) δ: 2.31 (s, 3H, $CH_3C(O)O$-Ph), 2.95 (s, 6H, $(CH_3)_2N$-Ph), 6.77 (d, 2H, $J^3 = 9.0$ Hz, H-3', H-5'), 7.14 (dd, 1H, $J^3 = 8.4$ Hz, $J^4 = 2.2$ Hz, H-6), 7.26 (d, 1H, $J^4 = 2.2$ Hz, H-8), 7.63 (d, 2H, $J^3 = 9.0$ Hz, H-2', H-6'), 7.76 (d, 1H, $J^3 = 8.5$ Hz, H-5), 8.11 (s, 1H, H-4; ^{13}C-NMR (100 MHz, d^6-DMSO) δ: 20.86, 39.84, 109.44, 111.58, 117.76, 118.57, 121.58, 126.00, 128.82, 129.11 136.46, 150.45, 151.90, 152.77, 159.74, 168.85; HRMS (ESI): Calc for $C_{19}H_{17}N_1O_4Na_1$ [M + Na]$^+$: 346.10553, found 346.10640.

3-(3-fluoro-4-hydroxyphenyl)-7-methoxy-2*H*-chromen-2-one (20). In the first step 2-fluoro-4-(7-methoxy-2-oxo-2H-chromen-3-yl)phenyl acetate was obtained. Yield 75%; ^{1}H-NMR (400 MHz, d^6-DMSO) δ: 2.35 (s, 3H, $CH_3C(O)O$-Ph), 3.88 (s, 3H, CH_3O-Ph), 6.99 (dd, 1H, $J^3 = 8.6$ Hz, $J^4 = 2.4$ Hz, H-6), 7.05 (d, 1H, $J^4 = 2.4$ Hz, H-8), 7.37 (t, 1H, $J = 8.3$Hz, H-6'), 7.62 (d, $J = 8.5$ Hz, 1H, H-5'), 7.68 (d, $J = 8.6$ Hz, 1H, H-5), 7.74 (dd, $J^{H-F} = 12.1$ Hz, $J^4 = 2.0$ Hz, H-3'), 8.31 (s, 1H, H-4); ^{13}C-NMR (100 MHz, d^6-DMSO) δ: 20.19, 55.97, 100.25, 112.79, 116.35 (d, $J^{C-F} = 20.3$ Hz), 121.02, 121.03, 123.83, 124.79 (d, $J^{C-F} = 3.2$ Hz), 129.86, 134.24 (d, $J^{C-F} = 7.7$ Hz), 137.20 (d, $J^{C-F} = 13.1$ Hz), 141.55, 153.00 ($J^{C-F} = 246$ Hz), 154.92, 159.65, 162.69, 168.19. In the second step 3-(3-fluoro-4-hydroxyphenyl)-7-methoxy-2*H*-chromen-2-one was obtained. Yield 70%; ^{1}H-NMR (400 MHz, d^6-DMSO) δ: 3.87 (s, 3H, CH_3O-Ph), 6.96-7.03 (m, 3H, H-6, H-8, H-5'), 7.41 (d, 1H, $J^3 = 8.4$, H-6'), 7.57 (dd, 1H, $J^{H-F} = 13.1$ Hz, $J^4 = 2.2$ Hz (H-H), 1H, H-2'), 7.66 (d, 1H, $J^3 = 8.4$, H-5), 8.18 (s, 1H, H-4), 10.09 (s, 1H, Ph-OH). ^{13}C-NMR (75.5 MHz, d^6-DMSO) δ: 55.91, 100.16, 112.61, 113.04, 115.95 (d, $J^{C-F} = 20$ Hz), 117.37 (d, $J^{C-F} = 3.3$ Hz), 121.78 ($J^{C-F} = 2.0$ Hz), 124.54 (d, $J^{C-F} = 3.0$ Hz), 126.08 (d, $J^{C-F} = 7.0$ Hz), 129.49, 139.62, 145.0 ($J^{C-F} = 13$ Hz), 150.46 (d, $J^{C-F} = 240$ Hz), 154.52, 159.87, 162.19; HRMS (ESI): Calc for $C_{16}H_{11}F_1O_4Na_1$ [M + Na]$^+$: 309.0539, found 309.0553.

3-(4-fluorophenyl)-6-methoxy-2H-chromen-2-one (21). Yield 58%; ^{1}H-NMR (400 MHz, d^6-acetone) δ: 3.87 (s, 3H, CH_3O-Ph), 7.19-7.33 (m, 5H, H-5, H-7, H-8, H-3', H-5'), 7.83 (dd, 2H, $J^{HF} = 5.4$ Hz, $J^{H-H} = 9.0$ Hz, H-2', H6'), 8.12 (s, 1H, H-4); ^{13}C-NMR (100 MHz, d^6-acetone) δ: 56.17, 111.34, 115.84 (d, $J^{C-F} = 22$ Hz), 117.85, 120.04, 121.04, 127.79, 131.62 (d, $J^{C-F} = 8$ Hz), 132.41 (d, $J^{C-F} = 3$ Hz), 140.82, 148.82, 157.13, 160.64, 163.72 (d, $J^{C-F} = 247$ Hz); HRMS (ESI): Calc for $C_{16}H_{11}F_1O_3Na_1$ [M + Na]$^+$: 293.05899, found 293.05850; elemental anal. for $C_{16}H_{11}F_1O_3$, calc C% 71.11, H% 4.10, found C% 71.10, H% 4.10.

3-(3-fluoro-4-hydroxyphenyl)-6-methoxy-2*H*-chromen-2-one (22). In the first step 2-fluoro-4-(6-methoxy-2-oxo-2H-chromen-3-yl)phenyl acetate was obtained. Yield 66%; ^{1}H-NMR (400 MHz, d^6-DMSO) δ: 2.33 (s, 3H, $CH_3C(O)O$-Ph), 3.82 (s, 3H, (CH_3O-Ph), 7.23 (dd, 1H, $J^3 = 9.0$ Hz, $J^4 = 3.0$ Hz, H-7), 7.30 (d, 1H, $J^4 = 3.0$ Hz, H-5), 7.35 (d, 1H, $J^3 = 9.2$ Hz, H-8), 7.61 (d, 1H, $J^3 = 8.5$ Hz, H-5'), 7.75 (dd, 1H, $J^{H-F} = 12.0$ Hz, $J^4 = 1.7$ Hz (H-H), 1H, H-3'), 8.30 (s, 1H, H-4); ^{13}C-NMR (100.6 MHz, d^6-DMSO) δ: 20.22, 55.69, 110.83, 116.67, 117.02, 119.66, 123.96,

125.10, 135.96, 141.18, 147.44, 151.78, 154.23, 155.70, 159.53, 168.21. In the second step 3-(3-fluoro-4-hydroxyphenyl)-6-methoxy-2*H*-chromen-2-one was obtained. Yield 71%; ^{1}H-NMR (400 MHz, d^6-DMSO) δ: 3.81 (s, 3H, (CH_3O-Ph), 7.02 (dd, 1H, J^3 = 9.2 Hz, H-6'), 7.18 (dd, 1H, J^3 = 9.0 Hz, J^4 = 3.0 Hz, H-7), 7.28 (d, 1H, J^4 = 2.9 Hz, H-5), 7.42 (d, 1H, J^3 = 8.4 Hz, H-5'), 7.57 (dd, 1H, J^{H-F} = 13.0 Hz, J^4 = 2.2 Hz (H-H), 1H, H-2'), 8.17 (s, 1H, H-4), 10.19 (s, 1H, Ph-OH); ^{13}C-NMR (100.6 MHz, d^6-DMSO) δ: 55.66, 110.59, 116.67, 117.02, 119.66, 123.96, 125.10, 135.96, 141.18, 147.44, 151.78, 154.23, 155.70, 159.53, 168.21. HRMS (ESI): Calc for $C_{16}H_{11}F_1O_4Na_1$ [M + Na]$^+$: 309.0539, found 309.0521.

3-(4-fluorophenyl)-6-methyl-2H-chromen-2-one (23). (Chauhan et al., 2016) Yield 74%; ^{1}H-NMR (400 MHz, d^6-DMSO) δ: 2.38 (s, 3H, CH_3-Ph), 7.27-7.35 (m, 3H, H-3', H-5', H-8), 7.43 (dd, 1H, J_3 = 8.5 Hz, J_4 = 2.1 Hz, H-7), 7.55 (d, 1H, J_4 = 1.4 Hz, H-5), 7.77 (dd, 2H, J^{HF} = 5.7 Hz, J^{H-H} = 9.0 Hz, H-2', H6'), 8.18 (s, 1H, H-4); ^{13}C-NMR (100.6 MHz, d^6-DMSO) δ: 20.26, 115.11 (d, J^{H-F} = 21.5 Hz), 115.64, 119.16, 125.76, 128.20, 130.70 (d, J^{H-F} = 8.4 Hz), 131.10 (d, J^{H-F} = 3.2 Hz), 132,61, 133.80, 140.48, 151.10, 159.82, 162.17 (d, J^{H-F} = 245 Hz); HRMS (ESI): Calc for $C_{16}H_{11}F_1O_2Na_1$ [M + Na]$^+$: 277.06408, found 277.06390; Elemental anal. for $C_{16}H_{11}F_1O_2$, calc C% 75.58, H% 4.36, found C% 75.42, H% 4.33.

3-(4-fluorophenyl)-6-hydroxy-2H-chromen-2-one (24). In the first step 3-(4-fluorophenyl)-2-oxo-2H-chromen-6-yl acetate was obtained and used as such for the next step. In the second step 3-(4-fluorophenyl)-6-hydroxy-2H-chromen-2-one was obtained. Yield 65%; ^{1}H-NMR (300 MHz, d^6-DMSO) δ: 7.04 (dd, 1H, J^3 = 8.8 Hz, J^4 = 2.9 Hz, H-7), 7.09 (d, 1H, J^4 = 2.8 Hz, H-5), 7.24-7.29 (m, 3H, H-3', H-5', H-8), 7.75 (dd, 2H, J^{HF} = 5.6 Hz, J^{H-H} = 8.9 Hz, H-2', H6'), 8.13 (s, 1H, H-4), 9.72 (s, 1H, HO-Ph); ^{13}C-NMR (75.5 MHz, d^6-DMSO) δ: 112.561, 115.03 (d, J^{H-F} = 21.5 Hz), 116.71, 119.78, 119.93, 125.80, 130.70 (d, J^{H-F} = 8.2 Hz), 131.18 (d, J^{H-F} = 3.2 Hz), 140.50, 146.35, 159.92, 162.17 (d, J^{H-F} = 246 Hz); HRMS (ESI): Calc for $C_{15}H_9F_1O_3Na_1$ [M + Na]$^+$: 279.04334, found 279.0444.

Monoamine Oxidase A and B

Both monoamine oxidase A (MAO-A) and B (MAO-B) protein and the reagents for the chromogenic solution of vanillic acid (4-hydroxy-3-methoxylbenzoic acid, 97% purity), 4-aminoantipyrine (reagent grade), horseradish peroxidase and the substrate tyramine hydrochloride (minimum 99% purity) as well as the potassium phosphate buffer, which was prepared using potassium phosphate dibasic trihydrate (≥99% ReagentPlus™) and potassium phosphate monobasic (minimum 98% purity, molecular biology tested), were purchased from Sigma-Aldrich (St. Louis, MO, USA) for the spectrophotometric assay.

The protocol for continuous spectrophotometric assay (Holt et al., 1997) was followed in the activity measurements. The assay was performed in 0.2 M potassium phosphate buffer pH 7.6 on 96-well plates (Nunc™ 96F microwell plate without a lid, Nunc A/S, Roskilde, DK) in 200 μl total volume. The chromogenic solution containing 1 mM vanillic acid, 500 μM 4-aminoantipyrine and 8 U/ml horseradish peroxidase in 0.2 M potassium phosphate buffer pH 7.6 was mixed anew for each measurement. 5 mM tyramine solution was used as the substrate. In order to determine the activity of both MAO-B and MAO-A, concentration series as duplicates were prepared. The protein was combined with the chromogenic solution and incubated 30 min at 37°C. The background signal was measured using multilabel reader (Victor™ X4, 2030 Multilabel Reader, PerkinElmer, Waltham, MA, USA) at A_{490} before reaching the total 200 μl volume by adding 20 μl of tyramine to final concentration of 0.5 mM on the plate. As a result, the final concentration of the chromogenic solution on the plate was 250 μM vanillic acid, 125 μM 4-aminoantipyrine and 2 U/ml horseradish peroxide. After adding the substrate, the plates were measured 300 times every 15 s using 1 s exposure time. The device was set to 37°C for the duration of the experiment.

Based on the activity measurement, suitable concentrations were chosen for both MAO-B and MAO-A to be used in the inhibition studies (Supplementary Figures S1, S2, and S5, **Table 1**, Supplementary Table S1). The experiment conditions should produce absorbance change of ~0.35 (Holt et al., 1997). With MAO-B, this was reached using 10 μl (equals 50 μg of protein with enzymatic activity 3.2 units per well) of the protein and running the experiment for 2 h (Supplementary Figures S1, S2, and S5, **Table 1**, Supplementary Table S1). MAO-A was significantly more active, providing absorbance change of >0.5 with 5 μl (equals 25 μg of protein with enzymatic activity 1.05 units per well) of protein and, consequently, the reaction maximum was reached already in 30 min (Supplementary Figure S5, **Table 1**, Supplementary Table S1). Thus, a wide panel of coumarin derivatives was analyzed at 10 μM (**Table 1,** Supplementary Table S1) and those 3-phenylcoumarin derivatives producing >70% inhibition were selected for further analysis (**Table 1**, **Figure 2**). The selected 24 candidates were measured as duplicates on a dilution series ranging from 50 μM to 1 nM, and based on the normalized measurement results, IC_{50} values were calculated (**Table 1**). The same wide panel of coumarin derivatives was additionally used to analyze the MAO-A inhibition at 100 μM (**Table 1,** Supplementary Table S1).

GRAPHPAD PRISM 5.03 (GraphPad Software Inc., CA, USA) was used to normalize the spectrophotometric assay data where the maximal signal was reached at the lowest concentration of 10^{-8} or 10^{-9} depending on the sample and the starting concentration of $5{\cdot}10^{-5}$ acted as the lowest point of signal. The measured data was then fitted on a curve using non-linear regression with the equation for log[inhibitor] vs. response. The IC50 values were therefore determined based on the curve fit. The fitted curves are shown on –log scale in Supplementary Figures S1, S2.

17-β-Hydroxysteroid Dehydrogenase 1

Inhibition of the 17-β-hydroxysteroid dehydrogenase 1 (HSD1) was determined by HPLC using recombinant human HSD1 proteins, produced in Sf9-insect cells, as described earlier (Messinger et al., 2009). The assay was performed in a final volume of 0.2 ml buffer (20mM KH2PO4, 1mM EDTA, pH 7.4) containing 0.1 mg/ml protein, 1 mM cofactor NADPH, 30 nM substrate estrone or estradiol, 800,000 cpm/ml of tritium labeled estrone ([3H]-E1) or estradiol ([3H]-E2) and inhibitor concentrations in the range of 0.1–5 mM. Triplicate samples were incubated for 25 min at RT. The reaction was stopped by addition of 20 ml 10% trichloroacetic acid per sample. After incubation the substrate and the product of enzymatic conversion [3H]-E1 and [3H]-E2, were separated and quantified by HPLC (Alliance 2790, Waters) connected to an online - counter (Packard Flow Scintillation Analyzer). The ratio of [3H]-E1 converted to [3H]-E2, or *vice versa*, determines the sample conversion percentage. Inhibition efficiencies were calculated by comparing the conversion percentages of the samples including inhibitors with those of conversion controls (without inhibitors).

Aromatase

Aromatase (CYP19A1) activity was measured as described previously (Pasanen, 1985) by using human placental microsomes and 50 nM [3H]-androstenedione as a substrate and inhibitor concentrations in the range of 60–1,000 nM. Aromatase activities were measured as released [3H]-H_2O in Optiphase Hisafe 2 scintillation liquid (Perkin Elmer, USA) with a Wallac 1450 MicroBeta Trilux scintillation counter (Perkin Elmer, USA). As a positive control for aromatase inhibition, 1 µM finrozole (generous gift from Olavi Pelkonen, University of Oulu, Finland) was used.

Cytochrome P450 1A2

Inhibition of CYP1A2 activity was determined with commercial heterologously expressed human CYP1A2 enzyme (Corning Inc., Corning, NY, USA) as described earlier (Korhonen et al., 2005). The metabolic activity was not in the scope of this particular study. The assay was adapted to the 96-well plate format. In each well, a 150 µL incubation volume contained 100 mM Tris-HCl buffer (pH 7.4), 4.2 mM MgCl2,1 µM 7-ethoxyresorufin, 0.5 pmol of cDNA expressed CYP1A2, 0-40 mM inhibitor, and a NADPH-generating system. All inhibitors were dissolved in ethanol, and the final concentration of ethanol was 2% in all incubations. The reaction was initiated by adding the NADPH-regenerating system after a 10 min preincubation at 37°C, and after a 20 min incubation, the reaction was terminated by the addition of 110 µL of 80% acetonitrile/20% 0.5 M Tris base. The formed fluorescence was measured with a Victor2 plate counter (Perkin-Elmer Life Sciences Wallac, Turku, Finland) at 570 nm excitation and 616 nm emission.

Estrogen Receptor

The pIC50 values for the derivatives (**Table 1**, Supplementary Table S1) were measured with green PolarScreen™ ER Alpha Competitor Assay (Life Technologies, CA, The United States of America) kit, following the manufacturer protocol as previously described (Niinivehmas et al., 2016). The final concentration of the compounds ranged from 0.0007 to 10 000 nM in the dilution series which were performed as duplicates. The molecules were combined with 25 nM ERα and 4.5 nM fluormone in the assay buffer and placed on black low volume 384-well assay plate with NBS surface (Corning, NY, The United States of America). After mixing the assay plate, it was incubated for 2 h in RT. The fluorescence polarization was measured using excitation wave length 485 and emission wave length 535 with bandwidths of 25/20 nm on a 2104 EnVision® Multilabel Plate Reader which had EnVision Workstation version 1.7 (PerkinElmer, MA, The United States of America).

Computational Methods

The small-molecule ligand structures were drawn in 3D and their tautomeric states at pH 7.4 were built using LIGPREP module in MAESTRO 2016-3 (Schrödinger, LLC, New York, NY, USA, 2016). The derivatives were docked to the X-ray crystal structure of MAO-B (PDB: 2V60) (Binda et al., 2007) with PLANTS 1.2 (Korb et al., 2009) using 10 Å radius and the C8 atom of inhibitor *C18* (PDB: 2V60) was used as the center. The R1-methoxy group rotamers of compounds **1**, **8**, **9**, **21**, **15**, **18**, and **22** were manually adjusted to indicate how the groups exploit the small hydrophobic niche in the cavity (green sector in **Figures 3A,B**). The 2D structures of the 3-phenylcoumarin scaffold and the 24 most potent inhibitor derivatives shown in **Figures 1E, 2** were drawn with BIOVIA DRAW 2016 (Dassault Systèmes, San Diego, CA, USA, 2016). **Figures 1A–D, 3–5** were prepared using BODIL (Lehtonen et al., 2004) and VMD 1.9.2 (Humphrey et al., 1996). The negative images of the MAO-B and MAO-A binding cavities shown in **Figure 3A** and C were outlined using PANTHER (Niinivehmas et al., 2011, 2015) and visualized with BODIL, MOLSCRIPT (Kraulis, 1991), and RASTER3D (Merritt and Murphy, 1994).

RESULTS AND DISCUSSION

Spectrophotometric Activity Measurements for Monoamine Oxidase B

All of the 52 derivatives were docked, synthetized and tested experimentally. Those 24 compounds that provided IC_{50} values below 10 µM were tested more thoroughly (**Table 1**). The fact that 24 of the synthesized derivatives with a wide variety of different R1-R7 groups (**Figure 2**) passed the 70% threshold indicates that the 3-phenylcoumarin is indeed a highly suitable scaffold for building MAO-B inhibitors. Notably, eight of these tested derivatives (**3**, **9–13**, **17**, and **23** in **Figure 2**) had been synthesized previously (Bhandri et al., 1949; Kirkiacharian et al., 1999, 2003; Prendergast, 2001; Vilar et al., 2006; Ferino et al., 2013; Chauhan et al., 2016; Dobelmann-Mara et al., 2017), however, this is the first time they are tested for MAO-B activity. The novel derivative **1** is the most potent inhibitor of the analog set with the IC_{50} value of 56 nM (**Figure 2**, **Table 1**); meanwhile, the rest of the tested derivatives are evenly distributed within a range of 0.1–10 µM (**Figure 2**, **Table 1**).

By focusing solely on the R1-R7 constituents of the derivatives (**Figures 1E, 2**) and the activity data (**Table 1**) it is possible to outline trends that determine which functional groups, positions or their combinations establish and weaken or improve the MAO-B inhibition.

Although the R1 and R2 groups in the coumarin ring are not necessarily required for establishing MAO-B inhibition (see **11**; **Figure 2**, Supplementary Figure S3F; **Table 1**), the activity measurements indicate that adding a methoxy, hydroxyl, acetoxy, methyl or even halogen group(s) into the ring can facilitate strong

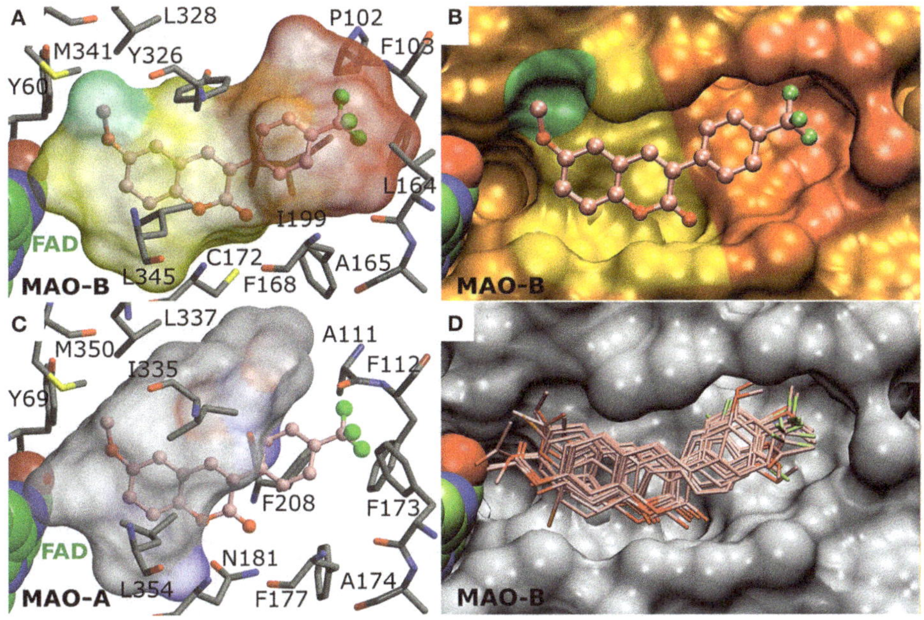

FIGURE 3 | The active site of monoamine oxidase B with docked 3-phenylcoumarin derivatives. **(A)** A negative image of the MAO-B active site shown as a transparent surface indicates the space available for inhibitor binding with docked derivative **1** (ball-and-stick model; **Figure 2**). **(B)** A cross section, showing half of the active site, displays the contours (opaque surface) that roughly match the inhibitor shape and conformation. The colored sectors highlight specific sections of the cavity dedicated to different aspects of the 3-phenylcoumarin derivative binding: 3-phenyl ring (orange), the R4-R7 groups of the 3-phenyl ring (red), coumarin ring (yellow), the hydrophobic niche occupied by the R1/R2-groups of the coumarin ring (green). **(C)** A negative image of the MAO-A active site shows that only two residue changes (Ile199→ Phe208; Leu164→ Phe173) are enough to prevent 3-phenylcoumarin analog binding. **(D)** The docked poses of the 23 most potent 3-phenylcoumarin derivatives show what space is collectively occupied by the new inhibitors. See **Figure 1** for details.

inhibition (**Table 1**). As a rule of thumb, introducing R1-methoxy group produces strong MAO-B inhibition (e.g., **1**; **Figure 2**; **Table 1**). In contrast, inserting for example a bulky R3 substituent such as acetoxy group weakens the inhibition considerably (26, 35, 47; Supplementary Figure S4; Supplementary Table S1). Whether the R1 or R2 position or any specific functional group in particular is favored depends on the composition of the 3-phenyl ring's R4-R7 constituents.

In fact, the activity data indicates that the R4-R7 substituents are vital for assuring strong MAO-B inhibition and without any 3-phenyl substituents, the activity is lost (41, 50, 52; Supplementary Figure S4, Supplementary Table S1). The most potent inhibitors were **1** (IC_{50} of ~56 nM; **Table 1**) and **2** (IC_{50} of ~138 nM; **Table 1**) housing R6-trifluoromethyl, but **3** (IC_{50} of ~141 nM; **Table 1**) with structurally similar R6-trifluoromethoxy group is almost equally potent. The combination of the R6-acetoxy and R7-fluorine groups in **6** (IC_{50} of ~189 nM) produces relatively strong inhibition. Furthermore, housing just one methoxy group at the R7 position (**8**; IC_{50} of ~230 nM) or two methoxy groups at both R5 and R7 positions (**9**; IC_{50} of ~255 nM) assures $<$ 300 nM inhibition.

The effects of the R4-R7 groups of the 3-phenyl ring and the R1-R3 groups of coumarin ring (**Figure 2**) for the derivative binding and inhibition are detailed below in a docking-based structure-activity relationship (SAR) analysis.

The Alignment of the 3-Phenylcoumarin Scaffold at the Active Site

The 3-phenylcoumarin derivative binding at the MAO-B active site is based on the premise that the coumarin and phenyl ring systems occupy roughly the same 3D space as the equivalent ring systems of the coumarin-based inhibitors co-crystallized with the enzyme (PDB: 2V60, 2V61; **Figures 1A–D**) (Binda et al., 2007). The fundamental difference between the 3-phenylcoumarin derivatives and those coumarin inhibitors with validated binding poses is that the coumarin alignment is reversed and the phenyl ring is attached to the C3-position instead of the C7-position (**Figures 1C,D**).

What is more, the "canonical" coumarin ring positioning inside the pocket is somewhat analogous to even simpler double ring constructs such as the indole of inhibitor isatin (PDB: 1OJA) (Binda et al., 2003). In fact, the hydrophobicity of the aromatic coumarin (yellow sector in **Figures 3A,B**) and 3-phenyl (orange sector in **Figures 3A,B**) rings is vital for establishing the MAO-B binding and it outweighs all other favorable interactions such as hydrogen or halogen bonding (*via* sigma hole) in importance (**Figure 4**). Thus, although the docking suggests variability in the coumarin and 3-phenyl ring positioning for the 3-phenylcoumarin derivatives due to different R1-R7 substituents, the hydrophobic interactions of the aromatic rings are highly similar between them (**Figure 3D**).

It is also noteworthy that the coumarin's C2-carbonyl is not facing the solvent based on the molecular docking simulations

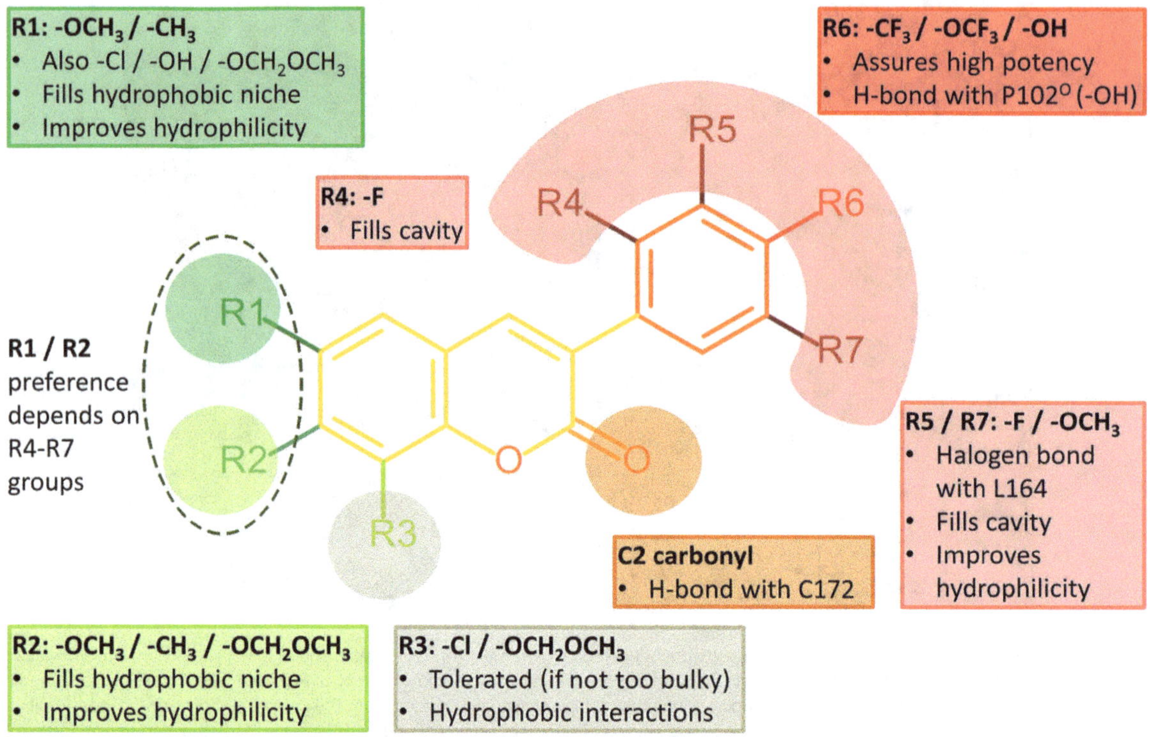

FIGURE 4 | Structure-activity relationship (SAR) analysis of the 3-phenylcoumarin derivatives.

(**Figure 3D**). Paradoxically, this does not matter, because the carbonyl group finds an atypical interaction partner from the thiol group of Cys172 side chain (**Figure 4**). Although the C2-carbonyl cannot form a full-fledged H-bond with the proton of the thiol group, the hydrophobic environment of the cavity likely enhances this ordinarily weak interaction between the two groups.

R6-Trifluoromethyl Packing Produces the Strongest Inhibition

Halogen substituents in the 3-phenyl ring ensure strong MAO-B inhibition (**Figure 4**). This makes sense with MAO-B, because despite their apparent electronegativity the halogen substituents actually improve the steric packing of small-molecules via persistent van der Waals interactions while also retaining the ability to act as a halogen bond donor. Both of these properties should assist inhibitor binding into the active site that is mostly hydrophobic (**Figures 3A,B**). Besides, the increased lipophilicity conveyed by the halogen substituents (logP values in **Table 1**) should assist the 3-phenylcoumarin derivatives in aggregating on the outer mitochondrial membrane on route to the MAO-B active site (**Figure 1A**).

The most potent derivative **1** (**Figure 2**, **Table 1**) has trifluoromethyl group at the R6 position in the 3-phenyl ring. The derivative is relatively flat when bound at the active site and the proximal R6-group cannot flex out of this plane (**Figure 5A**). The trifluoromethyl of **1** fits very snugly into the hydrophobic end of the cavity (red sector in **Figures 3A,B**). The high shape complementarity of this cavity part and the R6-trifluoromethyl of **1** is typical for this bulky moiety in drug compounds. Thus, the R6-group alignment of **1** is mostly relying on the collective potency of individually weak van der Waals interactions (**Figures 3A,B, 5A**).

Replacing the R6-trifluoromethyl of derivative **1** with a trifluoromethoxy in **4** (**Figure 2**) produces six times lower MAO-B inhibition (**Table 1**, Supplementary Figure S3B). This happens because the trifluoromethoxy already fills the available space almost optimally (**Figures 3A,B, 5A**) and elongating the substituent with an ether bond does not improve the fit (Supplementary Figure S3B). In fact, there is no extra wiggle room to fit the trifluoromethoxy (**Figures 3A,B**), if the 3-phenylcoumarin scaffold would be kept at the "canonical" position (**Figures 1C,D**). Hence, the coumarin ring of **4** pushes slightly closer to the cofactor. Although the binding site residues can adjust slightly in response to this shift, the realignment or rather misalignment of the scaffold (Supplementary Figure S3B) imposes an energetic cost that is reflected in the MAO-B inhibition (**Table 1**). In addition, depending on the rotamer pose of the R6-trifluorometoxy, a hydrogen bond could be bridged between a fluorine atom and the Pro102^{O} by a water molecule (not shown).

The Effects of Halogenation on the 3-Phenyl Ring Alignment

The chlorine and fluorine substituents of prior coumarin-based inhibitors form halogen bond with the Leu164^{O} based on

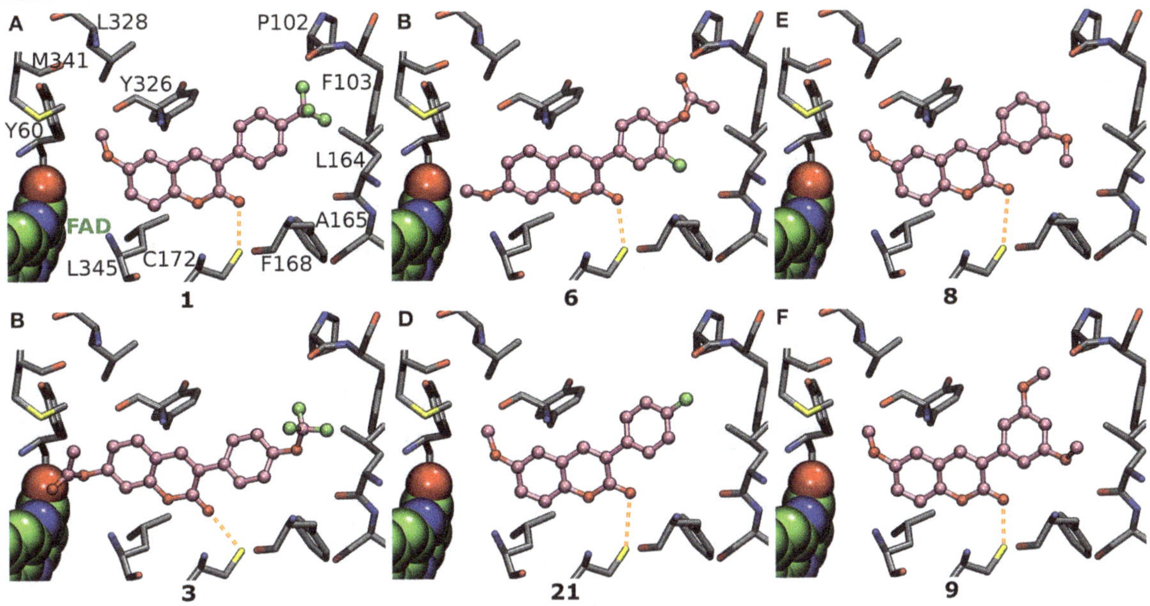

FIGURE 5 | The vital role of R4-R7 substituents of the 3-phenyl ring for the inhibition. Focusing on the 3-phenyl ring, the derivatives (ball-and-stick models with pink backbone) elicit strong MAO-B inhibition via **(A)** R6-trifluoromethyl (**1**; **Figure 2**; IC_{50} of 56 nM; **Table 1**), **(B)** R6-trifluoromethoxy (**3**; **Figure 2**; IC_{50} of 141 nM; **Table 1**), **(C)** R6-acetoxy and R7-fluorine (**6**; **Figure 2**; IC_{50} of 189 nM; **Table 1**), **(D)** R6-fluorine (**21**; **Figure 2**; IC_{50} of 433 nM; **Table 1**), **(E)** R7-methoxy (**8**; **Figure 2**; IC_{50} of 231 nM; **Table 1**), and **(F)** R5- and R7-methoxy (**9**; **Figure 2**; IC_{50} of 255 nM; **Table 1**) groups. See **Figure 1** for further details.

X-ray crystallography (PDB: 2V60, 2V61; **Figures 1A–D**; Binda et al., 2007). Accordingly, it is not surprising that those 3-phenylcoumarin derivatives with single halogen substituent at their 3-phenyl rings are also capable of blocking the MAO-B activity (**Figure 4**, **Table 1**).

Although it is known that fluorine is the poorest halogen bond donor (Cavallo et al., 2016), the R7-fluorine groups of **20** and **22** (**Figure 2**) could form halogen bond with the Leu164° (**Figures 6E,F**) similarly to the halogens of previously published inhibitors with validated binding modes (**Figures 1B–D**; Binda et al., 2007). In fact, the R7-halogen groups of **20** and **22** are inserted into the exact same position as the halogen groups of the established inhibitors (**Figure 1B** vs. **Figures 6E,F**). The MAO-B inhibition (**Table 1**) is reinforced further by the R6-hydroxyl group H-bonding with the Pro102^{O} (magenta dotted lines in **Figures 6E,F**). Because both **20** and **22** are bonding simultaneously with the Leu164^{O} and the Pro102^{O}, they elicit equivalent or stronger inhibition than derivatives **21** (**Figure 5D**), **23** (Supplementary Figure S3K), and **24** (Supplementary Figure S3L) that do not retain either one of these two interactions. Docking suggests that replacing the R6-hydroxyl with an acetoxy group prevents **6** (**Figure 2**) from forming direct halogen or hydrogen bonds (**Figure 5C**), but the R6-acetoxy and R7-fluorine could potentially connect via a water bridge with the Pro102^{O} (not shown). Despite this, the hydrophobic packing of the R6-acetoxy in **6** against the hydrophobic residues, mainly Phe103 (**Figure 5C**), is likely the reason behind doubling the inhibition in comparison to **20** (IC_{50} value of 391 vs. 189 nM; **Table 1**, **Figure 6E**).

Introducing fluorine to the R6 position of the 3-phenyl ring in derivatives **21**, **23**, and **24** (**Figure 2**) produces MAO-B inhibition ranging from 433 to 1,060 nM (**Table 1**). Due to the overall planarity of the 3-phenylcoumarin scaffold (**Figures 1C,D**), the R6-fluorine (**Figure 5D**, Supplementary Figures S3K,L), cannot take on the equivalent site occupied by the halogens of validated coumarin-based inhibitors that form halogen bond with the Leu164° (**Figure 1B**; Binda et al., 2007). In addition, the R6-fluorine is too limited in size to fill the end of the binding cavity as completely as for example the trifluoromethyl of **1** does (**Figures 3A,B**, **5A**). In addition, the R6-fluorine groups of derivatives **21**, **23**, and **24** (**Figure 5D**, Supplementary Figure S3K,L) reside within a suitable distance to form a halogen bond with the Pro102^{O} (3.6 Å), however, the available angles seem to rule out actual bonding.

Derivatives **15** and **16** (**Figure 2**) house three fluorine atoms at their 3-phenyl groups' R4, R6, and R7 positions (**Figures 6A,B**). In the case of **15** (**Figure 6A**), these halogen substituents assure an IC_{50} value that is almost 150 nM stronger than what is seen with derivatives housing only a single fluorine moiety at the R6 or R7 position (**21**, **23**, and **24**; **Figure 5D**, Figure S3K-L, **Table 1**). This is achieved by filling the hydrophobic cavity end (orange and red sectors in **Figure 3**) efficiently with the 3-phenyl ring and its fluorine moieties (**Figures 6A,B**). The fit is better for a 3-phenyl ring with the R5-trifluoromethyl than what is seen with the ring housing three separate fluorine substituents (**Figure 5A** vs. **Figure 6A**) and; accordingly, derivative **15** is not as potent MAO-B inhibitor as **1** (IC_{50} 292 vs. 56 nM; **Table 1**). In addition, depending on the 3-phenyl ring pose, the R4 or R7 fluorine

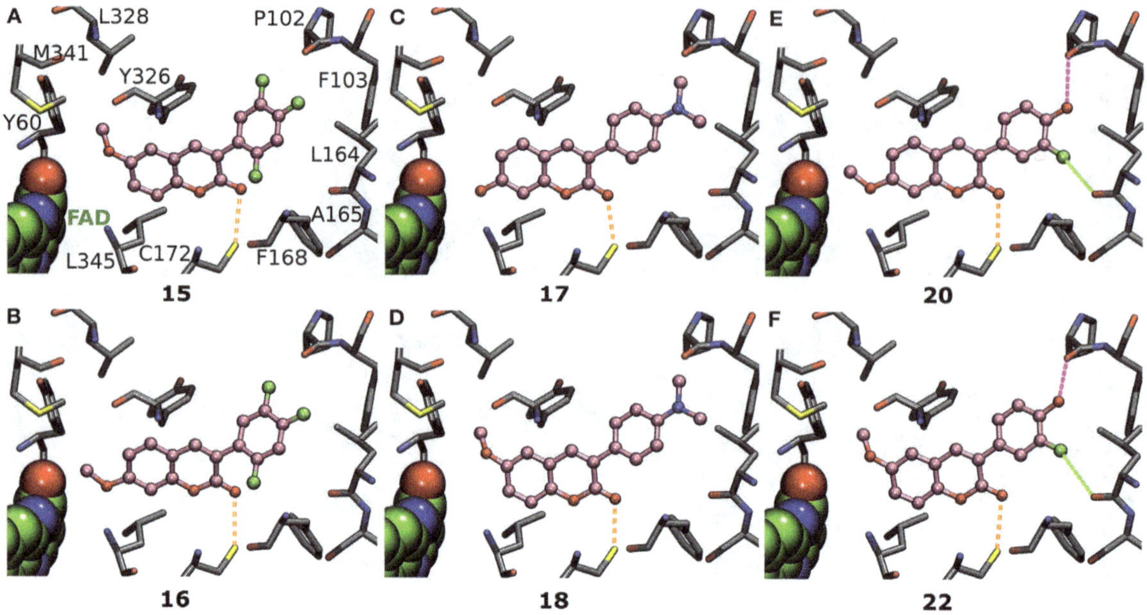

FIGURE 6 | The effects of R1 and R2 substituents are dependent on the 3-phenyl ring substituents. **(A)** Derivatives **15** (**Figure 2**; IC_{50} of 292 nM; **Table 1**) and **(B) 16** (**Figure 2**; IC_{50} of 1433 nM; **Table 1**) both have fluorine groups at R4, R6, and R7 positions, but switching the coumarin ring's R1-methoxy into the R2 position reduces the inhibition by whopping 1141 nM. In contrast, with **(C) 17** (**Figure 2**; IC_{50} of 384 nM; **Table 1**) and **(D) 18** (**Figure 2**; IC_{50} of 617 nM; **Table 1**), the R1-methoxy does not elicit as strong inhibition as the R2-hydroxyl due to the overall coumarin ring alignment dictated by the 3-phenyl's R5-dimethylamine. The R1/R2-methoxy switch produces a completely opposite effect for **(E) 20** (**Figure 2**; IC_{50} of 391 nM; **Table 1**) and **(F) 22** (**Figure 2**; IC_{50} of 831 nM; **Table 1**) than it did for **15** and **16** (panels **A,B**); namely, it lowered the inhibition by 440 nM (**Table 1**). For further details, see **Figures 1**, **4**.

groups could again potentially act as weak halogen bond donors to the Phe168^{O} or the Leu164^{O}, respectively (not shown).

The Effects of the Methoxy and Dimethylamine Groups for the 3-Phenyl Alignment

Derivatives with proximal methoxy groups (**Figure 2**), especially at the R7 position, assure relatively strong MAO-B inhibition (**Figure 4**) and produce at best 230 nM inhibition (e.g., **8** in **Figure 2**, **Table 1**).

Based on the docking, derivatives **8** and **11** (**Figure 2**) flip their R7-methoxy groups toward the Leu164° (**Figure 5E**, Supplementary Figure S3F), which is shielded from a clash with the methoxy group by forming intra-protein H-bond with the Phe168^{N} (not shown). Inserting an extra R5-methoxy into the 3-phenyl of **8** to produce otherwise identical derivative **9** (**Figure 2**) weakens the inhibition slightly (IC_{50} difference of 23 nM; **Table 1**), because the added methoxy group is unable to form particularly favorable interactions with the nearby Pro102° (**Figure 5F**). With derivatives **10** or **13** (**Figure 2**), the methoxy group is added to the phenyl ring's para position, and due to the planarity of the 3-phenylcoumarin scaffold, there is an energetic penalty for pushing the group toward either side of the cavity end (red sector in **Figures 3A,B**). Accordingly, to avoid a scaffold misalignment, the R6-methoxy group of **10** (and **13**) points directly toward the side chains of Phe103, Pro104, Trp119, and Ile199 (Supplementary Figures S3E,F), which, in turn, produces roughly 170 nM difference in the IC_{50} values with otherwise identical **8** (**Figure 5E**, **Table 1**) in favor of the R7-methoxy position.

A dimethylamine group at the 3-phenyl ring's para position (a.k.a. dimethylaniline; **Figure 2**) produces moderately strong MAO-B inhibition (**Table 1**) for derivatives **17** (**Figure 2**; IC_{50} value of 400 nM), **18** (**Figure 2**; IC_{50} value of 798 nM), and **19** (**Figure 2**; IC_{50} value of 955 nM). This is due to the ability of the R6-dimethylamine to fill the cavity end (red sector in **Figures 3A,B**) similarly to the R6-trifluoromethyl of **1** (**Figures 5A,B** vs. **Figures 6C,D**, Supplementary Figure S3J). The downside is that the bulkier R6-substituent cannot form halogen or hydrogen bonds with water or residues nor push against either side of the cavity and, most importantly, it causes unfavorable coumarin alignment. Accordingly, the R6-dimethylamine of derivatives **17–19** packs directly against the side chains of Phe103, Pro104, Trp119, Leu164, and Ile316 (**Figures 4C,D**, Supplementary Figure S3J).

Refining the Alignment via the R1–R3 Substituents of the Coumarin Ring

Inserting a functional group such as methoxy to the R1/R2 position of the coumarin ring (**Figure 2**), capable of forming both hydrophobic and hydrophilic interactions, generally improves the MAO-B inhibition (**Figure 4**, **Table 1**).

The benefits of this sort of dual-purpose group are evident when comparing the activity of otherwise identical derivatives with and without the proximal group; i.e., **11**, that lacks only the R1-methoxy of **8** (Supplementary Figure S3F vs. **Figure 5E**), produces significantly lower inhibition (IC_{50} value of 798 vs. 231 nM; **Table 1**). On one hand, the methyl of the R1-methoxy group of **8** (**Figure 5E**) packs into a hydrophobic niche formed by the side chains of Tyr60, Gln206, Tyr326, Leu328, Phe343, and Met341 (green sector in **Figures 3A,B**). On the other hand, the methoxy's oxygen increases the 3-phenyl ring's hydrophilicity and softens the clash of the coumarin ring with the solvent shielding the cofactor (**Figure 5E**).

Switching the R1-methoxy of **1** into the R2 position in **2** (**Figure 2**) makes the alignment of the coumarin ring more challenging, because the R2-methoxy is unable to occupy the same hydrophobic niche (green sector in **Figures 3A,B**) as the R1-methoxy (**Figure 4A** vs. Supplementary Figure S3A). Although the R1/R2 methoxy switch, by all means, does not prevent binding, it leads to ~80 nM reduction in the IC_{50} value (**Table 1**). Paradoxically, the opposite and considerably larger difference in inhibition is produced by the R1/R2 switch, when comparing the activity of derivatives **20** and **22** (**Figure 2**; **Table 1**). Accordingly, **20** with the R2-methoxy of (IC_{50} value of 391 nM; **Table 1**) provides twice as strong inhibition as **22** with the R1-methoxy (IC_{50} value of 831 nM; **Table 1**). The vast difference is caused by the coordinated R6/R7 interactions of the 3-phenyl ring, which pushes the coumarin ring closer to the Tyr326 side chain—a critical shift that is stunted by the R1-methoxy of **22** (**Figure 5E** vs. **Figure 5F**).

Replacing the R2-acetoxy of **3** (**Figure 2**) with the R1-methoxy in **4** (**Figure 2**) weakens the inhibition ~180 nM (**Table 1**). The coumarin ring of **4** is pushed closer to the cofactor due to the addition of the R6-trifluoromethoxy into the 3-phenyl ring (**Figure 5B** vs. Supplementary Figure S3B) and, in this new pose, the methyl of the R2-acetoxy is able to occupy the small hydrophobic niche (green sector in **Figures 3A,B**), meanwhile, exposing the acetoxy's oxygen atoms to the solvent (**Figure 3B**). However, substituting the R1-methoxy of **18** with the R2-acetoxy in **19** (**Figure 2**) does not improve the inhibition; instead, the IC_{50} value is reduced by ~250 nM (**Table 1**). This happens, because the R6-dimethylamine of **19** (Supplementary Figure S3J) is not forcing the scaffold to align close to the cofactor the same way as the R6-trifluoromethoxy does (**Figure 5B** vs. **Figures 6C,D**). In contrast, replacing the R1-methoxy of **18** with the R2-hydroxyl in **17** improves the inhibition (IC_{50} improvement of 234 nM; **Table 1**) by promoting water solubility near the cofactor (**Figure 6C** vs. **Figure 6D**).

The R6 and R7 interactions of **7** (**Figure 2**) are expected to remind closely those of **6** (Supplementary Figure S3D vs. **Figure 5C**), but its coumarin ring's R1- and R3-chlorine groups weaken the inhibition ~700 nM (**Table 1**). The R2-methoxy of **6** is able to play into the hydrophobic/hydrophilic dual nature of the cavity end facing the cofactor (**Figure 5C**) without occupying the small hydrophobic niche (green sector in **Figures 3A,B**). In this respect, the R1-chlorine is too bulky to occupy this specific niche although a methoxy group at the same position should be able to occupy the available space (e.g., **1** in **Figure 5A**).

Selectivity of the 3-Phenylcoumarin Derivatives

Determining the specificity and subtype selectivity of the 3-phenylcoumarin derivatives for MAO-B is needed to evaluate their true pharmacological potential. Unintended off-target effects with other proteins can render even the most promising drug candidates useless, ambiguous or even toxic. Here, the focus is put on MAO-A which has shared activity with MAO-B in deamination of dopamine and dietary amines tyramine and tryptamine. In addition, the effects of the derivatives are tested with a specific subset of enzymes, including HSD1, aromatase, CYP1A2, and ER, whose function is linked to different stages of estradiol action and metabolism. These particular enzymes were looked at with the derivatives, because they are known to have structurally similar ligands or even coumarin-based inhibitors based on prior studies and our upcoming study (Mattsson et al., 2014; Niinivehmas et al., 2016; Niinivehmas et al., unpublished results).

Monoamine oxidase A (MAO-A) is more prevalent than the subtype B in the gastrointestinal tract and, accordingly, the MAO-A inhibition can cause accumulation of tyramine from dietary sources. Because tyramine can displace neurotransmitters leading to potentially fatal hypertensive crisis, it is highly desirable to design MAO-B-specific inhibitors lacking MAO-A activity. The vast majority of the novel derivatives do not produce MAO-A inhibition at 100 μM despite the fact that it is ten times the concentration used in this study to determine MAO-B inhibition percentage (**Table 1**, Supplementary Table S1). Furthermore, only in those few cases where inhibition was detected, especially with the most potent MAO-B derivatives, it remains at moderate or close to non-existent level (**Table 1**). The strongest MAO-A inhibition was elicited by derivatives **42** and **43** (48.86 and 56.76%), but derivatives **27** and **45** (43.83 and 43.36%) are close runner-ups and next analogs down the list are already much weaker (Supplementary Figure S4, Supplementary Table S1). Notably, **1**, which is the most potent MAO-B inhibitor of the derivative set with the IC_{50} value of 56 nM, does not produce MAO-A inhibition at 100 μM (**Table 1**). The molecular basis for the lack of MAO-A activity is evident, when comparing the shape and size of the active sites of the two enzyme subtypes in the context of 3-phenylcoumarin binding (**Figure 3A** vs. **Figure 3B**).

17-β-hydroxysteroid dehydrogenase 1 (HSD1), which functions as the catalyst of the final reducing step in the estradiol biosynthesis, is often overexpressed in breast cancer and endometriotic tissue (Vihko et al., 2004; Dassen et al., 2007; Hanamura et al., 2014). Thus, specific inhibition of HSD1 has potential to reduce effective estradiol levels in the treatments. Although the synthesized 3-phenylcoumarin set contains several molecules that exhibit activity toward HSD1, the inhibition was generally very weak and the active compounds are not among the most potent MAO-B inhibitors. Of the 24 most potent MAO-B inhibitors, the strongest HSD1 inhibition could be recorded for **20** and **22** (46 and 54%; **Figure 2**, **Table 1**); however, considerably higher activity (48.20–83.90%) was seen with derivatives **30**, **31**, **33**, **38**, and **48** (Supplementary

Figure S4, Supplementary Table S1). Modest HSD1 inhibition (12–33%) was also elicited by **6**, **15**, **16**, **23**, **24** (**Figure 2**, **Table 1**) and **51** (Supplementary Figure S4, Supplementary Table S1). Importantly, derivative **1**, which is the most potent MAO-B inhibitor of the derivative set, does not inhibit HSD1.

Aromatase (CYP19A1) inhibition, which is important for blocking local estradiol synthesis for example in breast cancer treatment (Pasqualini et al., 1996), was not detected with the derivatives (**Table 1**, Supplementary Table S1). Although 3-phenylcoumarin should be able to sterically mimic the steroidal positioning at the active site (not shown), it would have to house a clear-cut H-bond acceptor at the R5/R7-position in the 3-phenyl to facilitate aromatase binding. This is, because X-ray crystallography shows that the Asp309 side chain is in neutral state at pH 7.4 and donating a proton to the carbonyl group of inhibitor androstenedione (PDB: 3EQM) (Ghosh et al., 2009). Inserting a hydroxyl group to the R5/R7 position could put an H-bond acceptor to this same location with the 3-phenylcoumarins (see **31**, **38**, **40**, **42**, **43**; Supplementary Figure S4, Supplementary Table S1). However, because the hydroxyl always has a dual role as an H-bond donor as well, any aromatase binding by the derivatives remains theoretical as it is prevented by a proton donor clash. The issue is described more thoroughly in our upcoming study (Niinivehmas et al., unpublished results).

Estrogen receptor (ER) agonists/antagonists or selective modulators are developed for infertility, contraception, hormone replacement, and ER positive breast cancer therapies. If the MAO-B inhibitors would function also as ER agonists, they could promote tumorigenesis in the breast tissue as a side effect. Unintended ER inhibition could also disturb natural estrogen levels or interrupt ER-targeted therapies. The measurements indicate that the 3-phenylcoumarin derivatives either are a hit or miss when considering ER inhibition. Although the ER activity could not be measured for all of the analogs due to running out of the synthesis products, the acquired results overwhelmingly support our prior findings stating that the R2-hydroxyl or the R6-hydroxyl/halogen is needed to prompt ER activity (Niinivehmas et al., 2016). This ER-specific effect is prominent with **12**, **20**, **22**, **27**, **28**, **29**, **30**, **39**, **40**, **41**, **44**, and **48** (**Table 1**, Supplementary Table S1, **Figure 2**, Supplementary Figure S4) and, moreover, ER activity is predicted for **17** and likely for **32** and **47** based on the well-established trend.

Cytochrome P450 1A2 (CYP1A2) catalyzes the oxidation of xenobiotics, especially polyaromatic hydrocarbons and steroid hormone-sized compounds such as 3-phenylcoumarins, into more soluble form for excretion (Zhou et al., 2010). Accordingly, it was prudent to get a rough estimate of the CYP1A2 inhibition levels for the novel 3-phenylcoumarin derivatives as well. In general, all of the derivatives inhibited CYP1A2 at some level (**Table 1**, Supplementary Table S1); however, typically the most potent CYP1A2 inhibitors such as **21–24** were less potent MAO-B inhibitors (**Table 1**). Similar to MAO-A, HSD1, and aromatase, the most potent MAO-B derivative **1** displayed only low CYP1A2 activity (IC_{50} value of 124 μM; **Table 1**).

Overall Assessment on the Druglikeness

As a whole, the selectivity analysis indicates that the cross-reactivity of 3-phenylcoumarins can be managed or even avoided via specific functional group substitutions without taking away the MAO-B activity. Coumarins in general do not belong to the PAINS (pan assay interference compounds) category as it is a privileged scaffold structure. Only derivative **50**, which is not a potent MAO-B inhibitor (Supplementary Table S1, Supplementary Figure S4), was recognized as a potential PAINS ligand by PAINS3 filter (or A filter) in CANVAS module in MAESTRO (Baell and Holloway, 2010). In the ChEMBL database, ~14,200 coumarin derivatives are included (observed online in 8.2.2018), which indicates that the scaffold can be tailored to target multitude of proteins. Despite this, the literature does not raise widespread concerns that the coumarin-based compounds in particular would cause harmful cross-reactivity or selectivity issues. The 24 active derivatives presented in this study (**Table 1**, **Figure 2**) have lower potency than some of the prior 3-phenylcoumarin compounds (Supplementary Figure S6, Supplementary Table S2) (Matos et al., 2009b, 2011a,b; Santana et al., 2010; Viña et al., 2012a); however, one has to be aware of fact that these results originate from different laboratories and activity assays and are, therefore, not fully comparable. To a degree this is the case even for the positive control pargyline (Fisar et al., 2010). Importantly, the new compounds follow closely the Lipinski rule of five regarding the logP value (logP $<$ 5) and remain in the logP range of 2–4. Moreover, the ligand-lipophilicity efficiency (LiPE) values of the new analogs suggest reasonable druglikeness (Freeman-Cook et al., 2013). What is more, derivative **1** clearly has the most promising selectivity profile of the derivatives for future consideration, because it is not only the most potent MAO-B inhibitor of the set but it is also selective against the other tested enzymes.

CONCLUSION

A broad set of 3-phenylcoumarin derivatives was designed using virtual combinatorial chemistry or rationally *de novo*, synthesized and tested for MAO-B inhibition potency using spectrophotometry (Supplementary Table S1). The results further validate prior studies suggesting that the 3-phenylcoumarin is a suitable scaffold for building potent small-molecule MAO-B inhibitors by functionalizing its ring systems. A moderate MAO-B inhibition could be achieved by inserting a wide variety of functional groups into the coumarin (R1–R3; **Figure 4**) or 3-phenyl (R4–R7; **Figure 4**) rings (Supplementary Table S1). Twenty-four of the derivatives (**Figures 2**, **3D**) were found to elicit >70% inhibition (**Table 1**, Supplementary Figures S1, S2). These promising derivatives inhibit the MAO-B at a ~100 nM to ~1 μM range (**Table 1**), while the most potent derivative **1** produces ~56 nM MAO-B inhibition. A molecular docking-based (**Figures 5**, **6**, Supplementary Figure S3) SAR analysis (**Figure 4**) describe the determinants of the MAO-B binding and inhibition at the atomistic level. Firstly, without any kind of the 3-phenyl substituents, no inhibition was detected. Although both hydrogen and halogen bonding can assist the 3-phenyl alignment and facilitate inhibition (**Figures 6E,F**, **Table 1**), the ability of the functionalized ring to fill the hydrophobic end of the binding cavity (red sector in **Figures 3A,B**) is the most important property for ensuring strong MAO-B inhibition (e.g., R6-trifluoromethyl of **1**; **Figure 5A**). Secondly, the SAR analysis reveals that a spot-on placement and composition of the coumarin ring's substituents can further enhance the MAO-B inhibition (**Figure 2**, **Table 1**), however, these effects are ultimately dependent on the scaffold alignment, which, in turn, depends on the 3-phenyl ring substituents (**Figure 4**). The cross-reactivity analysis focusing on MAO-A and a subset of estradiol metabolism-linked HSD1, aromatase, CYP1A2 and ER highlighted the potential of the 3-phenylcourmains, especially the most potent MAO-B derivative **1**, for producing selective MAO-B inhibition. Finally, the most potent 3-phenylcoumarin analogs presented in this study are estimated to operate at close to optimal ligand-lipophilicity efficiency—a feature highlighting their overall druglikeness.

AUTHOR CONTRIBUTIONS

SR: was responsible for the experimental testing regarding MAO-A and MAO-B; EMu: performed the MAO-A experimental analysis; SR: did the docking into MAO-B and prepared most of the figures; PAP: was responsible for the final SAR analysis; SK, ES, and JH: performed the organic synthesis; MA: did the PAINS screening; PK: performed the HSD1 measurements; NN, RJ, and HR: did the experimental analysis regarding CYP1A2; PH and MaP: executed the experimental analysis regarding aromatase; MiP: did preliminary screening for designing MAO-B ligands; SN, EMa, SK, and OTP: designed the molecules for the selected targets; SN, EMa, and OTP: designed the study. All the coauthors were involved in the manuscript preparation and approved the final version.

FUNDING

Academy of Finland is acknowledged for funding (OTP. Project No. 250311).

ACKNOWLEDGMENTS

The Finnish IT Center for Science (CSC) for computational resources (OTP; Project Nos. jyy2516 and jyy2585).

REFERENCES

Baell, J. B., and Holloway, G. A. (2010). New substructure filters for removal of pan assay interference compounds (PAINS) from screening libraries and for their exclusion in bioassays. *J. Med. Chem.* 53, 2719–2740. doi: 10.1021/jm901137j

Bhandri, P. R., Bose, J. L., and Siddiqui, S. (1949). 3-Phenylcoumarin series. I. Synthesis of some new members of the series. *J. Sci. Ind. Res.* 8B, 189–192.

Binda, C., Li, M., Hubalek, F., Restelli, N., Edmondson, D. E., and Mattevi, A. (2003). Insights into the mode of inhibition of human mitochondrial monoamine oxidase B from high-resolution crystal structures. *Proc. Natl. Acad. Sci. U.S.A.* 100, 9750–9755. doi: 10.1073/pnas.1633804100

Binda, C., Wang, J., Pisani, L., Caccia, C., Carotti, A., Salvati, P., et al. (2007). Structures of human monoamine oxidase B complexes with selective noncovalent inhibitors: safinamide and coumarin analogs. *J. Med. Chem.* 50, 5848–5852. doi: 10.1021/jm070677y

Borges, F., Roleira, F., Milhazes, N., Santana, L., and Uriarte, E. (2005). Simple coumarins and analogues in medicinal chemistry: occurrence, synthesis and biological activity. *Curr. Med. Chem.* 12, 887–916. doi: 10.2174/0929867053507315

Carradori, S., and Silvestri, R. (2015). New frontiers in selective human MAO-B inhibitors miniperspective. *J. Med. Chem.* 58, 6717–6732. doi: 10.1021/jm501690r

Catto, M., Nicolotti, O., Leonetti, F., Carotti, A., Favia, A. D., Soto-Otero, R., et al. (2006). Structural insights into monoamine oxidase inhibitory potency and selectivity of 7-substituted coumarins from ligand- and target-based approaches. *J. Med. Chem.* 49, 4912–4925. doi: 10.1021/jm060183l

Cavallo, G., Metrangolo, P., Milani, R., Pilati, T., Priimagi, A., Resnati, G., et al. (2016). The halogen bond. *Chem. Rev.* 116, 2478–2601. doi: 10.1021/acs.chemrev.5b00484

Chauhan, P., Ravi, M., Singh, S., Prajapati, P., and Yadav, P. P. (2016). Regioselective [small alpha]-arylation of coumarins and 2-pyridones with phenylhydrazines under transition-metal-free conditions. *RSC Adv.* 6, 109–118. doi: 10.1039/C5RA20954D

Dassen, H., Punyadeera, C., Kamps, R., Delvoux, B., Van Langendonckt, A., Donnez, J., et al. (2007). Estrogen metabolizing enzymes in endometrium and endometriosis. *Hum. Reprod.* 22, 3148–3158. doi: 10.1093/humrep/dem310

Dobelmann-Mara, L., Riedmueller, S., and Schraub, M. (2017). *Compounds for Optically Active Devices.* PCT Int. Appl. A1 20170302.

Edmondson, D. E., Mattevi, A., Binda, C., Li, M., and Hubálek, F. (2005). Structure and mechanism of monoamine oxidase. *Burger's Med. Chem. Drug Discov.* 11, 1983–1993. doi: 10.1002/0471266949.bmc111

Ferino, G., Cadoni, E., Matos, M. J., Quezada, E., Uriarte, E., Santana, L., et al. (2013). MAO Inhibitory activity of 2-arylbenzofurans versus 3-arylcoumarins: synthesis, *in vitro* study, and docking calculations. *ChemMedChem* 8, 956–966. doi: 10.1002/cmdc.201300048

Finberg, J. P. M., and Rabey, J. M. (2016). Inhibitors of MAO-A and MAO-B in psychiatry and neurology. *Front. Pharmacol.* 7:340. doi: 10.3389/fphar.2016.00340

Fisar, Z., Hroudová, J., and Raboch, J. (2010). Inhibition of monoamine oxidase activity by antidepressants and mood stabilizers. *Neuroendocrinol. Lett.* 31, 645–656.

Freeman-Cook, K. D., Hoffman, R. L., and Johnson, T. W. (2013). Lipophilic efficiency: the most important efficiency metric in medicinal chemistry. *Future Med. Chem.* 5, 113–115. doi: 10.4155/fmc.12.208

Gaweska, H., and Fitzpatrick, P. F. (2011). Structures and mechanism of the monoamine oxidase family. *Biomol. Concepts* 2, 365–377. doi: 10.1515/BMC.2011.030

Ghosh, D., Griswold, J., Erman, M., and Pangborn, W. (2009). Structural basis for androgen specificity and oestrogen synthesis in human aromatase. *Nature* 457, 219–223. doi: 10.1038/nature07614

Hanamura, T., Niwa, T., Gohno, T., Kurosumi, M., Takei, H., Yamaguchi, Y., et al. (2014). Possible role of the aromatase-independent steroid metabolism pathways in hormone responsive primary breast cancers. *Breast Cancer Res. Treat.* 143, 69–80. doi: 10.1007/s10549-013-2788-3

Holt, A., Sharman, D. F., Baker, G. B., and Palcic, M. M. (1997). A continuous spectrophotometric assay for monoamine oxidase and related enzymes in tissue homogenates. *Anal. Biochem.* 244, 384–392. doi: 10.1006/abio.1996.9911

Humphrey, W., Dalke, A., and Schulten, K. (1996). VMD: visual molecular dynamics. *J. Mol. Graph.* 14, 33–8, 27–8. doi: 10.1016/0263-7855(96)00018-5

Joao Matos, M., Vina, D., Vazquez-Rodriguez, S., Uriarte, E., and Santana, L. (2013). Focusing on new monoamine oxidase inhibitors: differently substituted coumarins as an interesting scaffold. *Curr. Top. Med. Chem.* 12, 2210–2239. doi: 10.2174/156802661121220008

Kirkiacharian, S., Chidiack, H., Philibert, D., Van De Velde, P., and Bouchoux, F. (1999). Binding affinity to steroid hormone receptors and antiproliferative action on MCF-7 cells of coumarinic derivatives and isoflavonoids. *Ann. Pharm. Fr.* 57, 332–339.

Kirkiacharian, S., Lormier, A. T., Resche-Rigon, M., Bouchoux, F., and Cerede, E. (2003). Synthesis and binding affinity of 3-aryl-7-hydroxycoumarins to human α and β estrogen receptors. *Ann. Pharm. Fr.* 61, 51–56.

Korb, O., Stützle, T., and Exner, T. E. (2009). Empirical scoring functions for advanced protein-ligand docking with PLANTS. *J. Chem. Inf. Model.* 49, 84–96. doi: 10.1021/ci800298z

Korhonen, L. E., Rahnasto, M., Mähönen, N. J., Wittekindt, C., Poso, A., Juvonen, R. O., et al. (2005). Predictive three-dimensional quantitative structure-activity relationship of cytochrome P450 1A2 inhibitors. *J. Med. Chem.* 48, 3808–3815. doi: 10.1021/jm0489713

Kraulis, P. J. (1991). MOLSCRIPT: a program to produce both detailed and schematic plots of protein structures. *J. Appl. Crystallogr.* 24, 946–950. doi: 10.1107/S0021889891004399

Lehtonen, J. V., Still, D.-J., Rantanen, V.-V., Ekholm, J., Björklund, D., Iftikhar, Z., et al. (2004). BODIL: a molecular modeling environment for structure-function analysis and drug design. *J. Comput. Aided. Mol. Des.* 18, 401–419. doi: 10.1007/s10822-004-3752-4

Lomize, M. A., Lomize, A. L., Pogozheva, I. D., and Mosberg, H. I. (2006). OPM: orientations of proteins in membranes database. *Bioinformatics* 22, 623–625. doi: 10.1093/bioinformatics/btk023

Matos, M. J., Terán, C., Pérez-Castillo, Y., Uriarte, E., Santana, L., and Viña, D. (2011a). Synthesis and study of a series of 3-arylcoumarins as potent and selective monoamine oxidase B inhibitors. *J. Med. Chem.* 54, 7127–7137. doi: 10.1021/jm200716y

Matos, M. J., Vazquez-Rodriguez, S., Uriarte, E., Santana, L., and Viña, D. (2011b). MAO inhibitory activity modulation: 3-Phenylcoumarins versus 3-benzoylcoumarins. *Bioorganic Med. Chem. Lett.* 21, 4224–4227. doi: 10.1016/j.bmcl.2011.05.074

Matos, M. J., Viña, D., Janeiro, P., Borges, F., Santana, L., and Uriarte, E. (2010). New halogenated 3-phenylcoumarins as potent and selective MAO-B inhibitors. *Bioorganic Med. Chem. Lett.* 20, 5157–5160. doi: 10.1016/j.bmcl.2010.07.013

Matos, M. J., Viña, D., Picciau, C., Orallo, F., Santana, L., and Uriarte, E. (2009a). Synthesis and evaluation of 6-methyl-3-phenylcoumarins as potent and selective MAO-B inhibitors. *Bioorganic Med. Chem. Lett.* 19, 5053–5055. doi: 10.1016/j.bmcl.2009.07.039

Matos, M. J., Viña, D., Quezada, E., Picciau, C., Delogu, G., Orallo, F., et al. (2009b). A new series of 3-phenylcoumarins as potent and selective MAO-B inhibitors. *Bioorg. Med. Chem. Lett.* 19, 3268–3270. doi: 10.1016/j.bmcl.2009.04.085

Mattsson, C., Svensson, P., and Sonesson, C. (2014). A novel series of 6-substituted 3-(pyrrolidin-1-ylmethyl)chromen-2-ones as selective monoamine oxidase (MAO) A inhibitors. *Eur. J. Med. Chem.* 73, 177–186. doi: 10.1016/j.ejmech.2013.11.035

Merritt, E. A., and Murphy, M. E. P. (1994). Raster3D Version 2.0. A program for photorealistic molecular graphics. *Acta Crystallogr. Sect. D Biol. Crystallogr.* 50, 869–873. doi: 10.1107/S0907444994006396

Messinger, J., Husen, B., Koskimies, P., Hirvelä, L., Kallio, L., Saarenketo, P., et al. (2009). Estrone C15 derivatives–a new class of 17beta-hydroxysteroid dehydrogenase type 1 inhibitors. *Mol. Cell. Endocrinol.* 301, 216–224. doi: 10.1016/j.mce.2008.10.022

Mokkila, S., Postila, P. A., Rissanen, S., Juhola, H., Vattulainen, I., and Róg, T. (2017). Calcium assists dopamine release by preventing aggregation on the inner leaflet of presynaptic vesicles. *ACS Chem. Neurosci. Acschemneuro.* 8, 1242–1250. doi: 10.1021/acschemneuro.6b00395

Niinivehmas, S. P., Manivannan, E., Rauhamäki, S., Huuskonen, J., and Pentikäinen, O. T. (2016). Identification of estrogen receptor α ligands with virtual screening techniques. *J. Mol. Graph. Model.* 64, 30–39. doi: 10.1016/j.jmgm.2015.12.006

Niinivehmas, S. P., Salokas, K., Lätti, S., Raunio, H., and Pentikäinen, O. T. (2015). Ultrafast protein structure-based virtual screening with Panther. *J. Comput. Aided Mol. Des.* 29, 989–1006. doi: 10.1007/s10822-015-9870-3

Niinivehmas, S. P., Virtanen, S. I., Lehtonen, J. V., Postila, P. A., and Pentikäinen, O. T. (2011). Comparison of virtual high-throughput screening methods for the identification of phosphodiesterase-5 inhibitors. *J. Chem. Inf. Model.* 51, 1353–1363. doi: 10.1021/ci1004527

Nurminen, E. M., Pihlavisto, M., Lázár, L., Pentikäinen, U., Fülöp, F., and Pentikäinen, O. T. (2011). Novel hydrazine molecules as tools to understand the flexibility of vascular adhesion protein-1 ligand-binding site: toward more selective inhibitors. *J. Med. Chem.* 54, 2143–2154. doi: 10.1021/jm200059p

Nurminen, E. M., Pihlavisto, M., Lázár, L., Szakonyi, Z., Pentikäinen, U., Fülöp, F., et al. (2010). Synthesis, *in vitro* activity, and three-dimensional quantitative structure–activity relationship of novel hydrazine inhibitors of human vascular adhesion protein-1. *J. Med. Chem.* 53, 6301–6315. doi: 10.1021/jm100337z

Orłowski, A., Grzybek, M., Bunker, A., Pasenkiewicz-Gierula, M., Vattulainen, I., Männistö, P. T., et al. (2012). Strong preferences of dopamine and l -dopa towards lipid head group: importance of lipid composition and implication for neurotransmitter metabolism. *J. Neurochem.* 122, 681–690. doi: 10.1111/j.1471-4159.2012.07813.x

Pasanen, M. (1985). Human placental aromatase activity: use of a C18 reversed-phase cartridge for separation of tritiated water or steroid metabolites in placentas from both smoking and non-smoking mothers *in vitro*. *Biol. Res. Pregnancy Perinatol.* 6, 94–99.

Pasqualini, J., Chetrite, G., Blacker, M., Feinstein, M.-C., Delalonde, L., Talbi, M., et al. (1996). Concentrations of estrone, estradiol, and estrone sulfate and evaluation of sulfatase and aromatase activities in pre- and postmenopausal breast cancer patients. *J. Clin. Endocrinol. Metab.* 81, 1460–1464.

Patil, P. O., Bari, S. B., Firke, S. D., Deshmukh, P. K., Donda, S. T., and Patil, D. A. (2013). A comprehensive review on synthesis and designing aspects of coumarin derivatives as monoamine oxidase inhibitors for depression and Alzheimer's disease. *Bioorganic Med. Chem.* 21, 2434–2450. doi: 10.1016/j.bmc.2013.02.017

Postila, P. A., Vattulainen, I., and Róg, T. (2016). Selective effect of cell membrane on synaptic neurotransmission. *Sci. Rep.* 6:19345. doi: 10.1038/srep19345

Prendergast, P. T. (2001). *Use of Flavones, Coumarins and Related Compounds to Treat Infections.* PCT Int. Appl., A2 20010118.

Santana, L., Orallo, F., Viña, D., Matos Joao Correia, P. C., Quezada, E., Yañes, J., et al. (2010). *Use of Derivates of 6-Substituted 3-Phenylcoumarins and Preparation of New Derivates.* Available online at: http://www.google.com.pg/patents/WO2010086484A1?cl=en

Serra, S., Ferino, G., Matos, M. J., Vázquez-Rodríguez, S., Delogu, G., Viña, D., et al. (2012). Hydroxycoumarins as selective MAO-B inhibitors. *Bioorganic Med. Chem. Lett.* 22, 258–261. doi: 10.1016/j.bmcl.2011.11.020

Shih, J. C., Chen, K., and Ridd, M. J. (1999). Monoamine oxidase: from genes to behavior. *Annu. Rev. Neurosci.* 22, 197–217. doi: 10.1146/annurev.neuro.22.1.197

Vihko, P., Härkönen, P., Soronen, P., Törn, S., Herrala, A., Kurkela, R., et al. (2004). 17β-Hydroxysteroid dehydrogenases - their role in pathophysiology. *Mol. Cell. Endocrinol.* 215, 83–88. doi: 10.1016/j.mce.2003.11.021

Vilar, S., Quezada, E., Santana, L., Uriarte, E., Yánez, M., Fraiz, N., et al. (2006). Design, synthesis, and vasorelaxant and platelet antiaggregatory activities of coumarin–resveratrol hybrids. *Bioorg. Med. Chem. Lett.* 16, 257–261. doi: 10.1016/j.bmcl.2005.10.013

Viña, D., Matos, M. J., Ferino, G., Cadoni, E., Laguna, R., Borges, F., et al. (2012a). 8-substituted 3-arylcoumarins as potent and selective MAO-B inhibitors:

synthesis, pharmacological evaluation, and docking studies. *ChemMedChem* 7, 464–470. doi: 10.1002/cmdc.201100538

Viña, D., Matos, M. J., Yáñez, M., Santana, L., and Uriarte, E. (2012b). 3-Substituted coumarins as dual inhibitors of AChE and MAO for the treatment of Alzheimer's disease. *Med. Chem. Commun.* 3, 213–218. doi: 10.1039/C1MD00221J

Youdim, M. B. H., Edmondson, D., and Tipton, K. F. (2006). The therapeutic potential of monoamine oxidase inhibitors. *Nat. Rev. Neurosci.* 7, 295–309. doi: 10.1038/nrn1883

Zhou, S.-F., Wang, B., Yang, L.-P., and Liu, J.-P. (2010). Structure, function, regulation and polymorphism and the clinical significance of human cytochrome P450 1A2. *Drug Metab. Rev.* 42, 268–354. doi: 10.3109/03602530903286476

13

How to Achieve Better Results Using PASS-Based Virtual Screening: Case Study for Kinase Inhibitors

Pavel V. Pogodin[1], Alexey A. Lagunin[1,2], Anastasia V. Rudik[1], Dmitry A. Filimonov[1], Dmitry S. Druzhilovskiy[1], Mark C. Nicklaus[3] and Vladimir V. Poroikov[1]*

[1] Department of Bioinformatics, Institute of Biomedical Chemistry, Moscow, Russia, [2] Department of Bioinformatics, Medical-Biological Department, Pirogov Russian National Research Medical University, Moscow, Russia, [3] Computer-Aided Drug Design Group, Chemical Biology Laboratory, Center for Cancer Research, National Cancer Institute, NIH, NCI-Frederick, Frederick, MD, United States

***Correspondence:**
Vladimir V. Poroikov
vladimir.poroikov@ibmc.msk.ru

Discovery of new pharmaceutical substances is currently boosted by the possibility of utilization of the Synthetically Accessible Virtual Inventory (SAVI) library, which includes about 283 million molecules, each annotated with a proposed synthetic one-step route from commercially available starting materials. The SAVI database is well-suited for ligand-based methods of virtual screening to select molecules for experimental testing. In this study, we compare the performance of three approaches for the analysis of structure-activity relationships that differ in their criteria for selecting of "active" and "inactive" compounds included in the training sets. PASS (Prediction of Activity Spectra for Substances), which is based on a modified Naïve Bayes algorithm, was applied since it had been shown to be robust and to provide good predictions of many biological activities based on just the structural formula of a compound even if the information in the training set is incomplete. We used different subsets of kinase inhibitors for this case study because many data are currently available on this important class of drug-like molecules. Based on the subsets of kinase inhibitors extracted from the ChEMBL 20 database we performed the PASS training, and then applied the model to ChEMBL 23 compounds not yet present in ChEMBL 20 to identify novel kinase inhibitors. As one may expect, the best prediction accuracy was obtained if only the experimentally confirmed active and inactive compounds for distinct kinases in the training procedure were used. However, for some kinases, reasonable results were obtained even if we used merged training sets, in which we designated as inactives the compounds not tested against the particular kinase. Thus, depending on the availability of data for a particular biological activity, one may choose the first or the second approach for creating ligand-based computational tools to achieve the best possible results in virtual screening.

Keywords: ChEMBL, bioactivity data, kinase inhibitors, SAR, PASS, virtual screening, classification, SAVI

INTRODUCTION

Discovery of novel pharmaceutical agents with improved safety and efficacy is the perpetual task of medicinal chemistry (Pammolli et al., 2011). In addition to the traditional methods of chemical synthesis and pharmacological studies of various drug-like substances, in recent years substantial attention has been paid to the analysis of the general chemical-biological space (Lipinski and Hopkins, 2004; Baell and Holloway, 2010; Bon and Waldmann, 2010; López-Vallejo et al., 2012; Deng et al., 2013; Medina-Franco et al., 2013; Buonfiglio et al., 2015; Rodriguez-Esteban, 2016; Horvath et al., 2017). Such approaches significantly increase the diversity of the studied chemical libraries as well as the chances to identify the pharmaceutical agents interacting with multiple molecular targets and causing additive or synergistic desired pharmacological action (Sidorov et al., 2015; Lauria et al., 2016).

Nowadays, available chemical libraries can be divided into four categories: (1) databases containing information about structure and properties of publicly disclosed chemical compounds, e.g., PubChem (Li et al., 2010; Wang Y. et al., 2014) and ChEMBL (Bento et al., 2014); (2) databases containing information about structure of commercially available chemical samples, e.g., ZINC (Sterling and Irwin, 2015); (3) databases of virtually generated structures comprehensively covering the particular chemical space, e.g., GDB-17 (Ruddigkeit et al., 2012); (4) databases of virtually generated, synthetically accessible, structures with data on starting materials and proposed synthetic routes, e.g., SAVI (Synthetically Accessible Virtual Inventory) (Pevzner et al., 2017). Although GDB-17 is one of the largest[1] currently known libraries of chemical structures containing 166.4 billion possible molecules up to 17 atoms of C, N, O, S, and halogen, SAVI looks more attractive for utilization in drug discovery because of the synthesability of its molecules. Furthermore, it was shown (Pevzner et al., 2017) that the overlap between the 93 million structures from PubChem with the 238 million SAVI database is only about 0.03%. Thus, SAVI represents a significant previously unexploited reservoir of novel structures, presumably useful for drug discovery.

To reveal the hidden pharmacological potential of the synthesizable molecules from SAVI, computer-aided virtual screening could be applied (Jorgensen, 2004; Nettles et al., 2006; Bajorath, 2014; Fujita and Winkler, 2016; Lee et al., 2016). Although structure-based methods are widely used now, ligand-based methods have important advantages (Leelananda and Lindert, 2016). In several case studies, machine learning approaches were shown to surpass the performance of both chemical similarity assessment and reverse docking (Anusevicius et al., 2015; Druzhilovskiy et al., 2016; Murtazalieva et al., 2017).

Thus, it is reasonable to analyze the probable biological activity of SAVI molecules using our computer program PASS that recently received high marks: "One of the earliest and most widely used examples of data-mining target elucidation is the continuously curated and expanded Prediction of Activity Spectra for Substances (PASS) software, which was assimilated from the bioactivites of more than 270,000 compound-ligand pairs" (Mervin et al., 2015). The PASS development started more than 25 years ago (Poroikov et al., 1993; Filimonov et al., 1995), and during this time its performance has continuously and significantly improved. PASS in its 2017 version predicts over 7,000 kinds of biological activity with an average accuracy of 94% based on the analysis of structure-activity relationships for more than 1 million known biologically active compounds.

Initially, in the PASS training set a molecule is designated as "active" if reliable information about some biological activity is found in a authoritative source (publication in a peer-reviewed journal, record in curated database, etc.); otherwise, it is designated as "(conditionally) inactive." This would seem to be a reasonable approach as it has been found that if the same set of chemical compounds is studied against the same molecular target in the three different assays, only 35% of active compounds completely coincided (Lipinski and Hopkins, 2004).

Since no one chemical compound has been tested for all known biological activities, this may appear to be the incorrect designation in some cases. However, it has been shown that PASS provides reasonable estimates of structure-activity relationships despite the incompleteness of information in the training set on both chemical structures and biological activities, due to the robustness of the Naïve Bayes approach in general (Rish, 2001; Rennie et al., 2003) and the MNA descriptors and the biological activity representation used in PASS in particular (Poroikov et al., 2000).

Quantitative data on structure and activity of many chemical compounds freely available from ChEMBL and PubChem databases allow one to consider alternative approaches for creating training sets that may improve the performance of machine learning methods. Such possibilities were recently considered in several studies (Heikamp and Bajorath, 2013; Smusz et al., 2013; Kurczab et al., 2014; Afzal et al., 2015; Mervin et al., 2015).

In this work we evaluated the PASS performance in virtual screening for kinase inhibitors with training performed using three approaches, which differ with respect to what compounds were selected as inactives: (1) only experimentally validated ("true") inactives; (2) combining true and conditionally inactives; (3) only conditionally inactives. The first and second approaches have the drawback that they require enough data on true inactives.

These training strategies are both related to the multi-label classification (Tsoumakas et al., 2010; Cherman et al., 2011; Afzal et al., 2015) and positive unlabeled learning (Kilic and Tan, 2012), because one and the same classifying object may simultaneously belong to several categories [have multiple labels, i.e., inhibit more than one kinase (Martin et al., 2011) in our case study] and the problem of inactives' selection may be solved using more than one method. In contrary to various approaches of inactives' selection described by the authors (Kilic and Tan, 2012), we used only straightforward approaches, since in chemoinformatics we

[1]The Danish biopharmaceutical company Nuevolution announced that it had created a library of 40 trillion unique molecules (C&EN, 2017, 95: 28–33); however, the web site (https://nuevolution.com/technology) states that the company enables DNA encoded synthesis of billions of chemically diverse drug-like small molecule compounds.

are forced to deal with extremely sparse data about ligand-protein interactions and, thus, introduction of data about target-to-target relations during the training may lead to strong overfitting.

The kinases were chosen for this study because of the strong family ties among kinases that manifest themselves through common structural features and predispose kinase inhibitors to polypharmacological action (Knight et al., 2010; Gani et al., 2015; Sidorov et al., 2015). Thus, the aforementioned differences in the training set formation may lead to visible changes in the virtual screening performance. Although this class of protein targets has a privileged place in contemporary drug discovery and there are thus many compounds that have been assayed against several or even numerous kinases (Fedorov et al., 2007; Gao et al., 2013; Christmann-Franck et al., 2016; Elkins et al., 2016), multitarget action is found only for a small and diverse subset of the whole chemical-biological space (Jasial et al., 2016).

Therefore kinases and their inhibitors represent an interesting and challenging case that provides useful insights into the influence of the multitarget action of chemical compounds on the success of virtual screening studies (Merget et al., 2017). Moreover, since the multitarget action is by definition an attribute of thoroughly studied compounds, such as FDA-approved drugs (Law et al., 2014), whereas most known compounds are not thoroughly studied, our results may be extrapolated to the target classes (Barelier et al., 2015; Munoz, 2017) less extensively studied compared to kinases, to help achieve better results in virtual screening of a huge chemical library.

MATERIALS AND METHODS

Brief Description of PASS

PASS (Filimonov et al., 2014) is a computer program for analysis of structure-activity relationships (SAR) that allows users to perform ligand-based virtual screening for ligands of multiple targets and/or compounds with desired biological activities (Abdou et al., 2017; James and Ramanathan, 2017; Stasevych et al., 2017; Yildirim et al., 2017). Structures of chemical compounds are represented in PASS as a set of 2D atom-centric substructural descriptors called MNA (Multilevel Neighborhoods of Atoms). It was previously shown that MNA descriptors are suitable for implementation in a wide range of qualitative (classification) SAR studies and reflect structural features important for ligand–target interactions (Filimonov et al., 1999). PASS predicts biological activity profiles for chemical compounds in standardized representation: uncharged, single-component, containing at least three carbon atoms, with molecular mass not exceeding 1,250 Da. The majority of drug-like molecules fulfill these conditions and clipping of the non-drug-like compounds allows us to avoid dealing with non-specific and atypical biological activities. The mathematical approach of PASS is based on a naïve Bayes classifier and its particular realization in PASS has been previously described in detail elsewhere (Filimonov et al., 2014).

The result of PASS prediction is a list of probable biological activities arranged in descending order of P_a-P_i values, where P_a is the probability of belonging to the class of "actives," while P_i is the probability of belonging to the class of "inactives". By default, P_a-$P_i > 0$ is considered as the cutoff for discrimination between "active" and "inactive" molecules. The result of PASS-based virtual screening for a chemical library is the list of molecules predicted as "actives"; and these could be recommended for biological testing.

Training and Test Datasets

Data Acquisition

Every dataset used in this study was formed based on the data contained in the ChEMBL database. We chose ChEMBL because this is one of the largest freely available sources of experimental bioactivity data, its data are well-organized and documented, they are easy to acquire (via graphical web interface or API), and easy to manipulate by setting-up a local version of the database. We used the list of protein kinases and their IDs that is available via the ChEMBL web interface by browsing targets by assigned protein classes to select the subset of targets for this case study.

The training set of chemical structures and activities of chemical compounds tested for inhibition of protein kinases was extracted from the 20th version of the ChEMBL database. The ChEMBL SQL-format file dump (dump itself and instructions are available from here: ftp://ftp.ebi.ac.uk/pub/databases/chembl/ChEMBLdb/releases/chembl_20/)was handled in MySQL, SQL queries and PHP scripts were used to manipulate the data and write them to external SD files. Basic validation and comparison of the virtual screening performance were executed using 5-fold cross-validation.

The external test sets contained data from the up-to-date 23rd version of ChEMBL on structures and activities not present in ChEMBL 20 (ftp://ftp.ebi.ac.uk/pub/databases/chembl/ChEMBLdb/releases/chembl_23/). ChEMBL 23 contains 1 154 583 new data on activities, among which we searched for those related to the targets involved in our study using the following procedure:

- We extracted the list of pairs of identifiers of chemical compounds and biological targets from both ChEMBL 20 and 23.
- Intersections between the lists (identical pairs) were excluded.
- We used the remaining pairs to perform virtual screening and compare the results obtained using the three aforementioned approaches.

Data Preparation

It is known that some noise and various contradictions are stored in, and migrate from one source of bioactivity data to another, along with correct records (Kramer and Lewis, 2012; Kalliokoski et al., 2013; Tiikkainen et al., 2013; Papadatos et al., 2015). Thus, it is necessary to filter the data before using them in order to eliminate incorrect data and records that are inconsistent with the goal of the virtual screening study (Fourches et al., 2016). To achieve this goal, we used the procedures described in our previous work (Pogodin et al., 2015) with slight differences, designed to reflect the peculiarities of the targets selected for this study.

Training data preparation

First, chemical structures were filtered to eliminate incorrect molecular representations and to provide PASS with unambiguous (in the given feature space of MNA descriptors) examples for training and validation. We used an in-house command-line utility (SDF-check) to check structures for PASS compatibility and remove unsuitable ones. In addition to this, we identified structures having different ChEMBL IDs, but the same sets of MNA-descriptors, i.e., equivalent structures. We treated such structures as a single one. Thus, data on their activities were joined together, and all structures except first one encountered were deleted from the set.

After the filtering and preparation of the structures, data on bioactivities were processed to remove unreliable and inconsistent data points. In this study we used the following endpoints: K_i, K_d, IC_{50}, Potency—assessed as concentration of compound that induces the given response; Activity, Inhibition and Residual Activity—assessed as response of the kinase, induced by the given concentration of the compound. In addition to duplicates and incomplete records, the following data were excluded:

- Records related to mutated kinases. Kinases with mutations can have different sensitivity to inhibitors, i.e., quantitatively they may really represent distinct targets, but in general they do not have their own ChEMBL IDs. This fact, taken together with the large number of different mutated forms, makes use of such data difficult and redundant in the context of this study.
- Records related to the (Q)SAR and docking studies of kinase inhibitory activity without experimental validation of the results provided. Unfortunately, calculated values of kinase inhibitory activities may be found in databases along with those measured experimentally, since data are collected automatically using text mining procedures. Even the subsequent curation of the collected data does not allow removal of all questionable data due to the large amount of diverse data. We searched for such records and excluded them, since semi-supervised learning (Rosenberg et al., 2007) was not planned to be studied in this work.
- Records where Activity, Inhibition, or Residual Activity values were provided for a concentration other than 1 μM.
- Records where activation of kinases was provided instead of inhibition.
- Records related to non-standard types of action: inhibition of unphosphorylated kinases (without ATP or prior to ATP addition), allosteric and covalent inhibition, substrate-competitive inhibition (PPI, [protein-protein interaction]). Such cases were excluded since structure-activity relationships for inhibitors of such types may differ (Cortés-Ciriano et al., 2015; Bosc et al., 2017) from the ATP-competitive inhibitors, which represent the majority of known inhibitors.
- Records where kinase inhibitory activities were assigned to the compounds on the basis of their influence on the phenotype of various cells and tissues. Biochemical studies are better suited for the purpose of our study, since they allow to precisely measure the effect of a chemical compound against the particular protein kinase.
- Data on inhibition of non-human kinases were also excluded.

Measurements assessed as response of the kinase (Activity, Inhibition, Residual Activity), induced by the given concentration of a chemical compound were transformed to Inhibition for convenience. The problem with the "Activity" records is their ambiguity. Such records may mean both Inhibition and Residual Activity. We clarified the meaning based on the content of the assay description field. Residual Activity and Inhibition are unambiguously connected (Residual Activity = 100 − Inhibition) and it was easier for us to deal with only one (Inhibition) type of measurement.

Records on the bioactivities were filtered semi-automatically, utilizing the content of the "Description" field from the "Assays" table. Distinct "Description" fields were reviewed and, in the cases of detection of ambiguous data, analogous records were found using suitable set of words or regular expressions. Thus, identified suspicious entries were inspected using the original publications and deleted, if the suspicions were confirmed.

To improve the validation reliability, we included in the study only those kinases that had at least 100 actives and 100 inactives (determined at the concentration 1 μM). These limitations also help with the creation of accurate classifiers, which may be used for their primary purpose: to search for novel kinase inhibitors. Attempts to balance sets in terms of actives to inactives ratio were not conducted, not in the least because the assessment of the difference in the quality of classifiers built on the training data with a different ratio of actives to inactives was of interest, since two of the studied approaches for the training set creation may be considered as a method to fight skewed training data distribution (Rennie et al., 2003).

After the filtering of the bioactivities, different measurements of the inhibitory activity were used to create overall qualitative assessments for each compound designating it as active or inactive against the particular kinase. As it was mentioned earlier, we had different types of data on activities in our set for some compounds. Within these types (percentage of kinase inhibition and compound concentration producing response), median values were calculated in case a given kinase-ligand pair had multiple assessments. If concentrations of compound were available and it was less than or equal to 1 μM, we designated it as active against the particular kinase. In cases where data on concentration of compound were absent we designated it as active if inhibition of the particular kinase produced by this compound was greater than or equal to 50%. Otherwise the compound was designated as inactive.

Initially we extracted from ChEMBL 458 863 records on kinase inhibition. After the completion of the all procedures described above we were left with 173 275 data points on kinase inhibitors evaluated relative to the cut-off value of 1 μM (62 309 on true actives and 110 966 on true inactives at given cut-off). These data characterize interactions of 55 162 compounds with one or more of 152 human protein kinases selected for this study. These kinases represent all major families of human kinases. Our data cover a significant portion of the human kinome and allow one to search for inhibitors for all kinase families (**Figure 1**).

External test data preparation

Preparation of the data for external test set was performed in the same way as for the training set data, except for the following differences:

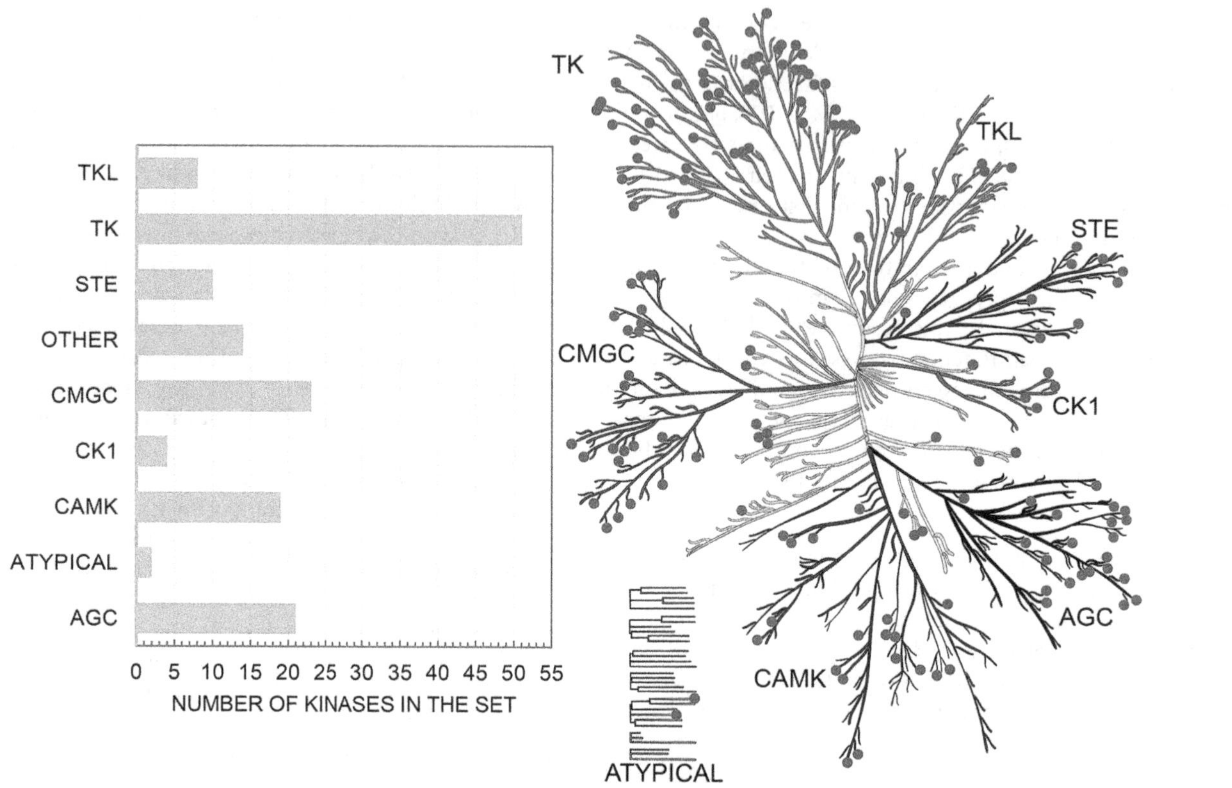

FIGURE 1 | Distribution of targets from the set over the human kinome tree. Illustration reproduced courtesy of Cell Signaling Technology, Inc. (www.cellsignal.com).

- Chemical data were not filtered, since done automatically by PASS.
- Potency was excluded from the list of the relevant activity types, since the majority of such activity records do not contain any data in the field "standard_relation."
- Activity was excluded from the list of the relevant activity types, since the majority of such activity records do not fulfill the requirement of absence of mutations, and/or compound concentration is not relevant to the selected cut-off.
- No minimum numbers for actives and inactives were imposed.

In total, we were able to identify 81 563 new activities against the kinases involved in this study in the 23rd version of ChEMBL. After filtering, 35 317 activities describing the action of 23 004 compounds against kinases remained.

Training set formation approaches

Filtered training set data on kinase inhibitors were stored in the local MySQL database and used to create three different training sets described below and presented in **Figure 2**. In addition, each training set was divided into the five non-overlapping and equivalent subsets for subsequent stratified 5-fold cross-validation (5-f CV).

Individual sets (I-sets)

The tested compounds for each kinase were sorted from the most active to the most inactive and, in this order, they were written to the five SD files: the first compound in the rank was placed into the first subset, the second compound into the second subset, the fifth compound into the fifth subset, the sixth then again into the first subset and so on; until each compound was placed into the each corresponding subset. The subsets were created in this way to be equivalent in terms of the total number of compounds and similar to each other in the degree of inhibitory activity of the placed compounds.

Merged actives and inactives set (MAI-set)

Then, we merged the first, second etc. subsets for each of the 152 kinases. If identical compounds were found in different subsets, only the structural formula was retained with all its kinase inhibiting activity data. As a result, we obtained 5 combined MAI-subsets, which were equivalent to the I-subsets because these subsets contained the same active compounds.

Merged actives set (MA-set)

This set was created in the same manner as MAI-set, but the true inactives were excluded.

Quality Metrics

We used the following metrics to evaluate the results of our ligand-based virtual screening of kinase inhibitors:

$$SENSITIVITY(RECALL) = TP/(TP + FN) \quad (1)$$

$$SPECIFICITY = TN/(TN + FP) \quad (2)$$

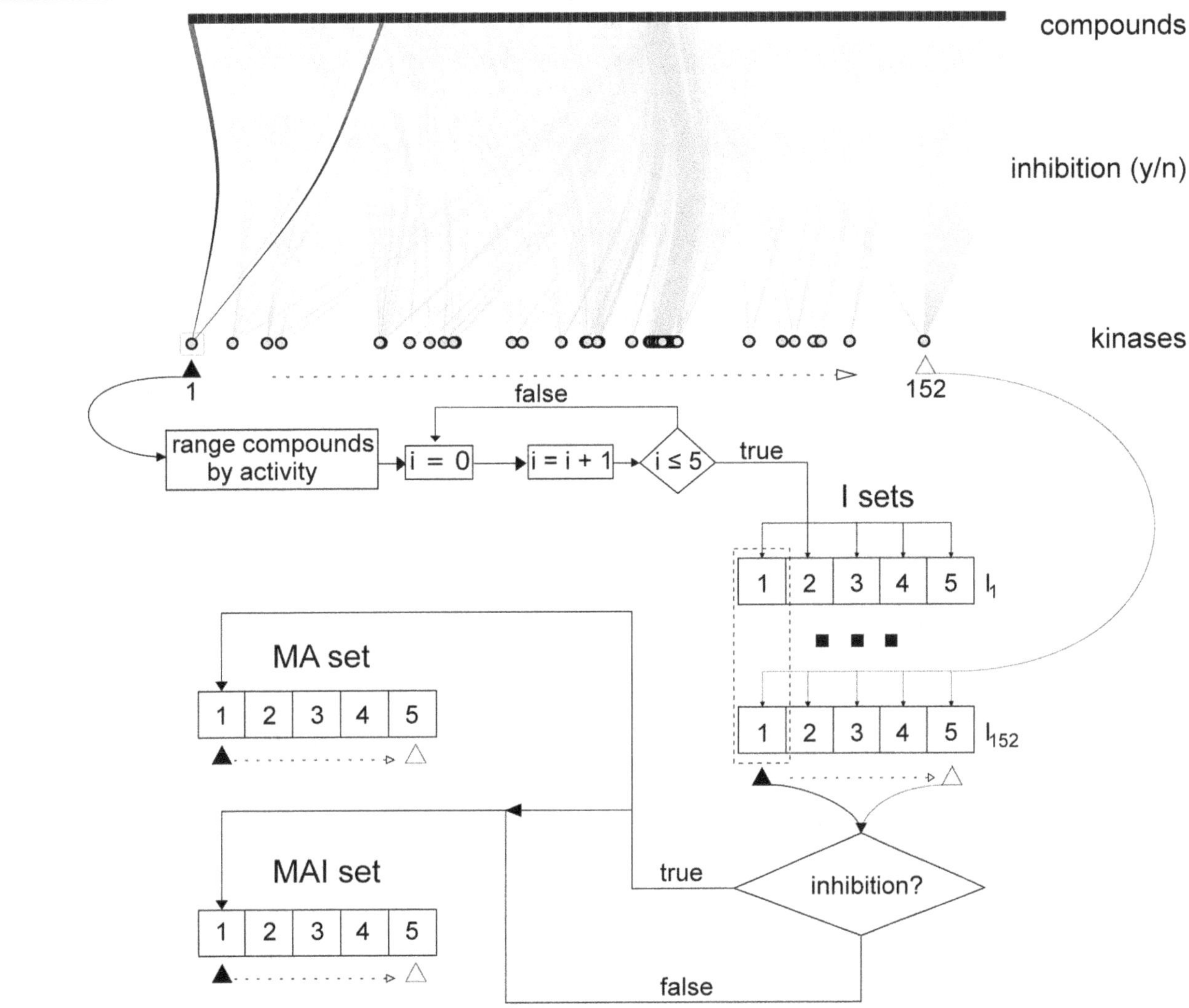

FIGURE 2 | Scheme describing how the training sets were created in accordance with the different approaches. Initial data on kinase inhibitors are represented via bipartite graph using all kinases and subset (~ 6 000) of tested compounds. Initially for 152 kinases 5x152 I-sets had been created; then, MA- and MAI-set were created as described in section Merged Actives and Inactives Set (MAI-set) and Merged Actives Set (MA-set).

$$BALANCED\ ACCURACY = \frac{1}{2} * \left(\frac{TP}{TP+FN} + \frac{TN}{TN+FP}\right) \quad (3)$$

$$PRECISION = TP/(TP+FP) \quad (4)$$

$$F1 = 2 * \frac{PRECISION * RECALL}{PRECISION + RECALL} \quad (5)$$

$$ROCAUC = P\left(Rank_{active_i} < Rank_{inactive_i}\right) \text{ in Uniform distribution} \quad (6)$$

$$BEDROC = P\left(Rank_{active_i} < Rank_{inactive_i}\right) \text{ in exponential Probability Density Function (PDF) with parameter } \alpha, \text{ IF } \alpha^{*}Ra << 1 \quad (7)$$

Metrics (1–6) are appropriate for the evaluation of the performance of the classification procedure, which determines the upper limits of the virtual screening quality under condition where every compound predicted as active is screened experimentally.

Boltzmann-Enhanced Discrimination of Receiver Operating Characteristic (BEDROC) (Truchon and Bayly, 2007) (Equation 7) represents the adaptation of ROC AUC metric to conditions under which detection of maximal number of TPs in a certain top fraction of the set is more important than general recognition. Thus, it is designed to evaluate the early detection rate, i.e., to assess the quality of virtual screening under the limitation that it is possible to evaluate experimentally only small fraction of top rated compounds from the whole library. Parameter α in the BEDROC AUC is inversely related to the size of the top fraction that will contribute to 80% of the score value while the other 20% will come from the assessment of the remaining part of the set. Values of α that were used in this study, and the corresponding top fractions of the sets, are given in **Table 1**.

TABLE 1 | Values of BEDROC parameter α and corresponding top fractions of sets.

Top fraction	BEDROC α	Actives rate	α * actives rate
1.00%	160.9	0.001	0.161
3.00%	53		0.054
5.00%	32.2		0.032
8.00%	20		0.020
10.00%	16.1		0.016
16.10%	10		0.010
20.00%	8		0.008

Performance Assessments

Stratified 5-Fold Cross-Validation

The training data had been divided into the five subsets in such a way that the average numbers of actives and inactives were approximately equal in all subsets (Refaeilzadeh et al., 2009). Four subsets from each set were used for the training, while one subset was used as the external test set. This procedure was repeated five times; each time a different subset was used as the external test set. The main differences from the standard 5-fold CV were:

- Corresponding individual subsets were always used as test, regardless of set type utilized for training.
- Compounds were placed into the subsets not on a random basis, but according to their degree of inhibitory activity.

The overall scheme for performance evaluation is given in **Figure 3**.

Such validation procedure provides reliable quality assessments for classifiers, since every compound in the test sets had experimental test results against a particular kinase. Besides, such an approach provides the conditions for comparison that are close to those observed in real research projects when one tries to find novel activity for a compound already included in the training set with some other activities. Such situations occur in drug repurposing projects or in *in silico* toxicological studies (Wang Y. J. et al., 2014).

The results of the predictions were assessed using the metrics described in the Materials and Methods section. Unfortunately, at least one of them, BEDROC, may suffer from saturation. To avoid this, the ration of actives to inactives for a set (Ra in Formula 7) must be low enough to fulfill the condition given in Formula 7.

The condition of low fraction of actives in the set seems acceptable and reasonable in the context of high throughput screening, which typically provides a number of hits below 5% (Murray and Wigglesworth, 2017). However, the data on kinase inhibitors from our set do not fulfill this condition. Thus, the saturation effect on BEDROC was expected to affect the results of our study. To avoid BEDROC saturation, we implemented the procedure of random sampling with replacement as realized in R package mlr (Bischl et al., 2016) applied to the prediction results. We undersampled the portions of actives and oversampled the portions of inactives for each kinase. Factors to under- and oversample actives and inactives were chosen in such a way that numbers of actives and inactives in the resampled set became equal to approximately 60 and 60 000, respectively (Formulae 8, 9). Thus, we maintained the same actives rate in the resampled sets, which was chosen to be approximately 0.001. This rate is low enough to calculate BEDROC values for each α level selected for this study without the risk of saturation.

$$Factor\ actives = 60/Number\ of\ actives \quad (8)$$

$$Factor\ inactives = 60\,000/Number\ of\ inactives \quad (9)$$

The resampling procedure was repeated 5 000 times for each type of sets and each kinase to achieve statistical significance in the subsequent assessment of differences between the results. BEDROC values were calculated on the resampled data using the R package enrichVS (http://cran.r-project.org/web/packages/enrichvs/index.html) for each resampled set. ROC AUC was also calculated using the R package pROC (Robin et al., 2011). To increase the speed of obtaining resampling results, we performed calculations in parallel mode using R package "parallel" (https://stat.ethz.ch/R-manual/R-devel/library/parallel/doc/parallel.pdf). Values of the classification quality metrics achieved in cross-validation and training set composition could be found in Supplementary Table 1.

Virtual Screening of the External Test Set

Prepared data from 23rd version of ChEMBL was used for forming the test sets according to the procedure used for preparation of the training I-sets. During the external validation (Chen et al., 2012) with these sets we calculated BEDROC values for the resampled prediction results. Values of the classification quality metrics achieved in external validation and training set composition could be found in Supplementary Table 2.

Comparison of the Results Obtained Using Different Training Approaches

The Tukey honest significant difference (HSD) test was used along with the analysis of variance to compare the quality of the created PASS classifiers based on the different types of training sets. These quality parameters include BEDROC for the resampled results; sensitivity, specificity, balanced accuracy, precision, F1 score and ROC AUC for the original results. The analysis was performed at a P-value < 0.05 using the functions "aov" and "TukeyHSD" from the R standard library. This provides the ranked lists for three PASS classifiers, which allows one to evaluate their performance.

RESULTS

Stratified 5-Fold Cross-Validation

All classification metrics values averaged over all kinases except the sensitivity values were slightly higher for the results achieved by classifiers trained on I-sets. Statistical analysis indicates that results obtained using the I-sets differ significantly from those obtained with the MA and MAI sets (**Figure 4**). The results of classifiers trained on the MA- and MAI-sets do not differ at the given level of significance from each other.

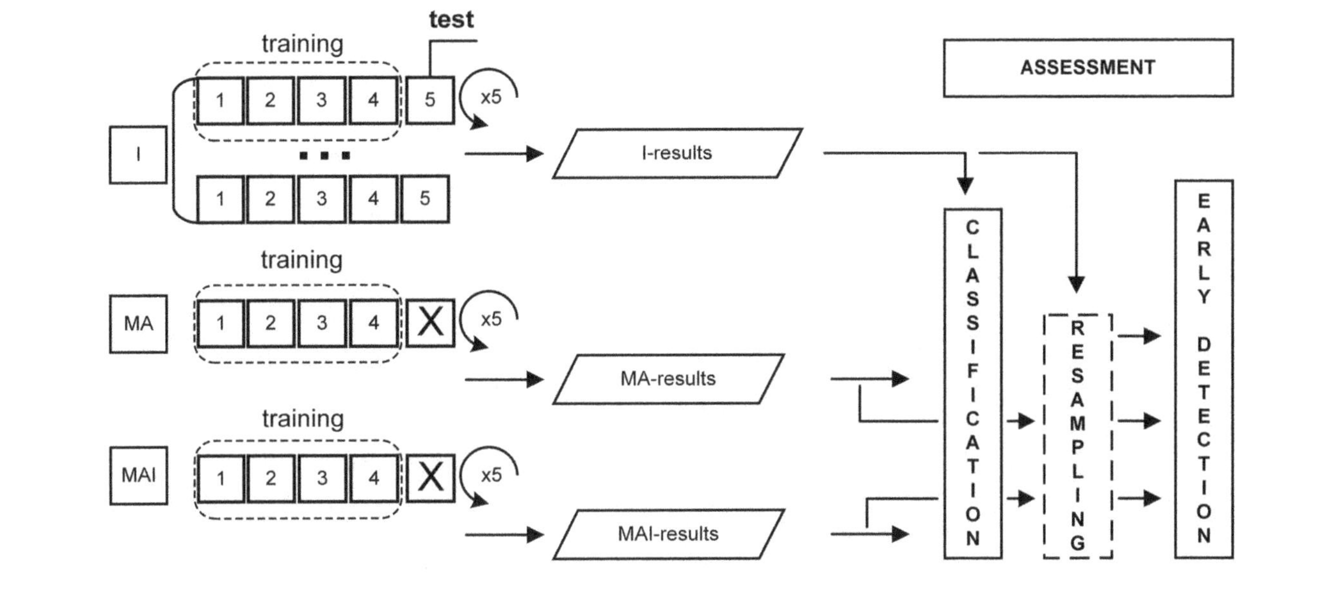

FIGURE 3 | Scheme for performance evaluation. I-subset was always used as a test set, thus corresponding MA- and MAI-subsets were just excluded from training.

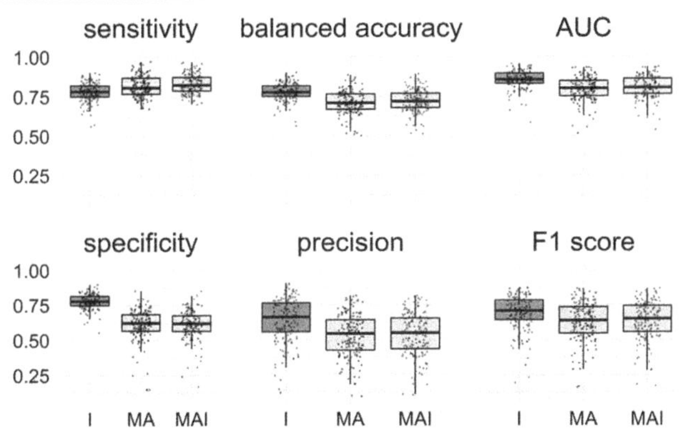

FIGURE 4 | Comparison of the results obtained using different types of sets. Results that are significantly different (*P*-value < 0.05) from one another are colored by distinct shades of gray. Results were obtained using stratified 5-f CV. Points correspond to the results achieved for the distinct kinases, shape of the points corresponds to the type of the training set.

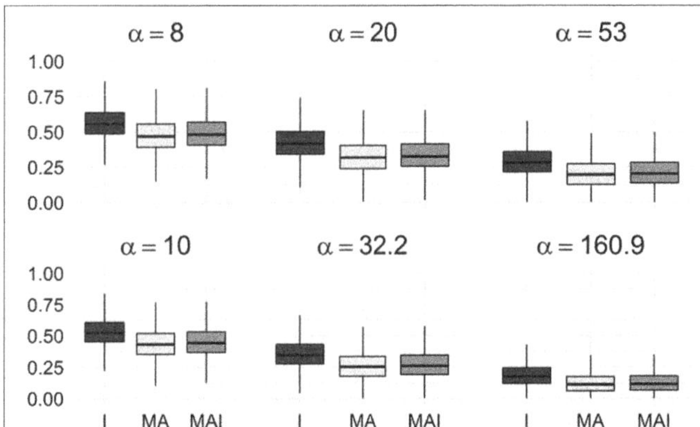

FIGURE 5 | Comparison of BEDROC values of resampled results for different kinases. In this case results obtained using different type of training sets were significantly different from each other (*P*-value < 0.05) for any value of α. Results were obtained using 5-f CV.

We used the resampled results to calculate values of BEDROC at different degrees of early recognition of TP (via varying values of α). These values were grouped according to the types of sets used for the training, and then averaged over the kinases in a manner similar to the way the original results were obtained. Statistical analysis of these data shows that classifiers trained on I-sets significantly outperform classifiers trained on MAI-sets and those, in turn, outperform classifiers trained on MA-sets (**Figure 5**) for any α value used in the study.

Also, using the resampled results, we were able not only to compare different approaches for the training by averaging values of the selected metrics across kinases, but to select the most adequate approach for each kinase individually. This was because after the resampling procedure repeated 5,000 times, we had enough data points to estimate the statistical significance. Such estimation was performed as follows: at the level of the *P*-value chosen earlier, less than 0.05, we found that for most of the kinases the best approach for training is to use I-sets; nonetheless, for some kinases it is better to use MA- or MAI-sets (**Figure 6**) according to our evaluation. In total, we depicted 13 kinases for which the classifiers trained using MA- or MAI-sets performed better in early recognition of TP at at least three levels of α.

Virtual Screening of External Test Set

Since we did not impose any limitations on the number of actives and inactives in our external test set, we were not able to calculate values for all the metrics for each kinase. We excluded such

Gene name	BEDROC α 8	10	20	32.2	53	160.9
EPHA2	■	■	■	■	■	■
DAPK3	■	■	■	■	■	■
PKN2	■	■	■	■	■	■
CDK9	■	■	■	■	■	■
PAK4		■	■	■	■	■
STK17A	■	■	■	■	■	■
HIPK2	■	■	■	■	■	■
MAP3K8	■	■	■	■	■	■
BTK			■	■	■	
MERTK			■	■	■	■
WEE1	■	■	■	■	■	■
LTK			■	■	■	
CDK8	■	■	■	■	■	■

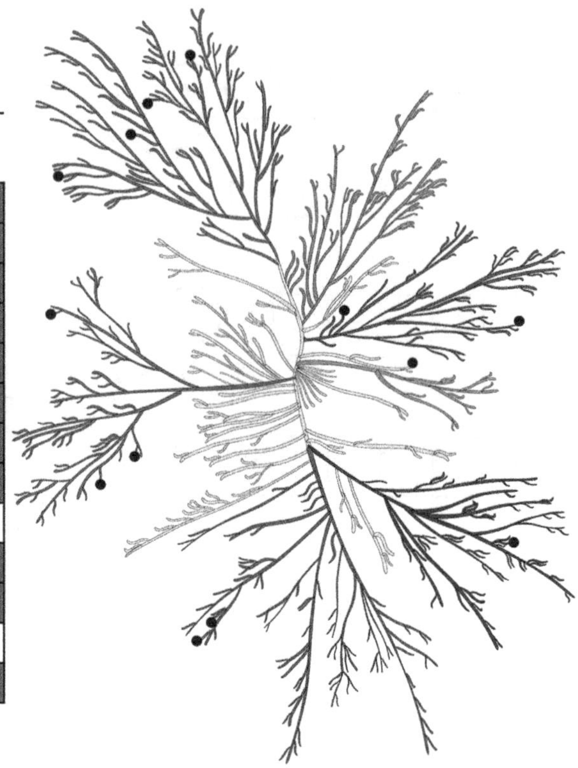

FIGURE 6 | Kinases for which inhibitors may be found at top ranks using MA- or MAI-training sets, according to the evaluation based on the resampling technique (P-value < 0.05). Empty cells correspond to the cases where I-sets still perform better. Illustration reproduced courtesy of Cell Signaling Technology, Inc. (www.cellsignal.com).

kinases before averaging the values of the classification metrics across the different training approaches, thus only results for 128 kinases were compared.

The main conclusions of the comparison of Specificity, Balanced Accuracy, and AUC values are similar to those obtained using 5-f CV: The training approach I provided significantly better results than those introducing conditionally inactives (MA and MAI). No significant difference for the other metrics was found (**Figure 7**).

To compare the earliness of actives detection achieved using different training approaches, we resampled results of the inhibitory activity prediction for each kinase and calculate BEDROC values. In this part of the study only results related to kinases having at least 20 actives and 20 inactives in the external test set were included. This restriction was imposed to exclude the influence of extreme cases, where only few actives and inactives exist. Despite the introduced restrictions, we were forced to change the resampling protocol in some cases; if the kinase had less than 60 actives, we used an oversampling procedure instead of undersampling to make sure we had 60 actives.

The main result of the comparison of BEDROC values was concordant to those obtained using 5-f CV: at each value of the criterion α, training using I-sets led to the better results than training performed using MA- or MAI-set, while MAI-sets outperformed MA-sets (**Figure 8**).

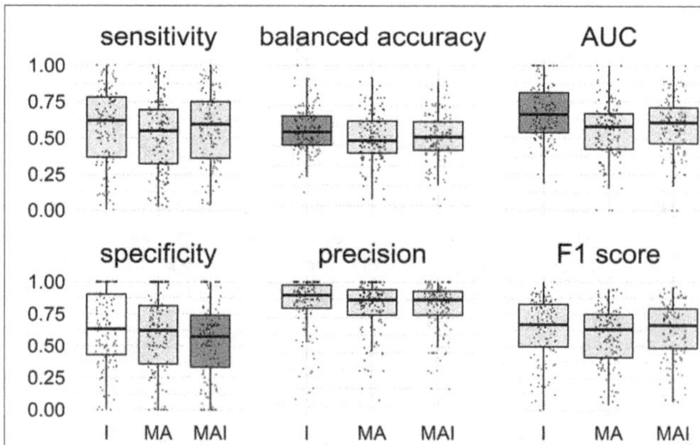

FIGURE 7 | Comparison of the results obtained using different types of sets. Results that are significantly different (P-value < 0.05) from one another are colored in distinct shades of gray. Results were obtained using external test set. Points correspond to the results achieved for the distinct kinases, the shape of the points corresponds to the type of the training set.

Correlations Between the Values of Metrics and Actives to Inactives Ratio in the Sets

We also analyzed the behavior of the employed accuracy metrics for different actives/inactives ratios, to be sure that they give an unbiased picture.

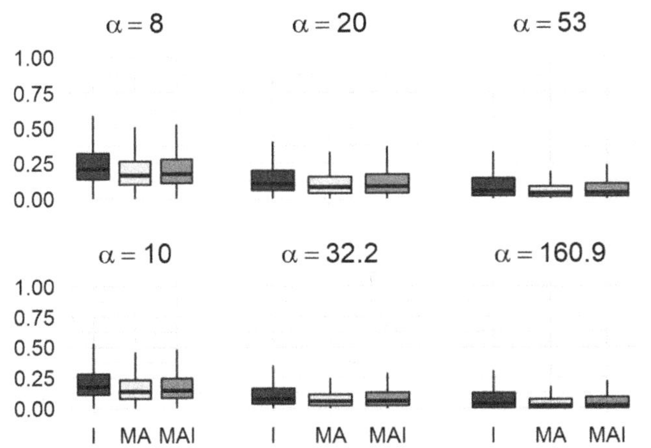

FIGURE 8 | Comparison of BEDROC values of the resampled results for distinct kinases. In this case results obtained using different type of training sets were significantly different from each other (*P*-value < 0.05) for any value of α. Results were obtained using the external test set.

Values of Precision and F1-score were found to show correlations with the actives to inactives ratio in the test sets. Thus, we conclude that sets' imbalance affects Precision and F1-score values, while the other metrics are significantly more robust (see Supplementary Figure 1), especially AUC and Balanced Accuracy.

Applicability Domain Estimation

To estimate the applicability domain, we calculated the values of the classification quality metrics for those cases where compounds had a certain number of new MNA-descriptors not found in the training set. In this case we merged the results over all kinases to obtain sufficient numbers of data points.

We showed that in the case of the results achieved using I-sets for training, the performance of the classifiers decreases linearly with increasing number of new MNA descriptors. In contrast to this, for the results achieved using MA- and MAI-sets for training, we were unable to find a strong dependence between the number of new MNA descriptors and the performance of the classifiers. Still, these results should be treated with caution, since the percentage of data points involved in this assessment decreases drastically with increasing number of new MNA descriptors, especially for the classifiers built using MAI- and MA-training sets (see **Figure 9**).

In the case of the classifiers built using I-sets for training we can judge that the applicability domain includes those compounds which have 4 or fewer new MNA descriptors, since the average balanced accuracy and AUC exceeded 0.7.

DISCUSSION

In contrast to the many contemporary studies in the field of the virtual screening, in this work no decoys (Irwin, 2008) were used to assess the enrichment achieved in virtual screening of large datasets. Instead, validation and subsequent comparison of the different training approaches were performed using only experimentally tested compounds, both actives and inactives. Today, due to the constant growth of available computational resources and amount of bioactivity data, it is possible to do this using 5-f CV and true external test sets. Moreover, since negative influence of the conditionally inactive compounds involved in training was shown, this makes us wonder: if conditionally inactives can do harm during training, are decoys good for testing? The exact answer is not known yet, but the risk of reaching wrong conclusions may be mitigated by using resampling-based approaches in parallel with, or instead of, decoys.

Our study represents a quantitative assessment of the trade-off between the initial requirements on the training data and the quality of PASS-based virtual screening. We have shown that the most efficient training approach for the ligand-based virtual screening system is to use the true actives and inactives for each target. This approach outperformed those where conditionally inactive compounds were introduced, in both classification quality and earliness of the detection. Moreover, in this case we observe a strong dependence of the performance depending on the number of new descriptors in the structures of the test compounds.

According to the analysis of the data from our training set, the higher the number of kinases for which compounds are tested, the more activities are found. Thus, using MA and MAI sets for training, some unknown actives could be treated as conditionally inactives (**Figure 10**). This may shed some light onto the problem of promiscuity of kinase inhibitors, which are often discussed as polypharmacological drugs. However, analysis of the content of bioactivity databases such as ChEMBL has shown that the average degree of promiscuity of such compounds is not so high (Hu et al., 2014). According to our results there is no contradiction between these points of view: kinase inhibitors tend to show promiscuity, but at the moment most of them have been studied against only a rather limited number of kinases.

Nevertheless, using MA and MAI approaches, it is possible to achieve good virtual screening results too, despite the softer requirements on the amount and quality of the training data. These approaches may be implemented in cases when only few active compounds are known, even in the absence of inactives, which helps expand the druggable target space and find new modes of action for existing molecular targets.

From this perspective it is surprising that we also found 13 kinases for which virtual screening may be performed more efficiently using training approaches introducing conditionally inactive compounds. This means that using machine learning it is easier to distinguish between inhibitors of these kinases and compounds tested against other kinases, than between their inhibitors and inactives at the given concentration cut-off. This fact can possibly be explained by the systematical shift in compounds selection for testing against these kinases. Also, it may indicate the importance of small structural changes in related targets leading to larger changes in inhibitor potency, since these 13 kinases are diverse, they belong to different families represented in our set and, in the case of other members of their families, introduction of the conditionally inactive compounds leads to the observed negative consequences. Thus, we show that virtual screening performance may benefit from the introduction of conditionally inactive compounds if these

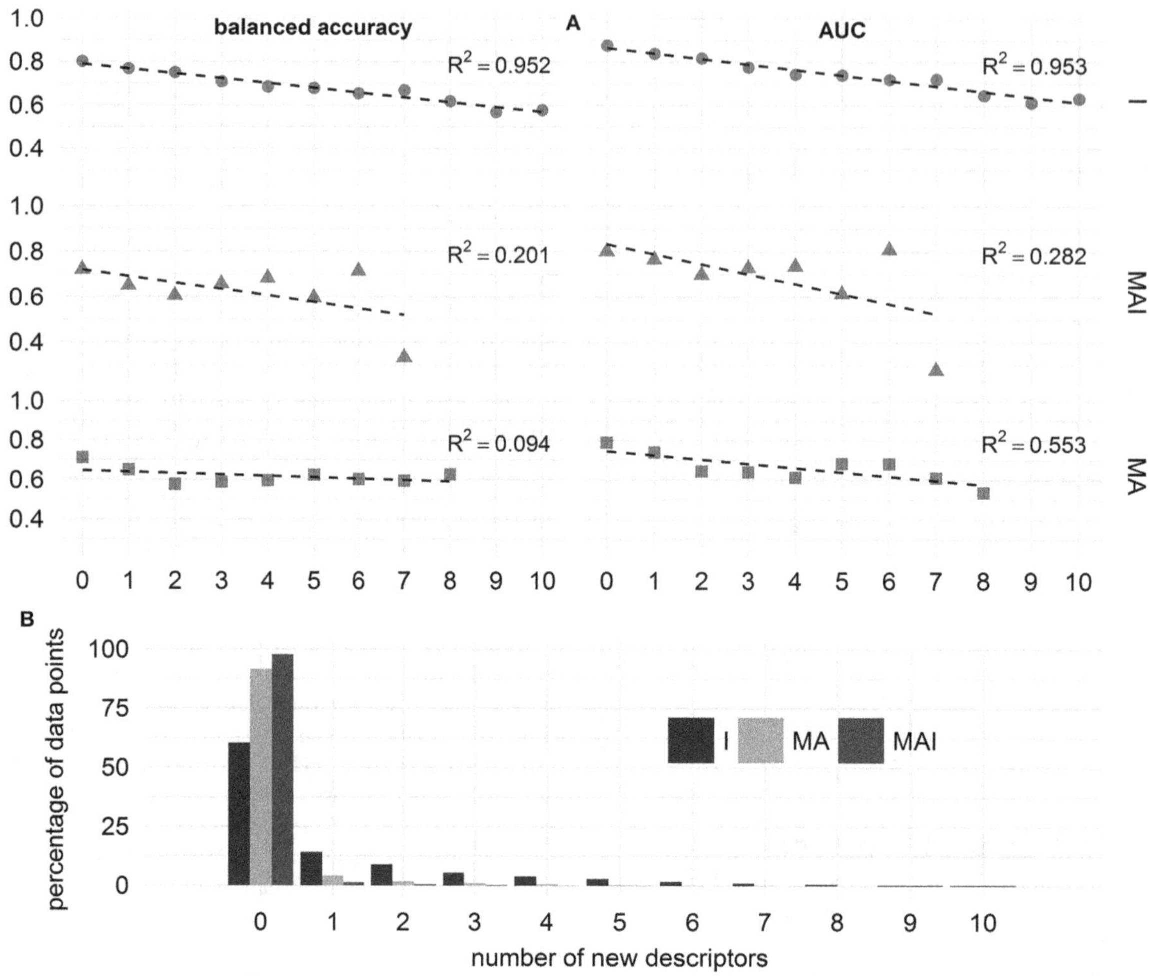

FIGURE 9 | Influence of the number of new descriptors in the structure of chemical compound on the quality of prediction. **(A)** Balanced accuracy and AUC assessed using different types of training sets. **(B)** Percentage of data points characterizing by the different number of new descriptors.

compounds are unfamiliar to the main target. Unfortunately, this knowledge is risky to apply to achieve better results in ligand-based virtual screening, since our knowledge on target-target relations mediated by common ligands are generally based on sparse training sets.

We obtained rather good results of both external (quasi prospective) and cross-validation. However, in case of data on kinase inhibitors extracted from ChEMBL, one initially deals with the pre-selected compounds studied in the appropriate biological activity area, which provides good predictivity, particularly using the approach based on individual sub-sets.

Big libraries like SAVI contain diverse and previously not investigated chemical structures, including compounds other than those possessing known ligand-related target signatures (Sidorov et al., 2015). To achieve the best predictivity for such library, it seems reasonable to make pre-selection with the standard PASS approach using conditionally inactive compounds. As we already mentioned above, PASS provides satisfactory results of prediction despite the incompleteness of data in the training set (Poroikov et al., 2000). Moreover, in this work, we showed that classifiers created using the merged training sets did not exhibit the significant dependence between the prediction quality and the number of new MNA descriptors contained in the predicted chemical structures.

Consequently, we propose two-steps procedure to analyze the big and diverse chemical libraries. At the first step, pre-selection is performed using the general classifier that took into account the conditionally inactives. At the second step, one may more thoroughly discriminate between the active hits and putatively inactive structures using the specific classifier that is based only on the real actives and inactives.

CONCLUSIONS

In this study, we compared the performance of three approaches for the analysis of structure-activity relationships that differ in their criteria for selecting "active" and "inactive" compounds for the training sets. We used the program PASS to build classifiers based on different subsets of kinase inhibitors extracted from ChEMBL 20 (for training and 5f-CV) and ChEMBL 23 (for external, quasi-prospective validation). The highest classification and early recognition quality was obtained by using individual

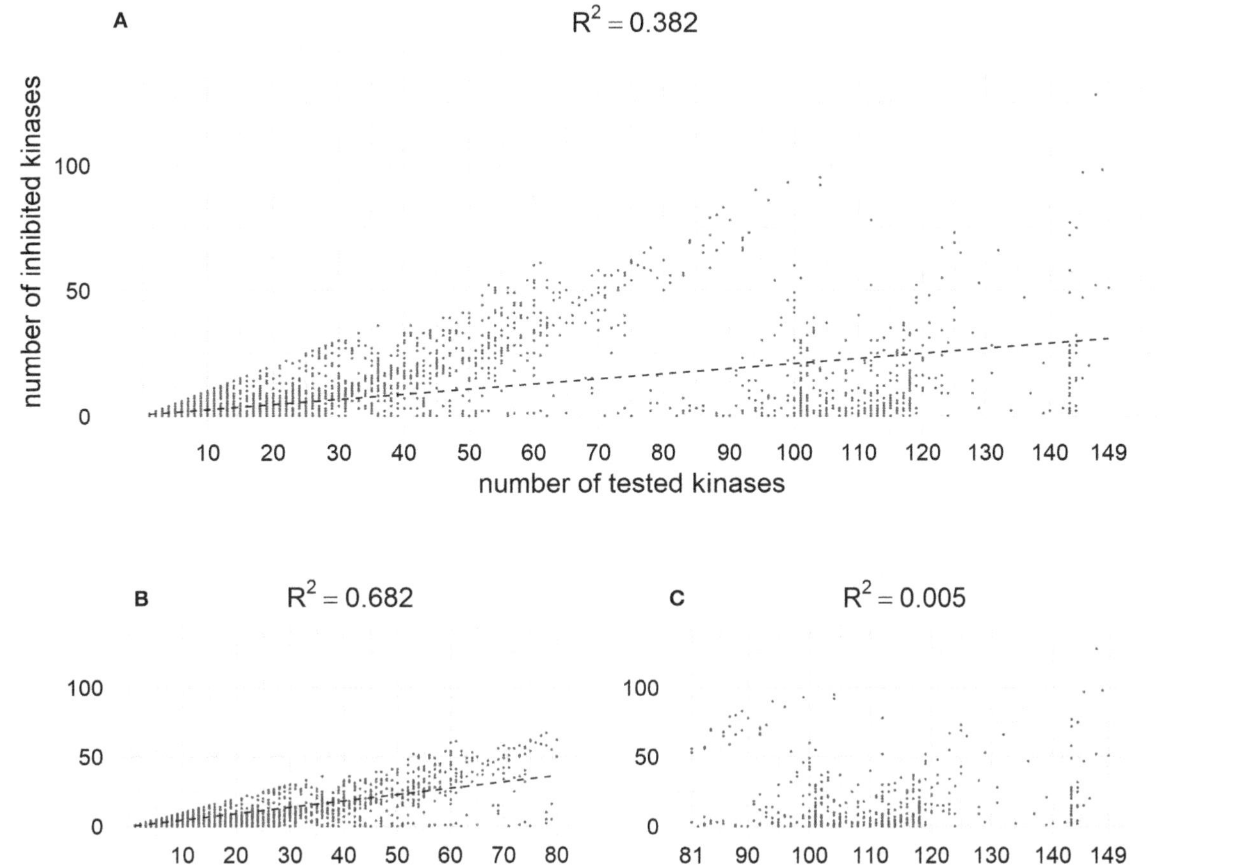

FIGURE 10 | Positive dependence between the number of tested kinases and number of inhibited kinases in the training set; **(A)** Relation for the whole set (weak); **(B)** Relation for the fraction of compounds tested against less than 80 kinases (moderate); **(C)** Relation for the fraction of compounds tested against more than 80 kinases (not observed). X-coordinates correspond to the number of chemical compounds against which compounds were tested, Y-coordinates corresponds to the amount of kinase against which compounds were found to be active at given cut-off (1 μM).

training sets for each kinase containing only experimental data. Nevertheless, other training strategies can provide acceptable results even in the absence of data on known inactives, which is often the case with the novel targets (Russ and Lampel, 2005; Nguyen et al., 2017). We assessed the applicability domain of our classifiers: while classifiers trained using individual sets expose strong dependence of the prediction quality on the predicted compounds' novelty, training strategies employing merged sets are much less sensitive to the novelty of predicted compounds.

Taken together these findings allow us to suggest that one can benefit most from using combinations of different training strategies when exploring huge chemical libraries containing diverse structures of unexplored chemical compounds.

AUTHOR CONTRIBUTIONS

All authors listed have made a substantial, direct and intellectual contribution to the work, and approved it for publication.

FUNDING

This work is supported by the Russian Foundation for Basic Research grant No. 17-54-30015-NIH_a.

REFERENCES

Abdou, W. M., Shaddy, A. A., and Kamel, A. A. (2017). Structure-based design and synthesis of acyclic and substituted heterocyclic phosphonates linearly linked to thiazolobenzimidazoles as potent hydrophilic antineoplastic agents. *Chem. Pap.* 71, 1961–1973. doi: 10.1007/s11696-017-0190-z

Afzal, A. M., Mussa, H. Y., Turner, R. E., Bender, A., and Glen, R. C. (2015). A multi-label approach to target prediction taking ligand promiscuity into account. *J. Cheminform.* 7, 1–14. doi: 10.1186/s13321-015-0071-9

Anusevicius, K., Mickevicius, V., Stasevych, M., Zvarych, V., Komarovska-Porokhnyavets, O., Novikov, V., et al. (2015). Design, synthesis, *in vitro* antimicrobial activity evaluation and computational studies of new N-(4-iodophenyl)-β-alanine derivatives. *Res. Chem. Intermed.* 41, 7517–7540. doi: 10.1007/s11164-014-1841-0

Baell, J. B., and Holloway, G. A. (2010). New substructure filters for removal of pan assay interference compounds (PAINS) from screening libraries and for their exclusion in bioassays. *J. Med. Chem.* 53, 2719–2740. doi: 10.1021/jm901137j

Bajorath, J. (2014). Improving data mining strategies for drug design. *Future Med. Chem.* 6, 255–257. doi: 10.4155/fmc.13.208

Barelier, S., Sterling, T., O'Meara, M. J., and Shoichet, B. K. (2015). The recognition of identical ligands by unrelated proteins. *ACS Chem. Biol.* 10, 2772–2784. doi: 10.1021/acschembio.5b00683

Bento, A. P., Gaulton, A., Hersey, A., Bellis, L. J., Chambers, J., Davies, M., et al. (2014). The ChEMBL bioactivity database: an update. *Nucleic Acids Res.* 42, D1083–D1090. doi: 10.1093/nar/gkt1031

Bischl, B., Lang, M., Kotthoff, L., Schiffner, J., Richter, J., Studerus, E., et al. (2016). mlr: Machine Learning in R. *J. Mach. Learn. Res.* 17, 1–5.

Bon, R. S., and Waldmann, H. (2010). Bioactivity-guided navigation of chemical space. *Acc. Chem. Res.* 43, 1103–1114. doi: 10.1021/ar100014h

Bosc, N., Wroblowski, B., Meyer, C., and Bonnet, P. (2017). Prediction of protein kinase-ligand interactions through 2.5D kinochemometrics. *J. Chem. Inf. Model.* 57, 93–101. doi: 10.1021/acs.jcim.6b00520

Buonfiglio, R., Engkvist, O., Várkonyi, P., Henz, A., Vikeved, E., Backlund, A., et al. (2015). Investigating pharmacological similarity by charting chemical space. *J. Chem. Inf. Model.* 55, 2375–2390. doi: 10.1021/acs.jcim.5b00375

Chen, B., Sheridan, R. P., Hornak, V., and Voigt, J. H. (2012). Comparison of random forest and Pipeline Pilot Naive Bayes in prospective QSAR predictions. *J. Chem. Inf. Model.* 52, 792–803. doi: 10.1021/ci200615h

Cherman, E., Monard, M., and Metz, J. (2011). Multi-label problem transformation methods: a case study. *CLEI Electron. J.* 14, 1–10.

Christmann-Franck, S., Van Westen, G. J., Papadatos, G., Beltran Escudie, F., Roberts, A., Overington, J. P., et al. (2016). Unprecedently large-scale kinase inhibitor set enabling the accurate prediction of compound-kinase activities: a way toward selective promiscuity by design? *J. Chem. Inf. Model.* 56, 1654–1675. doi: 10.1021/acs.jcim.6b00122

Cortés-Ciriano, I., Ain, Q. U., Subramanian, V., Lenselink, E. B., Méndez-Lucio, O., IJzerman, A. P., et al. (2015). Polypharmacology modelling using proteochemometrics (PCM): recent methodological developments, applications to target families, and future prospects. *Med. Chem. Commun.* 6, 24–50. doi: 10.1039/C4MD00216D

Deng, Z. L., Du, C. X., Li, X., Hu, B., Kuang, Z. K., Wang, R., et al. (2013). Exploring the biologically relevant chemical space for drug discovery. *J. Chem. Inf. Model.* 53, 2820–2928. doi: 10.1021/ci400432a

Druzhilovskiy, D. S., Rudik, A. V., Filimonov, D. A., Lagunin, A. A., Gloriozova, T. A., and Poroikov, V. V. (2016). Online resources for the prediction of biological activity of organic compounds. *Russ. Chem. Bull. Intern. Ed.* 65, 384–393. doi: 10.1007/s11172-016-1310-6

Elkins, J. M., Fedele, V., Szklarz, M., Abdul Azeez, K. R., Salah, E., Mikolajczyk, J., et al. (2016). Comprehensive characterization of the published kinase inhibitor set. *Nat. Biotechnol.* 34, 95–103. doi: 10.1038/nbt.3374

Fedorov, O., Marsden, B., Pogacic, V., Rellos, P., Müller, S., Bullock, A. N., et al. (2007). A systematic interaction map of validated kinase inhibitors with Ser/Thr kinases. *Proc. Natl. Acad. Sci. U.S.A.* 104, 20523–20528. doi: 10.1073/pnas.0708800104

Filimonov, D. A., Lagunin, A. A., Gloriozova, T. A., Rudik, A. V., Druzhilovskii, D. S., Pogodin, P. V., et al. (2014). Prediction of the biological activity spectra of organic compounds using the pass online web resource. *Chem. Heterocycl. Compd.* 50, 444–457. doi: 10.1007/s10593-014-1496-1

Filimonov, D. A., Poroikov, V. V., Karaicheva, E. I., Kazaryan, R. K., Boudunova, A. P., Mikhailovskiy, E. M., et al. (1995). Computer-aided prediction of biological activity spectra of chemical substances on the basis of their structural formulae: computerized system PASS. *Exp. Clin Pharmacol.* 58, 56–62.

Filimonov, D., Poroikov, V., Borodina, Y., and Gloriozova, T. (1999). Chemical similarity assessment through multilevel neighborhoods of atoms: definition and comparison with the other descriptors. *J. Chem. Inf. Comput. Sci.* 39, 666–670. doi: 10.1021/ci980335o

Fourches, D., Muratov, E., and Tropsha, A. (2016). Trust, but verify II: a practical guide to chemogenomics data curation. *J. Chem. Inf. Model.* 56, 1243–1252. doi: 10.1021/acs.jcim.6b00129

Fujita, T., and Winkler, D. A. (2016). Understanding the roles of the "two QSARs." *J. Chem. Inf. Model.* 56, 269–274. doi: 10.1021/acs.jcim.5b00229

Gani, O. A., Thakkar, B., Narayanan, D., Alam, K. A., Kyomuhendo, P., Rothweiler, U., et al. (2015). Assessing protein kinase target similarity: comparing sequence, structure, and cheminformatics approaches. *Biochim. Biophys. Acta* 1854, 1605–1616. doi: 10.1016/j.bbapap.2015.05.004

Gao, Y., Davies, S. P., Augustin, M., Woodward, A., Patel, U. A., Kovelman, R., et al. (2013). A broad activity screen in support of a chemogenomic map for kinase signalling research and drug discovery. *Biochem. J.* 451, 313–328. doi: 10.1042/BJ20121418

Heikamp, K., and Bajorath, J. (2013). Comparison of confirmed inactive and randomly selected compounds as negative training examples in support vector machine-based virtual screening. *J. Chem. Inf. Model.* 53, 1595–1601. doi: 10.1021/ci4002712

Horvath, D., Marcou, G., and Varnek, A. (2017). "Generative topographic mapping approach to chemical space analysis," in *Advances in QSAR Modeling*, ed K. Roy (Cham: Springer), 167–199.

Hu, Y., Gupta-Ostermann, D., and Bajorath, J. (2014). Exploring compound promiscuity patterns and multi-target activity spaces. *Comput. Struct. Biotechnol. J.* 9:e201401003. doi: 10.5936/csbj.201401003

Irwin, J. J. (2008). Community benchmarks for virtual screening. *J. Comput. Aided. Mol. Des.* 22, 193–199. doi: 10.1007/s10822-008-9189-4

James, N., and Ramanathan, K. (2017). Discovery of potent ALK inhibitors using pharmacophore-informatics strategy. *Cell Biochem. Biophys.* doi: 10.1007/s12013-017-0800-y. [Epub ahead of print].

Jasial, S., Hu, Y., and Bajorath, J. (2016). Determining the degree of promiscuity of extensively assayed compounds. *PLoS ONE* 11:e0153873. doi: 10.1371/journal.pone.0153873

Jorgensen, W. L. (2004). The many roles of computation in drug discovery. *Science* 303, 1813–1818. doi: 10.1126/science.1096361

Kalliokoski, T., Kramer, C., and Vulpetti, A. (2013). Quality issues with public domain chemogenomics data. *Mol. Inform.* 32, 898–905. doi: 10.1002/minf.201300051

Kilic, C., and Tan, M. (2012). Positive unlabeled learning for deriving protein interaction networks. *Netw. Model. Anal. Health. Inform. Bioinformatics* 1, 87–102. doi: 10.1007/s13721-012-0012-8

Knight, Z. A., Lin, H., and Shokat, K. M. (2010). Targeting the cancer kinome throuhg polypharmacology. *Nat. Rev. Cancer* 10, 130–137. doi: 10.1038/nrc2787

Kramer, C., and Lewis, R. (2012). QSARs, data and error in the modern age of drug discovery. *Curr. Top. Med. Chem.* 12, 1896–1902. doi: 10.2174/156802612804547380

Kurczab, R., Smusz, S., and Bojarski, A. J. (2014). The influence of negative training set size on machine learning-based virtual screening. *J. Cheminform.* 6:32. doi: 10.1186/1758-2946-6-32

Lauria, A., Bonsignore, R., Bartolotta, R., Perricone, U., Martorana, A., and Gentile, C. (2016). Drugs polypharmacology by *in silico* methods: new opportunities in drug discovery. *Curr. Pharm. Des.* 22, 3073–3081. doi: 10.2174/1381612822666160224142323

Law, V., Knox, C., Djoumbou, Y., Jewison, T., Guo, A. C., Liu, Y., et al. (2014). DrugBank 4.0: shedding new light on drug metabolism. *Nucleic Acids Res.* 42, 1091–1097. doi: 10.1093/nar/gkt1068

Lee, A., Lee, K., and Kim, D. (2016). Using reverse docking for target identification and its applications for drug discovery. *Expert Opin. Drug Discov.* 11, 707–715. doi: 10.1080/17460441.2016.1190706

Leelananda, S. P., and Lindert, P. (2016). Computational methods in drug discovery. *Beilstein J. Org. Chem.* 12, 2694–2718. doi: 10.3762/bjoc.12.267

Li, Q., Cheng, T., Wang, Y., and Bryant, S. H. (2010). PubChem as a public resource for drug discovery. *Drug Discov. Today* 15, 1052–1057. doi: 10.1016/j.drudis.2010.10.003

Lipinski, C., and Hopkins, A. (2004). Navigating chemical space for biology and medicine. *Nature* 432, 855–861. doi: 10.1038/nature03193

López-Vallejo, F., Giulianotti, M. A., Houghten, R. A., and Medina-Franco, J. L. (2012). Expanding the medicinally relevant chemical space with compound libraries. *Drug Discov. Today* 17, 718–726. doi: 10.1016/j.drudis.2012.04.001

Martin, E., Mukherjee, P., Sullivan, D., and Jansen, J. (2011). Profile-QSAR: a novel meta-QSAR method that combines activities across the kinase family to accurately predict affinity, selectivity, and cellular activity. *J. Chem. Inf. Model.* 51, 1942–1956. doi: 10.1021/ci1005004

Medina-Franco, J. L., Giulianotti, M. A., Welmaker, G. S., and Houghten, R. A. (2013). Shifting from the single- to the multitarget paradigm in drug discovery. *Drug Discov. Today* 18, 495–501. doi: 10.1016/j.drudis.2013.01.008

Merget, B., Turk, S., Eid, S., Rippmann, F., and Fulle, S. (2017). Profiling prediction of kinase inhibitors: toward the virtual assay. *J. Med. Chem.* 60, 474–485. doi: 10.1021/acs.jmedchem.6b01611

Mervin, L. H., Afzal, A. M., Drakakis, G., Lewis, R., Engkvist, O., and Bender, A. (2015). Target prediction utilising negative bioactivity data covering large chemical space. *J. Cheminform.* 7, 1–16. doi: 10.1186/s13321-015-0098-y

Munoz, L. (2017). Non-kinase targets of protein kinase inhibitors. *Nat. Rev. Drug Discov.* 16, 424–440. doi: 10.1038/nrd.2016.266

Murray, D., and Wigglesworth, M. (2017). "HTS methods: assay design and optimisation," in *High Throughput Screen. Methods*, eds J. A. Bittker and N. T. Ross (Cambridge: The Royal Society of Chemistry), 1–15.

Murtazalieva, K. A., Druzhilovskiy, D. S., Goel, R. K., Sastry, G. N., and Poroikov, V. V. (2017). How good are publicly available web services that predict bioactivity profiles for drug repurposing? *SAR QSAR Environ. Res.* 28, 843–862. doi: 10.1080/1062936X.2017.1399448

Nettles, J. H., Jenkins, J. L., Bender, A., Deng, Z., Davies, J. W., and Glick, M. (2006). Bridging chemical and biological space: "target fishing" using 2D and 3D molecular descriptors. *J. Med. Chem.* 49, 6802–6810. doi: 10.1021/jm060902w

Nguyen, D. T., Mathias, S., Bologa, C., Brunak, S., Fernandez, N., Gaulton, A., et al. (2017). Pharos: collating protein information to shed light on the druggable genome. *Nucleic Acids Res.* 45, D995–D1002. doi: 10.1093/nar/gkw1072

Pammolli, F., Magazzini, L., and Riccaboni, M. (2011). The productivity crisis in pharmaceutical R&D. *Nat. Rev. Drug Discov.* 10, 428–438. doi: 10.1038/nrd3405

Papadatos, G., Gaulton, A., Hersey, A., and Overington, J. P. (2015). Activity, assay and target data curation and quality in the ChEMBL database. *J. Comput. Aided. Mol. Des.* 29, 885–896. doi: 10.1007/s10822-015-9860-5

Pevzner, Y.U., Ihlenfeldt, W. D., and Nicklaus, M. (2017). Synthetically accessible virtual inventory (SAVI). in *Abstracts of the 253rd American Chemical Society National Meeting* (San-Francisco, CA: CINF), 141.

Pogodin, P. V., Lagunin, A. A., Filimonov, D. A., and Poroikov, V. V. (2015). PASS targets: ligand-based multi-target computational system based on a public data and naïve Bayes approach. *SAR QSAR Environ. Res.* 26, 783–793. doi: 10.1080/1062936X.2015.1078407

Poroikov, V. V., Filimonov, D. A., Borodina, Y. V., Lagunin, A. A., and Kos, A. (2000). Robustness of biological activity spectra predicting by computer program PASS for noncongeneric sets of chemical compounds. *J. Chem. Inf. Comput. Sci.* 40, 1349–1355. doi: 10.1021/ci000383k

Poroikov, V. V., Filimonov, D. A., and Boudunova, A. P. (1993). Comparison of the results of prediction of the spectra of biological activity of chemical compounds by experts and the PASS system. *Automat. Document. Mathemat. Linguist.* 27, 40–43.

Refaeilzadeh, P., Tang, L., and Liu, H. (2009). "Cross-Validation," in *Encyclopedia of Database Systems*, eds L. Liu and M. T. Özsu (Boston, MA: Springer), 532–538.

Rennie, J. D. M., Shih, L., Teevan, J., and Karger, D. R. (2003). Tackling the poor assumptions of naive Bayes text classifiers. *Proc. Twent. Int. Conf. Mach. Learn. (Seattle, WA)*, 20, 616–623. doi: 10.1186/1477-3155-8-16

Rish, I. (2001). "An empirical study of the naive Bayes classifier," in *IJCAI 2001 Workshop on Empirical Methods in Artificial Intelligence* (Seattle, WA), 41–46.

Robin, X., Turck, N., Hainard, A., Tiberti, N., Lisacek, F., Sanchez, J. C., et al. (2011). pROC: an open-source package for R and S+ to analyze and compare ROC curves. *BMC Bioinformatics* 12:77. doi: 10.1186/1471-2105-12-77

Rodriguez-Esteban, R. (2016). A drug-centric view of drug development: how drugs spread from disease to disease. *PLoS Comput. Biol.* 12:e1004852. doi: 10.1371/journal.pcbi.1004852

Rosenberg, C., Hebert, M., and Schneiderman, H. (2007). "Semi-supervised self-training of object detection models," in *7th IEEE Workshop on Applications of Computer Vision/IEEE Workshop on Motion and Video Computing Vision, WACV 2005* (Breckenridge, CO), 29–36.

Ruddigkeit, L., van Deursen, R., Blum, L. C., and Reymond, J. L. (2012). Enumeration of 166 billion organic small molecules in the chemical universe database GDB-17. *J. Chem. Inf. Model.* 52, 2864–2875. doi: 10.1021/ci300415d

Russ, A. P., and Lampel, S. (2005). The druggable genome: an update. *Drug Discov. Today* 10, 1607–1610. doi: 10.1016/S1359-6446(05)03666-4

Sidorov, P., Gaspar, H., Marcou, G., Varnek, A., and Horvath, D. (2015). Mappability of drug-like space: towards a polypharmacologically competent map of drug-relevant compounds. *J. Comput. Aided. Mol. Des.* 29, 1087–1108. doi: 10.1007/s10822-015-9882-z

Smusz, S., Kurczab, R., and Bojarski, A. J. (2013). The influence of the inactives subset generation on the performance of machine learning methods. *J. Cheminform.* 5:17. doi: 10.1186/1758-2946-5-17

Stasevych, M., Zvarych, V., Lunin, V., Deniz, N. G., Gokmen, Z., Akgun, O., et al. (2017). Computer-aided prediction and cytotoxicity evaluation of dithiocarbamates of 9,10-anthracenedione as new anticancer agents. *SAR QSAR Environ. Res.* 28, 355–366. doi: 10.1080/1062936X.2017.1323796

Sterling, T., and Irwin, J. J. (2015). ZINC 15 - Ligand discovery for everyone. *J. Chem. Inf. Model.* 55, 2324–2337. doi: 10.1021/acs.jcim.5b00559

Tiikkainen, P., Bellis, L., Light, Y., and Franke, L. (2013). Estimating error rates in bioactivity databases. *J. Chem. Inf. Model.* 53, 2499–2505. doi: 10.1021/ci400099q

Truchon, J. F., and Bayly, C. I. (2007). Evaluating virtual screening methods: good and bad metrics for the "early recognition" problem. *J. Chem. Inf. Model.* 47, 488–508. doi: 10.1021/ci600426e

Tsoumakas, G., Katakis, I., and Vlahavas, I. (2010). "Mining multi-label data," in *Data Mining and Knowledge Discovery Handbook*, eds O. Maimon and L. Rokach (Boston, MA: Springer), 1–19.

Wang, Y. J., Zhang, Y. K., Kathawala, R. J., and Chen, Z. S. (2014). Repositioning of tyrosine kinase inhibitors as antagonists of ATP-binding cassette transporters in anticancer drug resistance. *Cancers* 6, 1925–1952. doi: 10.3390/cancers6041925

Wang, Y., Suzek, T., Zhang, J., Wang, J., He, S., Cheng, T., et al. (2014). PubChem BioAssay: 2014 update. *Nucleic Acids Res.* 42, 1–8. doi: 10.1093/nar/gkt978

Yildirim, H., Bayrak, N., Tuyun, A. F., Kara, E. M., Çelik, B. Ö., and Gupta, G. K. (2017). 2, 3-Disubstituted-1, 4-naphthoquinones containing an arylamine with trifluoromethyl group: synthesis, biological evaluation, and computational study. *RSC Adv.* 7, 25753–25764. doi: 10.1039/C7RA00868F

14

In Silico Prediction of Chemical Toxicity for Drug Design Using Machine Learning Methods and Structural Alerts

Hongbin Yang, Lixia Sun, Weihua Li, Guixia Liu and Yun Tang*

Shanghai Key Laboratory of New Drug Design, School of Pharmacy, East China University of Science and Technology, Shanghai, China

***Correspondence:**
Yun Tang
ytang234@ecust.edu.cn

During drug development, safety is always the most important issue, including a variety of toxicities and adverse drug effects, which should be evaluated in preclinical and clinical trial phases. This review article at first simply introduced the computational methods used in prediction of chemical toxicity for drug design, including machine learning methods and structural alerts. Machine learning methods have been widely applied in qualitative classification and quantitative regression studies, while structural alerts can be regarded as a complementary tool for lead optimization. The emphasis of this article was put on the recent progress of predictive models built for various toxicities. Available databases and web servers were also provided. Though the methods and models are very helpful for drug design, there are still some challenges and limitations to be improved for drug safety assessment in the future.

Keywords: drug safety, chemical toxicity, drug design, machine learning, structural alerts

INTRODUCTION

Drug discovery and development is a long journey full of high risk. It is estimated that the attrition rate of drug candidates is up to 96% (Paul et al., 2010) and the average cost to develop a new drug reaches to 2.6 billion U.S. dollars in recent years (PhRMA, 2015). One of the major causes for the high attrition rate is drug safety, which accounts for 30% of drug failures (Giri and Bader, 2015). Even if a drug is approved in market, it could be withdrawn due to safety problems. Therefore, drug safety should be evaluated extensively as early as possible.

Usually, *in vitro* and *in vivo* tests are performed to investigate drug safety, including a variety of toxicities and adverse drug effects. In recent years, there are also some efforts to develop *in vitro* models such as "organ on a chip" to reduce cost (Huh et al., 2010, 2011). However, those approaches are still costly and time-consuming. In comparison of experimental approaches, computational methods have shown great advantages since they are green, fast, cheap, accurate, and most importantly they could be done before a compound is synthesized (Segall and Barber, 2014).

Till now, many computational models have been developed for drug safety assessment, which could be generally divided into three categories: qualitative classification, quantitative regression and read-across. As the first step of drug safety assessment, we only need to know a compound is toxic or non-toxic, highly toxic or slightly toxic, rather than its exact toxicity value, so classification models can be used. For a small number of chemical analogs, quantitative structure-toxicity relationship (QSTR) models can be derived for prediction of exact toxicity values. For those unique compounds, read-across is also a feasible approach to deduce certain toxicity endpoint from their similar structures with experimental toxicity values. These models have high accuracies especially in a local chemical space, and sometimes they can replace *in vitro* or *in vivo* assays for certain endpoints. Furthermore, structural alerts (SAs) can be derived from the models as keys for a compound to cause adverse effects on organs (Pizzo et al., 2015), which can be used in structural modification to reduce the risk by chemists.

In recent years, we have worked on drug safety assessment and developed a lot of predictive models for chemical toxicity with machine learning methods and structural alerts. A web server named admetSAR was also developed for publicly free access (Cheng et al., 2012b). In a previous paper published in 2013, we reviewed the advances and challenges of *in silico* prediction of chemical toxicity together with pharmacokinetic properties (Cheng et al., 2013a). Here, we would like to review the progress of *in silico* chemical toxicity prediction in recent 5 years, including methodologies of machine learning and structural alerts, and major toxicity endpoints in drug discovery and development (**Figure 1**). Available data sources and web servers were also mentioned. At last, challenges and future directions in this field were provided.

MODEL BUILDING WITH MACHINE LEARNING METHODS

The general procedure to build a predictive model contains roughly four steps: data collection, data description, model building, and model evaluation. Each step has its own requirements to guarantee the reliability and accuracy of the models.

Data Collection

The quality of experimental data is the most important in model building. Currently, there are numerous well-defined data available online, which greatly facilitates the construction of computational models by machine learning methods. In **Table 1**, we listed some widely used databases, including those linking chemical structures with safety outcomes, protein targets and/or biological pathways.

TOXNET is a comprehensive source that integrates several toxicity databases such as ToxLine and ChemIDplus (Fowler and Schnall, 2014). ACToR is a large database that aggregates data from thousands of public sources (Judson et al., 2008). DSSTox, a subset of ACToR, provides a high quality resource for toxicity prediction, including ToxCast and Tox21 data (Williams-DeVane et al., 2009). OECD established eChemPortal to provide chemical information including physicochemical properties, and toxicity. Many databases are contained in eChemPortal, such as ACToR and HSDB (Fonger et al., 2014). Some other toxicity databases include SuperToxic (Schmidt et al., 2009), T3DB (Wishart et al., 2015), and ToxBank (http://www.toxbank.net). We previously developed a web server admetSAR, which also contains toxicity data (Cheng et al., 2012b).

In addition to the phenotype data that are directly relevant to toxicity, databases on bioactivity, pathway and side effects are also important to toxicity prediction. Several bioactivity databases are free available, such as PubChem (Wang et al., 2009), ChEMBL (Gaulton et al., 2017), and BindingDB (Gilson et al., 2016). We developed a web server named MetaADEDB that integrates CTD (Davis et al., 2017), SIDER (Kuhn et al., 2010), and OFFSIDES (Tatonetti et al., 2012) with regard to the ADE of drugs (Cheng et al., 2013b,c).

Data Description

There are two ways to represent chemical structures as numeric features which can be processed by machine learning methods. One way is to use molecular descriptors, which can be calculated from chemical structures, physicochemical or topological properties. Currently thousands of continuous and discrete molecular descriptors can be obtained via chemoinformatics toolkits such as PaDEL-Descriptor (Yap, 2011), OpenBabel (O'Boyle et al., 2011), CDKit (Steinbeck et al., 2003), RDKit (Landrum, 2017), or web servers like E-Dragon (Tetko et al., 2005), ChemBCPP (Dong et al., 2017a), and ChemDes (Dong et al., 2015). Using numeric features may result in overfitting when the size of training set is small (Xue et al., 2004). Hence, feature selection should be done before model building, to reduce the risk of overfitting and enhance the performance of model (Sun et al., 2017).

The other way is to use molecular fingerprints, which represent a molecule as a binary string, such as MACCS, PubChemFP, and KRFP (Klekota and Roth, 2008). In a molecular fingerprint, lists of substructures or other kinds of patterns are predefined. If a specified pattern presents in a molecule, the corresponding bit in the binary string is set to "1," otherwise it will be set to "0." Comparing to molecular descriptors, these binary features are more interpretable because each bit corresponds to a specific substructure. In addition to the common fingerprints, custom patterns can also be used to enhance the predictability of the models (Yang et al., 2017b).

Single-Label Model Building

Machine learning methods are usually used to build the predictive models. There are many free and open access tools and development kits to fulfill this task. For example, Scikit-learn (Pedregosa et al., 2011) is a popular python toolkit for machine learning and TensorFlow (https://www.tensorflow.org) is a widely used python library for deep learning. WEKA (Frank et al., 2004), Orange (Demsar et al., 2013) and RapidMiner (https://rapidminer.com/) are machine learning toolboxes with GUI (Graph user interface).

Support vector machine (SVM), Random forest (RF), boost tree (BT), and k-nearest neighbor (kNN) are classic machine learning methods that are widely used in classification and regression models. SVM, also known as support vector classifier (SVC) or support vector regression (SVR) in particular tasks, is well-known for its high predictive performance and less risk of overfitting (Cortes and Vapnik, 1995). The basic idea of SVM is to construct a hyperplane in a high dimensional space with the largest distance to the nearest training data points (support

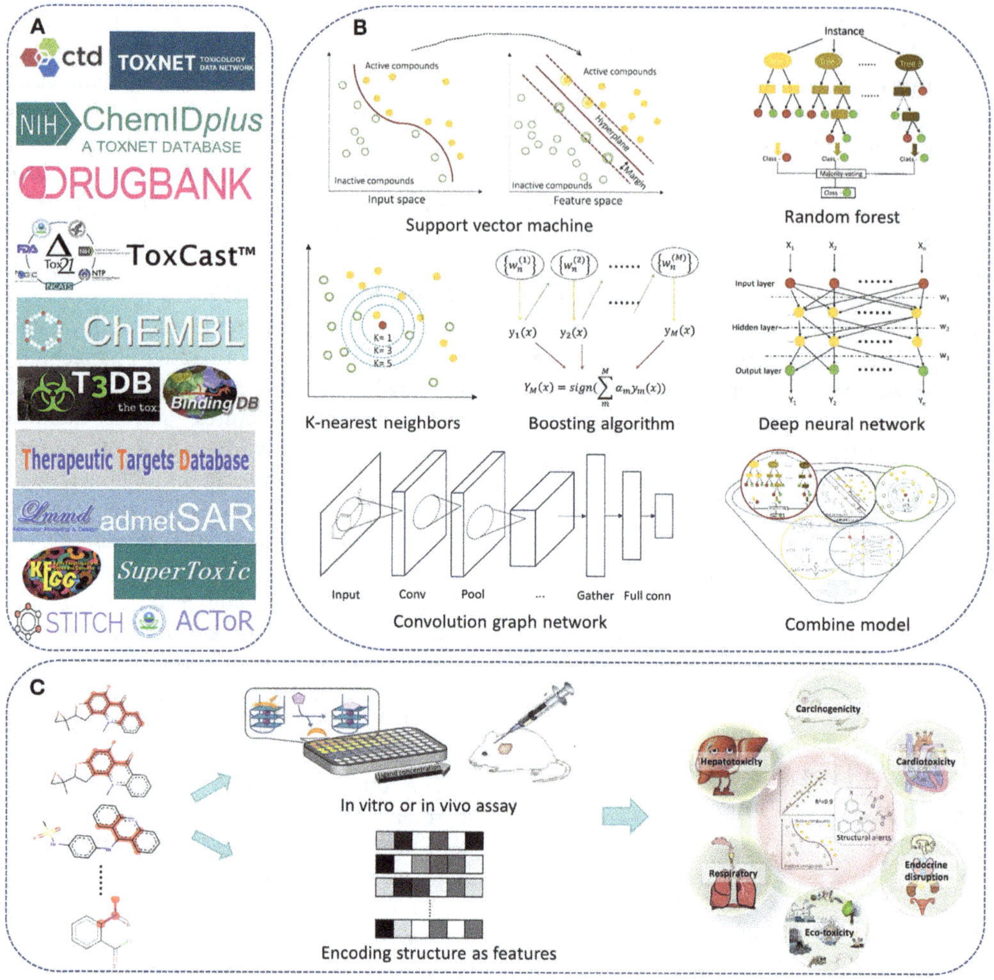

FIGURE 1 | The roadmap of *in silico* prediction of chemical toxicity with machine learning methods and structural alerts. **(A)** Examples of available data and web servers. **(B)** The state-of-the-art machine learning algorithms. **(C)** Scheme of building QSAR or structural alerts models for prediction of chemical toxicity.

vectors). RF and BT are derived from decision tree (Breiman, 2001; Elith et al., 2008). RF can be viewed as bagging many decision trees that use a random subset of features and combine them via a voting system. Different from RF, in which each tree is equal, BT dynamically adjusts the weight of each tree according to the mean error of prediction. kNN is one of the simplest algorithms (Cover and Hart, 1967). The creed of kNN is that compounds with similar structures have similar biological properties. In kNN, a sample is classified by the votes of the categories of its neighbors.

Sometimes, to enhance performance of prediction models, combination of these algorithms is applied. We developed a combined method using an artificial neural network (ANN) model to generate the final combination decision probability, which showed that the combined methods would be superior to "single" methods (Cheng et al., 2011b; Du et al., 2017; Sun et al., 2017).

Recently, deep learning (DL) has been applied in solving such challenging problems as computer vision and speech recognition (Deng et al., 2013; LeCun et al., 2015). Multilayer neural network (MNN) is one of the DL techniques. Different from common ANN that only has three layers including input layer, hidden layer and output layer (Shen et al., 2004), MNN contains more than one hidden layers and thus is more competent in large toxicological data with complex mechanisms. When the training set is large, it can perform better than ANN and above-mentioned classic machine learning methods (Mayr et al., 2016). However, more complex network indicates more weights to fit and more likely to be overfitting. Graph-convolutional networks (Duvenaud et al., 2015) and long short-term memory architectures (Altae-Tran et al., 2017) are recently developed to extract features from molecules based on atom features and show better performance in handling thousands of compounds or even more (Goh et al., 2017). DeepChem (https://deepchem.io) is an open source python library devoted to providing a high quality toolchain to facilitate the use of DL in drug discovery and other fields.

TABLE 1 | Data sources for prediction of chemical toxicity.

Database name	Type[a]	URL
TOXNET	CTA	https://toxnet.nlm.nih.gov/
ToxBank Data Warehouse	CTA	http://www.toxbank.net/data-warehouse
admetSAR	CTA	http://lmmd.ecust.edu.cn/admetsar1/
Pharmaco Kinetics Knowledge Base (PKKB)	CTA	http://cadd.zju.edu.cn/pkkb/
ToxCast	CTA	https://www.epa.gov/chemical-research/toxicity-forecasting
Tox21	CTA	https://tripod.nih.gov/tox21
CTD (Comparative Toxicogenomics Database)	CTA	http://ctdbase.org/
ECOTOX	CTA	https://cfpub.epa.gov/ecotox/
SuperToxic	CTA	http://bioinformatics.charite.de/supertoxic/
DSSTox	CTA	https://www.epa.gov/chemical-research/distributed-structure-searchable-toxicity-dsstox-database
ACToR	CTA	https://actor.epa.gov/actor/home.xhtml
T3DB	CTA	http://www.t3db.ca
eChemPortal	CTA	https://www.echemportal.org/echemportal/index.action
PubChem	CPI	http://pubchem.ncbi.nlm.nih.gov/
ChEMBLdb	CPI	https://www.ebi.ac.uk/chembldb/
BindingDB	CPI	http://www.bindingdb.org/bind/index.jsp
ChemProt	CPI	http://potentia.cbs.dtu.dk/ChemProt/
STITCH	CPI	http://stitch.embl.de/
DrugBank	CPI	http://www.drugbank.ca/
TTD	CPI	http://bidd.nus.edu.sg/group/cjttd/
IntAct	MI	http://www.ebi.ac.uk/intact/
SIDER	SE	http://sideeffects.embl.de/
MetaADEDB	SE	http://lmmd.ecust.edu.cn/online_services/metaadedb/
OFFSIDES	SE	http://www.pharmgkb.org
Chemical Effects in Biological Systems (CEBS)	SE	http://tools.niehs.nih.gov/cebs3/ui/
IntSide	SE	http://intside.irbbarcelona.org
Reactome	Pathway	http://www.reactome.org/
Pathway Commons	Pathway	http://www.pathwaycommons.org/
KEGG	Pathway	http://www.kanehisa.jp/
PharmGKB	Pathway	https://www.pharmgkb.org/

[a] *CTA, compound-toxicity association; MI, molecular interaction; SE, side effect; CPI, compound-protein interaction.*

Multi-Label Model Building

Unlike aforementioned single-label classification or regression models, multi-label classification (MLC) is a data mining approach in which each data instance can be assigned to multiple categories at once (Tsoumakas et al., 2010; Zhang and Zhou, 2014; Gibaja and Ventura, 2015). The demand for multi-label techniques is constantly growing in biology and genomics (Diplaris et al., 2005; Avila et al., 2009). The current algorithms used for this task are pretty new and many of them are still in an early stage of development.

There are three major approaches for multi-label learning: data transformation, method adaptation and ensembles of classifiers. The first one, including Binary Relevance (BR) (Godbole and Sarawagi, 2004), classifier chains (CC) (Read et al., 2011), and Label Powerset (LP) (Boutell et al., 2004), is to transform original multi-label dataset (MLD) to a set of binary datasets (BIDs) or one multi-class dataset (MCD) first, and then process them with traditional classification algorithms (Barot and Panchal, 2014). With the development of these frameworks for MLC, classification algorithms available for binary and multiclass data can be utilized as the underlying base classifier including SVM, ANN, decision tree, kNN, and so on. The second alternative aims for adapting existent algorithms to deal with multi-label data, such as multi-label C4.5 (Al-Otaibi et al., 2014), multi-label back-propagation (Zhang and Zhou, 2006), Rank-SVM (Wang et al., 2014), and multi-label kNN (Zhang and Zhou, 2007). Finally, the classification ensemble is also a widespread technique in multi-label field. For example, Ensemble of Classifier Chain (ECC) (Read et al., 2011), which consists of a set of CC with diverse label orders and then votes for the final prediction, is proposed to allow for the effect of chain order. Some other MLC methods based on the ensemble of multi-class classifiers were also proposed, such as EPS (Read et al., 2008), RAkEL (Tsoumakas and Vlahavas, 2007), and HOMER (Tsoumakas et al., 2008).

Model Evaluation

For regression models, three evaluation metrics, namely Pearson product moment correlation coefficient (R^2), mean absolute error (MAE) and root mean squared error (RMSE) are frequently used to estimate the performance of models. These parameters are defined as following:

$$R^2 = \left[\frac{\sum_1^N (x_i - \overline{x})(y_i - \overline{y})}{\sqrt{\sum_1^N (x_i - \overline{x})^2 \sum_1^N (y_i - \overline{y})^2}} \right]^2 \quad (1)$$

$$\text{MAE} = \frac{\sum_1^N |x_i - y_i|}{N} \quad (2)$$

$$\text{RMSE} = \sqrt{\frac{\sum_1^N (x_i - y_i)^2}{N}} \quad (3)$$

where x_i is the experimental value, y_i is the predicted value, $\overline{x}$, $\overline{y}$ are their corresponding means and N is the number of samples.

For traditional single-label binary or multiple classification models, most of the performance metrics are calculated based on the count of true positive (TP), true negative (TN), false positive (FP), and false negative (FN). Accuracy, sensitivity and specificity metrics can be calculated as the following equations to represent the overall predictive ability, the predictive accuracy for positive samples and the predictive ability for negative ones:

$$Accuracy = \frac{TP + TN}{TP + TN + FP + FN} \quad (4)$$

$$Sensitivity = \frac{TP}{TP + FN} \quad (5)$$

$$Specificity = \frac{TN}{TN + FP} \quad (6)$$

In addition to these computed from binary partition of labels, metrics these calculated from a confidence degree of being positive are also used like area under the receiver operating characteristic curve (AUC).

Comparing to the single-label classification patterns, multi-label classifiers can have multiple outputs for an instance, of which the predictions can be fully or partially correct. The multi-label performance metrics introduced there can be classified into two groups, i.e., example-based and label-based metrics (Tsoumakas et al., 2007; Zhang and Zhou, 2014). Here, five example-based metrics (subset accuracy, Jaccard similarity coefficient, hamming-loss, micro-precision, micro-recall) are described with mathematical formulations below.

$$SubsetAccuracy = \frac{1}{n} \sum_{i=1}^{n} [\![Y_i = Z_i]\!] \quad (7)$$

$$Jaccard\ Similarity\ Coefficient = \frac{1}{n} \sum_{i=1}^{n} \frac{|Y_i \cap Z_i|}{|Y_i \cup Z_i|} \quad (8)$$

$$Hamming\ Loss = \frac{1}{n}\frac{1}{k} \sum_{i=1}^{n} |Y_i \Delta Z_i| \quad (9)$$

$$Recall_{micro} = \frac{1}{n} \sum_{i=1}^{n} \frac{|Y_i \cap Z_i|}{|Y_i|} \quad (10)$$

$$Precision_{micro} = \frac{1}{n} \sum_{i=1}^{n} \frac{|Y_i \cap Z_i|}{|Z_i|} \quad (11)$$

where Y_i represents the real label-set of the *i*th instance, and Z_i the predicted one. n is the number of instances and k is the number of labels.

Furthermore, another example-based metric named ranking loss can be used. The ranking loss metric portrays how many times an irrelevant label is ranked above a relevant one according to their probabilities belonging to each label. As for label-based metrics, micro-AUC is the most commonly used one. It is also a ranking based metric similar to ranking loss. However, different from the ranking loss that compares the ranks for each example, micros-AUC counts the number of all the relevant-irrelevant pairs meeting the condition that the relevant label is ranked above irrelevant one (in which the labels are not necessarily for the same example).

METHODS FOR DETECTING STRUCTURAL ALERTS

Structural alerts (SAs) are key substructures responsible for certain toxicity. They are directly connected to toxicity and hence could be used for structural optimization by medicinal chemists to reduce the risk. In 1985, Ashby found strong associations between occurrence of some substructures or patterns and chemical mutagenicity to *Salmonella*, which was the first appearance of the concept of SA (Ashby and Tennant, 1988).

Till now, many methods and software have been developed for detecting SAs, such as SARpy (Ferrari et al., 2013), MoSS, Gaston, and MolFea. ToxAlerts is a web server that collects SAs defined by experts or identified by computational tools. It can predict toxicity according to the appearance of SAs (Sushko et al., 2012). Automatic detection of SAs by computational tools now becomes a hotspot as the development of cheminformatics and the explosion of available data (Lepailleur et al., 2013; Floris et al., 2017).

In a previous paper, we evaluated several methods for identification of SAs (Yang et al., 2017a). At present, the methods can be divided into three categories: fragment-based, graph-based, and fingerprint-based. Fragment-based methods, such as SARpy (Ferrari et al., 2013), cut the bonds of the molecules in dataset first to get all possible fragments. Then each fragment is evaluated according to their occurrence in toxic and non-toxic compounds. These methods have been used in detecting SAs for carcinogenicity (Golbamaki and Benfenati, 2016; Golbamaki et al., 2016). Graph-based approaches use subgraph searching algorithms, treating molecules as graphs that consist of a set of vertices and edges, to find the frequent patterns. MoSS uses depth-first search association rules to mine substructures (Borgelt and Berthold, 2002). Gaston is a stand-alone tool that uses a graph-based approach to obtain substructures from dataset (Kazius et al., 2006). Another graph-based method proposed by Ahlberg (Ahlberg et al., 2014) uses Atom Signature, a linear expression of a compound, to mined sub-signature as SAs. Fingerprint-based approaches do not obtain fragments from the dataset. Instead, the fragments are defined by different molecular fingerprints such as MACCS and SubFP (Shen et al., 2010). The selection of fingerprints may affect the final results of the identified SAs. Fingerprints such as Morgan, used by Bioalerts (Cortes-Ciriano, 2016) might lead to redundant SAs which are very similar and related to the same mechanism.

Information gain (IG) can also be used to evaluate the significance of a substructure. Compounds containing the substructure are categorized as toxic and others are categorized as non-toxic. IG is defined as the difference between the information entropy of original dataset and the weighted average information entropies of two datasets separated by a substructure (Sokolova and Szpakowicz, 2010). We previously used IG to detect privileged substructures whose occurrences have strong relevance to some endpoints (Shen et al., 2010).

PROGRESS IN TOXICITY PREDICTION

Carcinogenicity and Mutagenicity

Chemical carcinogenesis is of increasing importance in drug discovery for its serious effect on human health. Most of the predictive models use Carcinogenic Potency Database (CPDB) as the data source, which contains more than 1,500 chemicals with their labels (carcinogen or non-carcinogen) according to their TD_{50} values (Gold et al., 2005). Recently several publications shared their protocols to construct models to predict chemical carcinogenesis, including Naïve Bayes, kNN, probabilistic neural network, and SVM (Singh et al., 2013; Tanabe et al., 2013; Li et al., 2015; Zhang H. et al., 2016). Zhang et al. developed a web server, CarcinoPred-EL, for chemists to predict carcinogenicity online, in which Ensemble XGBoost was used to build the model (Zhang et al., 2017).

Due to its complicated mechanism and less available data, the predictive models based on phenotypic assays are not precise and reliable enough. It is an alternative to construct models based on *in vitro* assays. The mechanisms of carcinogenesis of chemicals can be categorized into: (1) genotoxicity, which are primarily caused by the mutagenicity of chemicals damaging DNA (Fan et al., in press); (2) non-genotoxic carcinogens acting through different specific mechanisms, which are more complicated (Golbamaki and Benfenati, 2016). Ames test devised by Bruce Ames is a well-known *in vitro* assay to detect mutagenic effects of chemicals. Currently more than 8,000 compounds with Ames mutagenicity are available. Both predictive models and structural alerts were promoted with these toxicity data in recent years (Kazius et al., 2005; Hansen et al., 2009; Xu et al., 2012; Yang et al., 2017a).

Acute Oral Toxicity

According to the exposure routes of chemicals, acute toxicity can be divided into oral, dermal and inhalation, among which acute oral toxicity is the most widely studied in computational prediction. It is often the first performed endpoint in drug discovery because any compounds causing acute toxicity will not be further considered for its strong hazardous to human health. Zhu et al. collected 7,385 compounds with LD_{50} values and built several models for prediction of chemical acute oral toxicity (Zhu et al., 2009). Based on the data set, several machine learning methods were developed and applied to construct classifiers and regression models to predict LD_{50} or their toxic categories (Li et al., 2014; Lei et al., 2016; Xu et al., 2017). Noticeably, the models built by Xu et al. have high performance in two test sets, more than 95% of accuracy for classification and 0.861 of R^2 for regression, and the model is free available in web server (http://www.pkumdl.cn/DLAOT/DLAOThome.php).

Cardiotoxicity

Blockade of the hERG (human ether-a-go-go related gene) potassium channel is the main adverse effect with regard to cardiotoxicity (Gintant et al., 2016). Several *in silico* models were developed according to the *in vitro* hERG blockage test in early screening assays. Our group recently developed an *in silico* model that used chemical category approaches to predict hERG blockage (Zhang et al., 2016b), in which 1,570 unique compounds were collected from ChEMBL database and early studies (Doddareddy et al., 2010; Wang et al., 2012). In addition to machine learning methods, combination with multiple pharmacophores can improve the predictive capabilities and the model would be more interpretable (Wang et al., 2016).

However, as the simplified *in vitro* approaches for detection of cardiac safety are less specific, the *in silico* models will also output the false-positive predictions that may result in unwarranted attribution of novel drug candidates (Gintant et al., 2016). Other categories such as contractile and structural cardiotoxicity should be considered and more *in vitro* or *in vivo* data should be used to construct sophisticated models.

Hepatotoxicity

Chemical hepatotoxicity in drug discovery, also termed "drug induced liver injury (DILI)," is the leading cause for drug failure or withdrawn from the market (Schuster et al., 2005). Due to its complicated mechanism and inconsistency in diverse patients, experimental detection of hepatotoxicity in preclinical and clinical trials is difficult.

Computational approaches to predict DILI of compounds are widely applied for their low cost and high efficiency. Hewitt reviewed the *in silico* models on DILI prediction from 2000 to 2015, including statistics-based methods and expert systems (Hewitt and Przybylak, 2016). Chemical or hybrid descriptors as features, and different machine learning methods such as linear discriminant analysis and ANN were used in these models to predict general or specific endpoints related to hepatotoxicity (Hewitt and Przybylak, 2016). Zhu constructed a human hepatotoxicity database for QSTR models using post-market safety data originated from FDA adverse event reporting system (Zhu and Kruhlak, 2014). Our group previously used molecular fingerprints and machine learning methods to build classification models with a data set containing 1,317 diverse compounds (Zhang et al., 2016a). Xu et al. used a deep learning method called undirected graph recursive neural networks (UGRNN) that encodes molecules into an undirected graph to build QSTR models (Xu et al., 2015). The performance was excellent compared to other models, up to 0.955 of AUC. More recently, Mulliner et al. classified the complex pathology of hepatotoxicity into 21 endpoints at three levels, with a large data set comprising 3,712 compounds. Then the specific models were combined into an optimized global human hepatotoxicity that has high sensitivity of 68% and excellent specificity of 95% (Mulliner et al., 2016).

Respiratory Toxicity

Respiratory toxicity is another toxicity category with complicated mechanisms. The most concerned endpoint is drug-induced interstitial lung disease (DILD), which can be classified into two categories in terms of their mechanisms: (1) cytotoxic lung injury and (2) immune-mediated (Matsuno, 2012). Another type of respiratory toxicity is respiratory sensitization, of which the mechanism is more complicated. There are still no good models for identification of respiratory sensitization (Mekenyan et al., 2014; Dik et al., 2015). The current QSTR studies tend to use phenotype data such as LD_{50}, LC_{50} or symptoms such as asthma as endpoints to represent the respiratory toxicity of a chemical, and the built models performed well enough (Jarvis et al., 2015; Lei et al., 2017).

Irritation and Corrosion

Risk assessment of eye and skin irritation/corrosion (EI/EC, SI/SC) is of importance in pharmaceutical and cosmetics industries. Though these endpoints might not be directly considered in drug discovery stage, *in silico* models for these endpoints are yet required since a lot of substances may cause irritation and corrosion and should be assessed, including the ocular and dermal pharmaceuticals and final products used in manufacturing, agriculture, and warfare (Wilhelmus, 2001; Kolle et al., 2017).

Verheyen et al. evaluated the existing QSTR models in Derek Nexus, Toxtree and Case Ultra for the prediction of skin and eye irritation/corrosion, and found that the performance of those models is unsatisfactory because of narrow applicability domain and low accuracy (Verheyen et al., 2017). However, using machine learning methods to predict eye injury was reported having high performance. For instance, Verma et al. build combined QSTR models by ANN and got 88% of sensitivity and 82% of specificity for EI (Verma and Matthews, 2015a), 96% of sensitivity and 91% of specificity for EC (Verma and Matthews, 2015b). Our group recently developed *in silico* models for EI/EC using machine learning methods and molecular fingerprints (Wang et al., 2017). In the paper, more positive data were manually collected from X-Mol (http://www.x-mol.com) and ChemIDplus and the performance is excellent, 94.6% of overall accuracy for EI and 95.9% for EC.

Endocrine Disruption

Chemicals interacting with nuclear receptors such as estrogen and androgen receptors (ER and AR) as off-targets or exposed in environment may cause endocrine disruption. These chemicals, called endocrine disrupting chemicals (EDCs), may interfere with the normal functions of these endogenous steroid hormones and lead to adverse health consequences such as tissue or organ proliferation, reproductive disorders, metabolic disorders, or even cancers (Colborn, 1995; Chawla et al., 2001; Grün and Blumberg, 2007).

For the specific mechanisms such as binding to ER, using *in silico* models to predict the bioactivity of chemicals and evaluate their risk of being EDCs is preferred for its high accuracy and less cost. We previously built *in silico* models for AR and ER binding using molecular fingerprints and machine learning methods and the best performance in the test set was 0.84 and 0.79, respectively (Chen et al., 2014). The Tox21 project also includes nuclear receptors assays which involve more diverse compounds (Hsieh et al., 2015). DeepTox, the winner of the "Tox21 Data Challenge," used deep neural network and obtained an excellent performance against other machine learning methods such as SVM (Mayr et al., 2016).

Previous studies on EDCs mainly focused on nuclear receptors. However, chemicals that do not directly interact with these receptors may also interfere through the pathway. For instance, aromatase (CYP19A1) is an important enzyme affecting the biosynthesis of estrogen and plays a key role in maintaining the balance between estrogen and androgen in many of the EDC-sensitive organs (Sonnet et al., 1998). Therefore, we recently built *in silico* models for prediction of aromatase inhibitors as potential EDCs using machine learning methods with molecular fingerprints (Du et al., 2017). The data used for training and test were collected from Tox21 and the best model had 0.84 of accuracy for the test set and 0.91 for the external validation set.

Eco-Toxicity

Pharmaceuticals and their metabolites exposed to the environment may affect the ecosystem since they are designed to be bioactive to creature (Halling-Sørensen et al., 1998). For instance, chemicals with binding affinities to hormone receptors may be EDCs of fishes or concentrate in fish body and finally reach to high-level animal bodies (He et al., 2017). To evaluate the environmental persistence of a chemical, biodegradation half-life is widely used as a common criterion (Raymond et al., 2001). We previously categorized chemicals as ready biodegradability and not ready biodegradability according to their biological oxygen demand (BOD) with a threshold of 60% and built several classification models. The best model used kNN with molecular descriptors and had a AUC of 0.873 in test set (Cheng et al., 2012a).

Fishes are usually used as model species to evaluate aquatic toxicity and avian species are widely used as model species to evaluate the terrestrial toxicity. Our group previously collected LC_{50} data of three fish species from ECOTOX database and built several local and global models (Sun et al., 2015). Recently, we reported a model focusing on the aquatic toxicity of pesticides and found that the molecule fingerprints performed different between local and global models (Li et al., 2017). For the avian species, several *in silico* models were developed including classification (Zhang et al., 2015) and regression (Mazzatorta et al., 2006; Toropov and Benfenati, 2006). In addition to the endpoints mentioned above, another commonly used model species for eco-toxicology is *Tetrahymena pyriformis* (Sauvant et al., 1999). Cheng et al. collected 1,571 unique chemicals with toxicity to *Tetrahymena pyriformis* and built several models of which the best performance was 92.6% for validation set (Cheng et al., 2011a).

SOFTWARE AND WEB SERVERS

Currently many software and web servers can predict chemical toxicity before synthesis. Drug design software suites such as Discovery Studio and Pipeline Pilot integrate toxicity prediction models to help filter compounds with risk of toxicity. But the endpoints are not as diverse as that in some toxicity-oriented commercial software including ADMET Predictor, Leadscope and Lhasa Derek, which take efforts primarily on predicting and alerting molecules with potential toxicity.

Free software or web servers are more preferred by academia, which can promote the development of high quality models and algorithms, and their applications in various fields including drug discovery. OCED Toolbox is an official suite for toxicity prediction and modeling using QSTR. Web servers are easier and lighter to use and will be preferred by outsiders of computational toxicology, such as medicinal chemists. Lazar is such a tool that can predict several toxicity endpoints with a user interface of drawing chemical structures (Maunz et al., 2013). ToxTree is an open source application that estimates toxic hazard by applying a decision tree approach (Patlewicz et al., 2008). Compared to QSTR-like models, ToxTree is more interpretable and the fragments (SAs) can guide the chemists in modification of the molecules. The performance of ToxTree, OECD Toolbox, and other commercial tools were compared in literature (Devillers and Mombelli, 2010; Mombelli and Devillers, 2010; Bhatia et al., 2015; Bhhatarai et al., 2016). Our group developed admetSAR that can also predict toxicity of compounds in SMILES format (Cheng et al., 2012b).

Web servers such as ChemSAR (Dong et al., 2017b) and ChemBench (Capuzzi et al., 2017) enable users to build custom models for particular use with machine learning methods and molecular descriptors. For chemists who have in-house data for some particular endpoints, it will be convenient to use these web servers to build predictive models to prioritize or substitute *in vitro* or *in vivo* tests.

PERSPECTIVES

Though *in silico* prediction of chemical toxicity has made a good progress in recent years, there are still some challenges and limitations to be improved. At first, data quality is still a big issue. Currently many toxicity data are obtained from high-throughput *in vitro* assays or *in vivo* tests on animals. For example, Tox21 and ToxCast provide the activity data of thousands of chemicals against hundreds of assays (Huang et al., 2016). While false positive and false negative data are inevitable in those assays, *in vivo* data from animals are also questionable to be used directly on humans. Therefore, more data from drug clinical trials and clinic applications are highly demanded.

Secondly, more computational methods should be developed to enhance the accuracy of the predictive models. For instance, read-across has gained wide attention recently because it can fill the gap of missing data (Shah et al., 2016). Meanwhile, some endpoints have complex mechanisms such as hepatotoxicity and respiratory toxicity, computational systems toxicology has emerged to use comprehensive data sources from gene to organ to understand the mechanisms of toxicity (Jack et al., 2013; Sauer et al., 2015). With the help of machine learning methods and cheminformatics techniques, more accurate models could be developed for toxicity prediction.

Thirdly, medicinal chemists are more interested in the relationship between substructures and chemical toxicity, which can guide the optimization of lead compounds. Using computational tools to identify SAs is a promising way. Current approaches of SA identification can only generate numerous but redundant substructures in terms of their frequency of occurrence, disregarding the chemical or biological mechanisms (Yang et al., 2017a). It is not difficult to obtain "potential" SAs for almost every endpoint with support of assay results, yet innovative protocol or framework is still required to further refine these substructures and explore the chemical mechanisms of toxicity.

AUTHOR CONTRIBUTIONS

YT, GL, and WL contributed conception and design of the study; HY wrote the first draft of the manuscript; HY and LS wrote sections of the manuscript. All authors contributed to manuscript revision, read and approved the submitted version.

ACKNOWLEDGMENTS

This work was supported by the National Key Research and Development Program of China (Grant 2016YFA0502304), the National Natural Science Foundation of China (Grants 81373329 and 81673356) and the 863 Project (Grant 2012AA020308).

REFERENCES

Ahlberg, E., Carlsson, L., and Boyer, S. (2014). Computational derivation of structural alerts from large toxicology data sets. *J. Chem. Inf. Model.* 54, 2945–2952. doi: 10.1021/ci500314a

Al-Otaibi, R., Kull, M., and Flach, P. (2014). "LaCova: a tree-based multi-label classifier using label covariance as splitting criterion," in *2014 13th International Conference on Machine Learning and Applications*, (Detroit, MI: Icmla), 74–79.

Altae-Tran, H., Ramsundar, B., Pappu, A. S., and Pande, V. (2017). Low data drug discovery with one-shot learning. *ACS Cent. Sci.* 3, 283–293. doi: 10.1021/acscentsci.6b00367

Ashby, J., and Tennant, R. W. (1988). Chemical structure, Salmonella mutagenicity and extent of carcinogenicity as indicators of genotoxic carcinogenesis among 222 chemicals tested in rodents by the U.S. NCI/NTP. *Mutat. Res.* 204, 17–115. doi: 10.1016/0165-1218(88)90114-0

Avila, J. L., Gibaja, E. L., and Ventura, S. (2009). Multi-label Classification with gene expression programming. *Hybrid Artif. Intell. Syst.* 5572, 629–637. doi: 10.1007/978-3-642-02319-4_76

Barot, P., and Panchal, M. (2014). Review on various problem transformation methods for classifying multi-label data. *Int. J. Data Min. Emerg. Technol.* 4, 45–52. doi: 10.5958/2249-3220.2014.00001.9

Bhatia, S., Schultz, T., Roberts, D., Shen, J., Kromidas, L., and Marie Api, A. (2015). Comparison of Cramer classification between Toxtree, the OECD QSAR Toolbox and expert judgment. *Regul. Toxicol. Pharmacol.* 71, 52–62. doi: 10.1016/j.yrtph.2014.11.005

Bhhatarai, B., Wilson, D. M., Parks, A. K., Carney, E. W., and Spencer, P. J. (2016). Evaluation of TOPKAT, toxtree, and derek nexus *in silico* models for ocular irritation and development of a knowledge-based framework to improve the prediction of severe irritation. *Chem. Res. Toxicol.* 29, 810–822. doi: 10.1021/acs.chemrestox.5b00531

Borgelt, C., and Berthold, M. R. (2002). "Mining molecular fragments: finding relevant substructures of molecules," in *Data Mining, (2002). ICDM 2003. Proceedings 2002 IEEE International Conference* (Maebashi: IEEE), 51–58.

Boutell, M. R., Luo, J. B., Shen, X. P., and Brown, C. M. (2004). Learning multi-label scene classification. *Pattern Recognit.* 37, 1757–1771. doi: 10.1016/j.patcog.2004.03.009

Breiman, L. (2001). Random forests. *Mach. Learn.* 45, 5–32. doi: 10.1023/A:1010933404324

Capuzzi, S. J., Kim, I. S., Lam, W. I., Thornton, T. E., Muratov, E. N., Pozefsky, D., et al. (2017). Chembench: A publicly accessible, integrated cheminformatics portal. *J. Chem. Inf. Model.* 57, 105–108. doi: 10.1021/acs.jcim.6b00462

Chawla, A., Repa, J. J., Evans, R. M., and Mangelsdorf, D. J. (2001). Nuclear receptors and lipid physiology: opening the X-files. *Science* 294, 1866–1870. doi: 10.1126/science.294.5548.1866

Chen, Y., Cheng, F., Sun, L., Li, W., Liu, G., and Tang, Y. (2014). Computational models to predict endocrine-disrupting chemical binding with androgen or oestrogen receptors. *Ecotoxicol. Environ. Saf.* 110, 280–287. doi: 10.1016/j.ecoenv.2014.08.026

Cheng, F., Ikenaga, Y., Zhou, Y., Yu, Y., Li, W., Shen, J., et al. (2012a). *In silico* assessment of chemical biodegradability. *J. Chem. Inf. Model.* 52, 655–669. doi: 10.1021/ci200622d

Cheng, F., Li, W., Liu, G., and Tang, Y. (2013a). *In silico* ADMET prediction: recent advances, current challenges and future trends. *Curr. Top. Med. Chem.* 13, 1273–1289. doi: 10.2174/15680266113139990033

Cheng, F., Li, W., Wang, X., Zhou, Y., Wu, Z., Shen, J., et al. (2013b). Adverse drug events: database construction and *in silico* prediction. *J. Chem. Inf. Model.* 53, 744–752. doi: 10.1021/ci4000079

Cheng, F., Li, W., Wu, Z., Wang, X., Zhang, C., Li, J., et al. (2013c). Prediction of polypharmacological profiles of drugs by the integration of chemical, side effect, and therapeutic space. *J. Chem. Inf. Model.* 53, 753–762. doi: 10.1021/ci400010x

Cheng, F., Li, W., Zhou, Y., Shen, J., Wu, Z., Liu, G., et al. (2012b). admetSAR: a comprehensive source and free tool for assessment of chemical ADMET properties. *J. Chem. Inf. Model.* 52, 3099–3105. doi: 10.1021/ci300367a

Cheng, F., Shen, J., Yu, Y., Li, W., Liu, G., Lee, P. W., et al. (2011a). *In silico* prediction of Tetrahymena pyriformis toxicity for diverse industrial chemicals with substructure pattern recognition and machine learning methods. *Chemosphere* 82, 1636–1643. doi: 10.1016/j.chemosphere.2010.11.043

Cheng, F., Yu, Y., Zhou, Y., Shen, Z., Xiao, W., Liu, G., et al. (2011b). Insights into molecular basis of cytochrome p450 inhibitory promiscuity of compounds. *J. Chem. Inf. Model.* 51, 2482–2495. doi: 10.1021/ci200317s

Colborn, T. (1995). Environmental estrogens: health implications for humans and wildlife. *Environ. Health Perspect.* 103 (Suppl. 7), 135–136.

Cortes, C., and Vapnik, V. (1995). Support-Vector Networks. *Mach. Learn.* 20, 273–297. doi: 10.1007/BF00994018

Cortes-Ciriano, I. (2016). Bioalerts: a python library for the derivation of structural alerts from bioactivity and toxicity data sets. *J. Cheminform.* 8:13. doi: 10.1186/s13321-016-0125-7

Cover, T., and Hart, P. (1967). Nearest neighbor pattern classification. *IEEE Trans. Inform. Theory* 13, 21–27. doi: 10.1109/TIT.1967.1053964

Davis, A. P., Grondin, C. J., Johnson, R. J., Sciaky, D., King, B. L., McMorran, R., et al. (2017). The comparative toxicogenomics database: update 2017. *Nucleic Acids Res.* 45, D972–D978. doi: 10.1093/nar/gkw838

Demsar, J., Curk, T., Erjavec, A., Gorup, C., Hocevar, T., Milutinovic, M., et al. (2013). Orange: data mining toolbox in python. *J. Mach. Learn. Res.* 14, 2349–2353. Available online at: https://orange.biolab.si/citation/

Deng, L., Hinton, G., and Kingsbury, B. (2013). "New types of deep neural network learning for speech recognition and related applications: an overview,"in *IEEE International Conference on Acoustics, Speech and Signal Processing* (Vancouver, BC), 8599–8603.

Devillers, J., and Mombelli, E. (2010). Evaluation of the OECD QSAR Application Toolbox and Toxtree for estimating the mutagenicity of chemicals. Part 1. Aromatic amines. *SAR QSAR Environ. Res.* 21, 753-769. doi: 10.1080/1062936X.2010.528959

Dik, S., Pennings, J. L., van Loveren, H., and Ezendam, J. (2015). Development of an *in vitro* test to identify respiratory sensitizers in bronchial epithelial cells using gene expression profiling. *Toxicol. In Vitro* 30(1 Pt B), 274-280. doi: 10.1016/j.tiv.2015.10.010

Diplaris, S., Tsoumakas, G., Mitkas, P. A., and Vlahavas, I. (2005). Protein classification with multiple algorithms. *Adv. Inform. Proc.* 3746, 448–456. doi: 10.1007/11573036_42

Doddareddy, M. R., Klaasse, E. C., Shagufta, Ijzerman, A. P., and Bender, A. (2010). Prospective validation of a comprehensive *in silico* hERG model and its applications to commercial compound and drug databases. *Chem. Med. Chem.* 5, 716–729. doi: 10.1002/cmdc.201000024

Dong, J., Cao, D. S., Miao, H. Y., Liu, S., Deng, B. C., Yun, Y. H., et al. (2015). ChemDes: an integrated web-based platform for molecular descriptor and fingerprint computation. *J. Cheminform.* 7:60. doi: 10.1186/s13321-015-0109-z

Dong, J., Wang, N.-N., Liu, K.-Y., Zhu, M.-F., Yun, Y.-H., Zeng, W.-B., et al. (2017a). ChemBCPP: a freely available web server for calculating commonly used physicochemical properties. *Chemometr. Intell. Lab. Syst.* 171, 65–73. doi: 10.1016/j.chemolab.2017.10.006

Dong, J., Yao, Z. J., Zhu, M. F., Wang, N. N., Lu, B., Chen, A. F., et al. (2017b). ChemSAR: an online pipelining platform for molecular SAR modeling. *J. Cheminform.* 9:27. doi: 10.1186/s13321-017-0215-1

Du, H., Cai, Y., Yang, H., Zhang, H., Xue, Y., Liu, G., et al. (2017). *In silico* prediction of chemicals binding to aromatase with machine learning methods. *Chem. Res. Toxicol.* 30, 1209–1218. doi: 10.1021/acs.chemrestox.7b00037

Duvenaud, D., Maclaurin, D., Aguilera-Iparraguirre, J., Gómez-Bombarelli, R., Hirzel, T., and Aspuru-Guzik, A. N., et al. (2015). *Convolutional Networks on Graphs for Learning Molecular Fingerprints. ArXiv e-prints [Online]*, (1509). Available online at: http://adsabs.harvard.edu/abs/2015arXiv150909292D (Accessed Sept 1, 2015).

Elith, J., Leathwick, J. R., and Hastie, T. (2008). A working guide to boosted regression trees. *J. Anim. Ecol.* 77, 802–813. doi: 10.1111/j.1365-2656.2008.01390.x

Fan, D., Yang, H., Li, F., Sun, L., Di, P., Li, W., et al. (in press). *In silico* prediction of chemical genotoxicity using machine learning methods and structural alerts. *Toxicol. Res.* doi: 10.1039/C7TX00259A

Ferrari, T., Cattaneo, D., Gini, G., Golbamaki Bakhtyari, N., Manganaro, A., and Benfenati, E. (2013). Automatic knowledge extraction from chemical structures: the case of mutagenicity prediction. *SAR QSAR Environ. Res.* 24, 631–649. doi: 10.1080/1062936X.2013.773376

Floris, M., Raitano, G., Medda, R., and Benfenati, E. (2017). Fragment prioritization on a large mutagenicity dataset. *Mol. Inform.* 36:1600133. doi: 10.1002/minf.201600133

Fonger, G. C., Hakkinen, P., Jordan, S., and Publicker, S. (2014). The National Library of Medicine's (NLM) Hazardous Substances Data Bank (HSDB): background, recent enhancements and future plans. *Toxicology* 325, 209–216. doi: 10.1016/j.tox.2014.09.003

Fowler, S., and Schnall, J. G. (2014). TOXNET: information on toxicology and environmental health. *Am. J. Nurs.* 114, 61–63. doi: 10.1097/01.NAJ.0000443783.75162.79

Frank, E., Hall, M., Trigg, L., Holmes, G., and Witten, I. H. (2004). Data mining in bioinformatics using Weka. *Bioinformatics* 20, 2479–2481. doi: 10.1093/bioinformatics/bth261

Gaulton, A., Hersey, A., Nowotka, M., Bento, A. P., Chambers, J., Mendez, D., et al. (2017). The ChEMBL database in 2017. *Nucleic Acids Res.* 45, D945–D954. doi: 10.1093/nar/gkw1074

Gibaja, E., and Ventura, S. (2015). A tutorial on multilabel learning. *Acm Comput. Surveys* 47, 1–38. doi: 10.1145/2716262

Gilson, M. K., Liu, T., Baitaluk, M., Nicola, G., Hwang, L., and Chong, J. (2016). BindingDB in 2015: a public database for medicinal chemistry, computational chemistry and systems pharmacology. *Nucleic Acids Res.* 44, D1045–D1053. doi: 10.1093/nar/gkv1072

Gintant, G., Sager, P. T., and Stockbridge, N. (2016). Evolution of strategies to improve preclinical cardiac safety testing. *Nat. Rev. Drug Discov.* 15, 457–471. doi: 10.1038/nrd.2015.34

Giri, S., and Bader, A. (2015). A low-cost, high-quality new drug discovery process using patient-derived induced pluripotent stem cells. *Drug Discov. Today* 20, 37–49. doi: 10.1016/j.drudis.2014.10.011

Godbole, S., and Sarawagi, S. (2004). Discriminative methods for multi-labeled classification. *Adv. Knowl. Discov. Data Min. Proc.* 3056, 22–30. doi: 10.1007/978-3-540-24775-3_5

Goh, G. B., Hodas, N. O., and Vishnu, A. (2017). Deep learning for computational chemistry. *J. Comput. Chem.* 38, 1291–1307. doi: 10.1002/jcc.24764

Golbamaki, A., and Benfenati, E. (2016). *In silico* methods for carcinogenicity assessment. *Methods Mol. Biol.* 1425, 107–119. doi: 10.1007/978-1-4939-3609-0_6

Golbamaki, A., Benfenati, E., Golbamaki, N., Manganaro, A., Merdivan, E., Roncaglioni, A., et al. (2016). New clues on carcinogenicity-related substructures derived from mining two large datasets of chemical compounds. *J. Environ. Sci. Health C Environ. Carcinog. Ecotoxicol. Rev.* 34, 97–113. doi: 10.1080/10590501.2016.1166879

Gold, L. S., Manley, N. B., Slone, T. H., Rohrbach, L., and Garfinkel, G. B. (2005). Supplement to the Carcinogenic Potency Database (CPDB): results of animal bioassays published in the general literature through 1997 and by the National Toxicology Program in 1997-1998. *Toxicol. Sci.* 85, 747–808. doi: 10.1093/toxsci/kfi161

Grün, F., and Blumberg, B. (2007). Perturbed nuclear receptor signaling by environmental obesogens as emerging factors in the obesity crisis. *Rev. Endocr. Metab. Disord.* 8, 161–171. doi: 10.1007/s11154-007-9049-x

Halling-Sørensen, B., Nors Nielsen, S., Lanzky, P. F., Ingerslev, F., Holten Lützhøft, H. C., and Jørgensen, S. E. (1998). Occurrence, fate and effects of pharmaceutical substances in the environment–a review. *Chemosphere* 36, 357–393. doi: 10.1016/S0045-6535(97)00354-8

Hansen, K., Mika, S., Schroeter, T., Sutter, A., ter Laak, A., Steger-Hartmann, T., et al. (2009). Benchmark data set for *in Silico* prediction of ames mutagenicity. *J. Chem. Inf. Model.* 49, 2077–2081. doi: 10.1021/ci900161g

He, J., Peng, T., Yang, X., and Liu, H. (2017). Development of QSAR models for predicting the binding affinity of endocrine disrupting chemicals to eight fish estrogen receptor. *Ecotoxicol. Environ. Saf.* 148, 211–219. doi: 10.1016/j.ecoenv.2017.10.023

Hewitt, M., and Przybylak, K. (2016). *In silico* models for hepatotoxicity. *Methods Mol. Biol.* 1425, 201–236. doi: 10.1007/978-1-4939-3609-0_11

Hsieh, J. H., Sedykh, A., Huang, R., Xia, M., and Tice, R. R. (2015). A data analysis pipeline accounting for artifacts in Tox21 quantitative high-throughput screening assays. *J. Biomol. Screen.* 20, 887–897. doi: 10.1177/1087057115581317

Huang, R., Xia, M., Sakamuru, S., Zhao, J., Shahane, S. A., Attene-Ramos, M., et al. (2016). Modelling the Tox21 10 K chemical profiles for *in vivo* toxicity prediction and mechanism characterization. *Nat. Commun.* 7:10425. doi: 10.1038/ncomms10425

Huh, D., Hamilton, G. A., and Ingber, D. E. (2011). From 3D cell culture to organs-on-chips. *Trends Cell Biol.* 21, 745–754. doi: 10.1016/j.tcb.2011.09.005

Huh, D., Matthews, B. D., Mammoto, A., Montoya-Zavala, M., Hsin, H. Y., and Ingber, D. E. (2010). Reconstituting organ-level lung functions on a chip. *Science* 328, 1662–1668. doi: 10.1126/science.1188302

Jack, J., Wambaugh, J., and Shah, I. (2013). Systems toxicology from genes to organs. *Methods Mol. Biol.* 930, 375–397. doi: 10.1007/978-1-62703-059-5_17

Jarvis, J., Seed, M. J., Stocks, S. J., and Agius, R. M. (2015). A refined QSAR model for prediction of chemical asthma hazard. *Occup. Med. (Lond).* 65, 659–666. doi: 10.1093/occmed/kqv105

Judson, R., Richard, A., Dix, D., Houck, K., Elloumi, F., Martin, M., et al. (2008). ACToR–Aggregated computational toxicology resource. *Toxicol. Appl. Pharmacol.* 233, 7–13. doi: 10.1016/j.taap.2007.12.037

Kazius, J., McGuire, R., and Bursi, R. (2005). Derivation and validation of toxicophores for mutagenicity prediction. *J. Med. Chem.* 48, 312–320. doi: 10.1021/jm040835a

Kazius, J., Nijssen, S., Kok, J., Bäck, T., and Ijzerman, A. P. (2006). Substructure mining using elaborate chemical representation. *J. Chem. Inf. Model.* 46, 597–605. doi: 10.1021/ci0503715

Klekota, J., and Roth, F. P. (2008). Chemical substructures that enrich for biological activity. *Bioinformatics* 24, 2518–2525. doi: 10.1093/bioinformatics/btn479

Kolle, S. N., van Ravenzwaay, B., and Landsiedel, R. (2017). Regulatory accepted but out of domain: *in vitro* skin irritation tests for agrochemical formulations. *Regul. Toxicol. Pharmacol.* 89, 125–130. doi: 10.1016/j.yrtph.2017.07.016

Kuhn, M., Campillos, M., Letunic, I., Jensen, L. J., and Bork, P. (2010). A side effect resource to capture phenotypic effects of drugs. *Mol. Syst. Biol.* 6:343. doi: 10.1038/msb.2009.98

Landrum, G. (2017). *RDKit.* Available online at: http://www.rdkit.org.

LeCun, Y., Bengio, Y., and Hinton, G. (2015). Deep learning. *Nature* 521, 436–444. doi: 10.1038/nature14539

Lei, T., Chen, F., Liu, H., Sun, H., Kang, Y., Li, D., et al. (2017). ADMET Evaluation in drug discovery. part 17: development of quantitative and qualitative prediction models for chemical-induced respiratory toxicity. *Mol. Pharm.* 14, 2407-2421. doi: 10.1021/acs.molpharmaceut.7b00317

Lei, T., Li, Y., Song, Y., Li, D., Sun, H., and Hou, T. (2016). ADMET evaluation in drug discovery: 15. Accurate prediction of rat oral acute toxicity using relevance vector machine and consensus modeling. *J. Cheminformat.* 8:6. doi: 10.1186/S13321-016-0117-7.

Lepailleur, A., Poezevara, G., and Bureau, R. (2013). Automated detection of structural alerts (chemical fragments) in (eco)toxicology. *Comput. Struct. Biotechnol. J.* 5:e201302013. doi: 10.5936/csbj.201302013

Li, F., Fan, D., Wang, H., Yang, H., Li, W., Tang, Y., et al. (2017). *In silico* prediction of pesticide aquatic toxicity with chemical category approaches. *Toxicol. Res.* 6, 831–842. doi: 10.1039/C7TX00144D

Li, X., Chen, L., Cheng, F., Wu, Z., Bian, H., Xu, C., et al. (2014). *In silico* prediction of chemical acute oral toxicity using multi-classification methods. *J. Chem. Inf. Model.* 54, 1061–1069. doi: 10.1021/ci5000467

Li, X., Du, Z., Wang, J., Wu, Z. R., Li, W. H., Liu, G. X., et al. (2015). *In silico* estimation of chemical carcinogenicity with binary and ternary classification methods. *Mol. Inform.* 34, 228–235. doi: 10.1002/minf.201400127

Matsuno, O. (2012). Drug-induced interstitial lung disease: mechanisms and best diagnostic approaches. *Respir. Res.* 13:39. doi: 10.1186/1465-9921-13-39

Maunz, A., Gütlein, M., Rautenberg, M., Vorgrimmler, D., Gebele, D., and Helma, C. (2013). lazar: a modular predictive toxicology framework. *Front. Pharmacol.* 4:38. doi: 10.3389/fphar.2013.00038

Mayr, A., Klambauer, G., Unterthiner, T., and Hochreiter, S. (2016). DeepTox: toxicity prediction using deep learning. *Front. Environ. Sci.* 3:80. doi: 10.3389/fenvs.2015.00080

Mazzatorta, P., Cronin, M. T. D., and Benfenati, E. (2006). A QSAR study of avian oral toxicity using support vector machines and genetic algorithms. *QSAR Comb. Sci.* 25, 616–628. doi: 10.1002/qsar.200530189

Mekenyan, O., Patlewicz, G., Kuseva, C., Popova, I., Mehmed, A., Kotov, S., et al. (2014). A mechanistic approach to modeling respiratory sensitization. *Chem. Res. Toxicol.* 27, 219–239. doi: 10.1021/tx400345b

Mombelli, E., and Devillers, J. (2010). Evaluation of the OECD (Q)SAR Application Toolbox and Toxtree for predicting and profiling the carcinogenic potential of chemicals. *SAR QSAR Environ. Res.* 21, 731–752. doi: 10.1080/1062936X.2010.528598

Mulliner, D., Schmidt, F., Stolte, M., Spirkl, H. P., Czich, A., and Amberg, A. (2016). Computational models for human and animal hepatotoxicity with a global application scope. *Chem. Res. Toxicol.* 29, 757–767. doi: 10.1021/acs.chemrestox.5b00465

O'Boyle, N. M., Banck, M., James, C. A., Morley, C., Vandermeersch, T., and Hutchison, G. R. (2011). Open Babel: an open chemical toolbox. *J. Cheminform.* 3:33. doi: 10.1186/1758-2946-3-33

Patlewicz, G., Jeliazkova, N., Safford, R. J., Worth, A. P., and Aleksiev, B. (2008). An evaluation of the implementation of the cramer classification scheme in the toxtree software. *SAR QSAR Environ. Res.* 19, 495–524. doi: 10.1080/10629360802083871

Paul, S. M., Mytelka, D. S., Dunwiddie, C. T., Persinger, C. C., Munos, B. H., Lindborg, S. R., et al. (2010). How to improve R&D productivity: the pharmaceutical industry's grand challenge. *Nat. Rev. Drug Discov.* 9, 203–214. doi: 10.1038/nrd3078

Pedregosa, F., Varoquaux, G., Gramfort, A., Michel, V., Weiss, R., Dubourg, V., et al. (2011). Scikit-learn: machine learning in python. *J. Mach. Learn. Res.* 12, 2825–2830. Available online at: http://scikit-learn.org/stable/about.html#citing-scikit-learn

PhRMA (2015). *2015 Biopharmaceutical Research Industry Profle.* Washington, DC: Pharmaceutical Research and Manufacturers of America.

Pizzo, F., Gadaleta, D., Lombardo, A., Nicolotti, O., and Benfenati, E. (2015). Identification of structural alerts for liver and kidney toxicity using repeated dose toxicity data. *Chem. Cent. J.* 9:62. doi: 10.1186/s13065-015-0139-7

Raymond, J. W., Rogers, T. N., Shonnard, D. R., and Kline, A. A. (2001). A review of structure-based biodegradation estimation methods. *J. Hazard. Mater.* 84, 189–215. doi: 10.1016/S0304-3894(01)00207-2

Read, J., Pfahringer, B., and Holmes, G. (2008). "Multi-label classification using ensembles of pruned sets," *ICDM 2008:* Eighth *IEEE International Conference on Data Mining, Proceedings* (Pisa), 995-1000.

Read, J., Pfahringer, B., Holmes, G., and Frank, E. (2011). Classifier chains for multi-label classification. *Mach. Learn.* 85, 333–359. doi: 10.1007/s10994-011-5256-5

Sauer, J. M., Hartung, T., Leist, M., Knudsen, T. B., Hoeng, J., and Hayes, A. W. (2015). Systems toxicology: the future of risk assessment. *Int. J. Toxicol.* 34, 346–348. doi: 10.1177/1091581815576551

Sauvant, M. P., Pepin, D., and Piccinni, E. (1999). Tetrahymena pyriformis: a tool for toxicological studies. A review. *Chemosphere* 38, 1631–1669. doi: 10.1016/S0045-6535(98)00381-6

Schmidt, U., Struck, S., Gruening, B., Hossbach, J., Jaeger, I. S., Parol, R., et al. (2009). SuperToxic: a comprehensive database of toxic compounds. *Nucleic Acids Res.* 37, D295-D299. doi: 10.1093/nar/gkn850

Schuster, D., Laggner, C., and Langer, T. (2005). Why drugs fail - A study on side effects in new chemical entities. *Curr. Pharm. Des.* 11, 3545–3559. doi: 10.2174/138161205774414510

Segall, M. D., and Barber, C. (2014). Addressing toxicity risk when designing and selecting compounds in early drug discovery. *Drug Discov. Today* 19, 688–693. doi: 10.1016/j.drudis.2014.01.006

Shah, I., Liu, J., Judson, R. S., Thomas, R. S., and Patlewicz, G. (2016). Systematically evaluating read-across prediction and performance using a local validity approach characterized by chemical structure and bioactivity information. *Regul. Toxicol. Pharmacol.* 79, 12–24. doi: 10.1016/j.yrtph.2016.05.008

Shen, J., Cheng, F., Xu, Y., Li, W., and Tang, Y. (2010). Estimation of ADME properties with substructure pattern recognition. *J. Chem. Inf. Model* 50, 1034–1041. doi: 10.1021/ci100104j

Shen, Q., Jiang, J. H., Jiao, C. X., Lin, W. Q., Shen, G. L., and Yu, R. Q. (2004). Hybridized particle swarm algorithm for adaptive structure training of multilayer feed-forward neural network: QSAR studies of bioactivity of organic compounds. *J. Comput. Chem.* 25, 1726–1735. doi: 10.1002/jcc.20094

Singh, K. P., Gupta, S., and Rai, P. (2013). Predicting carcinogenicity of diverse chemicals using probabilistic neural network modeling approaches. *Toxicol. Appl. Pharmacol.* 272, 465–475. doi: 10.1016/j.taap.2013.06.029

Sokolova, M., and Szpakowicz, S. (2010). *In Handbook of Research on Machine Learning Applications and Trends: Algorithms, Methods, and Techniques.* Hershey, PA: IGI Global.

Sonnet, P., Guillon, J., Enguehard, C., Dallemagne, P., Bureau, R., Rault S. Auvray P., et al. (1998). Design and synthesis of a new type of non steroidal human aromatase inhibitors. *Bioorg. Med. Chem. Lett.* 8, 1041–1044. doi: 10.1016/S0960-894X(98)00157-7

Steinbeck, C., Han, Y. Q., Kuhn, S., Horlacher, O., Luttmann, E., and Willighagen, E. (2003). The Chemistry Development Kit (CDK): an open-source Java library for chemo- and bioinformatics. *J. Chem. Inf. Comput. Sci.* 43, 493–500. doi: 10.1021/ci025584y

Sun, L., Yang, H., Li, J., Wang, T., Li, W., Liu, G., et al. (2017). *In silico* prediction of compounds binding to human plasma proteins by QSAR models. *ChemMedChem.* doi: 10.1002/cmdc.201700582. [Epub ahead of print].

Sun, L., Zhang, C., Chen, Y. J., Li, X., Zhuang, S. L., Li, W. H., et al. (2015). *In silico* prediction of chemical aquatic toxicity with chemical category approaches and substructural alerts. *Toxicol. Res.* 4, 452–463. doi: 10.1039/C4TX00174E

Sushko, I., Salmina, E., Potemkin, V. A., Poda, G., and Tetko, I. V. (2012). ToxAlerts: a web server of structural alerts for toxfic chemicals and compounds with potential adverse reactions. *J. Chem. Inf. Model.* 52, 2310–2316. doi: 10.1021/ci300245q

Tanabe, K., Kurita, T., Nishida, K., Lucić, B., Amić, D., and Suzuki, T. (2013). Improvement of carcinogenicity prediction performances based on sensitivity analysis in variable selection of SVM models. *SAR QSAR Environ. Res.* 24, 565–580. doi: 10.1080/1062936X.2012.762425

Tatonetti, N. P., Ye, P. P., Daneshjou, R., and Altman, R. B. (2012). Data-driven prediction of drug effects and interactions. *Sci. Transl. Med.* 4:125ra131. doi: 10.1126/scitranslmed.3003377

Tetko, I. V., Gasteiger, J., Todeschini, R., Mauri, A., Livingstone, D., Ertl, P., et al. (2005). Virtual computational chemistry laboratory–design and description. *J. Comput. Aided Mol. Des.* 19, 453–463. doi: 10.1007/s10822-005-8694-y

Toropov, A. A., and Benfenati, E. (2006). QSAR models of quail dietary toxicity based on the graph of atomic orbitals. *Bioorg. Med. Chem. Lett.* 16, 1941–1943. doi: 10.1016/j.bmcl.2005.12.085

Tsoumakas, G., Katakis, I., and Taniar, D. (2007). Multi-label classification: an overview. *Int. J. Data Warehousing Min.* 3, 1–13. doi: 10.4018/jdwm.2007070101

Tsoumakas, G., Katakis, I., and Vlahavas, I. (2008). "Effective and efficient multilabel classification in domains with large number of labels," in *Ecml/pkdd Workshop on Mining Multidimensional Data* (Ho Chi Minh City).

Tsoumakas, G., Katakis, I., and Vlahavas, I. (2010). "Mining Multi-label Data," in *Data Mining and Knowledge Discovery Handbook*, eds O. Maimon and L. Rokach. (Boston, MA: Springer), 667–685.

Tsoumakas, G., and Vlahavas, I. (2007). "Random k-labelsets: an ensemble method for multilabel classification," in *Proceedings of Machine Learning. ECML 2007* (Warsaw).

Verheyen, G. R., Braeken, E., Van Deun, K., and Van Miert, S. (2017). Evaluation of existing (Q)SAR models for skin and eye irritation and corrosion to use for REACH registration. *Toxicol. Lett.* 265, 47–52. doi: 10.1016/j.toxlet.2016.11.007

Verma, R. P., and Matthews, E. J. (2015a). Estimation of the chemical-induced eye injury using a weight-of-evidence (WoE) battery of 21 artificial neural network (ANN) c-QSAR models (QSAR-21): part I: irritation potential. *Regul. Toxicol. Pharmacol.* 71, 318–330. doi: 10.1016/j.yrtph.2014.11.011

Verma, R. P., and Matthews, E. J. (2015b). Estimation of the chemical-induced eye injury using a Weight-of-Evidence (WoE) battery of 21 artificial neural network (ANN) c-QSAR models (QSAR-21): part II: corrosion potential. *Regul. Toxicol. Pharmacol.* 71, 331–336. doi: 10.1016/j.yrtph.2014.12.004

Wang, J. R., Feng, J., Sun, X., Chen, S. S., and Chen, B. (2014). Simplified Constraints Rank-SVM for Multi-label Classification. *Pattern Recogn.* 483(Pt I), 229–236. doi: 10.1007/978-3-662-45646-0_23

Wang, Q., Li, X., Yang, H., Cai, Y., Wang, Y., Wang, Z., et al. (2017). *In silico* prediction of serious eye irritation or corrosion potential of chemicals. *RSC Adv.* 7, 6697–6703. doi: 10.1039/C6RA25267B

Wang, S., Li, Y., Wang, J., Chen, L., Zhang, L., Yu, H., et al. (2012). ADMET evaluation in drug discovery. 12. Development of binary classification models for prediction of hERG potassium channel blockage. *Mol. Pharm.* 9, 996-1010. doi: 10.1021/mp300023x

Wang, S., Sun, H., Liu, H., Li, D., Li, Y., and Hou, T. (2016). ADMET evaluation in drug discovery. 16. Predicting hERG Blockers by combining multiple pharmacophores and machine learning approaches. *Mol. Pharm.* 13, 2855–2866. doi: 10.1021/acs.molpharmaceut.6b00471

Wang, Y., Xiao, J., Suzek, T. O., Zhang, J., Wang, J., and Bryant, S. H. (2009). PubChem: a public information system for analyzing bioactivities of small molecules. *Nucleic Acids Res.* 37(Suppl. 2), W623–W633. doi: 10.1093/nar/gkp456

Wilhelmus, K. R. (2001). The Draize eye test. *Surv. Ophthalmol.* 45, 493–515. doi: 10.1016/S0039-6257(01)00211-9

Williams-DeVane, C. R., Wolf, M. A., and Richard, A. M. (2009). DSSTox chemical-index files for exposure-related experiments in ArrayExpress and Gene Expression Omnibus: enabling toxico-chemogenomics data linkages. *Bioinformatics* 25, 692–694. doi: 10.1093/bioinformatics/btp042

Wishart, D., Arndt, D., Pon, A., Sajed, T., Guo, A. C., Djoumbou, Y., et al. (2015). T3DB: the toxic exposome database. *Nucleic Acids Res.* 43, D928-D934. doi: 10.1093/nar/gku1004

Xu, C., Cheng, F., Chen, L., Du, Z., Li, W., Liu, G., et al. (2012). *In silico* prediction of chemical Ames mutagenicity. *J. Chem. Inf. Model.* 52, 2840–2847. doi: 10.1021/ci300400a

Xu, Y., Dai, Z., Chen, F., Gao, S., Pei, J., and Lai, L. (2015). Deep learning for drug-induced liver injury. *J. Chem. Inf. Model.* 55, 2085–2093. doi: 10.1021/acs.jcim.5b00238

Xu, Y., Pei, J., and Lai, L. (2017). Deep learning based regression and multiclass models for acute oral toxicity prediction with automatic chemical feature extraction. *J. Chem. Inf. Model.* 57, 2672-2685. doi: 10.1021/acs.jcim.7b00244

Xue, Y., Li, Z. R., Yap, C. W., Sun, L. Z., Chen, X., and Chen, Y. Z. (2004). Effect of molecular descriptor feature selection in support vector machine classification of pharmacokinetic and toxicological properties of chemical agents. *J. Chem. Inf. Comput. Sci.* 44, 1630–1638. doi: 10.1021/ci049869h

Yang, H., Li, J., Wu, Z., Li, W., Liu, G., and Tang, Y. (2017a). Evaluation of different methods for identification of structural alerts using chemical ames mutagenicity data set as a benchmark. *Chem. Res. Toxicol.* 30, 1355–1364. doi: 10.1021/acs.chemrestox.7b00083

Yang, H., Li, X., Cai, Y., Wang, Q., Li, W., Liu, G., et al. (2017b). *In silico* prediction of chemical subcellular localization via multi-classification methods. *Medchemcomm.* 8, 1225-1234 doi: 10.1039/C7MD00074J

Yap, C. W. (2011). PaDEL-descriptor: an open source software to calculate molecular descriptors and fingerprints. *J. Comput. Chem.* 32, 1466–1474. doi: 10.1002/jcc.21707

Zhang, C., Cheng, F., Li, W., Liu, G., Lee, P. W., and Tang, Y. (2016a). *In silico* prediction of drug induced liver toxicity using substructure pattern recognition method. *Mol. Inform.* 35, 136–144. doi: 10.1002/minf.201500055

Zhang, C., Cheng, F., Sun, L., Zhuang, S., Li, W., Liu, G., et al. (2015). *In silico* prediction of chemical toxicity on avian species using chemical category approaches. *Chemosphere* 122, 280–287. doi: 10.1016/j.chemosphere.2014.12.001

Zhang, C., Zhou, Y., Gu, S., Wu, Z., Wu, W., Liu, C., et al. (2016b). *In silico* prediction of hERG potassium channel blockage by chemical category approaches. *Toxicol. Res.* 5, 570–582. doi: 10.1039/C5TX00294J

Zhang, H., Cao, Z., Li, M., Li, Y., and Peng, C. (2016). Novel naive Bayes classification models for predicting the carcinogenicity of chemicals. *Food Chem. Toxicol.* 97, 141–149. doi: 10.1016/j.fct.2016.09.005

Zhang, L., Ai, H., Chen, W., Yin, Z., Hu, H., Zhu, J., et al. (2017). CarcinoPred-EL: novel models for predicting the carcinogenicity of chemicals using molecular fingerprints and ensemble learning methods. *Sci. Rep.* 7:2118. doi: 10.1038/s41598-017-02365-0

Zhang, M. L., and Zhou, Z. H. (2006). Multilabel neural networks with applications to functional genomics and text categorization. *IEEE Trans. Knowl. Data Eng.* 18, 1338–1351. doi: 10.1109/TKDE.2006.162

Zhang, M. L., and Zhou, Z. H. (2007). ML-KNN: a lazy learning approach to multi-label leaming. *Pattern Recognit.* 40, 2038–2048. doi: 10.1016/j.patcog.2006.12.019

Zhang, M. L., and Zhou, Z. H. (2014). A review on multi-label learning algorithms. *IEEE Trans. Knowl. Data Eng.* 26, 1819–1837. doi: 10.1109/TKDE.2013.39

Zhu, H., Martin, T. M., Ye, L., Sedykh, A., Young, D. M., and Tropsha, A. (2009). Quantitative structure-activity relationship modeling of rat acute toxicity by oral exposure. *Chem. Res. Toxicol.* 22, 1913–1921. doi: 10.1021/tx900189p

Zhu, X., and Kruhlak, N. L. (2014). Construction and analysis of a human hepatotoxicity database suitable for QSAR modeling using post-market safety data. *Toxicology* 321, 62–72. doi: 10.1016/j.tox.2014.03.009

15

Combined *In Vitro* and *In Silico* Studies for the Anticholinesterase Activity and Pharmacokinetics of Coumarinyl Thiazoles and Oxadiazoles

Aliya Ibrar[1], *Ajmal Khan*[2,3*], *Majid Ali*[2], *Rizwana Sarwar*[2], *Saifullah Mehsud*[1], *Umar Farooq*[2], *Syed M. A. Halimi*[4], *Imtiaz Khan*[5,6*] and *Ahmed Al-Harrasi*[3*]

[1] Department of Chemistry, Abbottabad University of Science & Technology, Havelian, Pakistan, [2] Department of Chemistry, COMSATS Institute of Information Technology, Abbottabad, Pakistan, [3] UoN Chair of Oman's Medicinal Plants and Marine Natural Products, University of Nizwa, Nizwa, Oman, [4] Department of Pharmacy, University of Peshawar, Peshawar, Pakistan, [5] Department of Chemistry, Quaid-i-Azam University, Islamabad, Pakistan, [6] School of Chemistry, Cardiff University, Cardiff, United Kingdom

***Correspondence:**
Ajmal Khan
ajmalchemist@yahoo.com
Imtiaz Khan
kimtiaz@hotmail.co.uk
Ahmed Al-Harrasi
aharrasi@unizwa.edu.om

In a continuation of our previous work for the exploration of novel enzyme inhibitors, two new coumarin-thiazole **6(a–o)** and coumarin-oxadiazole **11(a–h)** hybrids have been designed and synthesized. All the compounds were characterized by ^{1}H- and ^{13}C-NMR spectroscopy and elemental analysis. New hybrid analogs were evaluated against acetylcholinesterase (AChE) and butyrylcholinesterase (BuChE) in order to know their potential for the prevention of Alzheimer's disease (AD). In coumarinyl thiazole series, compound **6b** was found as the most active member against AChE having IC_{50} value of $0.87 \pm 0.09\,\mu$M, while the compound **6j** revealed the same efficacy against BuChE with an IC_{50} value of $11.01 \pm 3.37\,\mu$M. In case of coumarinyl oxadiazole series, **11a** was turned out to be the lead candidate against AChE with an IC_{50} value of $6.07 \pm 0.23\,\mu$M, whereas compound **11e** was found significantly active against BuChE with an IC_{50} value of $0.15 \pm 0.09\,\mu$M. To realize the binding interaction of these compounds with AChE and BuChE, the molecular docking studies were performed. Compounds from coumarinyl thiazole series with potent AChE activity (**6b**, **6h**, **6i,** and **6k**) were found to interact with AChE in the active site with MOE score of −10.19, −9.97, −9.68, and −11.03 Kcal.mol^{-1}, respectively. The major interactions include hydrogen bonding, π-π stacking with aromatic residues, and interaction through water bridging. The docking studies of coumarinyl oxadiazole derivatives **11(a–h)** suggested that the compounds with high anti-butyrylcholinesterase activity (**11e**, **11a,** and **11b**) provided MOE score of −9.9, −7.4, and −8.2 Kcal.mol^{-1}, respectively, with the active site of BuChE building π-π stacking with Trp82 and water bridged interaction.

Keywords: coumarin thiazoles, coumarin oxadiazoles, cholinesterase inhibition, molecular docking, MOE score

INTRODUCTION

Alzheimer's disease (AD), the most common cause of dementia, is a neurodegenerative disorder mainly characterized by progressive deterioration of memory and cognition (Terry and Buccafusco, 2003). One of the key therapeutic strategies adopted for primarily symptomatic AD is based on the cholinergic hypothesis targeting cholinesterase enzymes (acetylcholinesterase and butyrylcholinesterase; Cummings et al., 2007), two important enzymes from the group of serine hydrolases. Structurally, these serine hydrolases belong to the class of proteins known as the esterase/lipase family within the α/β-hydrolase fold superfamily (Cygler et al., 1993). The major role of AChE is the inhibition of the hydrolysis of acetylcholine in cholinergic synapses. Thus, blocking its metabolic activity and increasing the ACh concentration ultimately leading to a possible symptomatic treatment option for AD, whereas, the functional activity of butyrylcholinesterase (BChE) is less understood because it can hydrolyze ACh as well as other esters (Groner et al., 2007; Chiou et al., 2009). Butyrylcholinesterase has recently been considered as a potential target because it also plays an important role in regulating ACh level (Mesulam et al., 2002). AChE inhibitors currently approved as drugs for the treatment of Alzheimer's disease are donepezil, rivastigmine, galantamine, and tacrine (**Figure 1**). Although, donepezil is most commonly used AChE inhibitor, its Aβ formation inhibition activity is weak (Bartolini et al., 2003). In view of the limited number of cholinesterase inhibitors currently available for the treatment of AD, the search for new and potent inhibitors is of significant interest and a progressive area of current research.

Among oxygenated heterocycles, coumarin compounds have sustained efficacy as they inhibit both acetyl- and butyrylcholinesterase enzymes and help to slow down the formation of amyloid compounds (de Souza et al., 2016). Coumarins, both natural and synthetic demonstrate a wide spectrum of biological functions as they offer a wide range of structural changes on benzopyran ring. Activities like anti-tubercular (Manvar et al., 2011), anti-tumor (Maddi et al., 2007), anti-HIV (Kashman et al., 1992), anti-inflammatory (Ronad et al., 2010), anti-cancer (Olmedo et al., 2012), and anticoagulant (Martin-Aragón et al., 2001) have been reported. In addition, thiazole and oxadiazole skeletons are fundamentally important and versatile structural analogs of five-membered heterocyclic compounds. They show a vast majority of biological activities (Klimesová et al., 2004; Hang and Honek, 2005; Campiglia et al., 2009; Siddiqui et al., 2009; Jaishree et al., 2012; Romagnoli et al., 2012; Helal et al., 2013; Naveena et al., 2013; Venugopala et al., 2013; Yavari et al., 2014) in addition to be a part of numerous complex natural products like vitamin B1, penicillin (Shaker, 2006), and thiamine pyrophosphate, an important co-enzyme.

In the present study, two new coumarin-thiazole **6(a–o)** and coumarin-oxadiazole **11(a–h)** hybrids were synthesized and evaluated for their acetylcholinesterase (AChE) and butyrylcholinesterase (BuChE) inhibitory activity. Furthermore, the molecular docking studies on both series were also performed to explore their binding interactions.

RESULTS AND DISCUSSION

Chemistry

Two series of coumarinyl thiazoles **6(a–o)** and oxadiazoles **11(a–h)** were prepared with the aim to identify new and potent inhibitors of acetylcholinesterase and butyrylcholinesterase. Coumarinyl thiazole derivatives **6(a–o)** were accessed through a multi-component reaction approach which starts with the preparation of 3-(2-bromoacetyl)-2*H*-chromen-2-one **(3)** *via* base-catalyzed condensation of readily available starting materials (salicylaldehyde and ethyl acetoacetate) followed by bromination (**Scheme 1**; Ibrar et al., 2016). An acid-catalyzed one-pot reaction of intermediate **3**, different substituted acetophenones **(4)** and thiosemicarbazide **(5)** provided the title compounds **6(a–o)** in good yields (Ibrar et al., 2016).

In a second series, coumarinyl oxadiazole-2(3*H*)-thione conjugates **11(a–h)**, the central intermediate 3-(5-thioxo-4,5-dihydro-1,3,4-oxadiazol-2-yl)-2*H*-chromen-2-one **(8)** was prepared by the reaction of coumarinyl hydrazide **(7)** with carbon disulfide in ethanolic solution of KOH in good yield (Pattan et al., 2009). A one-pot reaction of compound **8**, paraformaldehyde **(9)** and different (aliphatic and aromatic) amines **(10)** gave the desired compounds **11(a–h)** in good yields (**Scheme 2**). The compounds were characterized by various spectroscopic techniques and full spectro-analytical data is described in our recent report (Ibrar et al., 2016).

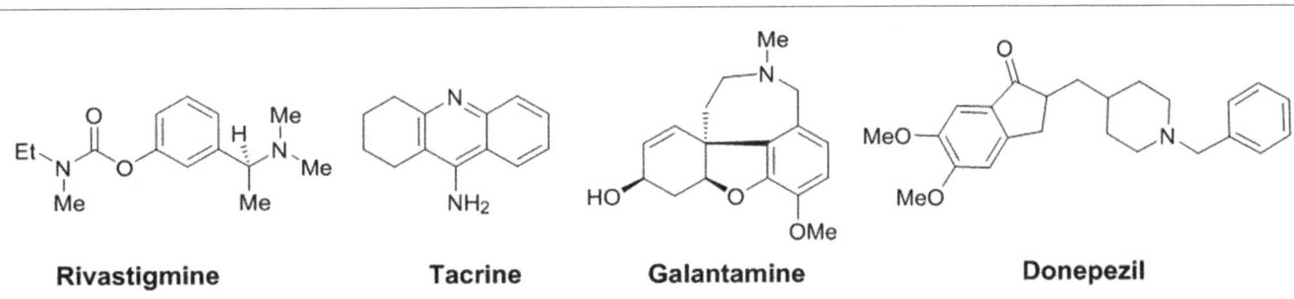

FIGURE 1 | Cholinesterase inhibitors used in AD therapy.

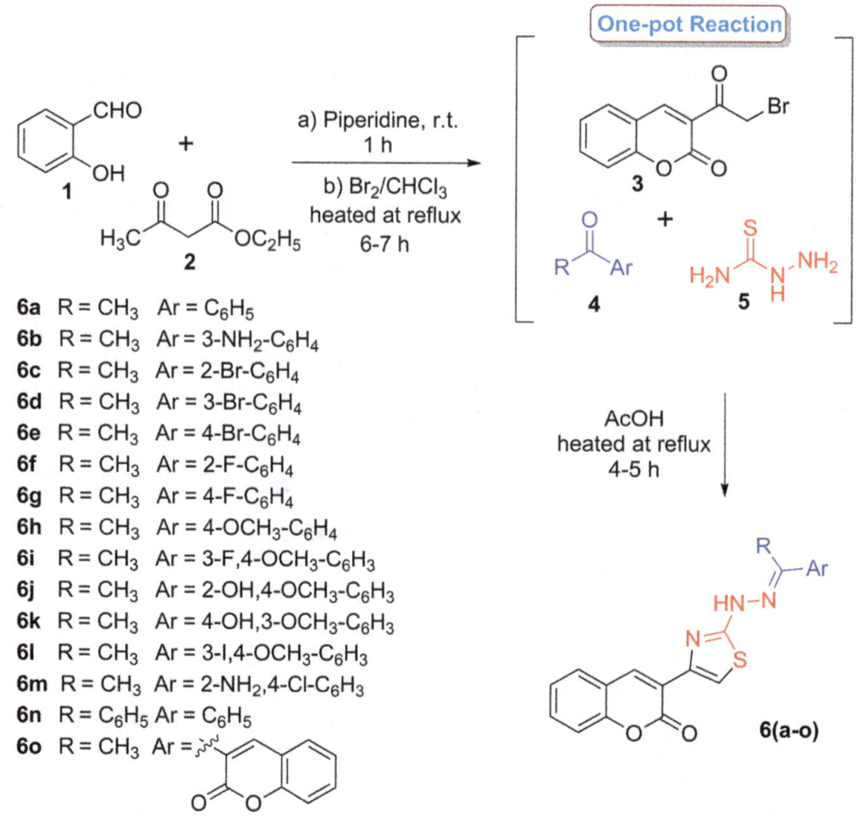

SCHEME 1 | One-pot multi-component synthetic protocol for the preparation of coumarinyl thiazole derivatives **6(a–o)**.

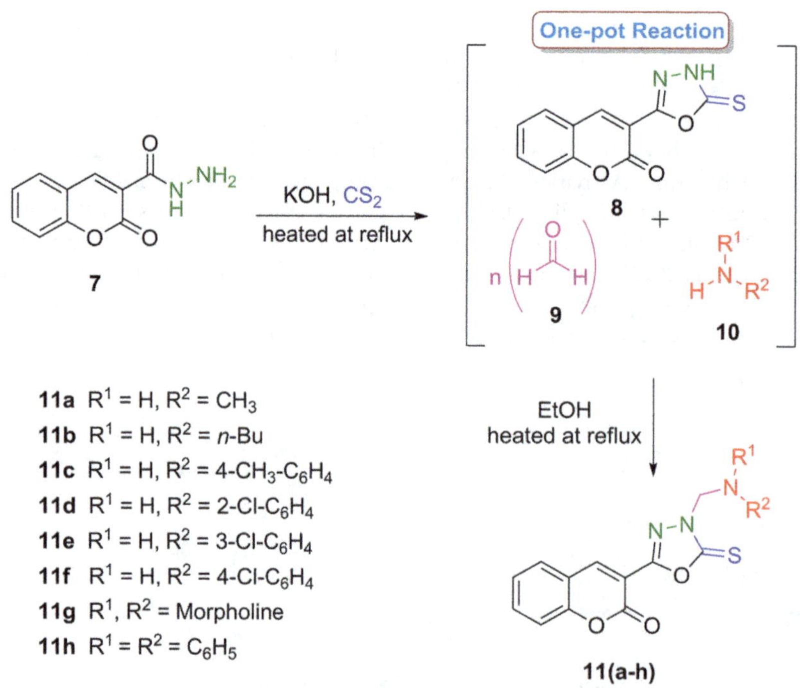

SCHEME 2 | One-pot multi-component synthetic protocol for the preparation of coumarin-oxadiazole-2(3*H*)-thione conjugates **11(a–h)**.

TABLE 1 | Inhibition potency of coumarinyl thiazoles **6(a–o)** against AChE and BuChE.

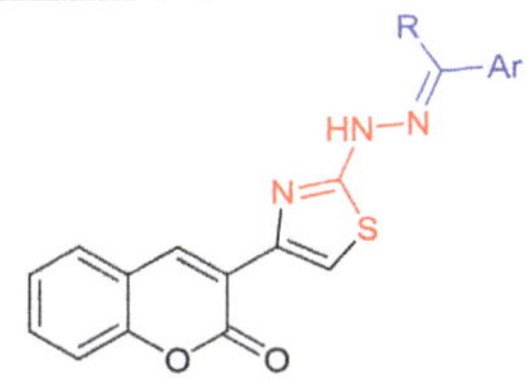

6(a-o)

Compound	Substituent (R)	Substituent (Ar)	AChE	BuChE	Selectivity for	
			IC_{50} (μM) ± SEM[a]		AChE	BuChE
6a	Me	Ph	16.91 ± 0.32	32.7 ± 2.08	1.93	0.51
6b	Me	3-NH_2-Ph	0.87 ± 0.09	31.22 ± 0.17	35.8	0.027
6c	Me	2-Br-Ph	21.19 ± 0.23	19.33 ± 1.42	0.91	1.09
6d	Me	3-Br-Ph	30.06 ± 1.73	15.16 ± 0.53	0.50	1.98
6e	Me	4-Br-Ph	33.42 ± 0.18	49.12 ± 0.12	1.47	0.68
6f	Me	2-F-Ph	23.06 ± 0.32	32.07 ± 1.21	1.39	0.71
6g	Me	4-F-Ph	36.34 ± 0.18	28.01 ± 0.21	0.77	1.29
6h	Me	4-OMe-Ph	1.08 ± 0.84	19.32 ± 0.11	17.8	0.055
6i	Me	3-F-4-OMe-Ph	2.34 ± 1.43	22.1 ± 1.08	9.44	0.105
6j	Me	2-OH-4-OMe-Ph	9.05 ± 0.23	11.01 ± 3.37	1.22	0.81
6k	Me	4-OH-3-OMe-Ph	5.86 ± 0.15	19.13 ± 1.32	3.29	0.303
6l	Me	3-I-4-OMe-Ph	13.84 ± 1.58	32.1 ± 1.08	2.32	0.42
6m	Me	2-NH_2-4-Cl-Ph	22.74 ± 0.16	37.17 ± 0.55	1.63	0.61
6n	Ph	Ph	11.19 ± 0.17	21.6 ± 3.09	1.94	0.51
6o	Me	Coumarin	10.1 ± 1.12	23.19 ± 0.29	2.28	0.43
Neostigmine	–	–	28.2 ± 2.01	16.1 ± 1.13	0.57	1.75
Donepezil	–	–	7.23 ± 0.13	0.03 ± 0.003	0.004	241

[a] *SEM, Standard mean error of three experiments.*

TABLE 2 | Inhibition potency of coumarinyl oxadiazoles **11(a–h)** against AChE and BuChE.

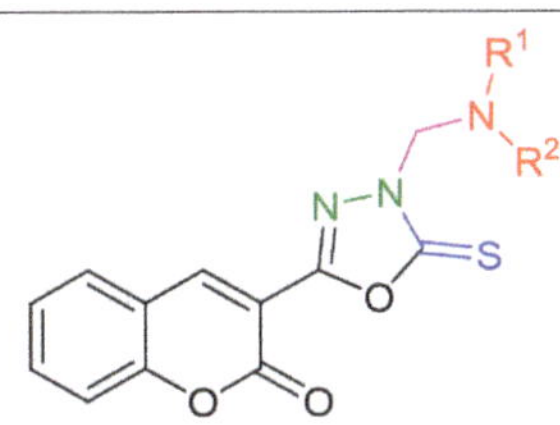

11(a-h)

Compound	Substituent (R^1)	Substituent (R^2)	AChE	BuChE	Selectivity for	
			IC_{50} (μM) ± SEM[a]		AChE	BuChE
11a	H	Me	6.07 ± 0.23	0.341 ± 0.06	0.056	17.8
11b	H	*n*-Bu	9.41 ± 0.55	0.77 ± 0.08	0.081	12.2
11c	H	4-Me-Ph	23.8 ± 0.94	8.01 ± 3.58	0.33	2.97
11d	H	2-Cl-Ph	16.6 ± 2.72	3.48 ± 1.58	0.20	4.77
11e	H	3-Cl-Ph	12.4 ± 0.08	0.15 ± 0.09	0.012	82.6
11f	H	4-Cl-Ph	18.6 ± 0.32	12.1 ± 1.08	0.65	1.53
11g	Ph	Ph	9.57 ± 1.42	4.54 ± 0.54	0.47	2.10
11h	Morpholine		12.2 ± 1.67	13.46 ± 0.41	1.09	0.91
Neostigmine	–	–	28.2 ± 2.01	16.1 ± 1.13	0.57	1.75
Donepezil	–	–	7.23 ± 0.13	0.03 ± 0.003	0.004	241

[a] *SEM, Standard mean error of three experiments.*

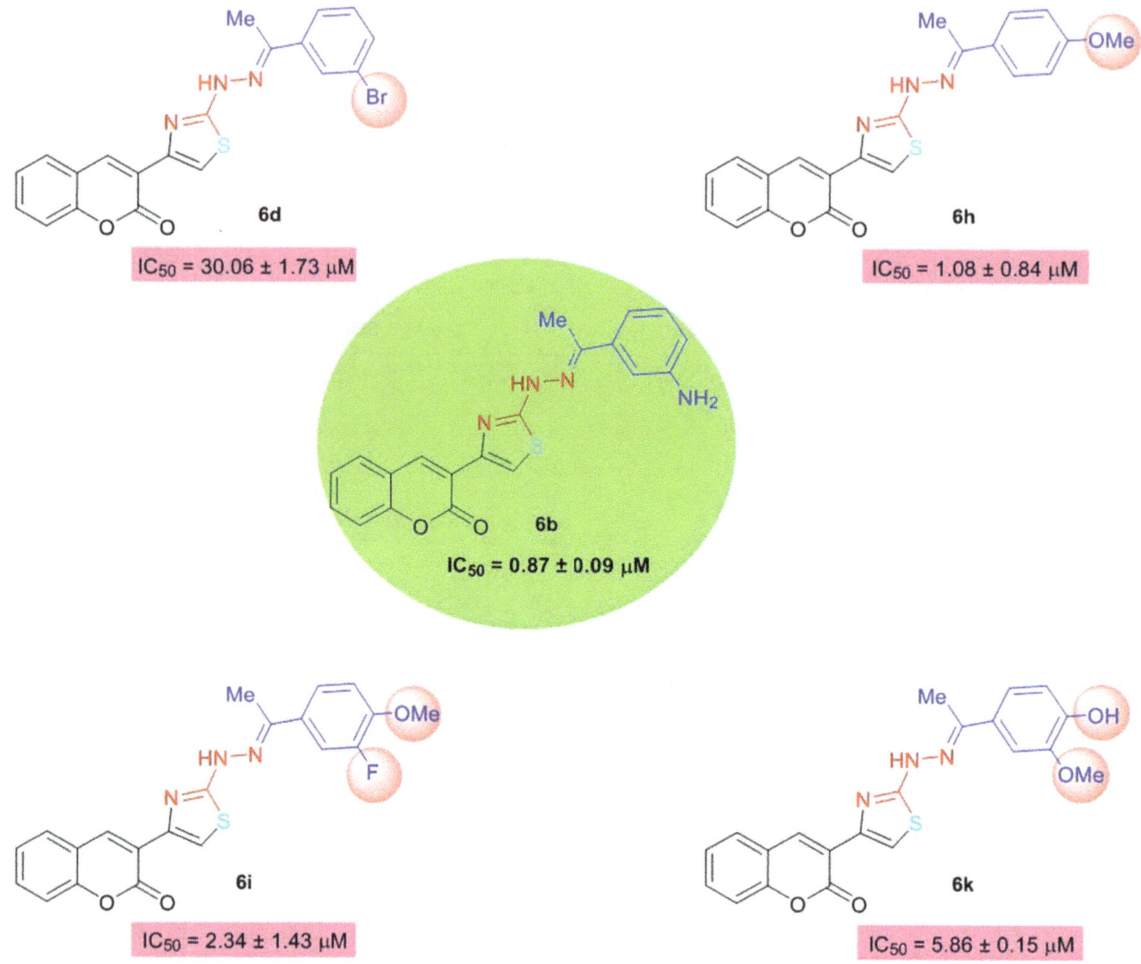

FIGURE 2 | Structure-activity relationship of compound **6b** with **6d**, **6h**, **6i**, and **6k**.

Pharmacology

The target compounds, coumarinyl thiazoles **6(a–o)** and coumarinyl oxadiazoles **11(a–h)**, were screened for their inhibitory activity against AChE and BuChE by Ellman's method. All the assays were carried out at micromolar level using neostigmine and donepezil as standard inhibitors having IC_{50} values of 28.2 ± 2.01 and 7.23 ± 0.13 μM for AChE, whereas 16.1 ± 1.13 and 0.03 ± 0.003 μM for BuChE, respectively. The results obtained for both series **6(a–o)** and **11(a–h)** are summarized in **Tables 1, 2**. The IC_{50} values revealed that most of the synthesized compounds displayed potent and selective inhibition toward cholinesterases.

Among them, **6b** of the coumarinyl thiazole series was found to be the strongest AChE inhibitor with an IC_{50} value of 0.87 ± 0.09 μM (**Table 1**, **Figure 2**). This compound inhibited AChE ~32-fold more strongly than the standard neostigmine, and nine-fold as effective against AChE as the second standard donepezil (IC_{50} = 7.23 ± 0.12 μM). The strong inhibitory potential of **6b** could be credited to the electron-donating amine group present at *meta*-position of the aryl ring. The introduction of a bromo group at the *meta*-position produced comparable results (**6d**; IC_{50} = 30.06 ± 1.73 μM) to the neostigmine. A slight decrease in the inhibition (IC_{50} = 1.08 ± 0.84 μM) was observed in case of compound **6h** having methoxy group at *para*-position but the inhibition was still 26-fold stronger than the standard neostigmine (**Figure 2**). However, compounds **6i** and **6k** bearing a double substitution at the aryl ring showed IC_{50} values of 2.34 ± 1.34 and 5.86 ± 0.15 μM, respectively. These compounds incorporate a combination of different electron-donating and electron-withdrawing groups which could potentially lead to increase the several folds in AChE inhibition than the neostigmine and comparable inhibition (in case of **6k**) to the donepezil (**Figure 2**). In the same series (**6a–o**), a slight decrease in the inhibition was observed in compounds **6j**, **6n**, **6o**, and **6l** as compared to the potent analogs, but the inhibition was still stronger compared to neostigmine.

On the other hand, in the coumarinyl oxadiazole series (**11a–h**), compound **11a** was found to be the most potent AChE inhibitor having IC_{50} value of 6.07 ± 0.23 μM (**Table 2**, **Figure 3**). This inhibitory potency might be attributed to an aliphatic methyl group substituted on the amine moiety. A slight decrease in the inhibition was observed when the methyl group

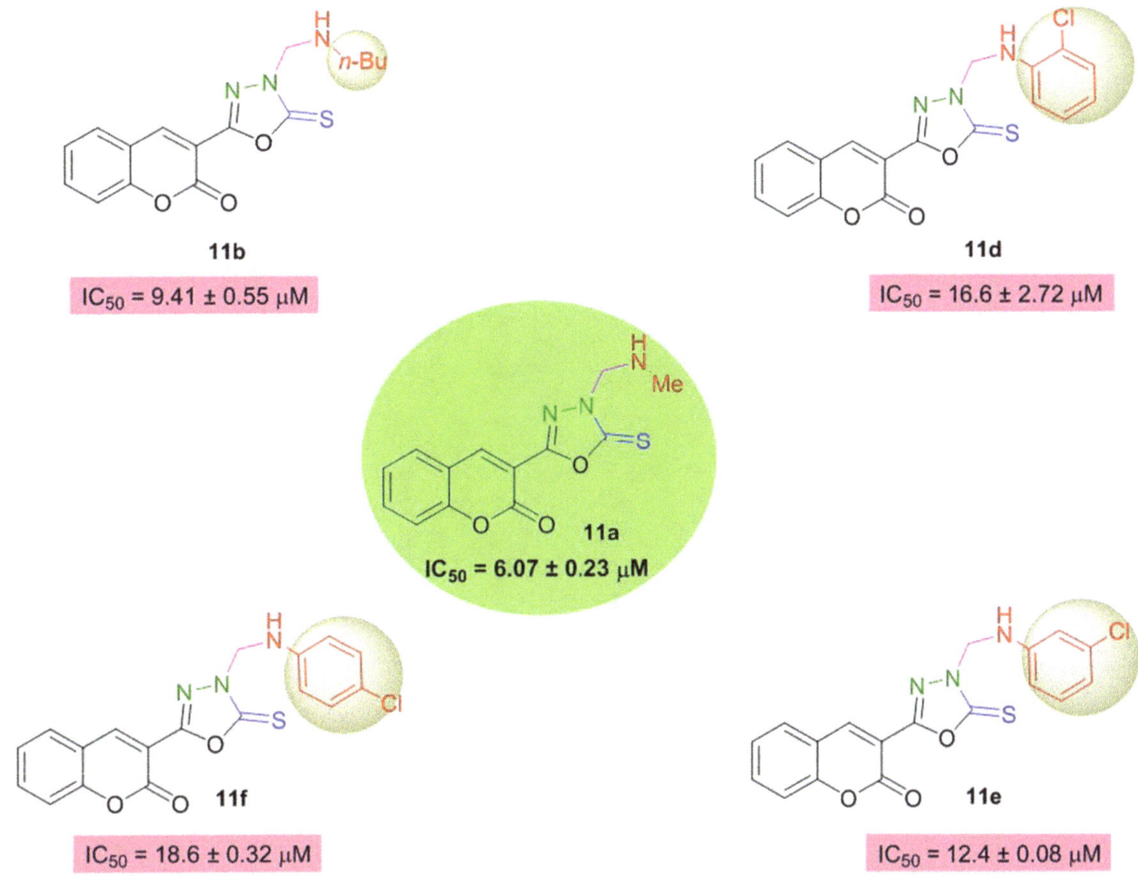

FIGURE 3 | Structure-activity relationship of compound **11a** with **11b** and **11d–f**.

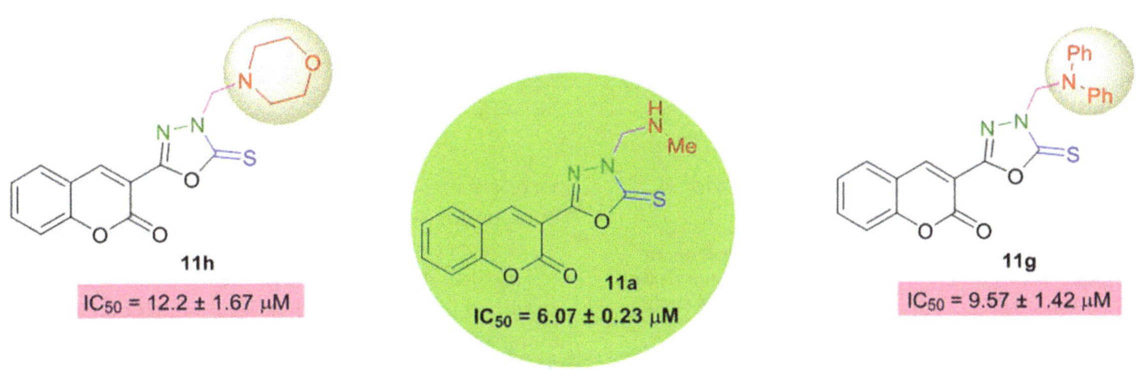

FIGURE 4 | Structure-activity relationship of compound **11a** with **11g** and **11h**.

was replaced by another aliphatic (*n*-Bu) group as revealed by compound **11b** (IC_{50} = 9.41 ± 0.55 μM). When these aliphatic groups were replaced by aromatic substitutions as in **11c–f**, reduced inhibition was observed (**Figure 3**).

Moreover, oxadiazole compounds with morpholine substituent (**11g**) and two phenyl groups (**11h**) were also found as moderate inhibitors of AChE with two- and three-fold higher inhibition as compared to neostigmine (**Figure 4**). Overall, among the tested compounds, coumarinyl thiazoles appeared as potent AChE inhibitors than the coumarinyl oxadiazoles.

All the synthesized analogs were also evaluated for butyrylcholinesterase inhibition and several compounds were found to possess potent inhibitory activity higher than

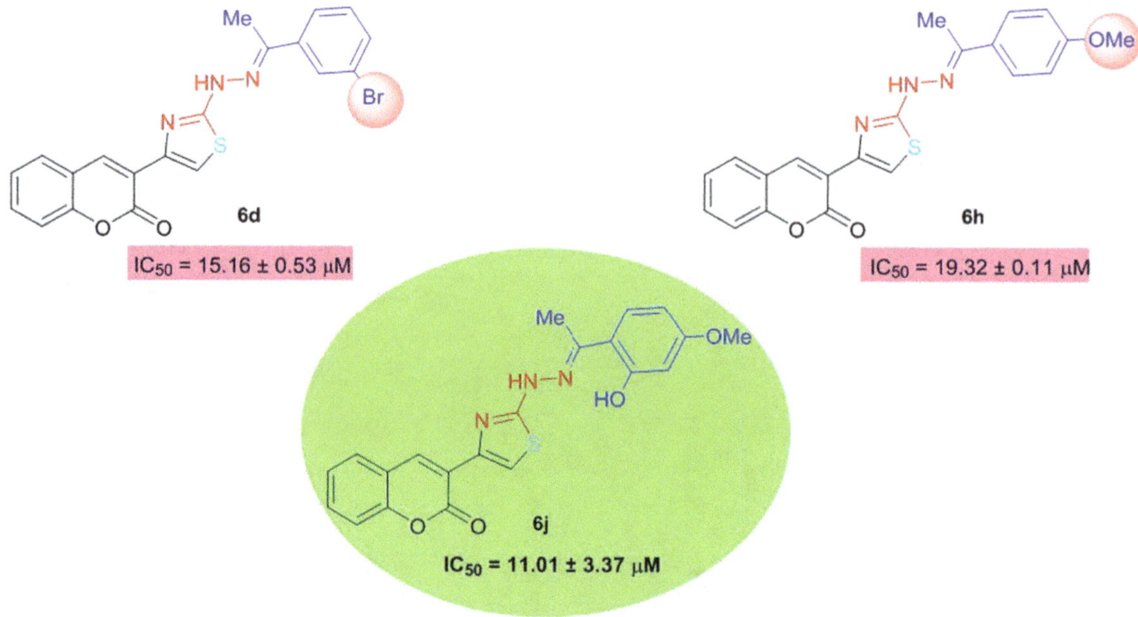

FIGURE 5 | Structure-activity relationship of compound **6j** with **6d** and **6h**.

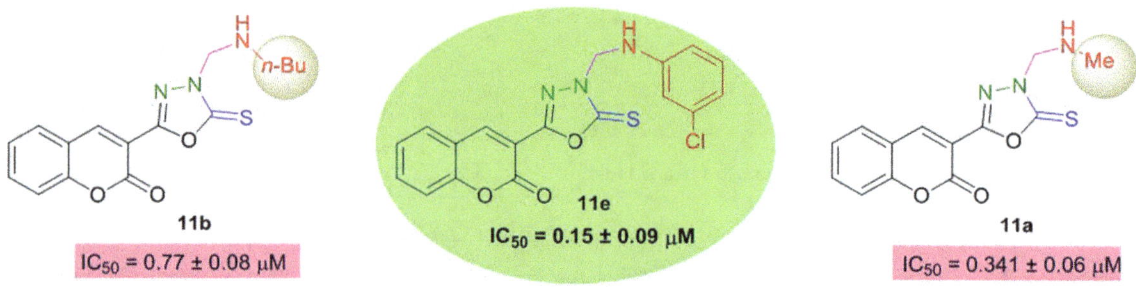

FIGURE 6 | Structure-activity relationship of compound **11e** with **11a** and **11b**.

TABLE 3 | MOE score of highly ranked coumarinyl thiazole and oxadiazole derivatives with the active site of AChE and BuChE.

Compound	MOE score (Kcal.mol^{-1}) with AChE (4EY7)	Compound	MOE score (Kcal.mol^{-1}) with BuChE (4BDS)
6b	−10.19	**11e**	−9.9
6h	−9.97	**11a**	−7.4
6i	−9.68	**11b**	−8.2
6k	−11.03	**11d**	−7.0
Neostigmine	−7.03	**Neostigmine**	−5.05
Donepezil	−9.14	**Donepezil**	−7.75

the standard neostigmine. Among the coumarinyl thiazoles, compound **6j** with dual electron-donating groups was the lead inhibitor with IC_{50} value of 11.01 ± 3.37 μM. Compounds **6d** and **6h** with *meta*-bromo and *para*-methoxy substituents were also moderate inhibitors of BuChE (**Figure 5**). The other compounds in the series showed weak inhibition for BuChE.

However, the coumarinyl oxadiazoles were strong inhibitors of BuChE. Compound **11e** bearing *meta*-chloro substituent inhibited the BuChE with an IC_{50} value of 0.15 ± 0.09 μM. This compound was about 107-fold more potent than neostigmine. The replacement of chloro phenyl with an aliphatic methyl and *n*-Bu group (**11a**; IC_{50} = 0.341 ± 0.06 μM, **11b**; IC_{50} = 0.77 ± 0.08 μM) directed a small decrease in the inhibition but the compounds were still several-folds more active than neostigmine (**Figure 6**). The other compounds in the series **11c, 11d, 11f, 11h,** and **11g** revealed significant inhibition more than the reference standard.

In general, among the synthesized analogs, the compounds from coumarinyl thiazole series (**6a–o**) were excellent AChE inhibitors than the two reference drugs neostigmine and donepezil while coumarinyl oxadiazoles (**11a–h**) showed strong inhibition for BuChE than the standard neostigmine. All in

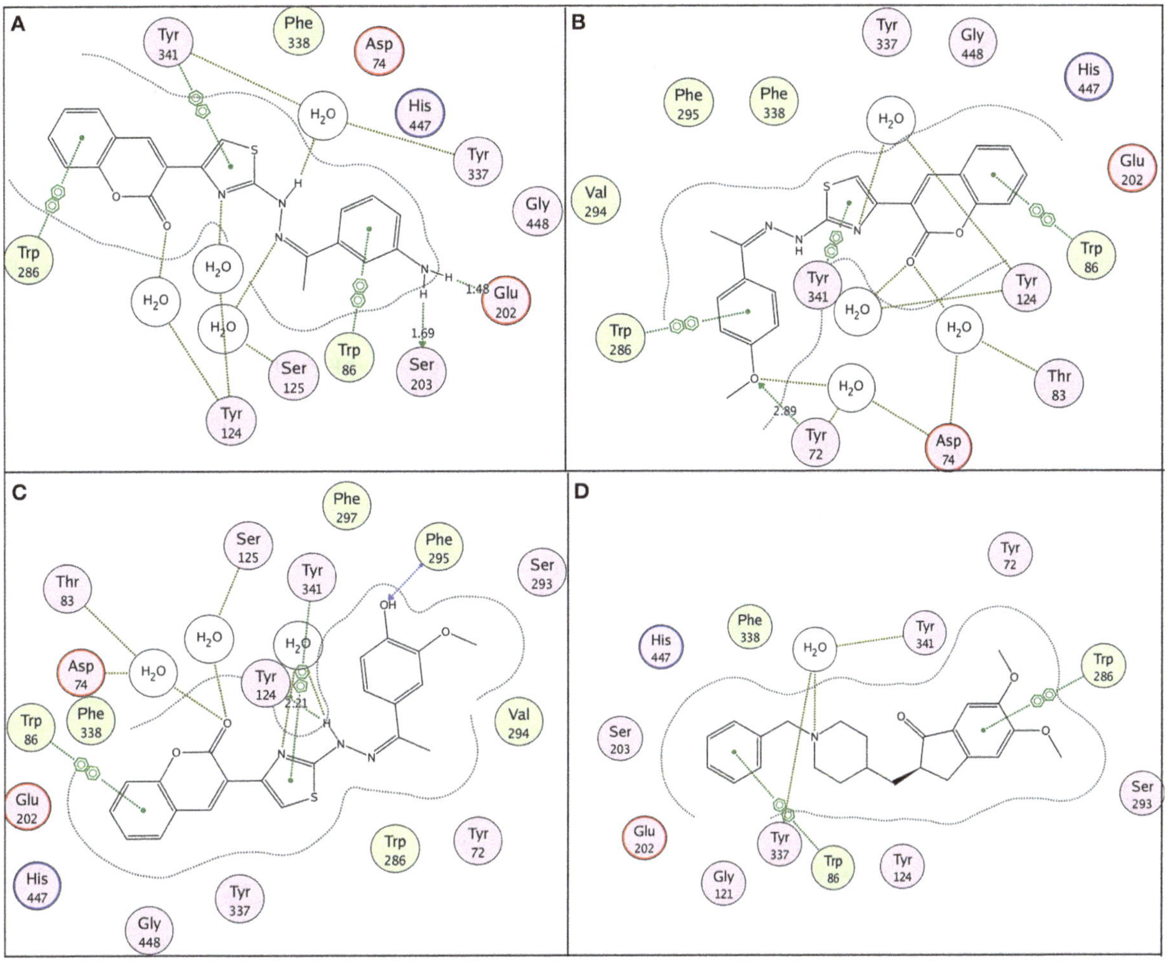

FIGURE 7 | 2D binding pose representation of compound **(A) 6b**, **(B) 6h**, **(C) 6k**, and **(D) donepezil** with the active site of AChE (4EY7) chain A.

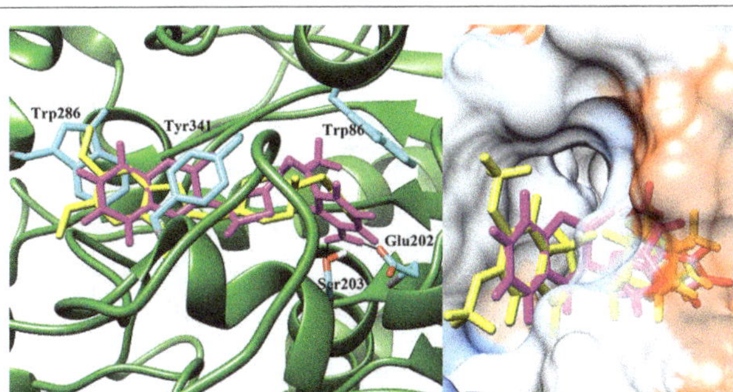

FIGURE 8 | (a) 3D ribbon model of AChE (4EY7) chain A (green) docked with compound **6b** (magenta) and co-crystalized ligand **donepezil** (yellow). Interacting residues shown in ball and stick model (cyan). Black solid lines represent hydrogen bonding. **(b)** Hydrophobic surface model and active site cavity of the enzyme bound with donepezil (yellow) and compound **6b** (magenta).

all, the target analogs proved to be very potent inhibitors of cholinesterase and by considering their strong inhibitory potential, these heterocyclic hybrid compounds hold great potential for the development of new targets for AD therapy.

Molecular Docking Studies

Possible binding modes of coumarinyl thiazole and oxadiazole derivatives were explored by MOE (Molecular Operating Environment) software. Molecular docking studies revealed that the thiazoles having high anti-acetylcholinesterase activity (**6b, 6h, 6i,** and **6k**) represented better interaction with the active site of AChE (4EY7) with MOE score of −10.19, −9.97, −9.68, and −11.03 Kcal.mol^{-1}, respectively, whereas oxadiazoles having high activity against butyrylcholinesterase (**11e, 11a,** and **11b**) represented better interaction with BuChE (4BDS) with MOE score of −9.9, −7.4, and −8.2 Kcal.mol^{-1}, respectively, as compared to reference ligands (neostigmine and donepezil) as shown in **Table 3**. Compound **6b** (IC_{50} = 0.87 ± 0.09 μM) demonstrated conventional hydrogen bonding with Glu202 (1.48 Å) and Ser203 (1.69 Å) due to amino group of aryl ring and π-π stacking with Trp86, Trp286, and Tyr341 along with water bridging with Tyr337, Tyr124, and Ser125 as shown in **Figure 7A**. The impact of amino group on the activity of compound was already mentioned earlier in the structure-activity relationship

(**Figure 2**). Compound **6h** ($IC_{50} = 1.08 \pm 0.84\,\mu M$) represented hydrogen bonding with Tyr72 (2.89 Å) and π-π stacking with Trp86, Trp286, and Tyr341 and Phe338 along with water bridging with Tyr72, Tyr124, and Thr83 as shown in **Figure 7B**. Compound **6i** ($IC_{50} = 2.34 \pm 1.43\,\mu M$) also demonstrated almost similar interactions (as with compound **6h**) except the length of hydrogen bond with Tyr72 (2.93 Å). Compound **6k** represented hydrogen bond with Tyr124 (2.21 Å), π-π stacking with Trp86 and Tyr341 (not with Trp286) and water bridging with Thr83, Ser125, and Asp74 as shown in **Figure 7C**. Reference compound (co-crystallized ligand) donepezil was also docked to compare and confirm our docking results where it was observed that it makes only π-π stacking with Trp86 and Trp286 along with water bridging with Tyr337 and Tyr341 as shown in **Figure 7D**. In agreement to the *in-vitro* results, molecular docking studies suggested that compounds **6b, 6h, 6i,** and **6k** represented better interaction than donepezil; (i) due to hydrogen bonding, (ii) due to extra π-π stacking with aromatic residues, and (iii) due to more interaction through water bridging as shown in **Figure 7**. Active site of the enzyme ribbon model (4EY7) and molecular docking comparison of the most active compound **6b** (magenta) with reference ligand donepezil (yellow) was depicted in **Figure 8a**, whereas hydrophobic surface and active site cavity of the enzyme docked with compound **6b** (magenta) was represented in **Figure 8b**.

According to molecular docking results, the highest ranked anti-butyrylcholinesterase compound **11e** ($IC_{50} = 0.15 \pm 0.09\,\mu M$) illustrated π-π stacking with Trp82 and interaction through water bridging with Asp70 and Ser79 as shown in **Figure 9A**. Compound **11a** ($IC_{50} = 0.34 \pm 0.06\,\mu M$) and **11b** ($IC_{50} = 0.77 \pm 0.08\,\mu M$) represented conventional hydrogen bonding with Glu197 (1.5 Å) and Ser198 (3.0 Å), respectively as shown in **Figures 9B,C**. However their low affinity binding poses also demonstrated π-π stacking with Trp82 and water bridging. Reference ligand donepezil represented π-π stacking with Trp82 and interaction through water bridging with Asp70,

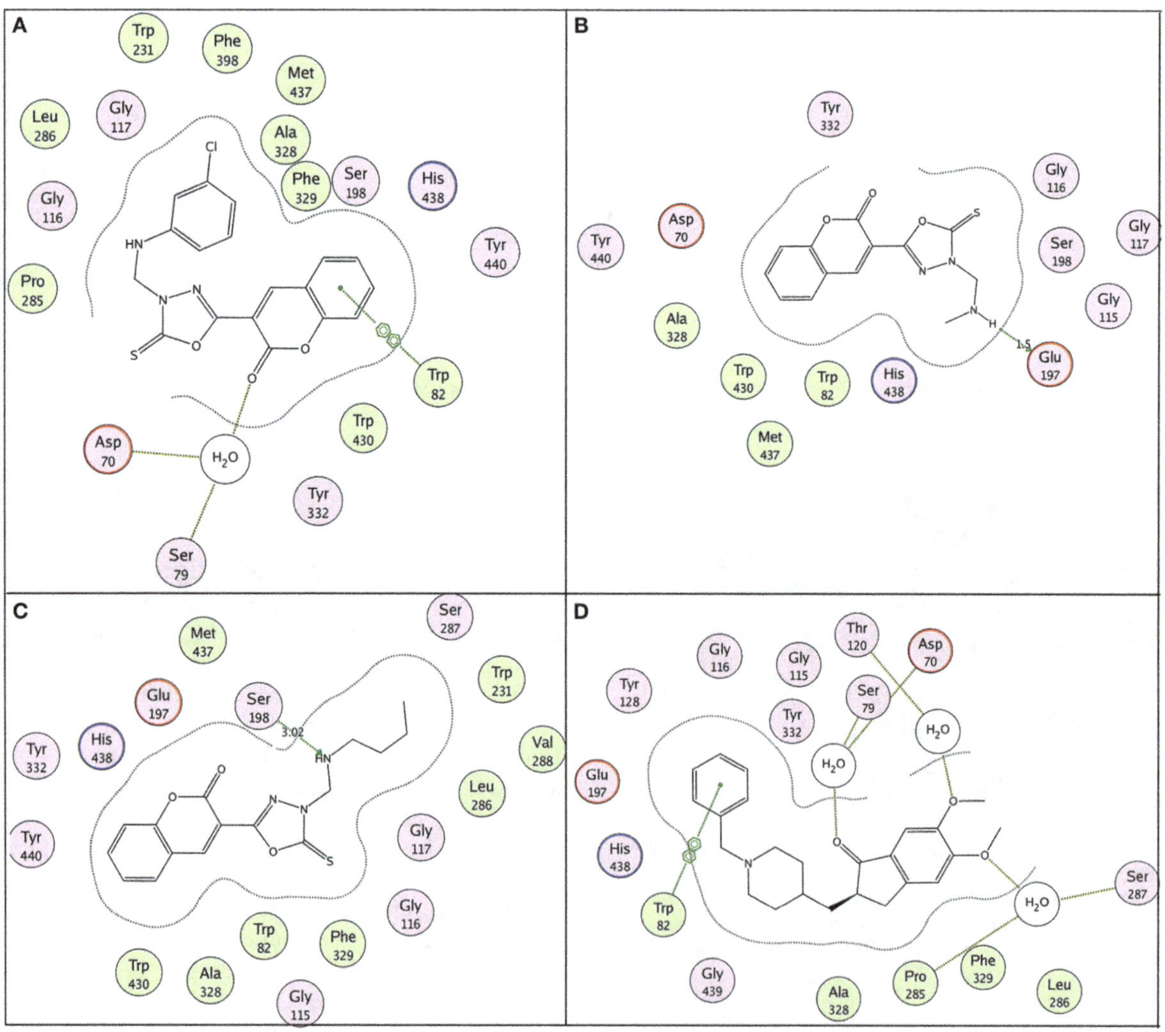

FIGURE 9 | 2D binding pose representation of compound **(A) 11e**, **(B) 11a**, **(C) 11b**, and **(D) donepezil** with the active site of BuChE (4BDS).

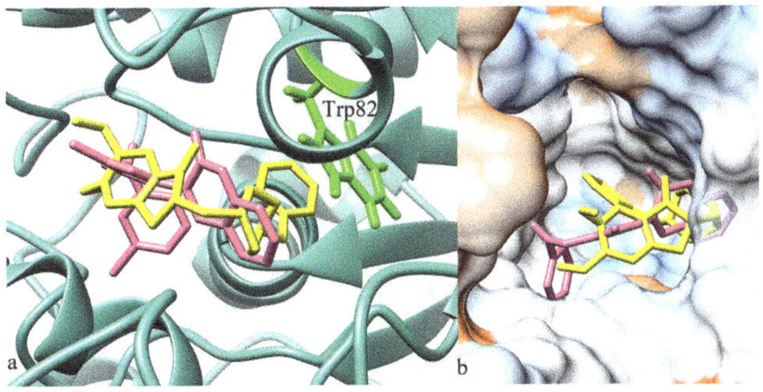

FIGURE 10 | (a) 3D ribbon model (blue) of BuChE (4BDS) docked with compound **11e** (pink) and reference ligand **donepezil** (yellow). **(b)** Hydrophobic surface and active site cavity of the enzyme bound with donepezil (yellow) and compound **11e** (pink).

TABLE 4 | Pharmacokinetics prediction of top ranked compounds.

Compound	MW	LogP	MR	HBD	HBA	nROT	tPSA	BBB	LD_{50}
6b	376.5	3.5	109	3	6	4	93	−ve	937.3
6h	391.4	4.5	110	1	6	5	77	+ve	523.0
6i	409.5	5.1	111	1	6	5	77	+ve	1,188
11a	289.3	1.4	77	1	6	3	73	+ve	N/A
11e	385.8	3.79	103	1	6	4	73	+ve	N/A

Ser79, Thr120, Ser287, and Pro285 as shown in **Figure 9D**. Docking comparison of compound **11e** (pink) with reference ligand donepezil (yellow) in the active site of BuChE (4BDS) ribbon model and surface model was depicted in **Figures 10a,b**, respectively.

Pharmacokinetics Prediction

Early prediction of *in-silico* ADMET properties of lead molecules has now realized as an effective tool in the drug discovery and development process. Therefore, Lipinski's criteria and oral rat LD_{50} value were estimated for top ranked active compounds by using TEST (Toxicity Estimation Software Tool) and Molinspiration online software. Top **five** compounds selected from coumarinyl thiazoles and oxadiazole (6b, 6h, 6i, 11a, and 11e) for the analysis and results were summarized in **Table 4**. Polar surface area (tPSA) values are important for the determination of blood brain barrier (BBB) penetration. According to Waterbeemd the cutoff value is 90 $Å^2$ or less. Almost all the compounds fulfilled the criteria except compound 6b with cutoff value slightly higher i.e., 93. Number of rotatable bonds (nROT) is an additional property that measures the flexibility of the molecule. The drugs that are BBB +ve, usually reported to have fewer nROT bonds. Another extension in RO5 to improve the prediction of drug-likeness is molar refractivity (MR) which should be 40–130. Oral rat LD_{50} was also predicted for these compounds and the compounds were found slightly toxic according to Hodge and Sterner scale. All the criteria were fulfilled by the compounds and no Lipinski's violation was found as shown in **Table 4**.

CONCLUSIONS

In summary, the present report clearly revealed that the new hybrid molecules show remarkable inhibition of AChE and BuChE enzymes. Compound **6b** from coumarinyl thiazole series was emerged as the most potent inhibitor of AChE, whereas **11e** from coumarinyl oxadiazole derivatives inhibited the BuChE with highest potency. Both the identified inhibitors follow Lipinski's RO5, slightly toxic and near the range of blood brain barrier crossing. In future, these compounds and their functionalized derivatives may be helpful in the development of potent drugs for Alzheimer's disease.

EXPERIMENTAL

Synthesis of Coumarinyl Thiazole 6(a–o) and Oxadiazole 11(a–h) Derivatives

The coumarinyl thiazole **6(a–o)** and oxadiazole **11(a–h)** analogs were prepared according to our recently published report (Ibrar et al., 2016).

Pharmacological Protocols

Methodology for Determining AChE and BuChE Inhibitory Activity

For the determination of cholinesterase inhibition, electric eel, and horse serum were used as source of AChE and BuChE, respectively. The Ellman's spectrophotometric method was used to determine the AChE and BuChE inhibitory activity with a slight modification (Ellman et al., 1961). The compounds with 1 Mm concentration were prepared in DMSO. Assay was carried out in 96 well-plate in triplicates. The reaction mixture comprised of 20 μL of buffer (tris HCl 50 mM, 0.02 M $MgCl_2.6H_2O$, 0.1 mM NaCl) at pH 8, 10 μL of the test compound, 10 μL enzyme acetylcholine or butyrylcholinesterase of 0.03 U/mL (500 U of AChE and 700 U/mg of BuChE). The contents were incubated for 10 min at 25°C followed by the addition of 1 mM of 10 μL of substrate acetylcholine iodide for AChE and butyrylthiocholine iodide for BuChE and incubated again at 25°C for 15 min. A 50 μL of 3 mM DTNB as a coloring agent was added and incubated at 25°C for further 10 min. The amount of product formed was measured by using micro plate reader (Bio-Tek ELx 800, Instruments Inc., Winooski, VT, USA) at 405 nm. The enzyme dilutions were made by using buffer of pH 8 (tris base 50 mM and having 0.1% BSA). The compounds which depict inhibitory activity more than 50% were further tested by making 9–12 serial dilutions in assay buffer and IC_{50} values were calculated by graph pad prism.

Molecular Docking

The molecular construction of the compounds was performed using ChemBioDraw Ultra 14 suite (PerkinElmer Inc.) and converted into 3D conformations by ChemBio3D (Mills, 2006). Molecular docking studies of the compounds were carried out using MOE (Molecular Operating Environment) software (ChemicalComputingGroup, 2008). The structures of the compounds were energy minimized using MMFF94x forcefield and gradient: 0.05. Crystal structures of the enzymes, acetylcholinesterase (PDB: 4EY7) and butyrylcholinesterase (PDB: 4BDS) were retrieved from Protein Data Bank (Berman et al., 2006). The co-crystallized ligands in the active site of AChE and BuChE, donepezil (PDB: E20), and Tacrine (PDB: THA) were taken as possible binding site. Ligand neostigmine was taken from PubChem (CID:4456) (Kim et al., 2015). The target proteins were prepared by the addition of hydrogen. All other parameters were used with the default settings. Donepezil and neostigmine were taken as reference ligands for comparison purposes. For each ligand 10 conformations were generated. The images in 2D were captured through MOE ligand binding interaction. 3D images were taken using UCSF Chimera 1.11 software (Pettersen et al., 2004).

AUTHOR CONTRIBUTIONS

All authors listed have made a substantial, direct and intellectual contribution to the work, and approved it for publication.

ACKNOWLEDGMENTS

Generous support from Higher Education Commission of Pakistan (project No. 21- 978/SRGP/R&D/HEC/2016) is gratefully acknowledged.

REFERENCES

Bartolini, M., Bertucci, C., Cavrini, V., and Andrisano, V. (2003). β-Amyloid aggregation induced by human acetylcholinesterase: inhibition studies. *Biochem. Pharmacol.* 65, 407–416. doi: 10.1016/S0006-2952(02)01514-9

Berman, H. M., Westbrook, J., Feng, Z., Gilliland, G., Bhat, T. N., Weissig, H., et al. (2006). "The protein data bank, 1999–," in *International Tables for Crystallography Volume F: Crystallography of Biological Macromolecules*, eds M. G. Rossmann and E. Arnold (Dordrecht: Springer), 675–684. doi: 10.1107/97809553602060000722

Campiglia, P., Scrima, M., Grimaldi, M., Cioffi, G., Bertamino, A., Sala, M., et al. (2009). A new series of 1, 3-Dihidro-Imidazo [1, 5-c] thiazole-5, 7-Dione derivatives: synthesis and interaction with Aβ (25-35) Amyloid Peptide. *Chem. Biol. Drug Des.* 74, 224–233. doi: 10.1111/j.1747-0285.2009.00853.x

ChemicalComputingGroup, M. (2008). *Molecular Operating Environment: Chemical Computing Group Montreal.* Quebec, QC.

Chiou, S. Y., Huang, C. F., Hwang, M. T., and Lin, G. (2009). Comparison of active sites of butyrylcholinesterase and acetylcholinesterase based on inhibition by geometric isomers of benzene-di-N-substituted carbamates. *J. Biochem. Mol. Toxicol.* 23, 303–308. doi: 10.1002/jbt.20286

Cummings, J. L., Doody, R., and Clark, C. (2007). Disease-modifying therapies for Alzheimer disease challenges to early intervention. *Neurology* 69, 1622–1634. doi: 10.1212/01.wnl.0000295996.54210.69

Cygler, M., Schrag, J. D., Sussman, J. L., Harel, M., Silman, I., Gentry, M. K., et al. (1993). Relationship between sequence conservation and three-dimensional structure in a large family of esterases, lipases, and related proteins. *Protein Sci.* 2, 366–382. doi: 10.1002/pro.5560020309

de Souza, L. G., Rennó, M. N., and Figueroa-Villar, J. D. (2016). Coumarins as cholinesterase inhibitors: a review. *Chem. Biol. Interact.* 254, 11–23. doi: 10.1016/j.cbi.2016.05.001

Ellman, G. L., Courtney, K. D., Andres, V. Jr, and Featherstone, R. M. (1961). A new and rapid colorimetric determination of acetylcholinesterase activity. *Biochem. Pharmacol.* 7, 88–95. doi: 10.1016/0006-2952(61)90145-9

Groner, E., Ashani, Y., Schorer-Apelbaum, D., Sterling, J., Herzig, Y., and Weinstock, M. (2007). The kinetics of inhibition of human acetylcholinesterase and butyrylcholinesterase by two series of novel carbamates. *Mol. Pharmacol.* 71, 1610–1617. doi: 10.1124/mol.107.033928

Hang, P. C., and Honek, J. F. (2005). Electronic structure calculations on the thiazole-containing antibiotic thiostrepton: molecular mechanics, semi-empirical and ab initio analyses. *Bioorg. Med. Chem. Lett.* 15, 1471–1474. doi: 10.1016/j.bmcl.2004.12.076

Helal, M. H., Salem, M. A., El-Gaby, M. S., and Aljahdali, M. (2013). Synthesis and biological evaluation of some novel thiazole compounds as potential anti-inflammatory agents. *Eur. J. Med. Chem.* 65, 517–526. doi: 10.1016/j.ejmech.2013.04.005

Ibrar, A., Tehseen, Y., Khan, I., Hameed, A., Saeed, A., Furtmann, N., et al. (2016). Coumarin-thiazole and-oxadiazole derivatives: synthesis, bioactivity and docking studies for aldose/aldehyde reductase inhibitors. *Bioorg. Chem.* 68, 177–186. doi: 10.1016/j.bioorg.2016.08.005

Jaishree, V., Ramdas, N., Sachin, J., and Ramesh, B. (2012). *In vitro* antioxidant properties of new thiazole derivatives. *J. Saudi Chem. Soc.* 16, 371–376. doi: 10.1016/j.jscs.2011.02.007

Kashman, Y., Gustafson, K. R., Fuller, R. W., Cardellina, J. H., McMahon, J. B., Currens, M. J., et al. (1992). HIV inhibitory natural products. Part 7. The calanolides, a novel HIV-inhibitory class of coumarin derivatives from the tropical rainforest tree, Calophyllum lanigerum. *J. Med. Chem.* 35, 2735–2743.

Kim, S., Thiessen, P. A., Bolton, E. E., Chen, J., Fu, G., Gindulyte, A., et al. (2015). PubChem substance and compound databases. *Nucleic Acids Res.* 44, D1202–D1213. doi: 10.1093/nar/gkv951

Klimesová, V., Zahajská, L., Waisser, K., Kaustová, J., and Möllmann, U. (2004). Synthesis and antimycobacterial activity of 1, 2, 4-triazole 3-benzylsulfanyl derivatives. *Il Farmaco.* 59, 279–288. doi: 10.1016/j.farmac.2004.01.006

Maddi, V., Mamledesai, S., Satyanarayana, D., and Swamy, S. (2007). Synthesis and antiinflammatory activity of substituted (2-oxochromen-3-yl) benzamides. *Indian J. Pharm. Sci.* 69, 847–849. doi: 10.4103/0250-474X.39452

Manvar, A., Bavishi, A., Radadiya, A., Patel, J., Vora, V., Dodia, N., et al. (2011). Diversity oriented design of various hydrazides and their in vitro evaluation against *Mycobacterium tuberculosis* H37Rv strains. *Bioorg. Med. Chem. Lett.* 21, 4728–4731. doi: 10.1016/j.bmcl.2011.06.074

Martin-Aragón, S., de las Heras, B., Sanchez-Reus, M. I., and Benedi, J. (2001). Pharmacological modification of endogenous antioxidant enzymes by ursolic acid on tetrachloride-induced liver damagein rats and primary cultures of rat hepatocytes. *Exp. Toxicol. Pathol.* 53, 199–206. doi: 10.1078/0940-2993-00185

Mesulam, M. M., Guillozet, A., Shaw, P., Levey, A., Duysen, E. G., and Lockridge, O. (2002). Acetylcholinesterase knockouts establish central cholinergic pathways and can use butyrylcholinesterase to hydrolyze acetylcholine. *Neuroscience* 110, 627–639. doi: 10.1016/S0306-4522(01)00613-3

Mills, N. (2006). *ChemDraw Ultra 10.0 CambridgeSoft, 100 CambridgePark Drive*, Cambridge, MA: Commercial Price: 1910fordownload, 2150 for CD-ROM; Academic Price: 710fordownload, 800 for CD-ROM: ACS Publications. Available online at: www. cambridgesoft. com

Naveena, C. S., Poojary, B., Arulmoli, T., Manjunatha, K., Prabhu, A., and Kumari, N. S. (2013). Synthesis and evaluation of biological and nonlinear optical properties of some novel 2, 4-disubstituted [1, 3]-thiazoles carrying 2-(aryloxymethyl)-phenyl moiety. *Med. Chem. Res.* 22, 1925–1937. doi: 10.1007/s00044-012-0195-7

Olmedo, D., Sancho, R., Bedoya, L. M., López-Pérez, J. L., Del Olmo, E., Muñoz, E., et al. (2012). 3-Phenylcoumarins as inhibitors of HIV-1 replication. *Molecules* 17, 9245–9257. doi: 10.3390/molecules17089245

Pattan, S. R., Rabara, P., Pattan, J. S., Bukitagar, A., Wakale, V., and Musmade, D. (2009). Synthesis and evaluation of some novel substituted 1, 3, 4-oxadiazole and pyrazole derivatives for antitubercular activity. *Indian J. Chem. Sec. B* 48, 1453–1456. Available online at: http://nopr.niscair.res.in/handle/123456789/6111

Pettersen, E. F., Goddard, T. D., Huang, C. C., Couch, G. S., Greenblatt, D. M., Meng, E. C., et al. (2004). UCSF Chimera—a visualization system for exploratory research and analysis. *J. Comput. Chem.* 25, 1605–1612. doi: 10.1002/jcc.20084

Romagnoli, R., Baraldi, P. G., Salvador, M. K., Camacho, M. E., Preti, D., Tabrizi, M. A., et al. (2012). Synthesis and biological evaluation of 2-substituted-4-(3′, 4′, 5′-trimethoxyphenyl)-5-aryl thiazoles as anticancer agents. *Bioorg. Med. Chem.* 20, 7083–7094. doi: 10.1016/j.bmc.2012.10.001

Ronad, P. M., Noolvi, M. N., Sapkal, S., Dharbhamulla, S., and Maddi, V. S. (2010). Synthesis and antimicrobial activity of 7-(2-substituted phenylthiazolidinyl)-benzopyran-2-one derivatives. *Eur. J. Med. Chem.* 45, 85–89. doi: 10.1016/j.ejmech.2009.09.028

Shaker, R. M. (2006). The chemistry of mercapto-and thione-substituted 1, 2, 4-triazoles and their utility in heterocyclic synthesis. *ARKIVOC* 9, 59–112. doi: 10.3998/ark.5550190.0007.904

Siddiqui, N., Arshad, M. F., and Khan, S. A. (2009). Synthesis of some new coumarin incorporated thiazolyl semicarbazones as anticonvulsants. *Acta Pol. Pharm. Drug Res.* 66, 161–167.

Terry, A. V., and Buccafusco, J. (2003). The cholinergic hypothesis of age and Alzheimer's disease-related cognitive deficits: recent challenges and their implications for novel drug development. *J. Pharmacol. Exp. Ther.* 306, 821–827. doi: 10.1124/jpet.102.041616

Venugopala, K. N., Krishnappa, M., Nayak, S. K., Subrahmanya, B. K., Vaderapura, J. P., Chalannavar, R. K., et al. (2013). Synthesis and antimosquito propertiesof 2, 6-substituted benzo [d] thiazole and 2, 4-substituted benzo [d] thiazole analogues against Anopheles arabiensis. *Eur. J. Med. Chem.* 65, 295–303. doi: 10.1016/j.ejmech.2013.04.061

Yavari, I., Malekafzali, A., and Seyfi, S. (2014). A synthesis of functionalized 2-imino-1, 3-thiazoles from tetramethylguanidine, isothiocyanates, and 2-chloro-1, 3-dicarbonyl compounds. *J. Iran. Chem. Soc.* 11, 285–288. doi: 10.1007/s13738-013-0299-0

16

How Diverse are the Protein-Bound Conformations of Small-Molecule Drugs and Cofactors?

Nils-Ole Friedrich [1]*, Méliné Simsir* [1,2] *and Johannes Kirchmair* [1]*

[1] *Department of Informatics, Center for Bioinformatics, Universität Hamburg, Hamburg, Germany,* [2] *Molécules Thérapeutiques In Silico, Université Paris Diderot, Sorbonne Paris Cité, Paris, France*

Correspondence:
Johannes Kirchmair
kirchmair@zbh.uni-hamburg.de

Knowledge of the bioactive conformations of small molecules or the ability to predict them with theoretical methods is of key importance to the design of bioactive compounds such as drugs, agrochemicals, and cosmetics. Using an elaborate cheminformatics pipeline, which also evaluates the support of individual atom coordinates by the measured electron density, we compiled a complete set ("Sperrylite Dataset") of high-quality structures of protein-bound ligand conformations from the PDB. The Sperrylite Dataset consists of a total of 10,936 high-quality structures of 4,548 unique ligands. Based on this dataset, we assessed the variability of the bioactive conformations of 91 small molecules—each represented by a minimum of ten structures—and found it to be largely independent of the number of rotatable bonds. Sixty-nine molecules had at least two distinct conformations (defined by an RMSD greater than 1 Å). For a representative subset of 17 approved drugs and cofactors we observed a clear trend for the formation of few clusters of highly similar conformers. Even for proteins that share a very low sequence identity, ligands were regularly found to adopt similar conformations. For cofactors, a clear trend for extended conformations was measured, although in few cases also coiled conformers were observed. The Sperrylite Dataset is available for download from http://www.zbh.uni-hamburg.de/sperrylite_dataset.

Keywords: bioactive conformational space, protein-bound ligand conformation, conformational variability, PDB, protein-ligand interaction, binding site, small-molecule drug, cofactor

INTRODUCTION

The protein-bound ("bioactive") conformations of ligands can differ substantially from those observed in solution, the gas phase and small-molecule crystal structures (Boström, 2001; Perola and Charifson, 2004; Seeliger and de Groot, 2010). Bioactive conformations can be distributed over large regions of the ligand's conformational space and can have considerable strain energy (Nicklaus et al., 1995; Boström et al., 1998; Boström, 2001; Perola and Charifson, 2004; Günther et al., 2006). For the application of 3D computational approaches such as docking or *de novo* design methods in drug discovery, the protein-bound conformations of small molecules need to be known or at least determinable (Brameld et al., 2008).

The Protein Data Bank (PDB) is the most comprehensive resource of experimental structural data on biomacromolecules and their interaction with small molecules (Berman et al., 2000). Currently, the PDB contains more than 100k structures of biomacromolecules that include a bound ligand. While the structural data available from the PDB are extremely valuable for the research of biomacromolecules and their interactions with small molecules, these data represent only a very small fraction of (known) interactions.

Sturm et al. (2012) investigated the relationship between the promiscuity of drug-like molecules and the molecular properties of ligands and their binding sites. In order to do so, they compiled a dataset of more than 1,000 protein-ligand complexes in which drug-like molecules are bound to at least two distinct proteins. They identified two major drivers of ligand promiscuity: the structural similarities of ligand binding sites (largely independent of the similarities of the overall protein sequences or folds) and the ability of ligands to adopt distinct binding modes for different proteins. The latter is facilitated by the conformational flexibility of ligands and/or the specific characteristics of their pharmacophoric features. In related work, He et al. (2015), analyzed the structures of 100 pharmaceutically relevant ligands bound to at least two different proteins (to which they bind with comparable *in vitro* affinities). Contrary to the common belief that ligand flexibility and promiscuity are correlated, no evidence for a distinct correlation was found within their dataset. In fact, for 59 out of the 100 investigated ligands, no significant changes between the conformers of ligands bound to different proteins were observed.

The relative abundance of available structural data on the conformation of protein-bound cofactors, and nucleotide cofactors in particular, has made them a primary subject of investigation. For example, Moodie and Thornton (1993) analyzed 65 structures of nucleotides bound to proteins and found them to bind predominantly in an extended conformation. In more recent work, Stockwell and Thornton (2006) analyzed the conformational variability of adenosine triphosphate (ATP), nicotinamide adenine dinucleotide (NAD) and flavin adenine dinucleotide (FAD) in a preprocessed set of more than 2,000 structures extracted from the PDB. Dym and Eisenberg (2001) compiled a set of 150 structures of FAD bound to 32 non-redundant flavoproteins. They found a clear correlation between the FAD-family fold, the shape of the cofactor binding site and the conformation of FAD. Bojovschi et al. (2012) investigated the conformational diversity of ATP/Mg:ATP in motor proteins based on a set of 159 X-ray structures extracted from the PDB. They found that ATP adopts a wide range of different conformations, with a preference for extended conformations in tight binding pockets (e.g., F1-ATPase) and compact conformations in motor proteins such as RNA polymerase and DNA helicase. The incorporation of Mg2+ was found to increase the conformational flexibility of ATP. They clustered the conformations of the individual ligands based on the similarity of their binding pockets and, in the case of ATP for example, identified 27 clusters with a mean intercentroid RMSD of more than 2 Å. The authors concluded that, within the individual protein superfamilies, the investigated ligands generally bind in a fairly conserved manner, although several exceptions were identified. In the case of ATP, most structures were found to have the ligand bound in an extended conformation. In few cases however, a conformation bent such that the terminal phosphate atoms are almost in van der Waals contact with the adenine ring was observed. Stegemann and Klebe (2012) explored the structural properties of six cofactors including an adenosine diphosphate moiety bound to a variety of different proteins with low sequence identity. They found that common binding pocket patterns sometimes only recognize parts of the cofactor and thereby induce similar conformations.

These and further studies have contributed substantially to the understanding of protein-bound ligand conformations. However, a major bottleneck is the limited quality (Liebeschuetz et al., 2012; Reynolds, 2014), quantity and diversity of the structural data that these studies are based on, in particular with respect to the uncertainty of atom coordinates that is inherent to crystallographic structures. Only recently, a robust and fully automated method for the assessment of the support of individual atom coordinates (as well as molecules) by the measured electron density (EDIA) has become available (Meyder et al., 2017). This allowed, for the first time, extraction of a complete subset of high-quality structures of protein-bound ligands from the PDB (Friedrich et al., 2017b). Prior to the development of the EDIA method, time-consuming manual inspection by human experts was required to assure the high quality of structural data, which limited the size of available datasets (see e.g., Warren et al., 2012).

In this work we assess the conformational variability of small molecules based on a complete set of high-quality structures of protein-bound ligands extracted from in the PDB, each of which is represented by at least ten high-quality X-ray structures. In total the conformational variability of 91 approved drugs and cofactors represented by 4,574 protein-bound conformations was assessed. The bioactive conformational space of 17 representative molecules was studied in detail.

MATERIALS AND METHODS

Dataset Compilation

The Sperrylite Dataset was extracted from the PDB using a workflow described previously (Friedrich et al., 2017a). It consists of 10,936 conformers of 4,548 unique small molecules. Ninety-one ligands in this dataset are represented by at least 10 structures, and these served as the basis of this analysis.

To ensure that all ligands with the same PDB ligand ID have identical stereochemistry, their isomeric smiles (generated with UNICON, Sommer et al., 2016) were compared in order to keep only the isomer with the most occurrences. The Approved Drugs subset of DrugBank (Wishart et al., 2017) was used to identify the approved drugs present in the Sperrylite Dataset.

RMSD, Rotatable Bonds and Sequence Identity Calculations

All RMSD values were calculated with NAOMI (Urbaczek et al., 2011), which selects the minimum heavy-atom RMSD for the best superposition of each pair of conformers, taking molecular symmetry into account via complete automorphism enumeration.

The number of rotatable bonds was calculated with RDKit (RDKit: Open-Source Cheminformatics, version 2015.09.1, 2015). The default definition was used, meaning that amide and ester bonds were not counted as rotatable bonds.

All-against-all sequence identity was determined with NCBI BLAST (Altschul et al., 1990; BLAST, version 2.2.31. https://blast.ncbi.nlm.nih.gov (accessed Jan 14, 2018); Camacho et al., 2009) and the sequence identity of individual pairs of proteins was measured with the Molecular Operating Environment (Molecular Operating Environment (MOE), version 2016.08; Chemical Computing Group Inc.: Montreal, QC, 2016) based on sequence and structural alignments.

Principal component analysis (PCA)-derived score plots of the alignments with the minimum median RMSDs were generated with R for each ligand.

Visualization

Visualization of the (i) alignments of ligand conformers (ii) alignments of protein structures and (iii) interactions of proteins and ligands were generated with Maestro (Schrödinger Release 2016-2: Maestro, Schrödinger, LLC, New York, NY, 2016), MOE (Molecular Operating Environment (MOE), version 2016.08; Chemical Computing Group Inc.: Montreal, QC, 2016) and LigandScout (LigandScout, version 4.2; Inte:Ligand GmbH: Vienna, Austria, 2017; Wolber and Langer, 2005), respectively.

For the sake of clarity, all hydrogens, only polar hydrogens or no hydrogens were included in the depictions on a case-by-case basis to avoid overcrowded figures.

RESULTS

The Sperrylite Dataset is a collection of all high-quality X-ray structures of small molecules bound to biomacromolecules that are contained in the PDB. The dataset includes 10,936 structures of 4,548 unique protein-bound ligands and was compiled with a recently developed cheminformatics pipeline that automatically (i) prepares the chemical structures of small molecules by taking into account the protein environment (in order to determine, e.g., the most likely tautomeric and protonation states); (ii) removes undesirable molecules such as crystallization aids as well as structures with topological and/or geometrical errors; and (iii) rejects structures of low quality (Friedrich et al., 2017a,b). Importantly, the procedure not only includes checks for resolution and DPI (Cruickshank, 1999), but also employs the recently developed EDIA method (Meyder et al., 2017) to assess the support of individual atoms of a structure by the electron density.

In this study the diversity of the protein-bound conformations of all ligands represented by at least 10 high-quality structures was investigated. This dataset consists of a total of 4,574 conformations of 91 unique ligands (an overview of all structures is provided in Scheme S1), including more than 30 nucleotides and 20 approved drug molecules. In an all-against-all comparison of the differences in conformation of each ligand as measured by RMSD, 81 of the 91 ligands had at least one conformer with an RMSD above 0.6 Å (which corresponds to the maximum positional uncertainty for atoms in the Sperrylite Dataset), and 69 had at least one conformer above 1 Å, meaning that they are clearly distinct. The correlation observed between the minimum median RMSD measured for all pairs of conformations and the number of rotatable bonds was (very) weak ($R^2 = 0.126$; Figure S1).

This work focuses on the analysis of the bioactive conformational space of a representative set of 17 approved drugs and cofactors (**Tables 1**, **2**; note that there is an overlap between cofactors and approved drugs). This set was compiled with the objective to include the most relevant and best-represented small molecules in a detailed analysis of individual ligands.

Definitions

In the following sections, "high-quality structures" refers to any structures matching the quality criteria defined in previous work (Friedrich et al., 2017b). Importantly, this term only refers to the quality of the protein-bound ligand, not the overall structure of the protein-ligand complex. Four-letter codes refer to PDB entries and three-letter codes in italics refer to PDB ligand identifiers.

Small-Molecule Drugs

Imatinib

Imatinib (*STI*) is an approved anti-cancer drug targeting Bcr-Abl and several other tyrosine kinases. The drug binds to the ATP-binding site, spanning almost the entire width of the protein (Reddy and Aggarwal, 2012). Imatinib locks the protein in a closed conformation, thus arresting the enzyme's functionality. The PDB lists 11 high-quality structures with imatinib, 10 thereof with the drug bound to one of three different tyrosine kinases (ABL1: 1IEP, 1OPJ, 3K5V, 3MS9, 3MSS, 3PYY; ABL2: 3GVU; c-Src: 2OIQ, 3OEZ) or a synthetic construct of tyrosine kinase AS (4CSV), a common ancestor of Src and Abl.

The accessible conformational space of imatinib, which has seven rotatable bonds, is large. However, the conformations observed for imatinib bound to any of these tyrosine kinases are similar (**Figures 1A,B**), which is reflected by the low maximum pairwise RMSD of just 0.3 Å and is in agreement with the findings of He et al. (2015). This conformational similarity can be explained by the highly conserved nature of the residues that form the ligand binding sites of these tyrosine kinases (the minimum pairwise sequence identity between these proteins is 45%; **Figure 1D**).

One high-quality structure of imatinib is a complex with human quinone reductase 2 (3FW1). This enzyme exists as a dimer with two active sites, each located in a deep pocket at the interface between the monomers (Foster et al., 1999; Winger et al., 2009). Quinone reductase 2 is structurally dissimilar to protein kinases. Imatinib binds to the enzyme active site in proximity to the isoalloxazine ring of the FAD cofactor (**Figure 1C**), thereby adopting a distinct, "horseshoe-like" conformation (Winger et al., 2009) that differs by at least 2.4 Å from any of the conformations observed with tyrosine kinases (**Figure 1A**).

TABLE 1 | Summary of approved drugs investigated in this work.

Name	No. of PDB entries	Protein names: No. of high-quality conformers	No. of Confs.[a]	Major observations
Imatinib (STI)	18	Tyrosine kinases: 10 Quinone reductase 2: 1	2	Conformers for different tyrosine kinases are similar, even for pairs of proteins with low sequence identity. A distinct conformation is observed in a complex with quinone reductase 2
Darunavir (017)	54	HIV-1 protease: 14	1	Conformers are highly similar, also those in complex with various different mutants of this protein
Acetazolamide (AZM)	29	Carboanhydrases: 9 Endochitinase: 1	n.d.[b]	It is likely that the ligand binds in a similar conformation to all proteins covered by the dataset (the experimental data do not allow a definitive conclusion)
Triclosan (TCL)	31	Enoyl-acyl carrier protein reductases: 11	1	All conformers are highly similar. The median RMSD is 0.1 Å and the maximum pairwise RMSD is below 0.6 Å
Ubenimex/bestatin (BES)	28	Aminopeptidases: 9 Leukotriene A-4 hydrolase: 2	3	Conformations observed for most (even distantly) related aminopeptidases and human leukotriene A-4 hydrolases are similar, with the exception of one conformation observed in complex with human aminopeptidase N
Biotin (BTN)	99	Streptavidin: 24 Avidin: 7 Biotin-protein ligase: 6 Others: 6	3	Conformations observed among the different complexes with core streptavidin are very similar. Two distinct conformers are observed in complex with biotin-protein ligase and biotin carboxylase
Sapropterin (H4B)	472	Total: 188	2	All but three conformers are extremely similar to each other (median RMSD smaller than 0.1 Å), even for distantly related proteins
Cholic acid (CHD)	74	Cytochrome c oxidase: 2 Ferrochelatase: 2 Alcohol dehydrogenase: 1 Others: 8	4	Due to the rigid steroid scaffold, the conformations observed for both ligands are all highly similar
Deoxycholic acid (DXC)	29	Cathepsin A: 11 Bet v1: 2 Others: 3	2	

[a] *No. of distinct bioactive conformations.*
[b] *The experimental data are insufficient to allow a definitive conclusion on the number of distinct bioactive conformations.*

Note that imatinib is known to bind to spleen tyrosine kinase (SYK) in an orientation that is different from that observed for Bcr-Abl and other tyrosine kinases (Alton and Lunney, 2008). A crystal structure of the imatinib-SYK complex exists (1XBB; Atwell et al., 2004) but is not part of the Sperrylite Dataset because of a poor electron density support of parts of the ligand facing the bulk water phase (Figure S2). The conformer of imatinib in complex with SYK has an RMSD of 2.5 Å to any of the other kinase-bound conformers but is similar to the imatinib conformation observed in the complex with quinone reductase 2 (RMSD = 1.3 Å).

Darunavir

Darunavir (*017*) is an antiretroviral drug approved for the treatment and prevention of human immunodeficiency virus (HIV) infections. The compound inhibits HIV-1 protease at picomolar concentrations by forming strong polar interactions with the target enzyme (King et al., 2004). Fourteen out of the 54 available structures with darunavir are of high quality, all of them being structures with darunavir bound to wild type or mutant HIV-1 protease. The mutations observed in the 14 high-quality structures introduce only subtle changes to the shape and chemical properties of the ligand binding environment. This is reflected in the high similarity of the protein-bound conformations of darunavir, where, among the high-quality structures, a maximum pairwise RMSD of just 0.2 Å was measured (Figure S3).

Acetazolamide

Acetazolamide (*AZM*) is an inhibitor of carbonic anhydrase and approved for the treatment of glaucoma, cardiac edema, idiopathic intracranial hypertension, epilepsy, and altitude sickness (Chakravarty and Kannan, 1994; Kaur et al., 2002). Ten out of the 29 structures of acetazolamide listed in the PDB are of high quality. Nine of these structures are with acetazolamide bound to one of six different human carbonic anhydrases (isoforms II, VII, IX, XII, XIII, and XIV, represented by PDB entries 3V2J, 3ML5, 3IAI, 1JD0, 3CZV, and 4LU3, respectively) or three different extremophilic bacteria carbonic anhydrases (*Sulfurihydrogenibium* sp., *Thermovibrio ammonificans*, and *Sulfurihydrogenibium azorense*, represented by PDB entries 4G7A, 4UOV, and 4X5S, respectively). The ligand binding pockets of all these carbonic anhydrase isozymes are highly similar (**Figure 2G**) and so are the conformations of acetazolamide observed for these complexes (**Figure 2A**). The protein-ligand complexes are stabilized by hydrogen bonds formed between the acetyl group of acetazolamide and the binding pocket (**Figure 2B**), with one exception, which is a complex with human carbonic anhydrase XII (1JD0). In that structure, the acetyl group of the ligand is rotated by about

TABLE 2 | Summary of cofactors and cofactor analogs investigated in this work.

Name	No. of PDB entries	Protein names: No. of high-quality conformers	No. of Confs.[a]	Major observations
Sinefungin (SFG)	70	Methyltransferase: 23 Others: 7	6	Three clusters of conformers are observed. The largest group includes 23 highly similar conformers and includes structures bound to proteins that share low sequence identity. The maximum RMSD measured for any of the sinefungin conformers is 3.6 Å
S-adenosylmethionine (SAM)	410	Methyltransferase: 92 Others: 31	24	A wide variety of conformations are observed, with a clear clustering into three distinct groups of conformers. Within these groups, a large number of similar conformers are observed, even when bound to proteins sharing low sequence identity. The maximum pairwise RMSD is 3.3 Å
S-Adenosyl-L-Homocysteine (SAH)	784	Methyltransferase: 284 RNA polymerase: 8 Others: 19	23	
Glutathione (GSH)	360	Glutathione transferase: 46 Others: 28	16	Most of the conformers have a pairwise RMSD between 0.6 and 1.6 Å, but the maximum pairwise RMSD is 3.6 Å
Adenosine monophosphate (AMP)	575	Total: 171	36	A wide variety of different conformers is observed. One distinct, extremely coiled conformer was observed in complex with an adenylate kinase-related protein. The maximum pairwise RMSD is 2.5 Å
Adenosine diphosphate (ADP)	1,810	Total: 462	81	The conformers are similar to those observed for AMP, despite the presence of an additional phosphate group. The median RMSD is 0.9 Å
Adenosine triphosphate (ATP)	1,079	Total: 218	76	ATP is observed in an extended conformation in most structures, but some conformers are extremely bent. The median and the maximum pairwise RMSDs are 1.6 and 3.9 Å, respectively
Flavin mononucleotide (FMN)	919	Total: 367	21	The overall median RMSD is 0.9. The all-against-all comparison revealed four groups of conformers, with peaks in the RMSD distribution at around 0.3, 1.2, 1.7, and 2.4 Å

[a]*No. of distinct bioactive conformations.*

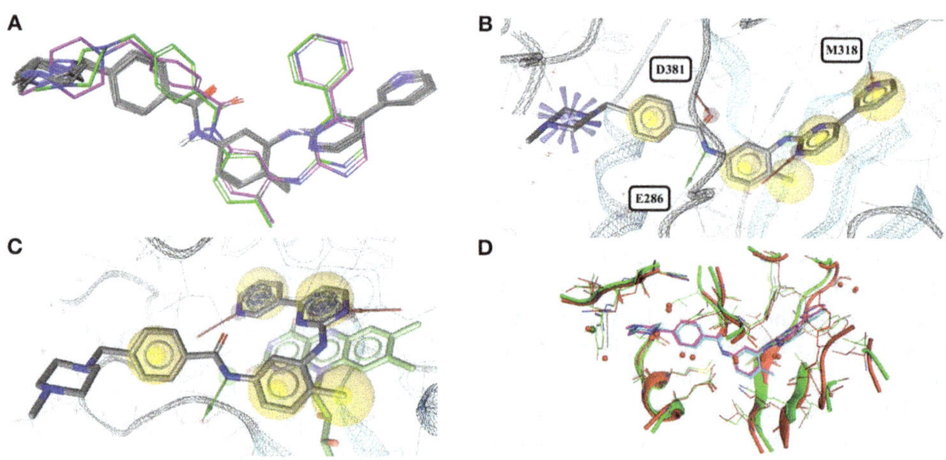

FIGURE 1 | (A) Ligand-based alignment of imatinib conformers observed in complex with three different tyrosine kinases (gray carbon atoms), human quinone reductase 2 (3FW1; violet carbon atoms) and human spleen tyrosine kinase (1XBB; green carbon atoms). **(B)** Imatinib bound to ABL1 (3MS9) in an extended conformation that is characteristic for the drug bound to tyrosine kinases. Red and green vectors indicate hydrogen bond donors and acceptors, respectively. Yellow spheres mark hydrophobic moieties involved in interactions with the protein, and blue astral centers indicate charge interactions involving a positively charged group on the ligand side. **(C)** Imatinib bound to human quinone reductase 2 in a conformation that is different from those characteristic of tyrosine kinases (3FW1; FAD with green carbon atoms). **(D)** Alignment of the binding sites of human ABL1 (3K5V; red) and c-Src (2OIQ; green). Despite a sequence identity of only 45%, the ligand binding sites of both proteins are almost identical.

140° as compared to any of the other structures (RMSD 0.9 Å; **Figure 2C**). A second, distinct conformation of acetazolamide is found in a complex with a different enzyme, endochitinase from *Saccharomyces cerevisiae* (2UY4) with a fundamentally different binding pocket. In that structure, the carbon-sulfur bond of the ligand is rotated by 120° (**Figure 2D**). The moieties in question are oriented toward the bulk water phase, freely rotatable, and not engaged in directed interactions with the protein. Also, the electron density maps do not allow a definitive conclusion on the orientation of these moieties (**Figures 2E,F**). It is therefore entirely possible that in reality all conformers of acetazolamide in the Sperrylite Dataset are nearly identical.

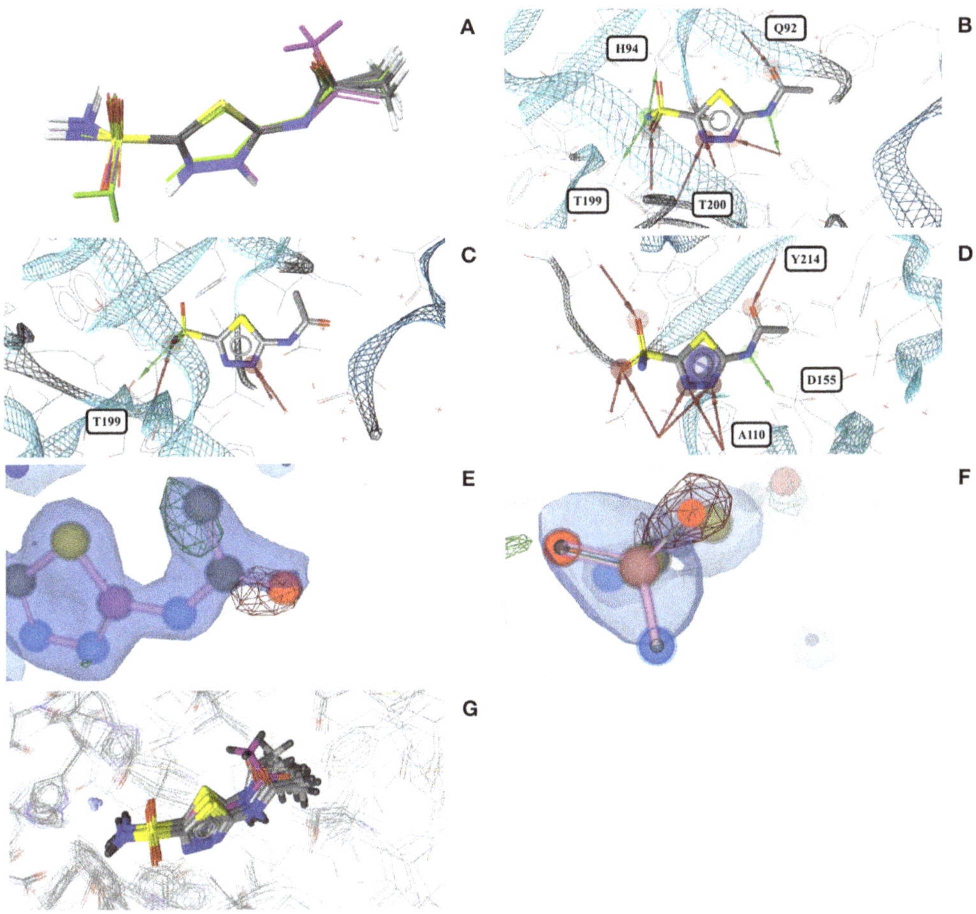

FIGURE 2 | (A) Ligand-based alignment of acetazolamide bound to different carbonic anhydrases (gray carbon atoms, except those of 1JD0, which are violet) and endochitinase (2UY4; green). **(B)** The acetyl group of acetazolamide forms hydrogen bond interactions with some carbonic anhydrases such as isozyme VII (3ML5) depicted here. **(C)** In a complex with human carbonic anhydrase XII (1JD0) the acetyl group of acetazolamide is rotated by about 140°. **(D)** In a complex with endochitinase (2UY4), the sulfonamide moiety of acetazolamide is rotated by about 120°. The support of atom positions by the measured electron density can be quantified by the EDIA score. For some of the atoms of the acetyl **(E)** and sulfonamide groups **(F)** of these structures the EDIA scores are below 0.8, meaning that their exact position is uncertain. The 2Fo-Fc, Fo-Fc(−ve) and Fo-Fc(+ve) sigma maps are shown in blue, red and green, respectively. It can therefore not be excluded that the acetyl group in **(C)** and the sulfonamide moiety in **(D)** are present in the same orientation that is observed in any of the other crystal structures. **(G)** Superposed binding pockets of the nine human and three extremophilic bacterial carbonic anhydrases.

Triclosan

Triclosan (*TCL*) is an antibacterial and antifungal agent inhibiting enoyl-acyl carrier protein reductases (ENR), which are key enzymes in the fatty acid elongation cycle. Its wide use as a disinfectant in cremes and consumer products (e.g., soaps, toothpaste, detergents) is a controversial topic nowadays (Buth et al., 2010; Carey and McNamara, 2014).

In all 31 structures of triclosan contained in the PDB, the ligand is bound to an ENR. The conformers of triclosan observed among the 11 high-quality structures with ENR I and ENR III are very similar (median RMSD 0.1 Å; maximum pairwise RMSD < 0.6 Å; **Figure 3A**). These include the structures of *Plasmodium falciparum* ENR I (2O2Y) and *Bacillus subtilis* ENR III (3OID) which, despite a sequence identity of just 14% and a highly flexible binding site region (when in the unbound state), show almost identical structural features in the presence of triclosan (Kim et al., 2011).

In an X-ray structure of triclosan bound to *Staphylococcus aureus* ENR I (3GR6; not included in the Sperrylite Dataset because of low EDIA scores), the hydroxyl group of all four instances of triclosan is modeled in a different orientation (RMSD 1.4 Å measured to any of the other conformations present in the dataset). The EDIA score for the oxygen atom of the hydroxyl group of the four instances of this conformer is just 0.11–0.27, and visual inspection of the electron density map confirms a lack of support of this conformation (**Figure 3B**). The characteristic hydrogen bonds formed between the phenolic hydroxyl group of triclosan and Y156 as well as NAD(P) (Heath et al., 1999; Levy et al., 1999; **Figure 3C**) are also missing in this model (**Figure 3D**). All of these observations taken together indicate a likely error in this structural model.

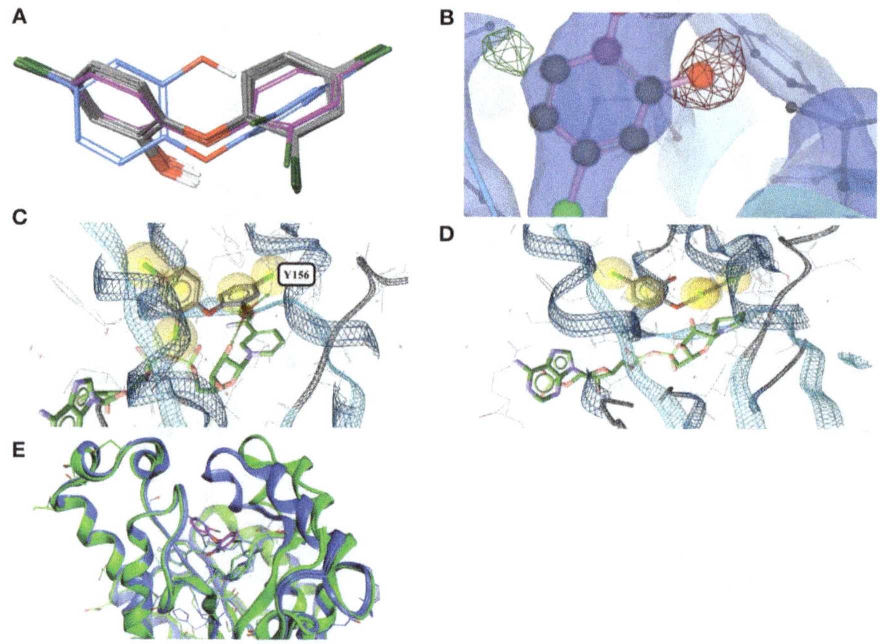

FIGURE 3 | (A) Ligand-based alignment of eleven conformers of triclosan present in the Sperrylite Dataset bound to ENRs, including the drug-resistant G93V mutant of ENR I (3PJF; violet carbon atoms) and an uncommon conformation observed in *Staphylococcus aureus* ENR I (3GR6; blue carbon atoms). The latter is not part of the Sperrylite Dataset because of a lack of support of the structural model by the electron density, as shown in **(B)**, with the 2Fo-Fc, Fo-Fc(–ve) and Fo-Fc(+ve) sigma maps in blue, red and green, respectively. **(C)** Interaction of triclosan and NAD (green carbon atoms), including the characteristic hydrogen bond between both molecules in the binding pocket of *E. coli* ENR I (1QG6). **(D)** Triclosan and NADP (green) bound to *Staphylococcus aureus* ENR I (3GR6). In this structural model, the characteristic hydrogen bond is missing because of the unusual position of the hydroxyl group. However, this conformation of triclosan lacks support by the measured electron density. **(E)** A G93V mutation in ENR I (green protein backbone; ligand with violet carbon atoms) induces a conformational shift of the flexible α-helical turn located in the proximity of triclosan. The complex of the WT protein and triclosan (4M89) is shown with the protein backbone and ligand in blue.

The largest deviations between conformers of triclosan within the Sperrylite Dataset were observed for the complex with a triclosan-resistant G93V mutant (3PJF) of ENR I from *Escherichia coli.* These deviations are related to small conformational changes of a flexible α-helical turn in close proximity to the ligand (**Figure 3E**), resulting in the weakening of some edge-to-face aromatic interactions near the ligand (Singh et al., 2011). The high-level resistance of this mutant is not caused by a substantial loss in binding affinity of the drug but is a consequence of the inability of the G93V mutant to form the high affinity ENR-NAD+-triclosan ternary complex that inhibits the wild type (Heath et al., 1999).

Ubenimex, Bestatin

Ubenimex, also known as bestatin (*BES*), is a competitive protease inhibitor under investigation for the treatment of acute myelocytic leukemia and lymphedema (Tian et al., 2017). The molecule inhibits aminopeptidases and has shown immunomodulatory and host-mediated antitumor activities (Urabe et al., 1993; Inoi et al., 1995; Sakuraya et al., 2000). It has been approved in Japan as an adjunct to chemotherapy agents against acute non-lymphocytic leukemia for decades and has been reported to inhibit the growth of malaria parasites (*Plasmodium falciparum*) *in vitro* (Nankya-Kitaka et al., 1998).

Twenty-eight structures of bestatin are listed in the PDB. All of the 11 high-quality structures are with bestatin bound to aminopeptidases. The ligand conformations observed in eight of these high-quality structures are very similar to each other (maximum pairwise RMSD = 0.8 Å), even though the proteins originate from three different bacteria (*E. coli*, *Pseudomonas putida* and *Vibrio proteolyticus*), the unicellular protozoan parasite *Plasmodium falciparum* and mouse, and their minimum pairwise sequence identity is only 3.3%.

In contrast, the structure of bestatin bound to human aminopeptidase N (4FYR) shows an extended ligand conformation that has an RMSD of 2.0 Å to any of the ligand conformers observed for the bacterial proteins (**Figure 4A**). The conformations of the drug bound to human leukotriene A-4 hydrolase differ only slightly from and have similar binding modes to the characteristic conformation observed for aminopeptidases mentioned above (RMSD = 1.0 Å for both 3FUH and 3FTX; **Figures 4B–D**).

Biotin

Biotin (*BTN*, vitamin B_7) is a water-soluble coenzyme for carboxylase enzymes and an approved drug for the treatment of dietary shortage or imbalance. There are 99 crystal structures including biotin listed in the PDB. The biotin conformers observed for the 43 high-quality structures can be assigned

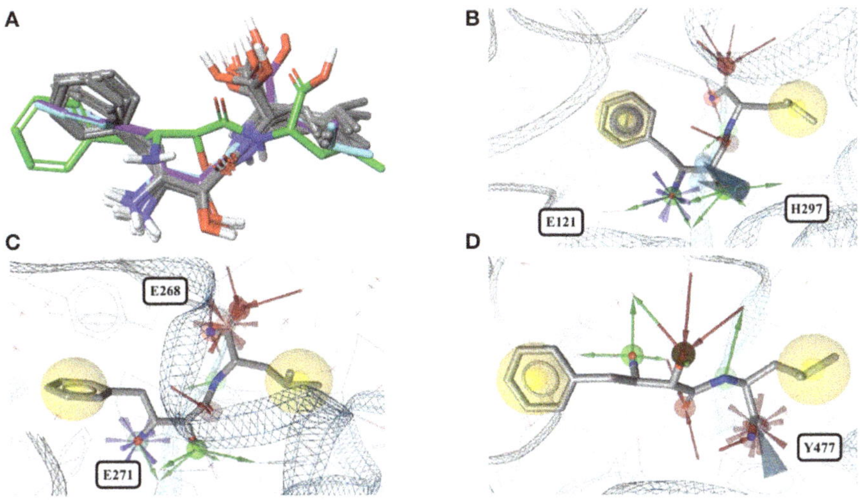

FIGURE 4 | (A) Superposition of all eleven conformers of bestatin in the Sperrylite Dataset. The carbon atoms of the conformers in complex with human aminopeptidase N (4FYR) and human leukotriene A-4 hydrolase (3FUH and 3FTX) are indicated in green, violet and cyan, respectively. The carbon atoms of all other structures are shown in gray. **(B)** Typical conformer of bestatin bound to aminopeptidases N from *E. coli* (2HPT). **(C)** A conformation that differs slightly from the characteristic conformation, observed in complex with human leukotriene A-4 hydrolase (3FUH shown here). **(D)** Uncommon, extended conformation of bestatin observed in complex with the human aminopeptidase N (4FYR).

to three distinct groups, indicated by gray, green and violet carbon atoms in **Figure 5A**. Twenty-four of the 43 structures are complexes with core streptavidin from different bacteria (both wild type and mutants). Streptavidin homotetramers have a very high affinity for biotin, one of the strongest non-covalent interactions known (Kd $\approx 10^{-14}$ to 10^{-16} M) (Laitinen et al., 2006). The protein-ligand complex stands out by a high degree of shape complementarity and an extensive network of hydrogen bonds formed between both binding partners. One of the 24 structures of biotin bound to core streptavidin (4GD9) shows the impact of the cutting of a binding loop on the conformation of the bound ligand (Figure S4; Le Trong et al., 2013). Another structure (2IZJ) shows subtle structural changes of the streptavidin-biotin complex induced by a low pH that stabilizes intersubunit salt bridges (**Figure 5A**; orange carbon atoms; Katz, 1997).

Six crystal structures of avidin from chicken (wild type and mutants) and one of engineered avidin (2C4I) are also included in the dataset. Avidin is loosely related to streptavidin, with an equally high affinity to biotin and a very similar binding site (Figure S4). As expected, biotin binds to this protein in a conformation that is very similar to those predominantly observed for complexes with streptavidin.

Biotin-protein ligase (1WPY, 2EJ9, 2EJF, 2DTH, 2FYK, and 2ZGW) and biotin carboxylase (3G8C) share very low structural similarity with streptavidin and with each other. The conformations observed for biotin bound to biotin-protein ligase (**Figure 5A**; violet carbon atoms) are virtually identical among each other but differ by an RMSD of 1.1 Å from the predominant conformation observed in the Sperrylite Dataset. In particular, the angle of the alkyl chain leaving the ring system differs by around 103° from that observed for biotin bound to streptavidin. A third conformer of biotin is observed in complex with *E. coli* biotin carboxylase (3G8C; **Figure 5A**; green carbon atoms), with an RMSD of 0.9 Å measured against any of the streptavidin-bound conformers. Despite substantial structural differences observed among the various different biotin-binding proteins, the non-covalent interactions formed between biotin and the target protein are largely conserved (**Figures 5B–D**).

Sapropterin

Sapropterin (tetrahydrobiopterin, *H4B*) is an approved drug for the treatment of tetrahydrobiopterin deficiency. It is an essential cofactor for the synthesis of nitric oxide and the hydroxylation of phenylalanine, tyrosine and tryptophan. The PDB counts 472 complexes with sapropterin, 188 of which are of high quality.

Of the high-quality conformers of sapropterin, all but three are extremely similar to each other (median RMSD of less than 0.1 Å; Figure S5A). All of these highly similar sapropterin conformers are bound to nitric oxide synthase, from five different species (human, rat, mouse, cattle and *Bacillus subtilis*). The exceptions are the conformers bound to human phenylalanine hydroxylase (1MMK, 1MMT and 1J8U), and differ by an RMSD of 0.7 Å from the conformer in human nitric oxide synthase (4D1N, Figure S5B). The sequence identity between human phenylalanine hydroxylase and human nitric oxide synthase is less than 15%. The slightly different conformer bound to phenylalanine hydroxylase is stabilized by hydrophobic interactions (Figure S5C).

Cholic Acid

Cholic acid (*CHD*) is one of the major bile acids produced from cholesterol in the liver. It is approved for the treatment of bile acid synthesis disorders and as an adjunctive treatment of peroxisomal disorders.

Thirteen of the 74 available crystal structures that include cholic acid are of high quality. Twelve thereof are from eukaryotic

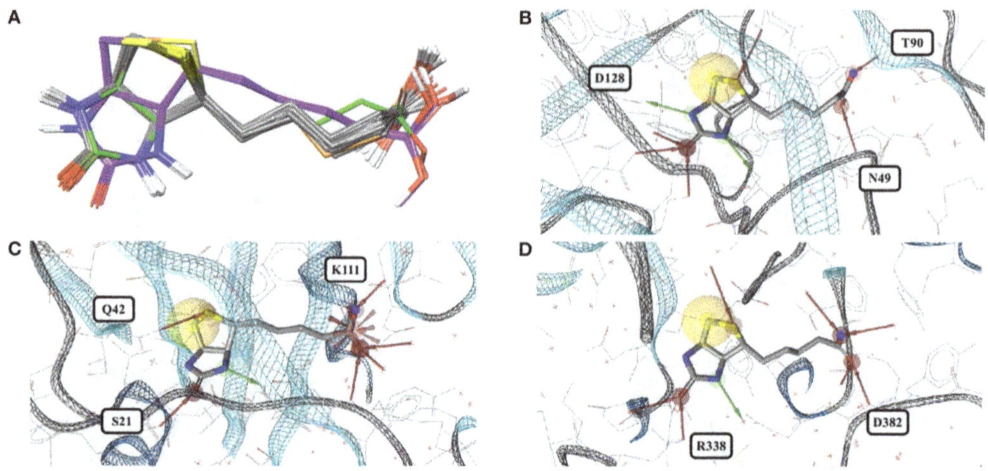

FIGURE 5 | (A) Superposition of 43 structures of biotin (BTN) bound to core streptavidin (gray carbon atoms), *E. coli* biotin carboxylase (3G8C; green carbon atoms), biotin-protein ligase (1WPY; violet carbon atoms), and streptavidin-biotin at low pH (2IZJ; orange carbon atoms). The binding modes observed for biotin in complex with **(B)** core streptavidin from *Streptomyces avidinii* (3WYP), **(C)** biotin-protein ligase from *Pyrococcus horikoshii* (1WPY) and **(D)** *E. coli* biotin carboxylase (3G8C) are very similar.

proteins, including alcohol dehydrogenase, ferrochelatase, cytochrome c oxidase and bile acid-binding proteins; one structure is of choloylglycine hydrolase from *Clostridium perfringens* (2RLC).

Some pockets of cholic acid-binding proteins can accommodate more than a single cholic acid molecule, as observed e.g., in structures of the chicken liver basic fatty acid-binding protein (1TW4) and the zebrafish liver bile acid-binding proteins (2QO5).

Given the rigid scaffold of steroids it is not surprising that, despite in part low sequence identity between the cholic acid-binding proteins, the observed ligand conformations (i.e., those bound to the deepest part of their respective binding pocket) are highly similar (median RMSD = 0.6 Å; **Figure 6A**). The maximum pairwise RMSD of 1.6 Å was measured between the conformation of cholic acid in the crystal structure of the G55R mutant of zebrafish liver bile acid-binding protein (2QO6) and in human mitochondrial ferrochelatase (3W1W).

Deoxycholic Acid

Deoxycholic acid (*DXC*), a metabolic byproduct of intestinal bacteria, is a steroid acid commonly found in the bile of mammals (Ridlon et al., 2016). Deoxycholic acid is a detergent that disturbs the integrity of biological membranes and is used to isolate membrane-associated proteins. Deoxycholic acid is approved for submental fat reduction, as a safer and less invasive alternative to surgical procedures for the treatment of lipomas (Duncan and Rotunda, 2011) and for improvements of aesthetic appearance.

Of the 29 entries deposited in the PDB, 18 are of high quality. Eleven of those structures are deoxycholic acid bound to cathepsin A and have a maximum pairwise RMSD of just 0.1 Å. Because of the rigid ligand core, deoxycholic acid also binds to structurally distinct proteins in very similar conformations (**Figure 6B**). Examples from the Sperrylite Dataset include two structures of *Betula pendula* Bet v1 (a major pollen allergen; 4A81 and 4A84), a structure of subunits I and II of cytochrome c oxidase (3DTU) from *Rhodobacter sphaeroides*, a structure of choloylglycine hydrolase from *Clostridium perfringens* (2BJF), a structure of the multidrug transporter MdfA (4ZP0) from *E. coli*, and even a conformer of deoxycholic acid bound to the interface of a dimer of the cell invasion protein SipD from *Salmonella enterica* (3O01; Chatterjee et al., 2011) The maximum pairwise RMSD (0.9 Å) was measured for the ligand conformers bound to a K9E mutant of cathepsin A (4HAJ) and salmonella invasion protein D (3O01), indicated by violet carbon atoms in **Figure 6B**.

Cofactors and Cofactor Analogs

The most abundant small molecules in the Sperrylite Dataset are cofactors and their analogs. The cofactors represented by at least 10 high-quality structures can roughly be grouped into three categories: sinefungin and its analogs (S-adenosylmethionine, SAM, and S-adenosylhomocysteine, SAH; **Figure 7**), adenosine phosphates (AMP, ADP, ATP; **Figure 8**), and three cofactors without analogs listed in the dataset (glutathione, flavin mononucleotide and sapropterin). The RMSD distributions (all-against-all comparisons) for the most relevant cofactors are reported in **Figure 9**.

Sinefungin and Analogs

Sinefungin

Sinefungin (*SFG*), an analog of the cofactor substrate SAM, inhibits a wide range of methyltransferases, thereby interfering with DNA synthesis (Pugh et al., 1978). It is an antifungal antibiotic and also a known effective inhibitor of the transformation of chick embryo fibroblasts by the cancer-causing *Rous sarcoma* virus (Vedel et al., 1978).

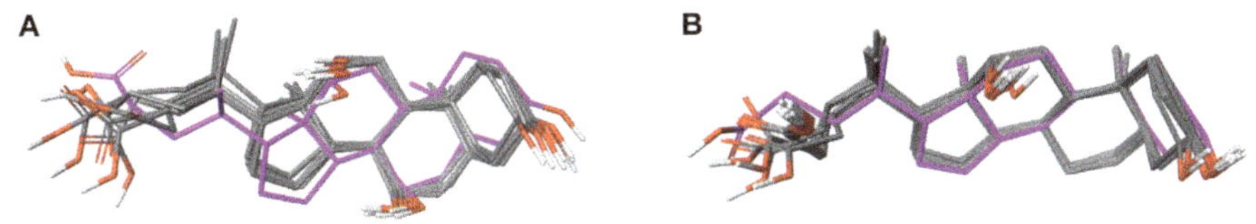

FIGURE 6 | (A) Ligand-based alignment of 13 structures of cholic acid bound to different eukaryotic proteins and choloylglycine hydrolase from *Clostridium perfringens* (2RLC; gray carbon atoms) and human mitochondrial ferrochelatase (3W1W; violet carbon atoms). **(B)** Ligand-based alignment of 16 structures of deoxycholic acid bound to structurally distinct proteins, including salmonella invasion protein D (3O01; violet carbon atoms).

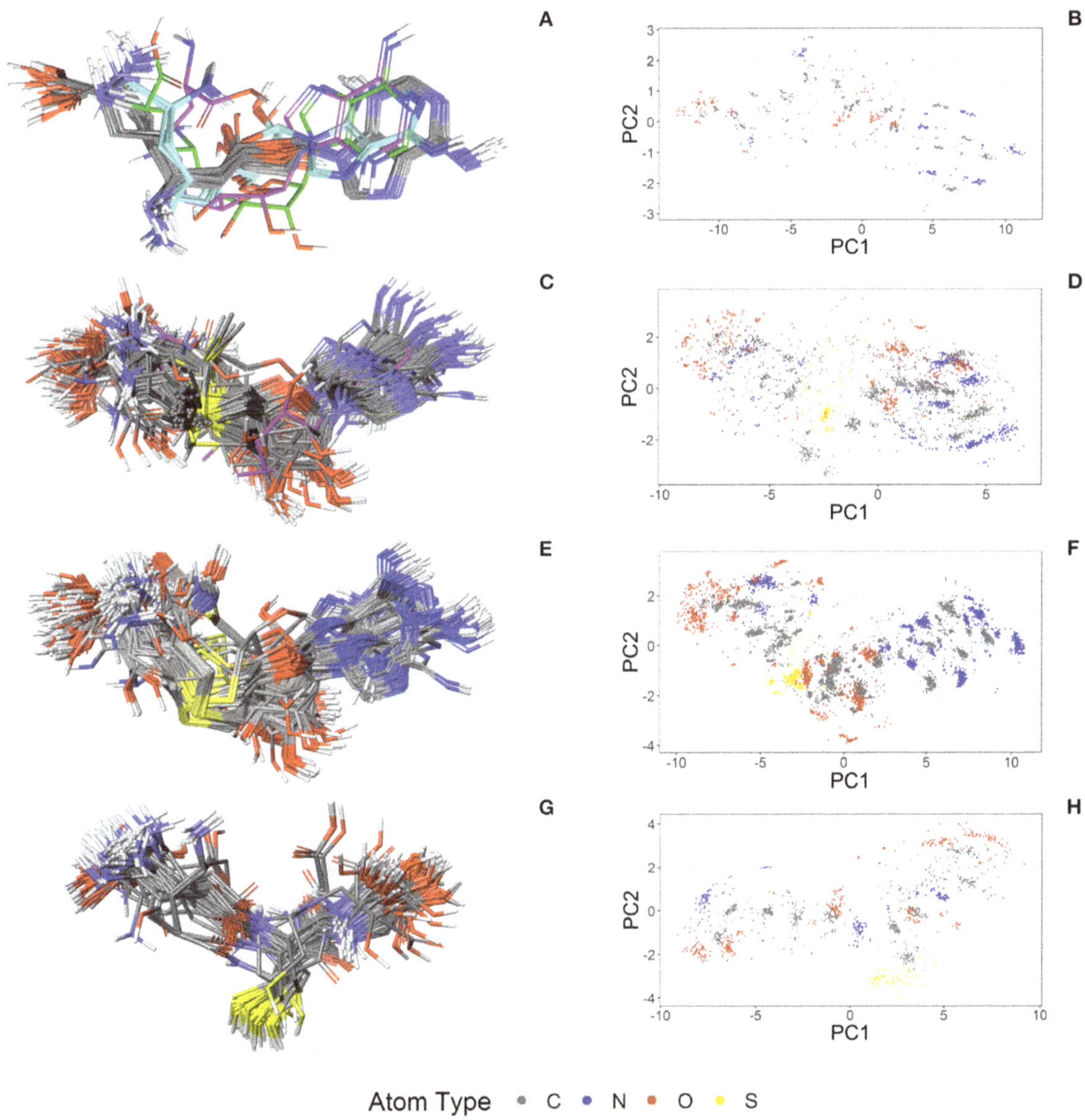

FIGURE 7 | Ligand-based alignment (left) and PCA-derived score plots (right) of **(A,B)** 30 structures of sinefungin bound to different methyltransferases (gray carbon atoms; these and all further color definitions in this caption are referring to the left panels only), ribosomal RNA small subunit methyltransferase NEP1 (3BBH; violet carbon atoms), tRNA (guanine-N(1)-)-methyltransferase (4YVH; green carbon atoms), SMYDs and SET7 lysine methyltransferase (3CBP, 3PDN, 3N71, 3QWW and 3RU0; cyan carbon atoms); **(C,D)** 123 structures of SAM bound to different methyltransferases (gray carbon atoms), tRNA(m1G37)methyltransferase (1UAK; violet carbon atoms) and yeast ribosome synthesis factor Emg1 (2V3K; green carbon atoms); **(E,F)** 311 structures of SAH and **(G,H)** 74 conformers of glutathione (GSH).

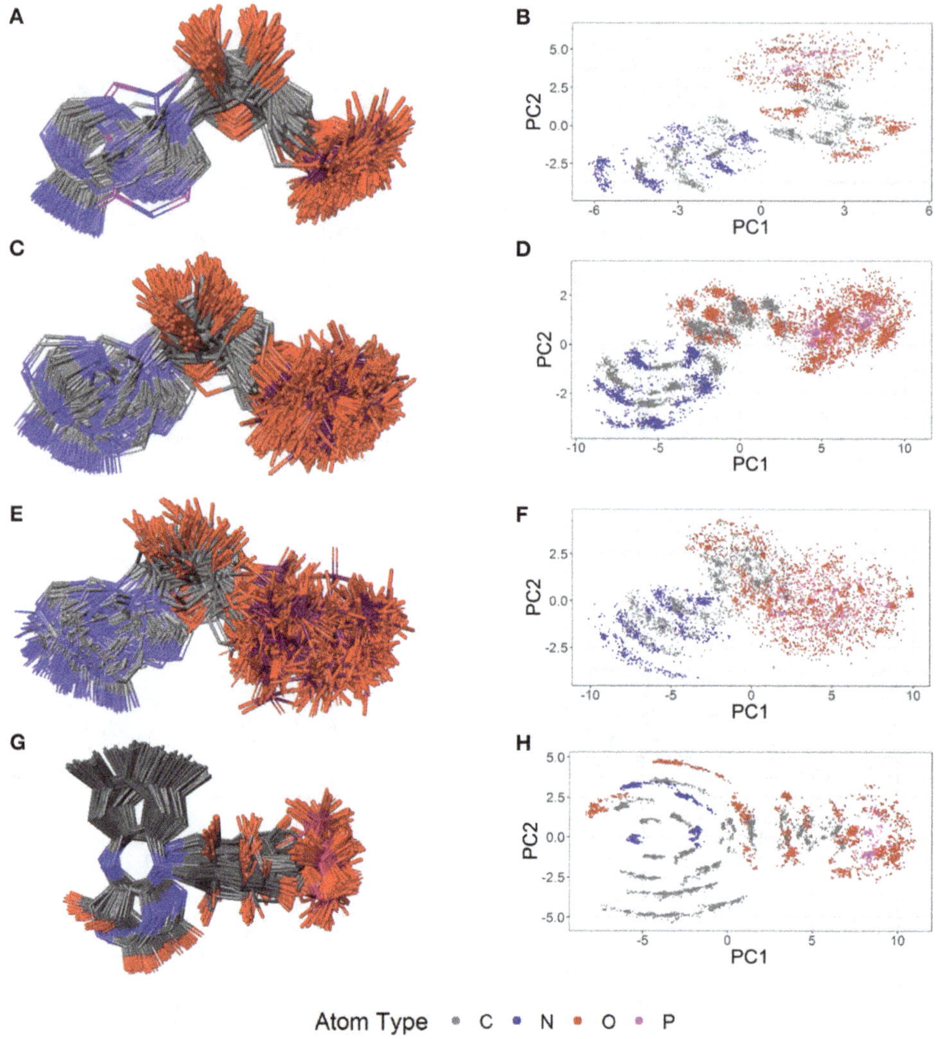

FIGURE 8 | Ligand-based alignment (left) and PCA-derived score plots (right) of **(A,B)** 171 conformers of AMP (conformer bound to adenylate kinase-related protein from *Sulfolobus solfataricus* in **(A)** with violet carbon atoms; 3LW7), **(C,D)** 462 conformers of ADP, **(E,F)** 218 conformers of ATP, and **(G,H)** 367 conformers of FMN.

The PDB lists 70 structures of sinefungin, all of them bound to methyltransferases. Thirty of these structures are of high quality. The observed conformers of sinefungin can be classified into three groups by an all-against-all comparison of their RMSDs (**Figure 9**). The largest group (**Figure 7A**; gray carbon atoms) includes 23 highly similar conformers (a representative example is given in **Figure 10A**) with a median RMSD of 0.5 Å, even though some of the proteins that these sinefungin molecules are bound to share low sequence identity (e.g., 30% for murine protein arginine N-methyltransferase 6 and the ribosomal protein L11 methyltransferase of *Thermus thermophilus*).

The second largest group consists of sinefungin conformers bound to the murine SET and MYND domains (SMYD) 1 (3N71) and 2 (3QWW), the human SMYD 3 (3PDN, 3RU0) and the SET7 lysine methyltransferase (3CBP), with RMSDs between 1.7 and 1.8 Å measured against the conformations representing the largest group (**Figure 7A**; cyan carbon atoms). Murine SMYD 1 (3N71) and human SET7 lysine methyltransferase (3CBP) have less than 15% sequence identity but bind sinefungin in very similar conformations (RMSD 0.3 Å).

Distinct conformations of sinefungin are observed for a complex with *Haemophilus influenzae* tRNA (guanine-N(1)-)methyltransferase (4YVH; **Figure 7A**; green atoms) and a complex with the ribosomal RNA small subunit methyltransferase NEP1 (3BBH, **Figure 7A**; violet carbon atoms, and **Figure 10B**) from *Methanocaldococcus jannaschii*, with RMSDs measured to the most abundantly observed conformation of 3.1 and 3.6 Å, respectively. In both cases the ligand conformation is stabilized by a hydrogen bond formed between the ligand's carboxyl group and the protein backbone.

S-Adenosylmethionine

SAM (*SAM*) is a cofactor that functions as a methyl donor in methyltransferases. It is essential for the methylation of proteins, DNA, lipids and small molecules. The bulk of SAM is generated in the liver, but all mammalian cells use it as an intermediate in the methionine-homocysteine cycle (Mato et al., 2013). SAM is also involved in the synthesis of many other endogenous metabolites. It has wide-ranging anti-inflammatory activity (Pfalzer et al., 2014) and, since its synthesis is depressed in chronic liver diseases, there has been considerable interest in its therapeutic use (Anstee and Day, 2012; Guo et al., 2015). S-adenosylmethionine is used as a drug for the treatment of depression, liver disorders, fibromyalgia, and osteoarthritis.

Four hundred ten structures listed in the PDB contain SAM. For example, almost all crystal structures of flavivirus methyltransferases contain SAM (because the molecule co-purifies with the enzymes (Noble et al., 2014). There are 119 high-quality SAM-containing structures present in the Sperrylite Dataset. Many of these conformers are similar, with an overall median RMSD of 0.6 Å (**Figures 7C,D**). Even conformers bound to proteins sharing a low sequence identity (e.g., 19% in the case of *Aeropyrum pernix* fibrillarin, 4DF3, and human NSUN5, 2B9E), have RMSDs of just 0.5 Å. The all-against-all RMSD comparison shows a partitioning into three groups that are mainly determined by the torsion angles between the adenine and the ribose and to the torsion angles including the sulfonium linkage (**Figure 7**). The highest RMSD measured between any pair of SAM conformers is 3.3 Å, which was measured for the ligand in complex with *Haemophilus influenzae* tRNA(m1G37)methyltransferase (1UAK; **Figure 7C**; violet carbon atoms) and with SAM methyltransferase from *Ruegeria pomeroyi* (3IHT).

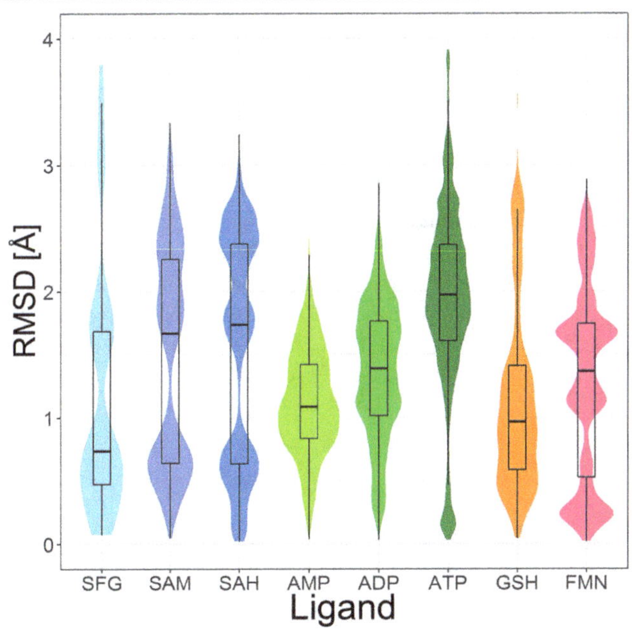

FIGURE 9 | Violin plot including box plots of the RMSD distributions of high-quality, protein-bound conformations of sinefungin (SFG), SAM, SAH, AMP, ADP, ATP, GSH and FMN. The width of each violin plot for a certain RMSD value indicates how often the specific value occurs in the pairwise comparison of all conformers.

S-Adenosyl-L-homocysteine

The strong product inhibitor SAH (*SAH*) is released in all SAM-dependent methyltransferase reactions (Tehlivets et al., 2013). The ratio of SAM to SAH controls the activity of methyltransferase enzymes ("methylation ratio"; Schatz et al., 1977).

The PDB lists 784 structures including SAH, of which an unusually high proportion (40%; 311 structures) is of high quality (**Figure 7**). These represent a highly diverse set of proteins from all three domains of organisms in nature. Most of the structures are of human (73 structures) and *Pyrococcus horikoshii* (72 structures) proteins.

Many of the SAH conformations are highly similar, with an overall median RMSD of 0.6 Å. The all-against-all RMSD comparison shows three groups of conformations and an overall spread very similar to that observed for SAM (**Figure 9**). As shown in **Figure 7**, the conformations observed for SAM and SAH are similar. Also, all conformations of sinefungin are closely represented by at least one conformation of SAM and SAH.

The largest difference observed among the SAH conformations was measured between a coiled conformer bound to *Haemophilus influenzae* tRNA (Guanine-N(1)-)-methyltransferase (1UAL) and a mostly stretched conformer bound to *E. coli* ribosomal RNA large subunit methyltransferase L (3V97) with an RMSD of 3.2 Å.

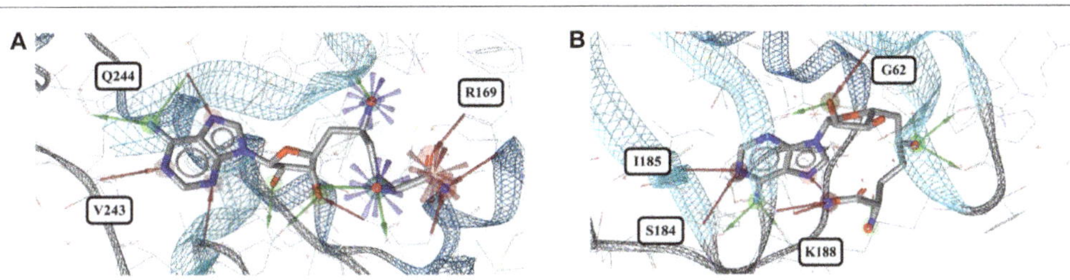

FIGURE 10 | (A) A typical conformer of sinefungin bound to human histone-arginine methyltransferase CARM1 (2Y1W) and **(B)** the coiled conformer in the ribosomal RNA small subunit methyltransferase NEP1 from *Methanocaldococcus jannaschii* (3BBH).

Glutathione

The tripeptide glutathione (GSH; *GSH*) is a cofactor of various different enzymes and a defensive reagent against toxic xenobiotics. Of the 360 entries with glutathione listed in the PDB, 74 structures are of high quality. These high-quality structures cover glutathione bound to 10 different proteins (**Figures 7G,H**). Most of the GSH conformers have a pairwise RMSD between 0.6 and 1.6 Å (**Figure 9**). The two most distinct conformers of glutathione observed in the Sperrylite Dataset are an unusually stretched conformer bound to a putative branched-chain amino acid ABC transporter from *Chromobacterium violaceum* (4PYR, **Figure 11A**) and an extremely coiled conformer bound to human mPGES-1 (4YL1, **Figure 11B**), with an RMSD of 3.6 Å. Nevertheless, their interaction patterns show similarities. Glutathione transferases are represented by 46 high-quality structures. These are mostly similar and have a median RMSD of less than 0.5 Å (**Figures 7G,H**).

Adenosine Phosphates

ATP functions as the most important molecule for intracellular storage and transport of chemical energy. It has many crucial roles in metabolism and is also a neurotransmitter. During metabolic processes, ATP is converted into adenosine diphosphate (ADP) and, subsequently, adenosine monophosphate (AMP), thereby releasing the stored energy.

Adenosine monophosphate

Out of the 575 complexes with AMP (*AMP*) found in the PDB, 171 conformers are of high quality. AMP has four rotatable bonds and the median RMSD measured between all high-quality conformers is 0.8 Å. The all-against-all comparison of AMP conformers results in a wide spread of the RMSD values (**Figure 9**). The flexibility of the molecule is mostly limited to the phosphate group (**Figures 8A,B**). The maximum RMSD of 2.5 Å was measured between an extremely coiled conformer bound to an adenylate kinase-related protein from *Sulfolobus solfataricus* (3LW7; **Figure 8A**, violet carbon atoms; **Figure 12A**) and the stretched conformer bound to NTPDasel from *Legionella pneumophila* (4BRN; **Figure 12B**).

Adenosine diphosphate

Out of the 1,810 entries including ADP (*ADP*) in the PDB, 462 conformers are of high quality. Despite an additional phosphate group and a total of six rotatable bonds, the conformational space covered by ADP is very similar to that covered by AMP (**Figures 8C,D**). This similarity is reflected in the median RMSD of 0.9 Å between the conformers of ADP and a similar overall spread in the all-against-all comparison (**Figure 9**). The two most different ADP conformers in the Sperrylite Dataset are those bound to tryptophanyl-tRNA synthetase from *Campylobacter jejuni* (3TZL; **Figure 13A**) and an Stt7 homolog from *Micromonas algae* (4IX6; **Figure 13B**), with an RMSD of 2.9 Å.

Adenosine triphosphate

Only 218 conformers out of the 1,079 structures of the PDB containing ATP (*ATP*) were of high quality. In all structures of ATP included in the Sperrylite Dataset, the N-glycosidic bond is found in an anti-orientation. With its eight rotatable bonds ATP is more flexible than the previously discussed adenosine

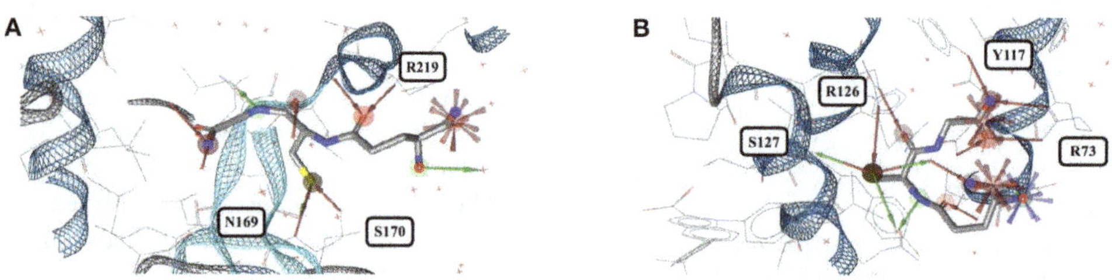

FIGURE 11 | (A) The most stretched conformer of glutathione bound to an ABC transporter from *Chromobacterium violaceum* (4PYR) and **(B)** an unusually coiled conformer of glutathione bound to human mPGES-1 (4YL1).

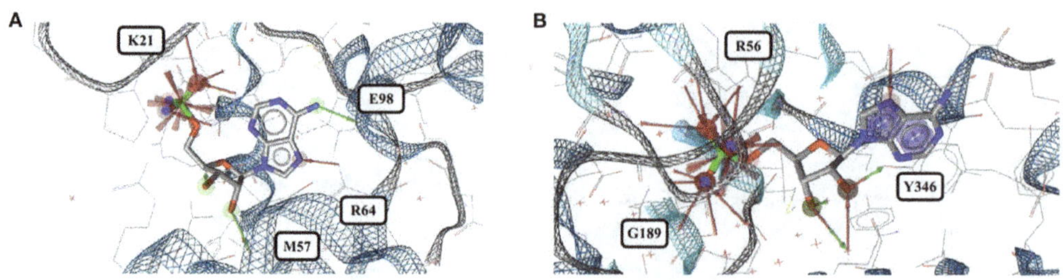

FIGURE 12 | (A) Unusually coiled conformer of AMP bound to adenylate kinase-related protein of *Sulfolobus solfataricus* (3LW7) and **(B)** the most stretched conformer in *Legionella pneumophila* NTPDase1 (4BRN).

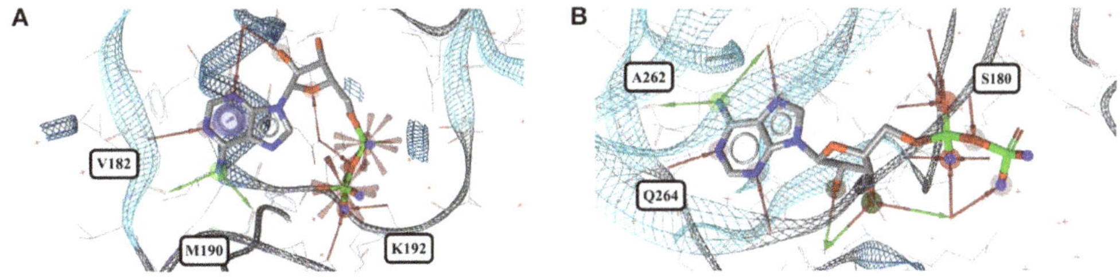

FIGURE 13 | The most distinct conformers of ADP in the Sperrylite Dataset are the coiled conformer from **(A)** tryptophanyl-tRNA synthetase from *Campylobacter jejuni* (3TZL; sodium ion in light blue) and **(B)** the stretched conformer from a Stt7 homolog from *Micromonas algae* (4IX6).

phosphates. This results in a median RMSD of 1.6 Å among the ATP structures of the Sperrylite dataset (as compared to a median RMSD of 0.9 Å measured for ADP) and a distinct spread of the RMSD values in the all-against-all comparison (**Figure 9**). The maximum pairwise RMSD was 3.9 Å, measured between ATP conformers from human lysyl-tRNA synthetase (3BJU) and *Drosophila melanogaster* Wiskott-Aldrich syndrome protein homology 2 (3MN6).

ATP is observed in an extended conformation in most structures (**Figures 8G,H**), which is in agreement with earlier studies (Moodie and Thornton, 1993; Stockwell and Thornton, 2006; Bojovschi et al., 2012; Stegemann and Klebe, 2012). As reported also by Stockwell and Thornton (Stockwell and Thornton, 2006), some conformers are bent to an extent that the terminal phosphate atoms are almost in van der Waals contact with the adenine ring. Examples of ATP in bent conformations include complexes with the aspartyl-tRNA synthetase from *Pyrococcus kodakaraensis* (1B8A; Figure S6) and the ribonucleotide reductase protein R1 from *E. coli* (3R1R).

Flavin Mononucleotide

Flavin mononucleotide (FMN; *FMN*) is the prosthetic group of various oxidoreductases (including NADH dehydrogenase), as well as a cofactor in biological blue-light photoreceptors (Froehlich et al., 2002; Schwerdtfeger and Linden, 2003). Blue-light receptors in plants (phototropins), for example, employ flavin mononucleotide as the chromophore for their light sensing function (He, 2002).

Its frequent occurrence as a prosthetic group and a cofactor result in flavin mononucleotide's presence in 919 structures deposited in the PDB, among which 367 conformers of FMN are of high quality. Despite having seven rotatable bonds, most structures show extended, similar conformations (**Figures 8G,H**), with a median RMSD of 0.9 Å. The all-against-all comparison reveals four groups of conformers, with peaks observed in the RMSD distribution around 0.3, 1.2, 1.7, and 2.4 Å (**Figure 9**). These peaks correspond to an accumulation of conformers with similar torsion angles of the side chain. The maximum RMSD of 2.9 Å was observed between the conformation of FMN in *E. coli* pyridoxine 5′-phosphate oxidase (1JNW) and in human glycolate oxidase (2RDU), with the sidechain bent into opposing directions.

CONCLUSIONS

The Sperrylite Dataset presented in this work is a complete subset of high-quality conformations of protein-bound ligands extracted from the PDB. This dataset resulted from a multi-step data processing and filtering procedure that, most importantly, also includes an automated approach for the evaluation of the support of individual atom positions by the electron density. The Sperrylite Dataset consists of a total of 10,936 high-quality structures of 4,548 unique ligands. Ninety-one of those ligands are each represented by a minimum of ten structures, and among these only a (very) weak correlation was observed between the number of rotatable bonds of a molecule and its overall variability (measured as the minimum median RMSD; $R^2 = 0.126$). Sixty-nine out of the 91 ligands had at least two distinct conformations (defined as RMSD above 1 Å).

A representative subset of 17 approved drugs and cofactors was analyzed in detail to determine the conformational variability of protein-bound conformations of small molecules. For all of the analyzed small-molecule drugs and some of the cofactors, a clear trend for the formation of few clusters of highly similar conformers was observed. Similar conformers were observed for proteins with similar binding sites, mostly independent of the overall protein sequence identity (which is in agreement with the findings of, e.g., Sturm et al., 2012). A particularly interesting example is imatinib, which was found to adopt highly similar conformations when binding to different tyrosine kinases (even to those sharing low overall sequence identity) but to adopt a distinct conformation upon binding to quinone reductase 2. For cofactors, a clear trend for extended conformations was observed, which is in agreement with previous works (Moodie and Thornton, 1993; Stockwell and Thornton, 2006; Bojovschi et al., 2012; Stegemann and Klebe, 2012). A few cases of strongly coiled conformers of cofactors were also observed. This result is well in line with earlier reports (Stockwell and Thornton, 2006).

It is clear that the currently available structural data on protein-bound ligands is still too limited to allow us to gain a full understanding of the bioactive space of small molecules. However, for several cofactors a large number of conformers observed in complex with dozens of proteins are available to date and provide valuable insight into the bioactive conformational space and the prevalence of bioactive conformations of small molecules. With an automated workflow for the extraction of high-quality ligand structures from the PDB in place, it is expected that the ever increasing amount of data will allow a more detailed understanding of, e.g., conformational preferences, ligand promiscuity, or the relationship between the bioactive conformational space of small molecules and the structural diversity of binding pockets.

AUTHOR CONTRIBUTIONS

JK and N-OF: conceived the work; N-OF and MS: conducted the computational studies. All authors contributed to the interpretation of the data and the writing of the manuscript. All authors have given approval to the final version of the paper.

ACKNOWLEDGMENTS

The authors thank Christina de Bruyn Kops for discussion and proofreading of the manuscript. MS was supported by the Erasmus+ Programme of the European Commission.

REFERENCES

Alton, G. R., and Lunney, E. A. (2008). Targeting the unactivated conformations of protein kinases for small molecule drug discovery. *Expert Opin. Drug Discov.* 3, 595–605. doi: 10.1517/17460441.3.6.595

Altschul, S. F., Gish, W., Miller, W., Myers, E. W., and Lipman, D. J. (1990). Basic local alignment search tool. *J. Mol. Biol.* 215, 403–410. doi: 10.1016/S0022-2836(05)80360-2

Anstee, Q. M., and Day, C. P. (2012). S-adenosylmethionine (SAMe) therapy in liver disease: a review of current evidence and clinical utility. *J. Hepatol.* 57, 1097–1109. doi: 10.1016/j.jhep.2012.04.041

Atwell, S., Adams, J. M., Badger, J., Buchanan, M. D., Feil, I. K., Froning, K. J., et al. (2004). A novel mode of Gleevec binding is revealed by the structure of spleen tyrosine kinase. *J. Biol. Chem.* 279, 55827–55832. doi: 10.1074/jbc.M409792200

Berman, H. M., Westbrook, J., Feng, Z., Gilliland, G., Bhat, T. N., Weissig, H., et al. (2000). The protein data bank. *Nucleic Acids Res.* 28, 235–242. doi: 10.1093/nar/28.1.235

Bojovschi, A., Liu, M. S., and Sadus, R. J. (2012). Conformational dynamics of ATP/Mg:ATP in motor proteins via data mining and molecular simulation. *J. Chem. Phys.* 137:075101. doi: 10.1063/1.4739308

Boström, J. (2001). Reproducing the conformations of protein-bound ligands: a critical evaluation of several popular conformational searching tools. *J. Comput. Aided Mol. Des.* 15, 1137–1152. doi: 10.1023/A:1015930826903

Boström, J., Norrby, P. O., and Liljefors, T. (1998). Conformational energy penalties of protein-bound ligands. *J. Comput. Aided Mol. Des.* 12, 383–396. doi: 10.1023/A:1008007507641

Brameld, K. A., Kuhn, B., Reuter, D. C., and Stahl, M. (2008). Small molecule conformational preferences derived from crystal structure data. A medicinal chemistry focused analysis. *J. Chem. Inf. Model.* 48, 1–24. doi: 10.1021/ci7002494

Buth, J. M., Steen, P. O., Sueper, C., Blumentritt, D., Vikesland, P. J., Arnold, W. A., et al. (2010). Dioxin photoproducts of triclosan and its chlorinated derivatives in sediment cores. *Environ. Sci. Technol.* 44, 4545–4551. doi: 10.1021/es1001105

Camacho, C., Coulouris, G., Avagyan, V., Ma, N., Papadopoulos, J., Bealer, K., et al. (2009). BLAST+: architecture and applications. *BMC Bioinformatics* 10:421. doi: 10.1186/1471-2105-10-421

Carey, D. E., and McNamara, P. J. (2014). The impact of triclosan on the spread of antibiotic resistance in the environment. *Front. Microbiol.* 5:780. doi: 10.3389/fmicb.2014.00780

Chakravarty, S., and Kannan, K. K. (1994). Drug-protein interactions. Refined structures of three sulfonamide drug complexes of human carbonic anhydrase I enzyme. *J. Mol. Biol.* 243, 298–309. doi: 10.1006/jmbi.1994.1655

Chatterjee, S., Zhong, D., Nordhues, B. A., Battaile, K. P., Lovell, S., and De Guzman, R. N. (2011). The crystal structures of the Salmonella type III secretion system tip protein SipD in complex with deoxycholate and chenodeoxycholate. *Protein Sci.* 20, 75–86. doi: 10.1002/pro.537

Cruickshank, D. W. (1999). Remarks about protein structure precision. *Acta Crystallogr. D Biol. Crystallogr.* 55, 583–601. doi: 10.1107/S0907444998012645

Duncan, D., and Rotunda, A. M. (2011). Injectable therapies for localized fat loss: state of the art. *Clin. Plast. Surg.* 38, 489–501, vii. doi: 10.1016/j.cps.2011.02.005

Dym, O., and Eisenberg, D. (2001). Sequence-structure analysis of FAD-containing proteins. *Protein Sci.* 10, 1712–1728. doi: 10.1110/ps.12801

Foster, C. E., Bianchet, M. A., Talalay, P., Zhao, Q., and Amzel, L. M. (1999). Crystal structure of human quinone reductase type 2, a metalloflavoprotein. *Biochemistry* 38, 9881–9886. doi: 10.1021/bi990799v

Friedrich, N.-O., de Bruyn Kops, C., Flachsenberg, F., Sommer, K., Rarey, M., and Kirchmair, J. (2017a). Benchmarking commercial conformer ensemble generators. *J. Chem. Inf. Model.* 57, 2719–2728. doi: 10.1021/acs.jcim.7b00505

Friedrich, N.-O., Meyder, A., de Bruyn Kops, C., Sommer, K., Flachsenberg, F., Rarey, M., et al. (2017b). High-quality dataset of protein-bound ligand conformations and its application to benchmarking conformer ensemble generators. *J. Chem. Inf. Model.* 57, 529–539. doi: 10.1021/acs.jcim.6b00613

Froehlich, A. C., Liu, Y., Loros, J. J., and Dunlap, J. C. (2002). White Collar-1, a circadian blue light photoreceptor, binding to the frequency promoter. *Science* 297, 815–819. doi: 10.1126/science.1073681

Günther, S., Senger, C., Michalsky, E., Goede, A., and Preissner, R. (2006). Representation of target-bound drugs by computed conformers: implications for conformational libraries. *BMC Bioinformatics* 7:293. doi: 10.1186/1471-2105-7-293

Guo, T., Chang, L., Xiao, Y., and Liu, Q. (2015). S-adenosyl-L-methionine for the treatment of chronic liver disease: a systematic review and meta-analysis. *PLoS ONE* 10:e0122124. doi: 10.1371/journal.pone.0122124

He, M. W., Lee, P. S., and Sweeney, Z. K. (2015). Promiscuity and the conformational rearrangement of drug-like molecules: insight from the protein data bank. *Chem. Med. Chem.* 10, 238–244. doi: 10.1002/cmdc.2014 02389

He, Q. (2002). White collar-1, a DNA binding transcription factor and a light sensor. *Science* 297, 840–843. doi: 10.1126/science.1072795

Heath, R. J., Rubin, J. R., Holland, D. R., Zhang, E., Snow, M. E., and Rock, C. O. (1999). Mechanism of triclosan inhibition of bacterial fatty acid synthesis. *Biol. Chem.* 274, 11110–11114. doi: 10.1074/jbc.274.16.11110

Inoi, K., Goto, S., Nomura, S., Isobe, K., Nawa, A., Okamoto, T., et al. (1995). Aminopeptidase inhibitor ubenimex (bestatin) inhibits the growth of human choriocarcinoma in nude mice through its direct cytostatic activity. *Anticancer Res.* 15, 2081–2087.

Katz, B. A. (1997). Binding of biotin to streptavidin stabilizes intersubunit salt bridges between Asp61 and His87 at low pH. *J. Mol. Biol.* 274, 776–800. doi: 10.1006/jmbi.1997.1444

Kaur, I. P., Smitha, R., Aggarwal, D., and Kapil, M. (2002). Acetazolamide: future perspective in topical glaucoma therapeutics. *Int. J. Pharm.* 248, 1–14. doi: 10.1016/S0378-5173(02)00438-6

Kim, K.-H., Ha, B. H., Kim, S. J., Hong, S. K., Hwang, K. Y., and Kim, E. E. (2011). Crystal structures of Enoyl-ACP reductases I (FabI) and III (FabL) from *B. subtilis. J. Mol. Biol.* 406, 403–415. doi: 10.1016/j.jmb.2010.12.003

King, N. M., Prabu-Jeyabalan, M., Nalivaika, E. A., Wigerinck, P., de Béthune, M.-P., and Schiffer, C. A. (2004). Structural and thermodynamic basis for the binding of TMC114, a next-generation human immunodeficiency virus type 1 protease inhibitor. *J. Virol.* 78, 12012–12021. doi: 10.1128/JVI.78.21.12012-12021.2004

Laitinen, O. H., Hytönen, V. P., Nordlund, H. R., and Kulomaa, M. S. (2006). Genetically engineered avidins and streptavidins. *Cell. Mol. Life Sci.* 63, 2992–3017. doi: 10.1007/s00018-006-6288-z

Le Trong, I., Chu, V., Xing, Y., Lybrand, T. P., Stayton, P. S., and Stenkamp, R. E. (2013). Structural consequences of cutting a binding loop: two circularly permuted variants of streptavidin. *Acta Crystallogr. D Biol. Crystallogr.* 69, 968–977. doi: 10.1107/S0907444913003855

Levy, C. W., Roujeinikova, A., Sedelnikova, S., Baker, P. J., Stuitje, A. R., Slabas, A. R., et al. (1999). Molecular basis of triclosan activity. *Nature* 398, 383–384. doi: 10.1038/18803

Liebeschuetz, J., Hennemann, J., Olsson, T., and Groom, C. R. (2012). The good, the bad and the twisted: a survey of ligand geometry in protein crystal structures. *J. Comput. Aided Mol. Des.* 26, 169–183. doi: 10.1007/s10822-011-9538-6

Mato, J. M., Martínez-Chantar, M. L., and Lu, S. C. (2013). S-adenosylmethionine metabolism and liver disease. *Ann. Hepatol.* 12, 183–189.

Meyder, A., Nittinger, E., Lange, G., Klein, R., and Rarey, M. (2017). Estimating electron density support for individual atoms and molecular fragments in X-ray structures. *J. Chem. Inf. Model.* 57, 2437–2447. doi: 10.1021/acs.jcim.7b00391

Moodie, S. L., and Thornton, J. M. (1993). A study into the effects of protein binding on nucleotide conformation. *Nucleic Acids Res.* 21, 1369–1380. doi: 10.1093/nar/21.6.1369

Nankya-Kitaka, M. F., Curley, G. P., Gavigan, C. S., Bell, A., and Dalton, J. P. (1998). *Plasmodium chabaudi* chabaudi and *P. falciparum:* inhibition of aminopeptidase and parasite growth by bestatin and nitrobestatin. *Parasitol. Res.* 84, 552–558. doi: 10.1007/s004360050447

Nicklaus, M. C., Wang, S., Driscoll, J. S., and Milne, G. W. (1995). Conformational changes of small molecules binding to proteins. *Bioorg. Med. Chem.* 3, 411–428. doi: 10.1016/0968-0896(95)00031-B

Noble, C. G., Li, S.-H., Dong, H., Chew, S. H., and Shi, P.-Y. (2014). Crystal structure of dengue virus methyltransferase without S-adenosyl-L-methionine. *Antiviral Res.* 111, 78–81. doi: 10.1016/j.antiviral.2014.09.003

Perola, E., and Charifson, P. S. (2004). Conformational analysis of drug-like molecules bound to proteins: an extensive study of ligand reorganization upon binding. *J. Med. Chem.* 47, 2499–2510. doi: 10.1021/jm030563w

Pfalzer, A. C., Choi, S.-W., Tammen, S. A., Park, L. K., Bottiglieri, T., Parnell, L. D., et al. (2014). S-adenosylmethionine mediates inhibition of inflammatory response and changes in DNA methylation in human macrophages. *Physiol. Genomics* 46, 617–623. doi: 10.1152/physiolgenomics.00056.2014

Pugh, C. S., Borchardt, R. T., and Stone, H. O. (1978). Sinefungin, a potent inhibitor of virion mRNA(guanine-7-)-methyltransferase, mRNA(nucleoside-2'-)-methyltransferase, and viral multiplication. *J. Biol. Chem.* 253, 4075–4077.

Reddy, E. P., and Aggarwal, A. K. (2012). The ins and outs of bcr-abl inhibition. *Genes Cancer* 3, 447–454. doi: 10.1177/1947601912462126

Reynolds, C. H. (2014). Protein-ligand cocrystal structures: we can do better. *ACS Med. Chem. Lett.* 5, 727–729. doi: 10.1021/ml500220a

Ridlon, J. M., Harris, S. C., Bhowmik, S., Kang, D.-J., and Hylemon, P. B. (2016). Consequences of bile salt biotransformations by intestinal bacteria. *Gut Microbes* 7, 22–39. doi: 10.1080/19490976.2015.1127483

Sakuraya, M., Tamura, J., Itoh, K., Kubota, K., and Naruse, T. (2000). Aminopeptidase inhibitor ubenimex inhibits the growth of leukaemic cell lines and myeloma cells through its cytotoxicity. *J. Int. Med. Res.* 28, 214–221. doi: 10.1177/147323000002800503

Schatz, R. A., Vunnam, C. R., and Sellinger, O. Z. (1977). S-Adenosyl-L-homocysteine in brain: regional concentrations, catabolism, and the effects of methionine sulfoximine. *Neurochem. Res.* 2, 27–38. doi: 10.1007/BF00966019

Schwerdtfeger, C., and Linden, H. (2003). VIVID is a flavoprotein and serves as a fungal blue light photoreceptor for photoadaptation. *EMBO J.* 22, 4846–4855. doi: 10.1093/emboj/cdg451

Seeliger, D., and de Groot, B. L. (2010). Conformational transitions upon ligand binding: holo-structure prediction from apo conformations. *PLoS Comput. Biol.* 6:e1000634. doi: 10.1371/journal.pcbi.1000634

Singh, N. J., Shin, D., Lee, H. M., Kim, H. T., Chang, H.-J., Cho, J. M., et al. (2011). Structural basis of triclosan resistance. *J. Struct. Biol.* 174, 173–179. doi: 10.1016/j.jsb.2010.11.008

Sommer, K., Friedrich, N.-O., Bietz, S., Hilbig, M., Inhester, T., and Rarey, M. (2016). UNICON: a powerful and easy-to-use compound library converter. *J. Chem. Inf. Model.* 56, 1105–1111. doi: 10.1021/acs.jcim.6b00069

Stegemann, B., and Klebe, G. (2012). Cofactor-binding sites in proteins of deviating sequence: comparative analysis and clustering in torsion angle, cavity, and fold space. *Proteins* 80, 626–648. doi: 10.1002/prot.23226

Stockwell, G. R., and Thornton, J. M. (2006). Conformational diversity of ligands bound to proteins. *J. Mol. Biol.* 356, 928–944. doi: 10.1016/j.jmb.2005.12.012

Sturm, N., Desaphy, J., Quinn, R. J., Rognan, D., and Kellenberger, E. (2012). Structural insights into the molecular basis of the ligand promiscuity. *J. Chem. Inf. Model.* 52, 2410–2421. doi: 10.1021/ci300196g

Tehlivets, O., Malanovic, N., Visram, M., Pavkov-Keller, T., and Keller, W. (2013). S-adenosyl-L-homocysteine hydrolase and methylation disorders: yeast as a model system. *Biochim. Biophys. Acta* 1832, 204–215. doi: 10.1016/j.bbadis.2012.09.007

Tian, W., Rockson, S. G., Jiang, X., Kim, J., Begaye, A., Shuffle, E. M., et al. (2017). Leukotriene B4 antagonism ameliorates experimental lymphedema. *Sci. Transl. Med.* 9:eaal3920. doi: 10.1126/scitranslmed.aal3920

Urabe, A., Mutoh, Y., Mizoguchi, H., Takaku, F., and Ogawa, N. (1993). Ubenimex in the treatment of acute nonlymphocytic leukemia in adults. *Ann. Hematol.* 67, 63–66. doi: 10.1007/BF01788128

Urbaczek, S., Kolodzik, A., Fischer, J. R., Lippert, T., Heuser, S., Groth, I., et al. (2011). NAOMI: on the almost trivial task of reading molecules from different file formats. *J. Chem. Inf. Model.* 51, 3199–3207. doi: 10.1021/ci200324e

Vedel, M., Lawrence, F., Robert-Gero, M., and Lederer, E. (1978). The antifungal antibiotic sinefungin as a very active inhibitor of methyltransferases and of the transformation of chick embryo fibroblasts by *Rous sarcoma* virus. *Biochem. Biophys. Res. Commun.* 85, 371–376. doi: 10.1016/S0006-291X(78)80052-7

Warren, G. L., Do, T. D., Kelley, B. P., Nicholls, A., and Warren, S. D. (2012). Essential considerations for using protein-ligand structures in drug discovery. *Drug Discov. Today* 17, 1270–1281. doi: 10.1016/j.drudis.2012.06.011

Winger, J. A., Hantschel, O., Superti-Furga, G., and Kuriyan, J. (2009). The structure of the leukemia drug imatinib bound to human quinone reductase 2 (NQO2). *BMC Struct. Biol.* 9:7. doi: 10.1186/1472-6807-9-7

Wishart, D. S., Feunang, Y. D., Guo, A. C., Lo, E. J., Marcu, A., Grant, J. R., et al. (2017). DrugBank 5.0: a major update to the DrugBank database for 2018. *Nucleic Acids Res.* 46, D1074–D1082. doi: 10.1093/nar/gkx1037

Wolber, G., and Langer, T. (2005). LigandScout: 3-D pharmacophores derived from protein-bound ligands and their use as virtual screening filters. *J. Chem. Inf. Model.* 45, 160–169. doi: 10.1021/ci049885e

Permissions

All chapters in this book were first published by Frontiers; hereby published with permission under the Creative Commons Attribution License or equivalent. Every chapter published in this book has been scrutinized by our experts. Their significance has been extensively debated. The topics covered herein carry significant findings which will fuel the growth of the discipline. They may even be implemented as practical applications or may be referred to as a beginning point for another development.

The contributors of this book come from diverse backgrounds, making this book a truly international effort. This book will bring forth new frontiers with its revolutionizing research information and detailed analysis of the nascent developments around the world.

We would like to thank all the contributing authors for lending their expertise to make the book truly unique. They have played a crucial role in the development of this book. Without their invaluable contributions this book wouldn't have been possible. They have made vital efforts to compile up to date information on the varied aspects of this subject to make this book a valuable addition to the collection of many professionals and students.

This book was conceptualized with the vision of imparting up-to-date information and advanced data in this field. To ensure the same, a matchless editorial board was set up. Every individual on the board went through rigorous rounds of assessment to prove their worth. After which they invested a large part of their time researching and compiling the most relevant data for our readers.

The editorial board has been involved in producing this book since its inception. They have spent rigorous hours researching and exploring the diverse topics which have resulted in the successful publishing of this book. They have passed on their knowledge of decades through this book. To expedite this challenging task, the publisher supported the team at every step. A small team of assistant editors was also appointed to further simplify the editing procedure and attain best results for the readers.

Apart from the editorial board, the designing team has also invested a significant amount of their time in understanding the subject and creating the most relevant covers. They scrutinized every image to scout for the most suitable representation of the subject and create an appropriate cover for the book.

The publishing team has been an ardent support to the editorial, designing and production team. Their endless efforts to recruit the best for this project, has resulted in the accomplishment of this book. They are a veteran in the field of academics and their pool of knowledge is as vast as their experience in printing. Their expertise and guidance has proved useful at every step. Their uncompromising quality standards have made this book an exceptional effort. Their encouragement from time to time has been an inspiration for everyone.

The publisher and the editorial board hope that this book will prove to be a valuable piece of knowledge for researchers, students, practitioners and scholars across the globe.

List of Contributors

Xiaobing Deng
Peking–Tsinghua Center for Life Sciences, Peking University, Beijing, China
Center for Quantitative Biology, Academy for Advanced Interdisciplinary Studies, Peking University, Beijing, China

Xiaoling Zhang and Qi Shen
Center for Quantitative Biology, Academy for Advanced Interdisciplinary Studies, Peking University, Beijing, China

Bo Tang
BNLMS, State Key Laboratory for Structural Chemistry of Unstable and Stable Species, College of Chemistry and Molecular Engineering, Peking University, Beijing, China

Hongbo Liu
Peking–Tsinghua Center for Life Sciences, Peking University, Beijing, China

Ying Liu
Center for Quantitative Biology, Academy for Advanced Interdisciplinary Studies, Peking University, Beijing, China
BNLMS, State Key Laboratory for Structural Chemistry of Unstable and Stable Species, College of Chemistry and Molecular Engineering, Peking University, Beijing, China

Luhua Lai
Peking–Tsinghua Center for Life Sciences, Peking University, Beijing, China
Center for Quantitative Biology, Academy for Advanced Interdisciplinary Studies, Peking University, Beijing, China
BNLMS, State Key Laboratory for Structural Chemistry of Unstable and Stable Species, College of Chemistry and Molecular Engineering, Peking University, Beijing, China

Yanyan Diao, Disha Wang, Yi Tong, Xia Wang, Lili Zhu, You Yang, Xiuqin Hu, Jing Jiang, Shoude Zhang, Shiliang Li, Yufang Xu, Jin Huang and Honglin Li
Shanghai Key Laboratory of New Drug Design, State Key Laboratory of Bioreactor Engineering, School of Pharmacy, East China University of Science and Technology, Shanghai, China

Lei Shan and Weidong Zhang
Department of Phytochemistry, School of Pharmacy, Second Military Medical University, Shanghai, China

Doris E. Braun and Ulrich J. Griesser
Institute of Pharmacy, University of Innsbruck, Innsbruck, Austria

Muhammad Akram and Daniela Schuster
Institute of Pharmacy - Pharmaceutical Chemistry and Center for Molecular Biosciences Innsbruck (CMBI), University of Innsbruck, Innsbruck, Austria

Watcharee Waratchareeyakul
Department of Chemistry, Faculty of Science and Technology, Rambhai Barni Rajabhat University, Chanthaburi, Thailand

Joerg Haupenthal
Department of Drug Design and Optimization, Helmholtz Institute for Pharmaceutical Research Saarland, Saarbrücken, Germany

Rolf W. Hartmann
Department of Drug Design and Optimization, Helmholtz Institute for Pharmaceutical Research Saarland, Saarbrücken, Germany
Department of Pharmacy, Pharmaceutical and Medicinal Chemistry, Saarland University, Saarbrücken, Germany

Irene Maffucci, Xiao Hu, Valentina Fumagalli and Alessandro Contini
Dipartimento di Scienze Farmaceutiche, Sezione di Chimica Generale e Organica "Alessandro Marchesini," Università degli Studi di Milano, Milan, Italy

Mariela Bollini, Emilse S. Leal and Gabriela A. Fernández
Laboratorio de Química Medicinal, Centro de Investigaciones en Bionanociencias, Consejo Nacional de Investigaciones Científicas y Técnicas, Ciudad de Buenos Aires, Argentina

Natalia S. Adler, María G. Aucar and Claudio N. Cavasotto
Laboratory of Computational Chemistry and Drug Design, Instituto de Investigación en Biomedicina de Buenos Aires, Consejo Nacional de Investigaciones Científicas y Técnicas, Partner Institute of the Max Planck Society, Ciudad de Buenos Aires, Argentina

María J. Pascual, Fernando Merwaiss and Diego E. Alvarez
Instituto de Investigaciones Biotecnológicas, Universidad Nacional de San Martín, Consejo Nacional de Investigaciones Científicas y Técnicas, San Martín, Argentina

Max Hirte, Nicolas Meese, Michael Mertz, Monika Fuchs and Thomas B. Brück
Werner Siemens Chair of Synthetic Biotechnology, Department of Chemistry, Technical University of Munich, Munich, Germany

Jinxuan Li, Jing-Yi Chen, Ya-Lin Deng, Qian Zhou, Yinuo Wu, Deyan Wu and Hai-Bin Luo
School of Pharmaceutical Sciences, Sun Yat-sen University, Guangzhou, China

Linjiang Tong and Hua Xie
Division of Anti-tumor Pharmacology, State Key Laboratory of Drug Research, Shanghai Institute of Materia Medica, Chinese Academy of Sciences, Shanghai, China

Wenchao Lu, Rukang Zhang, Hao Jiang and Cheng Luo
Drug Discovery and Design Center, CAS Key Laboratory of Receptor Research, State Key Laboratory of Drug Research, Shanghai Institute of Materia Medica, Chinese Academy of Sciences, Shanghai, China
Department of Pharmacy, University of Chinese Academy of Sciences, Beijing, China

Huimin Zhang
Drug Discovery and Design Center, CAS Key Laboratory of Receptor Research, State Key Laboratory of Drug Research, Shanghai Institute of Materia Medica, Chinese Academy of Sciences, Shanghai, China
School of Life Science and Technology, ShanghaiTech University, Shanghai, China

Hongbin Huang, Yuquan Zhou, Suling Chen and Shangkang Mai
Key Laboratory for Medical Molecular Diagnostics of Guangdong Province, Dongguan Scientific Research Center, Guangdong Medical University, Dongguan, China
The Second School of Clinical Medicine, Guangdong Medical University, Dongguan, China

Guigui Zhang, Chenru Lin, Yutong Lin and Zunnan Huang
Key Laboratory for Medical Molecular Diagnostics of Guangdong Province, Dongguan Scientific Research Center, Guangdong Medical University, Dongguan, China
School of Pharmacy, Guangdong Medical University, Dongguan, China

Sanna Rauhamäki, Pekka A. Postila, Sanna Niinivehmas, Mira Pasanen, Mira Ahinko and Elina Multamäki
Computational Bioscience Laboratory, Department of Biological and Environmental Science & Nanoscience Center, University of Jyväskylä, Jyväskylä, Finland

Sami Kortet and Emmi Schildt
Computational Bioscience Laboratory, Department of Biological and Environmental Science & Nanoscience Center, University of Jyväskylä, Jyväskylä, Finland
Department of Chemistry & Nanoscience Center, University of Jyväskylä, Jyväskylä, Finland

Elangovan Manivannan
Computational Bioscience Laboratory, Department of Biological and Environmental Science & Nanoscience Center, University of Jyväskylä, Jyväskylä, Finland
School of Pharmacy, Devi Ahilya University, Madhya Pradesh, India

Pasi Koskimies
Forendo Pharma Ltd., Turku, Finland

Niina Nyberg, Pasi Huuskonen, Markku Pasanen, Risto O. Juvonen and Hannu Raunio
School of Pharmacy, University of Eastern Finland, Kuopio, Finland

Juhani Huuskonen
Department of Chemistry & Nanoscience Center, University of Jyväskylä, Jyväskylä, Finland

Olli T. Pentikäinen
Computational Bioscience Laboratory, Department of Biological and Environmental Science & Nanoscience Center, University of Jyväskylä, Jyväskylä, Finland
MedChem.fi, Institute of Biomedicine, University of Turku, Turku, Finland

Pavel V. Pogodin, Anastasia V. Rudik, Dmitry A. Filimonov, Dmitry S. Druzhilovskiy and Vladimir V. Poroikov
Department of Bioinformatics, Institute of Biomedical Chemistry, Moscow, Russia

Alexey A. Lagunin
Department of Bioinformatics, Institute of Biomedical Chemistry, Moscow, Russia
Department of Bioinformatics, Medical-Biological Department, Pirogov Russian National Research Medical University, Moscow, Russia

Mark C. Nicklaus
Computer-Aided Drug Design Group, Chemical Biology Laboratory, Center for Cancer Research, National Cancer Institute, NIH, NCI-Frederick, Frederick, MD, United States

Hongbin Yang, Lixia Sun, Weihua Li, Guixia Liu and Yun Tang
Shanghai Key Laboratory of New Drug Design, School of Pharmacy, East China University of Science and Technology, Shanghai, China

Aliya Ibrar and Saifullah Mehsud
Department of Chemistry, Abbottabad University of Science & Technology, Havelian, Pakistan

Ajmal Khan
Department of Chemistry, COMSATS Institute of Information Technology, Abbottabad, Pakistan
UoN Chair of Oman's Medicinal Plants and Marine Natural Products, University of Nizwa, Nizwa, Oman

Majid Ali, Rizwana Sarwar and Umar Farooq
Department of Chemistry, COMSATS Institute of Information Technology, Abbottabad, Pakistan

Syed M. A. Halimi
Department of Pharmacy, University of Peshawar, Peshawar, Pakistan

Imtiaz Khan
Department of Chemistry, Quaid-i-Azam University, Islamabad, Pakistan
School of Chemistry, Cardiff University, Cardiff, United Kingdom

Ahmed Al-Harrasi
UoN Chair of Oman's Medicinal Plants and Marine Natural Products, University of Nizwa, Nizwa, Oman

Nils-Ole Friedrich and Johannes Kirchmair
Department of Informatics, Center for Bioinformatics, Universität Hamburg, Hamburg, Germany

Méliné Simsir
Department of Informatics, Center for Bioinformatics, Universität Hamburg, Hamburg, Germany
Molécules Thérapeutiques In Silico, Université Paris Diderot, Sorbonne Paris Cité, Paris, France

Index

www.ingramcontent.com/pod-product-compliance
Lightning Source LLC
LaVergne TN
LVHW082145200926
848484LV00008B/2110
* 9 7 9 8 8 8 7 4 0 0 1 6 7 *